Herbal Medicine
keys to
Physiomedicalism

including

Pharmacopoeia

The information presented in the Practitioners Pharmacopoeia is intended for qualified Medical Herbalists, Naturopaths and Doctors only. If you think that you have a health concern or illness then consult your qualified Medical Herbalist. The writer advises that no self-treatment be undertaken. No responsibility is accepted for self diagnosis or treatment using methods described in this work.
Every effort has been made to establish the correct references. Apologies are given for those references which inadvertently have been missed.
No part of this work is to be reproduced or stored in any form whatsoever without written permission of the author.

Acknowledgements
Grateful appreciation are given to Barbara Walsh, Bill Parkinson, Brenda Cooke, Christopher Hedley, Graham Price and Kerry Caldock for their time spent in proof reading and tolerance of my moods while creating this manuscript. To the teachers and pupils of Talipanan Mangyan School, Oriental Mandoro, Philippines Merlin Turville - Petre for his inventive artistry.

Dedicated to my sons who gave me encouragement and help with the computer.

Feedback
Comments on this work are welcomed to the address below.

Published by the Faculty of Physiomedical Herbal Medicine [FPHM].
16 Grosvenor Road, Newcastle, Staffs ST5 1LW, England.

ISBN   0 – 9545518 – 0 - X

Important note
Hubbard says be certain that you understand the words. The only reason a person gives up a study or is unable to learn is because they have gone past a misunderstood word. Confusion or inability to learn comes after a word that was not understood. If the material becomes confusing there will be a word just earlier that you have not understood. Find the misunderstood word and get it defined. A glossary of definitions will be found at the back of the book.

Introduction - do not pass this by without reading it
A theory is only as good as it works and it works, as long as it explains observed data and predicts new material, which will be found in fact to exist.
  Socrates said 'I cannot teach anybody anything, I can only make them think.'

Physiomedicalism is the primary system of herbal therapeutics used by herbalists. Lately, there are various schools of herbalism, which will seek to turn away from the natural, tried and trusted physiomedical system, towards empiricism. This work brings together modern scientific theory and conventional herbal practice with philosophical balance.
Complex as the subject of physiomedical herbal medicine may appear to be, it is important for us to make a careful enquiry to assess our heritage. Following this introduction, various texts are quoted. In the writer's view, the texts serve us in the quest for a system of useful philosophy for the herbalist to use with patients/clients. It does not say there is only one way or another that may be better for the herbalist. The physiomedical system has proven itself to be of value in practice.
Where practical methods have been used with success by herbalists through the ages, an avid herbalist will not "throw out the baby with the bath water" when searching or researching new ideas or historical aspects of herbalism. All aspects will be used to compliment one another.

Once the herbalist has a sure footing upon which to build, there can be no question of a new philosophy, only a rearrangement of existing facts and some incorporation of renewed ideas and themes.

Even new words may be substituted for the present language that you use. Is it to the advantage of the patient to learn another system of philosophy where physiomedicalism works well? Further knowledge can be brought into the physiomedical philosophy to enlarge the existing framework that you already possess. Often it is the herbalist's lack of knowledge that makes them seek other ideas or other systems.

Two other philosophies spring to mind while researching for this work: namely Ayurvedic and Tibetan. It is no surprise that these two systems of medicine prove that the physiomedicalists had it right from the first. It has been the writers attempt to disprove physiomedicalism but time and again the facts just keep getting confirmed. Confirmation of existing facts appears in the research and writings of authors and herbalists of standing.

Central to physiomedicalism is typology also known as habitus type or somatotype - an individuals bodily frame upon which the physical constitution is built, is identical to the Ayurvedic, Tibetan and Physiomedical systems. Vasant Lad [258] explains - Ayurveda has three constitutions: Vata, Pitta and Kapha: known as monotypes [pure types], dual and triple types are mixtures of the constitutions, thus giving nine constitutional types in all. It also proves there is no such thing as a pure constitution. Thurston [13] quotes Galen's constitutions; Sanguine etc. and further quotes Powel's binary sub types making ten in all. Tibetan medicine teaches, says Gerti Samel [259], that there are three energies and these are principles known as rlung [wind], mkhrispa [bile] and badkan [phlegm]. These represent movement, fluid and warmth respectively. It also fits in perfectly with Culpeper's medicine as mkhrispa relates to hot disorders – those associated with the sun, and badkan with cold disorders associated with the moon. Cold disease requires hot medicine. Thomson the first physiomedicalist, says heat or the lessening of cold is the cause of disease - cold promotes disease causation and obstructions to the circulation with end organ disruption and consequent toxin overload. Priest [6] says 'the secret of good therapy is to recognise the limitations of functional flexibility and vital resource inherent in the particular constitution under treatment hence the importance of typological assessment as a background to specific treatment'.

Physiomedicalism has been in existence for around 300 years, in that short amount of time it has raised the profile of herbalism. Tremendous advances have been made using the physiomedical system it has proved itself in the consulting room. The system of herbalism currently gives the vitalistic approach, required by the patient and practitioner alike. Physiomedicalism gives to the patient and herbalist the complete framework for the patient to be healed. To the healer, the knowledge of comprehensive, effective treatment.

It is a great shame that more research has not been put into the philosophical concept of herbalism. Some say that herbalists need no philosophy in order to practice. Perhaps we could merely throw together any herbs and hope for a desired result. With the balance of probability, one may get a certain degree of success. Results of treatment will not be holistic or remotely patient centred; at worst it could be damaging to the body. A disturbing influence is obtained with herbs if an incorrect prescription is given to the patient.

To those looking merely at the plant constituent theory as a basis for their treatment:
Chemistry is very reductionist, very little progress is being made in the reductionist analysis of complexity of synergy which is regarded as the central plank of modern medical herbalism. Increasing dependence upon chemical science if not counter balanced poses a threat to physiomedical philosophy. Plant chemistry can be a valuable servant to herbal practice and the knowledge of prescribed herbal medicines. Herbal chemistry has been known about for over 150 years.

A comprehensive approach, to the patient, will be found by using physiomedicalism. Physiomedicalism offers a certain advantage over empirical methods of herbal treatment. There are subtle differences in the way herbalists view and treat a patient using the physiomedical system. Medical herbalists treat the patient not the disease. Some universities offering herbal courses teach the treatment of disease only, with little consideration of the tissue state to be treated. Kill the infection say the medical doctors. Medical herbalists agree it is necessary to limit the infective process as well as cleanse the tissue, also known as detoxification. Holistic treatment must address the elimination processes. The eliminatory organs are frequently at fault when disease is encountered. Hypercholesterolaemia is a complicated disorder and is an effect of and a frequent finding in disorders of the liver, gall bladder, pancreas, thyroid or nervous system. There are genetic and dietary factors to be considered too.

Physiomedical terminology is different from any empirical approach; full explanations are given in the text.

Three basic principles that will be encountered are **Relax - Astringe - Stimulate**.

Once these principles are understood, it is relatively easy with Physiomedicalism. Various chapters of this book will discuss the therapeutic approach to the patient. Look at the physiomedical approach to the patient and apply the rules of holism. Research is justified when looking for proof of efficacy within a particular syndrome or efficacy of treatment. The study of causes together with physiology enables practitioners to comprehend the requirement for patient orientated treatment. The requirement enables considerable clarity in management and subsequent treatment of the case. Within herbal medical circles treatment is to be [1] of a safe standard [2] correctly administered and [3] effective for the patient.

The Practitioners Pharmacopoeia covers 420 herbal medicines. The monograph material is written from a research base of [a] practitioner involvement, [b] case histories, [c] herbal books - see bibliography, [d] the writer's qualifications and clinical experience as a Medical Herbalist, Naturopath and Iridologist, [e] pharmaceutical books - BP, Codex, BNF, Martindale's and the BHP. When further research is required to evaluate the information it is suggested that one attempts to disprove the value of information given in these pages rather than the writer trying to prove the contents of this work. Edward de Bono explains 'the analysis of data is not enough we also need to speculate and to use provocative hypotheses if we are to rapidly develop skills'. He further argues our hypothesis is a scaffold upon which to organise and seek new information. Hypotheses can be provocative and speculative says de Bono. In this manner one is not limited by research methods but there is a greater amount of freedom to pursue and be speculative.

What this book is about
This work has six categories:
1] Physiomedical approach to the patient - Vital chi force. Contract, Relax, Stimulate.
2] Aetiology and Pathology. Pathophysiology. Prognosis. Elimination.
3] Bodily system conditions - diseases and herbal medical treatments
4] Naturopathy - nutrition, fasting, hydrotherapy, diets. Vitamins and minerals.
5] Practitioners pharmacopoeia - 420 monographs. Pharmacy. Pharmacology.
6] Emergency herbal medicine

Many abbreviations will be found particularly in prescriptions and the Pharmacopoeia, a glossary of terms will be found in the pharmacy chapter.

CONTENTS

Factors influencing the vasomotor system.
Vasa privata. Vasa publica

Comments by Dr Lindlahr, Dr Greer.
Too much relaxation of:
Muscle. Organ. Circulation – capillary. Nerves.
Too much Tension of:
Muscles. Organs. Circulation. Nerve. Nerve and muscle. Secretory organs.
Evaluation of the case
Contraction and relaxation of tissue.
Tone and trophic state

Posture. Symptom variability. Relapse. Disease stages.
Chronic inflammatory activity.

Diagnosis - concepts and principles. Impact and reaction within the tissues.
Miasms. Typology.
How long will it take to get better? Acute and chronic cases. Curing a patient

Functional adjustments. Trophorestoration.. Active and passive hyperaemia

Vital force in prognosis. Exciting aetiology. Predisposing aetiology.
Trophorestoration. Factors to be assessed in prognosis.
Vaccinations [See Chapter 6]. Genetics. Crisis.
Getting the patient better. Conclusions. Law of cure. Proximate causes of death.

Cook's explanation. Remedial impressions. Functional actions. Drug interactions.
Combining remedies. Herbal constituents. Active compounds in plants.

Cook's definition of disease. Thurston's definition of disease.
Why do symptoms appear? Pyrexia. Inflammation. Congestion. Irritation. Pain.
Vertical & horizontal assessment. Bodily organ system and cellular relationships

Pharmacy continued
Oral compounds. External prescriptions – dressings, plasters, inhalations, liniments, pessaries, sprays, suppositories. [See also dermatology].

Bioavailability. Remedy form
What are medicines. Pharmacokinetics.
Whole fresh plant extracts. Standardisation. Healing agents.
Long term healing effects. Detoxification. Toxic effects.
Finding the correct dose
Prescribing and dispensing, contra indications.
Sterilisation techniques.

Materia medica monographs of 420 herbal medicines
Each monograph is written in the following order:

1] Remedy name. 2] Constituents. 3] Primary action. 4] Therapeutic class.
5] Medicinal indications. 6] Tissue conditions. 7] Cautions. 8] External use.
9] Preparations. 10] Dosage and mode of application.
A page 436. B 513. C 531. D 605. E 618. F 644.
G page 651. H 674. I 692. J 696. K 700. L 701. M 721.
N page 743. O 748. P 756. Q 814. R 815. S 837. T 887.
U page 910. V 918. W 938. Y 939. Z 940. Medical astrology 946

Acute medical emergencies with herbal medication

Amino acids. Anti oxidants. Dairy produce. Enzymes.
Mineral [daily allowance] DA. Oils. Vitamin DA. Trace elements.

Marketing, Accountancy.

A quick reference guide to dosing

1
Historical Aspects of herbal writers throughout the ages

What this Chapter is about
Various authors and notable people are mentioned here, as principal contributors to the world of herbal medicine. It is not intended to give an exhausted list of people or books written on herbalism.
The following account gives brief acknowledgements of importance.

Egyptians
To our recent knowledge, discovery of medicine, first came from the Egyptians and is generally ascribed to the god Thoth or Hermes, who published six books on physic, the first of which was on Medicine and Surgery. Egyptian gods and goddesses were especially skilled in medicine and the art of healing. Osiris is a god of vegetation and skilled in the knowledge of plants. Isis is the ancient mother goddess. In the Ebers papyrus she addresses Isis: 'O Isis, thou great magician, heal me, and deliver thou me from all bad, evil and typhonic things and deliver thou me from every kind of fatal sickness and from diseases caused by devils and from impurity of every kind.' Isis was taught by Thoth and by the use of secret names she could vanquish evil, destroy poisons and raise the dead.

Virtually all herbal knowledge and evidence of medicines come from the following papyri.

[1] Ebers papyrus [pub. by Stern at Leipzig in 1875].
[2] The Great Medical papyrus at Berlin [No 3032] published by
                                        Brugsch & Wreszinski].
[3] The Medical papyrus in the British Museum [no. 10059].
[4] The Hearst papyrus [pub. Wrezinski in 1912].
[5] The Kahun papyrus [pub. by Griffith].
[6] The Edwin Smith papyrus.

Ebers papyrus - purchased by Professor George Ebers in 1862 it contains about 700 herbal remedies. William Smythe [Smith] also purchased a papyrus - they give the medical conditions for which herbs were used at this time. It is most unfortunate that the only surviving medical texts are the following:

The very same substances used in Egypt are found in Babylonian, Greek, Syrian and European herbals of later dates. Many oils were used for healing and for embalming purposes for the dead. There were 7 holy oils and examples of these oils are inscribed on tablets and can be seen in the British museum [nos. 6122, 6123, 29421]. Henna seems to pop up with frequent occurrence in the texts. [109]

1

Herbal Medicine - Keys

Shen Nung 2800 B.C.
Listed are 366 herbs in the *Pen Tsao* - the herbal Chinese materia medica. [1]

Aesculapius 1250 BC
Some say he learnt his herbalism from Cheiron. An ancient tradition says Aesculapius was a native of Memphis in Egypt who emigrated to Greece, where he introduced the knowledge of medicine into that country.

Susrata Samhita 560 – 480BC
An Indian herbal text from around the time of Budda containing around 700 medicinal plants.

Hippocrates 460 - 361 B.C.
He derived a great deal of his learning from the Egyptians. His emphasis was for an holistic approach. Treatment was with dietetics [food], hydrotherapy, hygiene and herbal medicine. He stressed balance of the mental, emotional and physical body, disease was a disturbance of this balance. The Hippocratic Collection was published in eight volumes during the 20th century by Loeb Classical library. The ruined Asclepion hospital in Kos, through which many doctors passed through, is receiving a revival through the International Federation of Kos [IHFK]. The site next to the original hospital will house meeting rooms and lecture theatres [386].

Diocles Carystius –380 BC.
Around the 4th century B.C. a pupil of Aristotle, known as Diocles from Carystius wrote *Rhizotomika* the first Greek herbal - The Rhizotomika contained lists of herbs with their properties [2].

Theophrastus 372 - 285 B.C.
He wrote *Historia Plantarum*. He mentions 500 different plants and sought to develop scientific botany. It was a standard textbook of the time and continued to be so for hundreds of years. His knowledge of plants was acquired during his travels.

Crataeus
Wrote his herbal in the first century B.C.. He was physician to Mithridales VI eupador, king of Pontus. [2]

Dioscorides 60 A.D.
Wrote - *De Materia Medica* in the 1st century A.D.. It was an authoritive reference book and established a common text of plant description, medicinal qualities, preparation and dosage. Over 500 medical plants were described.

Historical aspects

Pliny 60 A.D.
Pliny was Roman he wrote his a number of volumes of natural history, maintaining there was a herb for every disease.

Galen 150 A.D.
Galen learnt from Hippocratic teaching, that health was one in which the four humours of blood, bile, phlegm and choler were equally balanced. That there were four elements - air, fire, water and earth and that these elements expressed in individuals as four temperaments, sanguine, choleric, phlegmatic & melancholic. It was the herbalist's duty to ascertain the particular humoral imbalance and then to prescribe the correct herb to counteract it. Galen remarked long ago that symptoms accompany diseases as a shadow follows the substance, and the presence of the shadow certifies the existence of the substance.

Apuleius Platonicus
This popular Herbarium was written in the fifth century. It was a household book and had been translated from the Latin.

Avicenna [Abou Ibn Sina]. 980 A.D. - 1037 A.D.
The prince of physicians and one of the most remarkable men of the Arab world. He was author of an herbal encyclopaedia; *The Canon of Medicine.*

Salerno 980AD
Salerno was where a Greek school of medicine flourished for around 300 years.

Hildegard of Bingen 1090 -1179
A Benedictine abbess of the monastery in Bingen, Germany.
She wrote two treatises on medicine and natural history, known in English as the *Book of Simple Medicine* [Physica] and the *Book of Composed Medicine [Causae et Curae]*. Medicinal uses of more than 200 herbs along with a catalogue of 47 diseases.
Hildegard adopted the concept of the four humours.

Herbal Medicine - Keys

Anglo Saxon herbalists
Albertus magnus. Died 1280
A botanist and physician. He wrote about plants used as medicines.

Bald
Bald wrote the **Leech book** in three volumes; the word Leech means doctor. In the book conditions were vividly detailed with remedies to treat them.
Modern copies of Leech have been published: *Leechdoms, Wortcunning and starcraft of early England*. Thomas O' Cockayne. Holland press 1961. *Leechcraft – Early English Charms*. Stephen Pollington. Anglo Saxon books 2001.

Herbarium – a popular Latin medical work of the early middle ages. Modern copy by Hubert Jan de Vriend, *The Old English Herbarium*, early English text society 1984.

Witchcraft in 17th Century England
Through the fifteenth to seventeenth centuries Europe passed through a 'witch craze.' It was not only men who were tried as witches, 10% of those being accused of witchcraft in England were men. In Scotland the figure rises to 20% and a similar level was found in Europe. Most of the trials and executions occurred in the early seventeenth century. Over a period of 200 years nearly 100,000 women were executed for witchcraft. In 1542 during Henry the eighths reign a statute was passed. Witchcraft was punishable by death this was later repealed. Matthew Hopkins a self appointed witchfinder who over one and a half years was able to murder around 200 witches. Hopkins made a tidy sum for himself. Stowmarket paid him £23, the average daily wage was 6d [3 pence]. In 1512 legal status was granted to doctors prior to this all treatment of the sick was carried out by women.

Henry VlII
Granted a royal charter to herbalists in 1496. This charter would help prevent herbalists being persecuted or tried as witches.

Bartholomew.
A Professor of theology in Paris. His first herbal was printed in Basle in 1470, an English copy was produced in 1495 and ran into many editions.

Jerome of Brunswick [1528]
'A most excellent and perfect homish apothecarye or homely physick booke for all the grefes and diseases of the bodye'. *'The vertuose book of distyllacyon'* covered chemistry and essential oils of plants. He was army surgeon in 1475.

Historical aspects

Hieronymus Bock [1498 – 1554]
Bock was an early German pharmacologist, botanist and physician. His masterly book was the *New Kreuterbuch*, published in 1539.

Paracelsus [1493 – 1541]
Paracelsus wrote 'In medicine we should never lose heart and never despair. For each ill there is a remedy that combats it. Thus there is no disease that is inevitably mortal. All diseases can be cured without exception.' 'The nature and force of a disease must be discovered by their cause and not by their symptoms....for we must not merely extinguish the smoke of the fire - but the fire itself.' 'The herbalist should direct this thought to the origin of the disease, and not only to that which his eyes see.' Smoke is only the symptom of the fire, not the fire itself
The body has four kinds of taste - bitter, sour, sweet and salty.
Everything bitter is hot and dry   i.e. choleric – bad tempered.
Everything sour is cold and dry   i.e. melancholic – given to brooding.
Everything sweet is cold and moist i.e. phlegmatic – slothful.
Everything salty is hot and moist   i.e. sanguine – spirited, boyant and lively.

Doctrine of signatures
'We......discover everything that lies hidden in the mountains by external signs and correspondences, and thus do we find all the properties of herbs'. There is nothing that nature has not signed in such a way that a man may discover its essence....the form shows what a given herb is.'[4]

There are several herbals written during the middle ages.
Writers include: Bancks [1525], Brunfells [1530].

Theodor Dorsten [Frankfurt 1540]
Botanicon continens herbarum usus in medicinis.

Leonard Fuchs [1501 – 1566]
A German botanist and doctor, he translated and adapted the books of Galen and Hippocrates. His book *De historia stirpium* contains 516 woodcuts of plants.

Codice Badiano, or Badianus manuscript written in the Aztec language
[Natuatl] by Martinus de la Cruz in 1552. It contains descriptions of 184 plants used by Indian physicians. 272, 1994, 7 [1] 27-33

Herbal Medicine - Keys

Turner [1568]
A London herbalist he published - '*New Herball*'. He studied plants scientifically and his work reveals considerable knowledge. His description of plants are meticulously accurate. [3]

John Gerrard [1597]
From Nantwich, Cheshire. His Herbal was known as '*The general history of plants*'. He quotes from Dioscorides, Hypocrites and Galen.

Rembert Dodoens [1517 – 1585]
He wrote *New herbal' or historie of plants*

William Cole
Published a book on the medicinal use of plants in medicine. Cole was a famous herbalist of his day. Later on he published his investigations into the use of plant juices preserved with honey or wine. [2]

Thomas Johnson
An enlarged and amended version was published in 1633. Gerards Herbal contained 2765 illustrations of plants.

Culpeper [1616 – 1654]
His most well known work is '*The Complete Herbal and English physician.*' The Physical directory was published in 1649. *The 'English Physician Enlarged'* was an authoritative text. There have been many reprints of Culpepers books over the years.

Thomas Sydenham [1624 –1689]
An English physician who worked upon opium as a treatment.

John Parkinson [1640]
Published a *Theatrum botanicum*: the theatre of plants. It contained descriptions of the medicinal use of 3800 plants. He refers to Pliny in this work.

Jacob Theodorus [Basle 1664]
New volkommenlich - Krauter Buch

Robert Lovell [1665]
Pambotanologia or a complete herbal.

Nicholas Lemery [1700]
Published *Pharmacopoeia.*

Historical aspects

Linnaeus [1707 – 1778]
He classified plant names and the L after a plant signifies his trademark.

John Wesley
The first edition of *'Primitive Physic'* was available in 1747. It was an assertion Wesley said, 'of the right of every man of common sense; to prescribe to himself or his neighbour'.
Wesley was a Methodist preacher; he saved many lives using herbalism and thus turned much misery into happiness for the sufferers of disease. [9]

William Withering
A Staffordshire doctor published his work on Foxglove in 1785.

Samuel Thomson [1769 – 1843]
Published - *Narrative of the life and medical times of Samuel Thomson* in 1822 and *New guide to health* in 1825. Both books ran into ten editions.
Physiomedicalism commenced in North America with Thomson, he stated that cold or the lessening of heat was the cause of all disease and by restoring heat a cure was produced. Disease was caused by obstruction.

Herman Kohler
Published *Medicinal Pflanizen* [Medicinal plants] by 1887. It contains many beautiful illustrations of medicinal plants.

A.I. Coffin. M.D.
Wrote - *Botanic Guide to Health*: around 1860, forty one editions were published. He was one of the original founders of the N.I.M.H. He came to London in the early 19th century to lecture on the methods of Samuel Thomson. Coffin had practices in Leeds, Manchester and London.

During the 1850's, many new societies emerged - for example, the Peoples Medico - Botanic Association [based in London], and the British Thermo - Botanic Association [based in Birmingham]. Those leaders who hoped that herbalists might be included in the proposed Medical [registration] Acts, sought national unity to improve their case. In 1853 the National Medical Reform League was formed in London. Skelton, in Leeds, was asked to take part, but tried instead to extend his Friendly United Medico - The Botanic Sick and Burial Society. Skelton's later move to London Probably facilitated the foundation of the National Association of Medical Herbalists. From 1877 to 1888, a northern - based society of United Medical Herbalists of Great Britain attracted many established practitioners.

Herbal Medicine - Keys

These associations were considerably different from the mid - century organisations. The Medical act of 1858 had excluded herbalists, but herbalism became increasingly popular as a form of retailing. The number of herbalists listed in Manchester directories grew from two in 1852 to 171 in 1891, most of them in working class areas. The leaders of herbalism, endeavoured to raise the educational level of retailers. The new associations came to require courses of study and qualifying examinations. In 1890, after the National Association had absorbed the United Medical Herbalists, the new leadership tried to gain a Charter of Incorporation that would have enabled them to register and control herbal practice in England [10].

John Skelton
Wrote - *Science and Practice of Botanic Medicine* in 1870.

Wooster Beach M.D.
He founded the Reformed Medical College of New York in 1829 and published *American Practice* in 1842.

National Institute of Medical Herbalists was founded in 1864. It was dedicated to encourage the study and knowledge of herbal medicine. Professional journal started in 1888

William H. Cook
Cook published: *Physiomedical Dispensatory* [1869]. *Science and Practice of Medicine* [1879]. *Woman's book of health* [1902].

Jacob Redding
Medical professor at the Physiomedical college Indiana. He demonstrated the difference in the actions of herbs on white blood corpuscles.

T.J. Lyle
In 1897 Lyle published *Physiomedical therapeutics and materia medica*. He was Professor of therapeutics and materia medica at the physiomedical college, Chicago.

J.H. Greer
Wrote *Physician in the house* in 1897. He was Physician - in - chief, at the Harvard Medical Institute, Chicago.

J.M. Thurston
Tied in together, all the previous knowledge of the other physiomedicalists in his book '*Philosophy of Physiomedicalism*' it was published in 1900.

Historical aspects

William Fox. M.D.
In 1924 *'Family Botanic Guide'* was published. It gave a clear explanation of botanic practice, as well as a treatise of Samuel Thomson's theory of disease and Thomson's life history. [5]

M. Grieve
In 1931 *'A Modern Herbal'* was published. An encyclopaedic herbal with recipes.

A. Barker and A. Hall
Jointly edited by two herbalists. *The National Botanic pharmacopoeia* was printed in 1932.

A.W. & L.R. Priest
Herbal Medication is the most up to date physiomedical text published. It gives practical theory and remedies to physiomedical standards. Published in 1985. Reprinted NIMH 1999.

Review of physiomedical writers
Brief reviews of the important writers on physiomedicalism follows in this Chapter. Emphasis is upon each of the writer's contribution to improving standards of physiomedical philosophy and practice.

Thomson
Concentrated on elimination of accumulated toxins through the skin and alimentary tract. He used emetics and enema together with diaphoretics.

Wooster Beach
He defined fever and inflammation, which he says is either reconstructive or eliminative.
Elimination of toxins and equalisation of the circulation was his therapeutic regime. He observed the role of circulation in producing congestion.

John Skelton
Skelton's work concentrated upon the condition and impoverishment of the blood which led to chronic disease.

William Cook
Aimed to balance the physiology of the body. The level of contraction and relaxation being the primary cause of most diseases.
T. J. Lyle
Explains the physiomedical concept: relax - astringe - stimulate. Materia medica was included in this work.

Herbal Medicine - Keys

J.M. Thurston

Thurston saw the autonomic nervous system [ANS] as the controller of the viscera. If the A.N.S. is balanced, the bodily organs act in harmony together. Thurstons theorem and principia explain that the Vital force is always supportive in it's attempts to improve health. It is a force that always heals and strengthens it may perform inadequately depending upon the conditions within the tissues. Explanations are given on temperaments, vasomotor function, etc..

A & L Priest

An updated handbook for concise determination of physiomedical conditions. A useful materia medica is found within its pages.

Summary

Physiomedical ideas and hypothesis are suggested in this chapter as the way to treat the patient, not the disease. Writers quoted in this text offer considerable experience in their treatment of patients using herbal medication.

2
Philosophy of Physiomedicalism

What this Chapter is about
Physiomedical therapeutics may be clearly distinguished from empirical approaches. Physiomedical principles have been laid down for herbal use since Thomson's era.
Concise physiomedical herbalism is founded upon a system of enlightened therapeutic knowledge. It was Samuel Thomson who gave early insight and application of physiomedical principles.

Physiomedical philosophy offers a clear and ready system of therapeutics that can be used in the consulting room. It is a useful and practical approach that can give the herbalist clear insight into how to treat a patient. "The greatest enemy of any science is a closed mind" explains Dr. J. Rozencwajg, MD, PhD. Berman and Flannery give an updated account of the American Botanic movement from Thomson to Lloyd – an pharmacological history of herbal medicine [383].

What is Physiomedicalism?
Physiomedicalism is a science, in which the herbalist makes a diagnosis, from the presenting symptoms, history and examination of the patient. The diagnosis of any bodily condition will always reflect the level of vital force, physiological disturbance and the tissue state within the body. Tissue conditions are the first area for consideration by the physiomedicalist. Typology and bodily types are important factors in the assessment of the patient.

The physiomedical assessment is concerned with regulating physiological equilibrium and to reverse pathological changes. It places major emphasis upon the role of the blood, endocrine glands and ANS, as these are the mechanisms through which the organism is influenced from every level of higher function. The influences of various conditioning factors affecting the body may be seen long before disease emerges. The predispositions toward any particular type of disease disturbance arise because of the tendencies latent in the type of physique or type of personality and the study of these tendencies is referred to as typology. Typology sections in Chapter 10 carry these ideas forward.

Thurston's definition of Physiomedicalism.
'A medical philosophy founded on the theorem of vital force or energy inherent in the living matter of tissue cells, whose aggregate expression in health and disease are the functional activities of the organism whose inherent tendency is **integrative and constructive, resistive, eliminative and reconstructive to inimical invasions and disease causations'** [13].

Herbal Medicine - Keys

For a starting point to the philosophy of Physiomedicalism, we must look at the works of the early physiomedicalists.

The first of the pioneers is **Samuel Thomson,** he lived between 1769 - 1843.
He said 'the cause of all disease was due to cold [reduction in heat] in the body' [6]. Improve the level of thermotaxis [heat production] and the disease would be cured. Natural diffusion of heat through the body by using *Capsicum* would resolve any obstructive condition. The distribution of heat through the bodily tissues will clear any inhibiting effect of disease.
Thomson called obstruction 'canker', a white mucus coating, which attached itself to the stomach and bowel. It caused disease putrefaction and death [2].

Herbal medicine was used to open obstructions, promote perspiration and revive the digestive system. Thomson says: 'excite and maintain a due degree of heat and action through the system in every form of disease'. His recipe for curing all disease was this formula - to give *Capsicum* in every case. *Capsicum* would provide the stimulus for healing the patient. Thomson saved many lives during those times when fever, colic, quinsy, dysentery and chest ailments were common.

Thomson used the principle of stimulus to heat production, to promote removal of obstruction at the tissue level. He used other means such as emesis, vapour baths and stimulants to remove surface encumbrance.
[Note that surface refers to internal as well as external surfaces[.

The term obstruction refers to a condition that is either toxic, thermal or bacteriological. Fever is the vital response to any obstruction within tissues [12].

Thomson was granted a patent in 1813.
His patient was specified as - a system of practice, it applied:
[a] Stimulants
[b] Steam/vinegar baths in fever.
[c] Apply astringents to remove canker
[mucus and ulcerations in the alimentary tract].

Treatment would consist of the following.
He advised an emetic and purgative for a patient, this would remove the mucus conditions in the gastro intestinal tract. A hot steam bath would encourage the fever process; afterwards the patient would be given a digestive tonic.

Philosophy of Physiomedicalism

Thomson formulated six preparations

No 1. *Lobelia* Sig 2.5ml with no 2. Removes obstructions in the system. Give 3-8 doses for effect. Small doses first then increase as required.

No 2. *Capsicum* Sig 2.5-5ml. Retains internal heat and causes free perspiration.

No 3 aa *Myrica, Nymphaea, Pinus canadensis*. Scours the gastro intestinal tract and removes canker. Canker is a tendency to disease in any locality internal or external with ulcerations and tendency to putrefaction.
An alternative prescription is *Rhus aromatica, Rubus, Hamamelis*.

No 4. *Chelone, Populus tremuloides, Myrica, Hydrastis aa.*
The bitters restore digestion, create appetite, relieve indigestion and headache.

No 5. *Poplar bark and Myrica* 500g aa, *ground peach meats* 250g or *Cherry stone meats* 250g. Add aq 4 litres, sugar 1750g. Alcohol 4000ml. Sig 15ml TDS.
Used for dysentery it would strengthen the stomach and intestine.

No 6. *Commiphora, Capsicum*. Sig 5-10ml alone or add this amount to the bottle of medicine. Use for full central stimulation; asphyxia, drowning, rheumatic drops, remove pain, to prevent mortification, and promote a natural heat. [110]

Dr Wooster Beach.
He founded the Reformed Medical College of New York in 1929.
Beach describes several important physiomedical concepts in his book – *American Practice*, published in 1842.
Beach saw and criticised the current practice of orthodoxy.
'The increase in chronic disease is the result of secondary effects, which occur from suppressed and inadequately treated patients'. Beach said, the herbalist must

'observe nature's reactions closely and follow her indications'

Beach states:
[a] 'Health cannot exist without a natural and uniform balance between the nervous, circulatory and organic systems - it is a matter of surprise that physiologists have never noticed the connection between the nervous and circulatory systems'.
[b] 'Disease is obstruction. Use herbal medicines that will assist nature to remove the obstructions.
[c] 'The herbalist must assist nature to throw off morbid matter and thereby restore health to the patient'.
[d] Disease was intrinsic to the body.

Herbal Medicine - Keys

Two factors are required to produce a disease:

[a] the predisposition of the body towards the disease process and
[b] the application of the exciting cause [e.g. infection, chill etc]

Beach formulated three principles of herbal therapy.
[a] Assist the excretions - through improved elimination of waste matter.
[b] Restore thermotaxis [level of heat and cold] within the body. Achieve thermotaxis by improving circulatory function. Revived capillary circulation will relieve any deeper congestion of blood.
[c] Equalise the circulation.

Thermotaxis is related to circulatory function. Bodily levels of thermotaxis are balanced by using the capillary circulation. If congestion of blood in organ areas is present it will be adjusted through the capillary circulation.

Current disorders will indicate some deficiency in the local circulation. Once a current circulatory deficiency persists the area in question becomes irritated.

Irritated conditions result from blood becoming trapped in one area, irritation is the effect. Blood effusion to one location would impede the local circulation. The tissues would then retain their waste - which is unable to be removed.

Beach says
'When the balance of circulation is lost in the system; when the blood becomes unequal, or is driven from one part of the body to another from the influence of cold *or any other cause,* morbid excitement or a deviation from healthy action is the consequence. It has been almost invariably the case, if one part of the system has suffered from disease, particularly inflammatory, the opposite part of the system has been unusually cold'.

The treatment for irritated and inflamed conditions, consisted of bathing the skin, to recall the blood to the surface, by the application of heat and/or sudorifics. [6]

Beach describes inflammation and fever:
'Did practitioners know the nature and design of inflammation their treatment would be different. In fever it is produced by an increased action of the heart and arteries to expel acrid and noxious humours and should be promoted until the irritating matter is dislodged from the system. This should be effected by inducing perspiration to produce a natural degree of heat or inflammation that must be excited by internal/external remedies. Fever is nothing neither more nor

less than a wholesome and salutary effort of nature to throw off some morbific matter' [to remove toxins].

Fever arises as the body [a] tries to clear morbid waste [toxins] and [b] equalises the circulation.

Sometimes there is too much heat. It may then become necessary to lessen the hyper pyrexia and the accompanying arterial excitement by using [a] tepid sponging & [b] steam bath with *Nepeta cataria* herb added.

Eruptive diseases are due to deficient capillary circulation of the skin and organ congestion. Once the capillary circulation diminishes as a result of a disease process, the blood is driven to deeper levels and will congest in the organs. Beach tells us to bathe the body with warm water and give diaphoretics.

Typhoid fever
Bathe the whole surface skin with cold applications according to the temperature of the body. Give diaphoretic medicines, to return the eruptions to the skin surface [6]. Excessively stimulating diaphoretics [*Capsicum*] would aggravate the condition and is contra - indicated.

Pain or inflammation
[a] Where a stomach disorder or coated tongue are found administer an emetic.
[b] Use a steam bath with Catnep, Pennyroyal, Spearmint and Tansy.
[c] Give an infusion of Catnep [6].
When there is coldness of the body, stomach or bowel pain with weak pulse use stimulants.

Chronic disease
[a] Disordered stomach or furred tongue - requires an emetic.
[b] The next day give a purgative.
[c] Once the bowel has evacuated - give bitters and tonics.
[d] Bathe the whole body in a weak solution of soda crystals [Epsom salts], to clear the skin of viscid matter, which is obstructing the perspiration.
Repeat the course once or twice a week according to the indications.

John Skelton published his book, *Science and Practice of Medicine in 1870.*
Skelton's primary area of consideration was the blood. All disease originated in or from the blood. Treatment would aim to restore the blood to its original healthy condition [6].
These days, Physiomedicalism views the blood as a separate tissue for treatment. Herbalists use Vasotonic alterative to treat various blood conditions.

Herbal Medicine - Keys

Skelton says: 'The immediate cause of suffering was the gradual but constant deterioration of the blood from impure air and exhaustion by day, bad ventilation by night, and want of attention to the ordinary requirements of life'.
Skelton is saying here, that the underlying cause of disease is a deterioration of the blood condition.

Throughout the 726 pages of Skelton's work, many conditions are mentioned, together with the herbal treatments of that period - some are covered elsewhere in this work.

W.H. Cook

Around 700 pages of text make up *'Science and Practice of Medicine'*; it was published in 1879. Cook starts by saying 'The work here offered to the profession is an attempt to harmonise therapeutics with physiology'. Cook was Professor of Science and Medicine, Materia Medica, and Nervous Diseases at the College of Medicine, Chicago.

Cook says, 'any therapy must aim at a restoration of abnormal tissues, to the standard from which they have departed, that disturbances of function, which resulted from the abnormal conditions of the tissues, will cease when the normal tissue conditions have been restored'. For therapeutics must be the handmaiden to physiology and only by studying pathology in comparison with physiology can we hope to develop an accurate therapy. [6,11]

'An attempt to cure disease without definite principles or laws is *empiricism*; and while empiricism may occasionally be successful, it gives no relation between cause and effect, and can inspire no confidence as to future results - in the health of the patient'.
Physiomedicalism is thus clearly distinguished from the empirical approach.

Dr Jacob Redding

Redding made careful and exhaustive examinations of living leukocytes under the microscope, observing the different reactions that occurred under the influence of non poisonous herbal agents and poisonous drugs. In an article published in the Physiomedical journal, July 1881, Redding gives an account of the effects of *Capsicum* on living white blood cells. They presented a spherical form and which the granules [microzymas of Bechamp] rapidly moved in every direction, enabling the cell to move along with vigour and energy never before observed. Changes of form were observed which were at first slow but become more vigorous. The movement across the slide was fast but the cell was not seen to be exhausted at all. A similar experiment using Lobelia indicated that the agent produced the greatest degree of relaxation in the blood cells, which became as if

Philosophy of Physiomedicalism

dead and without movement at first but later gradually recovered their normal activity and vitality, none the worse for the effect of this herbal agent. Minute amounts of strychnine and morphine created a dead and dreary cell mass. Strychnine and morphine are agents that tend to be destructive and lethal to cells.

Dr T. J. Lyle

His book *Physiomedical Therapeutics and Materia Medica* was published in 1932. Some 44 pages are devoted to physiomedical principles with the remainder outlining herbal remedies in physiomedical concepts.

Lyle says '**Disease is defective physiology**'.

Treatment aims:
[a] Avoid all toxic and irritant agents during treatment.
[b] True medicine acts in harmony with the vital force.
[c] To restore health - create the opposite condition of that existing e.g. Congestion: apply heat and relieve the circulation using circulatory stimulation.

Dr Joseph. M. Thurston

The **Philosophy of Physiomedicalism** was published in 1900. It gives full details of the nature of disease, their aetiology and how to treat physiomedically. The Theorem and Principia of medicine are given in full. The term vital force is explained in an easy to understand language for herbalists. Health and disease are clearly defined. Changes from health, towards disease and disorder should be recognised and treated with herbalism.

Vasomotor function is the way that the autonomic and circulatory systems are intimately connected, to one another, and is described by Thurston. Some quotations in this text will help the aspiring physiomedicalist to understand the approach to patient treatment. Certain sentences may require to be read a number of times in order that they may be digested.

Modern scientific theory

Scientific thinking comes from the analysis of all the evidence collected. It should be for you to try to prove that any hypothesis previously formed in the mind is wrong. It is doubtful that the collection and prior analysis of evidence would produce a reasonable hypothesis. When you analysed the evidence did this produce new ideas or confirm existing ideas? It follows that the mind can only see what it is prepared to see.

Scientific procedure based upon Bechamp's theories must insist the absolute science of medicine is to **treat the patient**, not the disease.

Dr Lyle explains 'in all cases of either extra or depressed vital effort, carefully diagnose the conditions present that cause the vital force to put forth such efforts for its relief.'

> **'A diagnosis of the conditions present will furnish you with the indications for scientific medication'**
>
> [Lyle p17]

Summary
Physiomedical writers believe in the concept of a vital force as true healer of the body. Tissues become toxic when the body is unable to adequately eliminate toxins and impurities. Many acute symptoms are the result of the vital force trying to clear tissue toxins, resulting in the symptom complexes of disease.

Research is usually required to validate any theory. Students are taught in their courses to prove it with statements and quote authorities. There are many pieces of research by so-called authority figures who are sufficiently unqualified but their statements appear to carry weight because of their position in society rather than their knowledge. It is narrow minded and blinkered thinking that presumes no ideas or statements are to be valued because a statement cannot be verified scientifically.

Edward De Bono states 'ask the question and try to disprove the theory'. It is suggested that the reader do this - attempt to disprove the physiomedical theories explained in this work. The materia medica section containing remedies used in practice accepts the facts of remedy activity. Activity can be checked from any pharmacology book. Bibliography contains the herbal books used in this work as references.

3
Principles of treatment

What this Chapter is about
In treating chronic illness the following factors are of importance - degenerative, toxic and enervated states. Chronic illness refers to conditions that are of a long-standing nature. Many acute illnesses have their basis in a chronic syndrome. Chronic conditions often have a genetic background.

Four secondary conditions are covered in this chapter:
[a] acidity and uric acid
[b] catarrh
[c] cholesterol disturbances [See also Chapter 20 Cardiovascular system].
[d] toxic conditions.
All reflect general systemic disturbances with their resultant encumbrances upon the tissues.

Organ weakness known as hypotrophic states will determine the effectiveness of functional action and therefore the ability of the organ to perform its work.

1] Encumbrance
Assess the level of **encumbrance** within the tissues from a thorough case history e.g. tonsillectomy and appendicectomy indicate toxic reabsorption. Cholecystitis and cholelithiasis suggest reabsorption of biliary pigments. Stomach and pancreatic disturbance is often associated with disorders of the liver and gall bladder. It is often found that long standing biliary trouble tends to disturb the breakdown of cholesterol that ultimately accumulates in the blood vessels.
Encumbrance reflects the requirement for tissue cleansing. A history of papules, pustules, mucus/catarrhal discharge, sinus disturbances, inflammatory disturbances, operations, these all indicate a condition of encumbrance within the tissues.
2] Vitality
The state of vitality, especially the vital reserves, which must be drawn on in any disordered condition including emergency or acute illness when the body is attempting to improve health. **Vitality levels** are measured through the pulse and blood pressure together with the level of symptoms indicating the resistive strength of the vital force.
3] Organ weakness
Hypotrophic organ weakness particularly eliminative organ weakness and circulatory disturbances.

These three factors must be related to each other in any attempt to improve health matters. Development of a treatment plan for the patient depends upon a diagnosis of the tissue condition rather than treatment of the disease.

Alterative action - Vasotonic alteratives are blood cleansers.
Avoid any deep alterative changes while there remains any deficiency in the eliminative systems or in the circulatory system.
Evaluate the patient, in terms of their circulatory function as shown by the balance of **heat and cold**. That is the distribution of blood within the tissues. Is the patient warm in all parts? What is the pulse level and the blood pressure? Disturbance will often show the need for circulatory rebalancing.

Elimination
Heal the organs of elimination [secernants] before deep tissue cleansing takes place. Treat the [secernants] liver, gall bladder, intestines, kidneys and skin, as all eliminated toxins must be removed from the body by one avenue or another. Carefully assess any particular organ or system weakness before stimulating any activity that would throw extra strain upon that system. The most important precautions here are to avoid stressing the heart or lungs when these organs are in a weakened condition by stimulating an eliminative crisis by powerful alterative medicines.
Remember that it is wise to hasten slowly with treatment that involves blood and tissue cleansing.

Elimination

The secernants are the organs of elimination, liver, gallbladder, intestines, skin and kidneys.

Disturbance of an organ of elimination creates:
[1] Accumulation of toxins
[2] Enlargement of the organ [eventually organ congestion]
[3] Reabsorption of the uneliminated secretion or toxic matter.

Disturbance of the eliminative organs [secernants] result in circulatory obstructions, i.e. capillary congestion and engorgement. Eliminative organs are maintained in health by capillary activity. Local obstruction will result in a damming back of the blood to other blood vessels. Liver involvement creates portal engorgement with blood pooling in the small and large intestine, stomach and spleen. Adjustment of the capillary circulation is via vasomotor control of the blood vessels involved - either over-contraction or over-relaxation of those blood vessels.

Principles of Treatment

Blood pools in one area [hyperaemia] together with an ischaemia in another part of the body. There is a specific amount of blood for circulation and increase in one area means a decrease in another. Acute disease brings more blood to the area of disturbance e.g. inflammation [active hyperaemia].

Remedial agents required to produce a cleansing action are called Vasotonic alteratives. As vasotonics cleanse the blood of impurities the cell is encouraged to rid itself of impurities; cellular function is thus improved. Most organ remedies are also gently alterative in their action.

Blood and tissue cleansing must always allow for the level of assumed toxicity. If is important to understand that 50% of cell volume waste can only be encouraged to clear into a 5% of blood volume. Slow release of impurities would prevent a bottleneck to elimination. When elimination is promoted too quickly it will cause an excess of impurities to be cast into the blood. The excess impurities are particularly dangerous, where there is an inability of the secernants to rid the impurity quickly. No major blood cleansing action is advised until the secernants are eliminating adequately.

Priority is given to strengthen organs that are weak or under functioning.

Secretory deficits are treated by
1] balancing: the vasomotor function via relaxation or toning
2] stimulating the tissue cells for cleansing [Vasotonic alterative, immune supportives].
3] toning the tissue.
4] circulatory disturbances: remove obstructions and equalise, e.g. *Angelica archangelica, Zingiber.*
5] nerve adjustment requires either toning or a relaxing influence.

Secondary conditions frequently observed are:
Acidity
Catarrh
Infection
Inflammation
Toxicity/autotoxaemia

The above conditions commonly present the great majority of the effects of disease processes found in the patient. A cause for the above effects should be sought. Many conditions can be helped with changes to diet and enhancement of nutritional levels of amino acids, fats, carbohydrates, vitamins, minerals and trace elements.

Herbal Medicine - Keys

Acidity [uric acid]

It is the constantly changing environment of cellular activity, tissue activity, nerve function and blood condition that affect the individual levels of tissue acidity.

The blood acid level constantly varies depending upon:
1] The kinds of food being eaten
2] Cellular activity
3] Blood acid level
4] Levels of stress and nerve function
5] The ability of the body to eliminate the residual acid from the blood and hence the tissues, with dependency on hepatic and renal system clearance.

1] Foodstuffs

Acid is produced from metabolic activity. Dietary acid is produced from meat, particularly red meat, also coffee, tea, refined white sugar white bread and vinegar. Stimulants like coffee, tea and alcohol cause acid to move from the blood to the tissues. Excess accumulation of acid eventually creates depression, lassitude, fatigue and headache. Sufferers crave more stimulants in an attempt to overcome the above symptoms which then creates more acid and further symptoms. Reduction of acid forming substances enables the blood to clear the excess acid. Changes made in the diet support the reduction of blood acid. When the blood is cleared of excess acid, over time, the whole body benefits. In severe cases a dietary regime is needed, possibly with fasting or mono food diets.

Correct mineral therapy is required to support the tissue elimination of acid e.g. Sodium phosphate taken as a mineral tissue salt in acidic conditions.

2] Cell activity

Cellular activity creates the acid that then finds its way into the blood to be eliminated. Cellular fluids have a normal alkaline range of pH 7.2 to 7.5. Any reduction in these levels towards one of acid creates changes in the cellular environment. Excess uric acid causes inflammation of cellular tissue. Unpleasant body odour could indicate the elimination of acids through the skin this is known as a vicarious elimination.

3] Blood acid

The blood is detoxified by the liver and filtered by the kidneys. Excess amounts of acid can be eliminated via the skin if the load through the kidneys is excessive. When the blood acid increases to dangerous levels the acid is often redirected into the musculoskeletal system. It will be noticed that once this occurs there will be a temporary improvement in the patient's condition - symptoms improve under these homeostatic measures. The body has moved the acid to where it will do the least harm. The muscle and joint areas have now become pools for the acid. Eventually the patient will complain of rheumatics and the so-called arthritis syndrome develops. Rheumatic symptoms show that uric acid is causing a chronic inflammatory condition within the muscles and bones that requires reduction of acid levels to alleviate the situation. Continued acidity destroys cartilage and creates chronic pain. Reduction of acid levels may not occur quickly under treatment, the condition must be controlled first before any symptoms improve.

4] Stress and nerve hyperfunction
Neurone activity at the dendrites creates waste uric acid at transmitter sites from amino acids L - aspartic and L - glutamic acids. Following neurotransmitter action enzymes are required to break down the transmitter chemical. In health this is cleared automatically. Excitability of nerve cells; long continued anxiety, worry and stress create further blood acid. Nerve excitability becomes a major cause of acid build-up and frequently the body is unable to eliminate the high levels of acid so produced.

5] Elimination of acid
Hypofunction of the renal system commonly throws acid back into the blood where it may show at some period of seemingly unrelated acute illness. The beginnings of rheumatic and arthritic troubles are felt once blood uric acid levels are excessive. During diabetic keto acidosis and starvation the eliminative force of respiratory and renal systems spring into action to remove excess acid and maintain acid - base balance in the tissues. Typically the breath smells sweet in ketosis.

6] Stomach acidity
Hyperchlorhydria is often associated with an increase of general acidity within the tissues. Reduction of stomach acid supports the overall process of reducing excessive blood acid levels. Apple cider vinegar is alkaline when taken orally.

Remedies which have an affinity to clear acid residue:
General cleansers - apple cider vinegar - diluted with 3 parts water and a little honey added if necessary. Medicinal charcoal and Lemon juice are antacid and have alkalising effects.
Stomach – Hyper/hypochlorhydria – *Agrimonia, Artemesia absinthium, Carum carvi, Chamomilla, Cinnamomum, Erythraea, Filipendula, Fumaria, Gentiana, Jateorrhiza, Melissa, Menyanthes, Taraxacum rad,*
Dec. Jam. Sarsae Co. [Compound decoction of Jamacian Sarsparilla].
Biliary system/hepatic/cholagogue – Taraxacum rad, Berberis species, Dioscorea, Peumus.

Herbal Medicine - Keys

Diuretics for the kidneys – Agropyron, Apium, Zea.
Blood and cellular herbs are alterative/antacid/astringent - Cimicifuga, Filipendula, Guaiacum, Salix alba, Menyanthes, Populus tremuloides, Smilax, Teucrium species.

Catarrh

Mucus is a normal secretion within the body and maintains a protective function for mucous membranes. Excessive mucus production occurs when the mucous membrane becomes disordered due to a variety of factors.

Excessive mucus production arises from:
- Infection
- Inflammation
- Injury to tissues e.g. ulcers
- Irritations to the mucous membrane e.g. allergies, dust, hay fever, smoke inhalation.
- Vicarious elimination of blood impurities in the form of catarrh.

When the blood is cleansed and detoxified little excess mucus exists. It is when blood toxins or impurities become excessive that catarrh arises. Catarrh is the overflow of toxins from the blood. Using the analogy of a bucket – as the bucket fills no symptoms emerge, it is not until the bucket is full and overflows that we encounter symptoms. Stopping the catarrh and drying it up is inadequate treatment. What about the bucket full of impurities, that also must be emptied, this always takes time to achieve. Excess mucus is most often the result of eliminative disorder.

As the disorder clears excessive mucus subsides. When mucus persists astringent medicines are used which dry up excessive mucus; they contain tannin which is also antiseptic. Where the cause is infective then vasotonic alterative antimicrobials are used which have a stronger action to limit an infective process.

Never use too strong astringents where infection is present, as they risk drying the infection into the membrane and thereby delay recovery.
Salty tasting mucus suggests renal disorder possibly from a urinary infection or urinary congestion.

Medicines used to clear catarrh depend on the causative factors:
Nasal catarrh - Calendula, Eucalyptus, Euphrasia, Ephedra.
Bronchial catarrh - Agrimonia, Armoracea, Eucalyptus, Hyssopus, Marrubium, Symphytum.

Principles of Treatment

Stomach atony - Agrimonia, Gentiana.
Intestinal atony - Hamamelis, Plantago, Polygonum, Uncaria.
Renal atony - Capsella, Solidago.
General anticatarrhals – Althea, Capsicum, Glechoma hederacea, Hydrastis, Ocimum.
Infective catarrh: treated with antimicrobial and antiseptic Vasotonic alterative - Allium, Baptisia, Berberis vulgaris, Commiphora, Echinacea, Hydrastis, Phytolacca, Sambucus, Solidago, Tabebuia, Thymus, Ulmus, Uncaria.

Infection see Chapter 6
Inflammation see Chapter 6

Cholesterolaemia

Cholesterol is a necessary component for health. It is necessary to reduce and if possible eliminate bad cholesterol [**LDL** cholesterol] in the diet. LDL cholesterol is responsible for Hyperchoesterolaemia.
Bad cholesterol is produced from saturated animal fats - fat on meat, excessive animal fat intake leads to immune depression, the skin of poultry, margarine, refined sugar, cream, hydrogenated vegetable oils, etc. must be removed from the diet in order for the good fats [**HDL**] to predominate in the diet. [See Chapter 20].

Hypothyroid conditions can increase blood cholesterol. Hypoglycaemia and diabetes create cholesterol disturbances as part of the disease process.

Essential fatty acids [EFA's] linoleic and linolenic acids occur in plants and help protect against autoimmune disease, cancer, heart disease, etc. Essential fatty acids are polyunsaturated fats. They serve to function as components of cellular membranes, nerve cells and prostaglandins. They are found in Borago, Oenothera [Evening primrose oil] and blackcurrants.

Treatment scheme to reduce cholesterol
Increase the amount of fibre in the diet. Fruit, green and root vegetables are good as they contain fibre that breaks down cholesterol.
During normal metabolism any excess homocysteine derived from the breakdown of the amino acid methionine can be eliminated with the use of the following:
Chromium has a balancing effect upon blood lipids and glucose levels.
Folic acid – corrects methionine metabolism.
Betaine hydrochloride - corrects methionine metabolism.
Vitamin B5 [pantothenic acid] - supports transport of fats to and from cells.
Vitamin B6- corrects methionine metabolism.
Vitamin B3 [Niacin] - lowers fibrinogen, LDL. and tryglycerides.
Vitamin C – oxygenation of the blood and tissues.

Anticholesterolaemic medicines
Acacia goetzei, Albizia anthelmintica/lebbeck, Allium [fresh is better than the oil], Andrographis paniculata, Angelica sp., Berberis sp., Betula, Capsicum, Centella, Cimicifuga, Commiphora, Corchorus oliturius [saluyot], Crataegus, Curcuma longa, Ganoderma, Mentha piperita, Momordia charantia [ampalaya], Moringa oleifera [malunggay], Panax, Plantago - 5g BD, Tilia, Trigonella, Viscum, Vitex negundo [lagundi], Yucca, Zanthoxylum, Zingiber.
[Cholesterol-lowering benefit of supplement confirmed by study.
P. C. Colmenares. Manilla bulletin. Health & Science. 26 March 2003].
Herbal treatment must always attend to the thyroid, pancreatic, liver and gall bladder function, blood and nervous system as they effect the amount of cholesterol within the blood.
Cholagogues and choleretics are used to promote bile secretion and excretion.
Relaxing cholagogues: Eupatorium perfoliatum, Carduus, Leptandra, Taraxacum, Silybum.
Tonic hepatics: Agrimonia, Berberis species, Hydrastis, Iris and Myrica.
Pancreas supportives – Chionanthus, Iris.

Toxicity/autotoxaemia

What is a toxin?
A toxin is any damaging influence that could affect the cell. Autotoxaemia means the absorption from a toxic focus i.e. from a leaky gut, chronic infective conditions i.e. tonsillitis. Toxins and impurities are carried from the toxic focus by the bloodstream to a group of cells anywhere within the body and settle [are tolerated] or eliminated often in the form of furunculosis, abscess, pustules etc.

Where do toxins come from?
Toxins can occur from chemicals in foods and most certainly from synthetic drugs.
Organ damage and poor trophic response within an organ encourages inability to remove the impurities, which cause encumbrance and toxin build-up.

Intestine
The intestine can leak toxins [abnormal, immature proteins] into the blood setting up allergic reactions.
Liver
A main action of the liver is to detoxify the blood. Liver activity is affected by the health of the intestine, gall bladder and nervous system.
Kidneys
Renal action is affected by the blood pressure level. Hypotension diminishes renal activity. Skin activity affects the kidneys. Under functioning skin increases the

amount of blood that can become congested in the deeper tissues. Sallow, dry, hypotrophic skin is devoid of blood and is a frequent accompaniment to poor capillary activity of the skin.

Summary

Many common conditions often arise from deeper organ disturbances. Catarrh from intestinal disorders - constipation, IBS, renal disturbances, poor skin function, diet etc. Assess the condition of the eliminative organs together with the diet and treat accordingly. [See Chapter 11].

4
Vitality and the Vital Force

What this Chapter is about
Vitality and Vital force are terms often confused when put side by side. They mean two quite different things. Vitality, reserve vital energy and life tenacity are terms used to consider the prognosis of the patient. Vital force encompasses Chi in a more modern concept however the principles all remain the same throughout this work. Consideration is given to their relevance in herbal practice.

Vitality means **an individuals hold on life** [Oxford dictionary]. Thurston says **'vitality** relates to the force and vigour of vital action as manifest by the general functional activities.' An individual has a level of vigour that is part of their personality. One may be said to be vigorous, full of pep and energy. Vitality levels are dependent upon a healthy functioning of the CNS. The vital and vigorous types are less susceptible to disease aetiology. Priest says vitality is a measure of vital expenditure [6].

Vital force is a term used by physiomedicalists to explain the amount of energy within the tissues and organs of the body. Vital force is the **cellular energy** present in the cell mitochondria.

Liebig gives his comments on the vital force. 'It is a great and comprehensive law of matter that it's particles possess no self activity, no inherent power of originating motion when at rest.' 'Motion must be imparted by some extraneous cause.' 'The vital force is manifested in the form of resistance, in as much as by its presence in the living tissues, their elements acquire the power of withstanding the disturbance and change in their form and composition which external agents tend to produce - a power which as chemical compounds, they do not possess.' 'The laws of life cannot be investigated in an organised being which is dead or dying' [6].

The vital force is 'a form of energy ordering the movement of matter at an organic level
Vitality builds up the frame, repairs it and maintains it's motions, this power also resists the influences of destruction and preserves the body against other forces that incline it to decay' explains Cook [11].

Vitality is strong when the individual feels healthy, robust and glowing together with the absence of emotional disorder. Negative emotions such as fear, worry or depression all deplete the vitality. Depletion of vitality induces illness and may provoke disease conditions. Some individuals maintain a very strong hold on life.

Vitality and the Vital Force

Even in the presence of severe disease such people keep on struggling never giving in to illness. Where depleted vitality is encountered frequent illness is found. In some of these individuals when one condition clears another condition replaces it. There may not be enough vital force to remove the causative condition permanently. Lowered vitality is considered a **primary cause of disease**. [42]

Typology [somatotype] enables the herbalist to assess the levels of potential energy within the body. Asthenic typology types expend their energy rapidly due to ANS instability. Pyknic types have more direct control over their energy because of greater ANS stability. Typology supports the view of ANS balance in the individual [See typology Chapter 10].

Vital resistance. 'The resistive and eliminative capacity of vital force as manifest in the individual under exposure to disease causations' [Thurston]. Vital resistance enables the cell to resist disease.

Reserve vitality. 'The reserve vital energy remaining in the cell during the functional activities in health and disease' [Thurston]. Resting or potential energy is held in the tissues as *reserve energy*. In disease conditions the potential energy becomes kinetic energy and some is utilised to ward off disease.

Life tenacity. Is expressed as 'one's will to live'. 'The persistence with which an individual clings to life under adverse environments and severe disease conditions'. [Thurston p185].
The attributes vital force, vital resistance, etc. if related to the constitution [typology and level of trophicity] will be valuable when making a forecast as to the patient's prognosis.

Flower remedies for the emotions are found useful in such cases of depleted vitality with emotional disorder. Rebalancing with flower remedies allows vitality to flow unobstructed through the body. The Bach flower remedy Olive is used for mental and physical exhaustion, Hornbeam for the weary and being unable to cope with the daily workload. [See Chapter 25].

Negative feelings create a constriction to the flow of vitality resulting in a holding of emotion to certain organ areas. Fear binds to the kidneys and gastro intestinal tract. Depression binds to the liver and gall bladder. Excitability affects the heart. The area of emotional hold upon the organ [called holding points] depends upon the specific characteristics of the patient. A constitutional or familial tendency would produce effects upon the tissue or organ area. Genetic predispositions create these same disturbances. Sufficient negative emotional excitation would be required for symptoms to emerge. Some individuals could become ill in a short space of time where a lowered threshold of response is found. Careful history taking gives useful information on the predispositions toward the effect negative feelings have together with the effects of such emotions. Iridology gives information for assessment of the holding points of disease. Disorders of the emotions and actual physical disease disperses through the ANS as [sympatheticotonia/parasympatheticotonia]. Over excitability of the ANS creates disturbed physiology in the end organ.

The theorem and principia of medicine
Extracted from Philosophy of Physiomedicalism 1900. Professor J. Thurston.

Theorem
'The living organism is essentially a vital realm dominated by the vital force. All functional operations of the organism in health or disease are the expressions of vital action in the living matter of tissue cells. This vital force manifests only through the cell. It is endowed with integrating and developmental instincts and from the basic cell builds up the organism and maintains its functional integrity. Vital force through living cells is always resistive, eliminative and reconstructive in intent and purpose when inimical substances, forces or influences invade the vital domain. Vital force is an energy that resides within the cell. It always attempts to heal and preserve the integrity of the organism.'

Principia
'The human organism has integrative, constructive and regenerative instincts. The living organism is a systematic and purposeful aggregation of tissue cells each cell developed with activity by the vital force. The vital force working within the cell takes in nutrients that are synthesised for cellular use. Vital force is a living energy and manifests itself through the resistive activity of the cells. This Physiomedical philosophy looks upon disease as an enforced departure of vital activities from the normal standard of functional integrity because of invasion of the tissue cells by extrinsic [extracellular] inimical influences. The primary effect of such invasion is always manifest upon the cell.'

'The **functional changes**, such as the exaggerated or depressed and lowered functional activity are the consequences as **secondary effects** they follow the primary disturbance of the cell.'

Vital force is always **resistive, eliminative and reconstructive** in its efforts to heal the body says Thurston. **Resisting** disease is a primary function of the vital force. Most symptoms are produced because of this feature, e.g. cough, diarrhoea, pain, skin rash, etc. An attempted elimination of toxins by the tissues occurs with the above complaints. Most acute disease is of this nature and should not be

Vitality and the Vital Force

suppressed. **Elimination** of waste and toxins is a functional necessity to preserve health. **The vital force undertakes reconstruction of and repair of tissue**, for example; a cut heals and leaves a scar. Chronic conditions, for example ME [myalgic encephalomyelitis] occur because there is an insufficient level of vital force to heal the nerve cells. This leaves the tissues depleted and exhausted. Trophorestorative medication is then required to encourage cellular activity and improve trophic response. Many chronic diseases fall into the hypotrophic category.

Vital force Chi energy is the energy within the cell. It is the directive conscience of the cell. It governs cellular activity. Giving positive restorative food and medicines can increase the actual amount of vital force available. The vital force utilises the nutrient material given to it. No food or medicine can have any effect upon a dead cell. The difference between a live cell and a dead cell - is the vital force. Vital action is always aroused in an attempt to resist disease.

Vital chi energy is present in the cell **mitochondrial** organelles of which there are many within each cell. Classes of medicines called stimulants stimulate cellular energy. No amount of stimulants can produce vital force. It is the stimulant that **draws energy from the cell.**

To stimulate [the vital force] means local or general functional activity is increased whereby the supply of vital force to a part is focussed with the stimulant and it's carrier remedy.

Consideration needs to be made on the strength of stimulus in a prescription. If a strong herb like *Capsicum* is given inappropriately e.g. too early in pyrexia, it can raise the level of vital force too quickly before the tissues have completed their work. This may leave the tissue encumbered and the causative factors persisting. When Capsicum or other strong stimulant are used too early they deplete rather than arouse the vital force to heal. When required pyrexia is enhanced with *Achillea, Zanthoxylum or Zingiber* - they increase the temperature. Chronic conditions require stimulation.

If the patient presents with an acute illness while under treatment, the new condition is treated immediately. When symptoms abate or the resistance becomes tardy this is the time to use more stimulation to cellular function and further arouse the secernants [eliminative organs] to promote elimination.

Typology [bodily physique] is a guide to the amount of vital force available for healing.

Symptoms are the direct result of the vital force in action. The vital force is always trying to do its best to preserve the cell from damage by eliminating impurities. Symptoms reflect the tissue state, whereby treatment encourages a healthy state of function. Sometimes symptoms are robust this is always a good sign. Symptoms guide us to the area of disturbance reflect the vital force in action, they are not the disease itself. A decline in the activity of symptoms can indicate reduced vital power and calls for stronger stimulation. Chronic disease will **deplete** the vital chi force. Healing can only fully take place where sufficient vitality and vital force are present. Modern medicine seeks to suppress the symptoms of the vital force. Using antipyretics in fever, anti inflammatories in inflammation and painkillers for pain these suppress symptoms. Physiomedical treatment is centred towards the cell in all treatments.

Observation of the vital chi force within the body will require an analysis of the following:

a] **A normal vital effort**
b] **A vital effort in disease resistance**
c] **A vital effort under the influence of remedial measures**   [Lyle. P2]

A **normal vital effort** is healthy action within the tissues. Normal vital action is found when the body clears all waste from the tissues without the appearance of symptoms.

Vital effort in disease resistance encroachment requires that more vital energy be used to clear the disease process, whereupon latent vital energy springs into action and becomes kinetic energy available for healing. It is during this stage symptoms may arise.

Under the influence of remedial measures the vital force is directed towards the disturbed tissue. It uses the medicine to bring about elimination of toxins and repair of cells.

The vital force has three levels of function:

Positive   Tolerant   Negative

A **Positive** vital force is found in a healthy individual and is eliminative and reconstructive. A robust level of vital action is found whenever disease attempts to gain a hold. Vital action is quick to bring about a normalisation of tissue activity and function, often without the effects of any symptoms. Absences of symptoms require a certain amount of discrimination to decide whether the patient is healthy or unwell. It may be decided the condition is being sufficiently dealt with by the vital force and little treatment is required except to restrict the food intake. Less food means an increased level of vital energy in the tissue. When no food is taken all vital energy is diverted to detoxifying the tissues. Other guides of functional activity of the vital force are: typology, tongue diagnosis,

Vitality and the Vital Force

pulse and blood pressure readings, skin examination - colour, tone and temperature are useful **indicators** of vital activity within the tissues.
A **Tolerant** vital force reflects depletion of cellular energy. It is unable to remove the disease cause and must therefore tolerate it. Toleration of disease conditions will give rise to **encumbrance**. Encumbrance hinders the movement of toxins from the tissue.
A **Negative** vital force within the tissues confirms a depleted level of energy that is ineffective in removing encumbrance, this leads to chronic symptoms. Long standing disease reflects the negative vital state. In the negative vital state symptoms are of a lower grade than in the acute condition.

Assessment of the vital force is made by a study of the symptoms and signs. Children often have a higher level of vitality when compared with an adult - fewer encumbrances of the tissues from toxins are found in children. Encumbrance depletes both vitality and vital force this leads to symptom expression.

The freer the flow of life forces the greater the vitality of the patient. Vital force is converted from a reserve [potential energy], which it gives out as required during disease [kinetic energy] conditions. Inimical influences disturb cellular activity, as a result the vital force becomes a less efficient dispenser of energy under adverse conditions of the tissues. Disease is an unbalanced and disturbed polarity wherein the affected molecular activity of the cellular environment is disturbed. The cell in disease has a lowered vibratory activity. As the vibratory activity is lowered so the cellular activity becomes disturbed. This leads to encumbrance and toxins in the cell. Depleted vital force occurs in incorrect feeding habits, negative thinking and overindulgence of all kinds.
Vitality and the vital force are stimulated by stimulants for example *Capsicum, Cochleria, Myrica, Szygium, Zanthoxylum, Zingiber and tonics.* These medicines stimulate the vital force to action, removing obstruction and encouraging healthy functional action of the tissue cells. Depleted vitality may require longer-term alteratives [Vasotonic alterative] to clear the tissues of encumbrance and toxins. Pathology of the tissue or an encumbrance will require careful assessment before deep cleansing takes place. The patient may need gentle tonics in order to strengthen them **before** any deep cleansing is undertaken.
Herbalists always work with the vital force, encouraging healing and detoxification of the tissue. An understanding of the vital force will help to medicate in a scientific manner.

How to **enhance vitality and the vital chi force**.
Vital force enhancement: correct feeding habits, calm nerves, relaxation, correct breathing and herbal medication.

Herbal Medicine - Keys

Whole foods are of the order when organic and fresh. Foods with a balance of proteins, carbohydrates and fats sufficient minerals and vitamins are necessary for good health. Foods lightly cooked by steaming or stir-fry best preserves the nutrients.

A healthy nervous system will not be over excitable or depressed in its function. Depressed nerve function robs the nerve of its vitality, as does anxiety.
An aid to relaxation is found by deep **breathing**. Lindlahr mentions deep breathing to balance the body. Most Yoga teachers advise deep breathing. Deep breathing settles anxiety and rebalances the emotions together with the vital force. It gives one a feeling of well being [increased vitality] and found when the body and mind are calm.

Flower remedies can be used to remove a negative feeling which block happiness. A frequent finding in chronic disease is decreased vitality and a negative vital force. Both conspire to aggravate the disease process and feelings of hopelessness within the patient. Flower remedies release blocks within the emotions. Flower remedies and tissue salts assist the vital force to heal the body and mind. It is the disordered vibration accompanying a disease that if matched by the appropriate remedy of the same or similar vibration will alleviate the condition. An electromagnetic current within the body directly linking the nervous and circulatory systems is influenced by herbal and vibrational remedies e.g. tissue salts, herbal and flower remedies. Herbal medicine will enhance the vitality of the patient.

1] **Long standing anxiety depletes the vital force** which in turn leads to a depressed function or exhaustion of the nerves at the level of the CNS. Nervines restore depleted vitality, help to rebalance nerve action, reduce anxiety or remove depression. [See Chapter 25]

2] **Chronic tissue encumbrance can deplete the vitality**. An understanding of the vital force and the vitality level supports treatment in a scientific way.
The vital chi force is the healing force of the cell it has various levels that require to be interpreted before undertaking treatment. Vitality and vigour give an estimation of the individual's personality. Using typology as a guide we are able to assess the level of the vital force available and to make certain prognostic recommendations as to treatment and lifestyle for the patient. Emotional disorders require flower remedies.
Nervine medicines are used when a condition of undue nerve distress is encountered.

Vitality and the Vital Force

Disease is a tissue state

'Any substance or influence that will change the normal vital standard of functional potency in the living matter of cells must secondarily and proportionately pervert the functional integrity and harmony of the organised tissues and structures within the body. It follows no substance can alter the functional activity except as it changes the conditions of the cell. If conditions are normal then normal physiology follows. If a substance produces abnormal conditions in the cell it is **inimical** to the cell and perverted functional cellular activity will result. When the cell is invaded by any abnormal influence it will increase the functional activity to elevate eliminative functions. The altered vital action must always ensue from some extrinsic inimical influence' Thurston.

Symptoms can arise from two sources
[1] functional secondary effects within the tissues as a result of disturbance within the cell
[2] the vital force resisting disease will produce effects on any of three levels:

[a] Cell level
[b] Within the whole body at a level within the capacity to adapt and heal
[c] Where the body produces symptoms because is under greater threat

Other effects that occur such as inflammation, fever, irritation and pain always follow changes within the cell. These effects are functional aberrations and not disease but are symptoms and signs of an abnormal tissue state.

Summary
The revival of Thurston's principia calls us to demand a readjustment of old truths and principles to a basic hypothesis that will admit of perfect harmony and rational continuity of each and every known fact into an exact and **scientific system** of medicine.

5
Functional associations and functional changes

What this chapter is about
The physiomedical system is based upon using the cell mitochondria as the focus of energy. This is where the vital force resides. Cellular function takes up and uses nutrients. When a problem arises in the body it is the single cell that has become disturbed and has affected other cells in a circumscribed area. Functional disturbance follows disturbed cellular function. Disturbances of function create symptoms as disease progresses. Functional change implies a change in cellular activity away from a contracted or relaxed condition towards pathology. Primary change is the excess contracted or relaxed condition of tissues from normal health towards pathological change. Pathology means the tissue has progressed towards a more permanent change in the tissue structure. A change in tissue structure eventually carries the disease tissue into a congestive phase. Congestive conditions require stimulants.

The body functions as a complete organism and recognises that no single organ could be disturbed without imparting some disturbance to other areas. The nervous and circulatory systems receive impressions as disease patterns become established. Both the circulatory and nervous systems are dependent upon one another. When the nerves of any part become excited, the activity of the local circulation is increased for example a transient blush called up by emotion.

The nerves transmit impressions of disease. These nerves when irritated by disease encroachment, proclaim the fact. They are never content to keep it to themselves, the local ganglia are stimulated to function. The affected nerve carries the impulse through the nerve innervation to effector end plates:

[a] **First to contiguous parts**
[b] **Then to organs associated in a common purpose**
[c] **Lastly to the organism at large**

Indirect functional effects can occur with disease conditions that affect the primary tissue. Symptoms result from the secondary disturbance of the primary disorder such as a cough; from a mitral valve lesion, urethral irritation from the kidney, comedones from impure blood, etc. Tissues can become over relaxed or over contracted in their function. Over contraction or over relaxation of the tissue is known as the functional state.
Disease encroachment rallies the vital force to resist disease. Medicine should be prescribed for the cause of the suffering. Treatment of pain may be needed to allay suffering as pain can cause depletion of the vital force and delay recovery.

Functional Associations & Functional Changes

Pain may also become a cause of disease - a pathocausative. Pain can cause mental distress and thereby further the patients suffering.

Mixed tissue states

Reflected conditions occur frequently within the tissues. A disorder can throw the burden of encumbrance upon another organ area. Some systems are intimately connected as the following shows:

- Lung disease can accompany disease from the liver/gall bladder or stomach.
- Renal disease and lung disease may occur together.
- Renal and skin function affect one another.
- Bladder disorders can affect hearing and ear disorders. See ear/bladder line in Iridology.
- Duodenal disorders can affect pancreatic activity and bile flow.
- Intestinal and skin diseases are often found e.g. acne.
- Intestinal pathology causes autointoxication [reabsorption of toxins].
- Pancreatic disease and hepatic/gall bladder disturbance often coincide
- Nerve disease can be affected from retained secretions of bile/uric acid. Nervous disorders affect immunity e.g. long continued stress and depression depletes vital energy.

Reflex associations

- Giving a laxative can ease throat disorders such as halitosis, soreness, and tonsillitis.
- Cholesterol disturbances can result from disturbed diet, anxiety, hypothyroid also from a disturbed pancreas, liver and gall bladder.
- Anxiety effects cholesterol levels.
- Stomach inactivity can be eased with the use of an emetic and cathartic.
- Relieve the liver in renal trouble thereby aiding kidney function.
- Diarrhoea is often nature's way and is homeostatic in that offensive waste is removed by clearing the bowel.
- Diarrhoea and constipation could occur from liver disorders that is from a lack of secretion and excretion of bile.
- Constipation will irritate the kidneys from absorption of toxins.
- Urethral irritation is aggravated if bowel or hepatic disturbance is present. Retained biliary pigment always affects the condition of the blood and eventually the kidneys and bladder attempt to carry off the waste this causes infections and irritable conditions within the genito urinary system.
- Kidney and adrenal activity are effected by the emotions. Diuresis is often increased with a panic attack.
- Vaginal and uterine irritation may progress from a bladder disturbance; that is from mucus membrane surfaces or organs in close proximity with one another

Cellular environments

The cell is effected in its function by:

1] Cell membrane permeability
2] Intracellular fluid
3] Extracellular fluid, lymph and autoimmune components
4] The blood
5] Nerve innervation
6] Endocrine secretions.

Treatment aims to restore the cell to its healthful condition

Cell membrane

The cell membrane is permeable to molecules entering or leaving the cell. Sodium and potassium are important minerals. The sodium pump within the cell tends to displace the more important potassium leading to cellular oedema.

Intracellular fluid

The fluid within the cell is subject to toxicity when inadequately detoxified.

Extracellular fluid, lymph and autoimmune components

The tissue fluid surrounds all cells it carries nutrients and also impurities.

Blood

Vasotonic alterative medicines effect the condition of the blood. These also effect the tissue fluid and lymph. Blood carries nutrients and impurities and its condition is determined by the ability of the liver to detoxify and the kidneys to filter out deleterious material from the blood.

Blood volume is effected through the vasomotor control to the cell and organs including the endocrine glands [see vasomotor].

Nerve mineral effects

Mineral balance is often crucial particularly in acute conditions. Potassium and sodium balance affect the fluid levels within the body and each individual cell. Calcium and magnesium are antagonists and balance bone deposition and nerve relaxation. Checking the diet for sufficient amounts of these minerals is a necessity.

Endocrine glands

The thyroid, parathyroid, testes, ovaries and adrenals are the endocrines and have important effects. Glandular activity creates hormones which in turn effect cellular activity. Hypothyroidism is a frequent finding. Adrenal over activity is common and leads to exhaustion. The fertility cycle determines ovarian activity.

Summary

Once disease becomes established within the tissues, the disease process will eventually effect other tissues and organs. For example a genetic predisposition towards hyperchoesterolaemia will be encouraged in an Asthenic whose nervous system is delicate. Tension that effects the gall bladder will eventually affect the

Functional Associations & Functional Changes

liver too this encourages hyperchoesterolaemia with consequent atherosclerosis. The blood vessels develop cholesterol plaques, these plaques will narrow the lumen of the artery, and this process affects all arteries. Coronary and cerebral vessels carry greater risk of obstruction from sclerosis. Disease can encroach along several different channels at the same time.

6
Pathology

What this Chapter is about? [See also Prognosis Chapter 12]
Cook says 'always keep your mind untainted of that mediaeval absurdity which to this day would make disease consist of some physical presence or bodily entity to be assailed and driven forth as if it were a personality that had crept into the system with the condition of health as the central line departures from this standard must be in one direction or the other'.

What is pathology?
Pathology is the study of the progression of disease together with their aetiology and effects. Temperament and typology habitus [somatotype - body types] can detrimentally affect visceral function. Specific visceral hypotrophicity account for many chronic conditions. Tissue changes occur when affected by local or systemic disturbances.

Florence Nightingale, a famous nurse insisted

'There are no specific diseases only specific disease conditions'

The following method of examining pathology shows:
- The general characters of structural change more or less common to all tissues.
- The complexity of such changes in organs made up of compound tissues and different structures.
- The progressive degeneration of structures from the simple primitive changes to their final decomposition.

Cook says 'It is impossible to dissociate these changes from the acts of the vital force in progress during any stages of disease. Pathology cannot be studied except, as the laws of physiology are associated with it'. The nature of the tissue changes is reflected through functional actions of the organ tissue. The influence that the tissue changes exert upon the functions is observed in pathological conditions.

Cook tells us to assess functional departures of the body from the healthy state in disease conditions. This departure is called **pathologic physiology** and is known as the study of disordered functions [11]. Disease consists in an abnormal condition of the tissues in consequence of which the functions of the tissues are incorrectly performed.

Pathology

[a] The diseased changes in a structure progress through a series more or less regularly - highly variable in acute conditions and with wide variation as to time in chronic disorders.

[b] The secretions and excretions are changed according to the altered nature of the tissues.

[c] Changes of a more or less permanent character may take place in the structures producing changes in the normal degree of sensibility, circulation and general activity e.g.. hypertrophy, atrophy, liquefaction, fatty degeneration, infiltration, new growths.

[d] The continuance of disease is a period of perpetual warfare between the vital force and the physical forces. The oscillations in the symptoms make known the preponderance of chances in favour of life or death. The more fully, firmly and steadily the functions of a part are carried on, the more favourable are the chances of recovery. Feebleness, curtailment or irregularities in the functions are unfavourable as they mark a diminished vital control.

[e] The vital force as it attempts to remove diseased conditions present fluctuations of a more or less even character. When the vital struggle is feeble these ebbs and flows of excitability will be noticed but little - they are also indistinct in most chronic conditions.

[f] The greater and more constant the disturbances of function, the more serious the disease. When the functional disturbances are long continued, becoming more irregular and allowing fewer intervals of rest the departure from health is greater [11].

Cook states 'All functional processes are due to the vital force they are actions belonging to vitality. Their imperfect action is a consequence of the changed condition of the structures. It is important this principle is kept in mind for it places before us the fact that disease is a condition and not an action. It enables discrimination between the operations of life and those of death. **Do not view the vital symptoms of disease as being the disease itself'** [11].

'Vital efforts always aim to restore health' [Cook]

Cook says 'Assess the functional state of the tissue in terms of over relaxation or over contraction. Tissues left untreated eventually result in organic changes of the tissues and organs'

Aetiology

Aetiology is either **primary** or **secondary**. Primary causation with or without secondary effects is dependent upon the level of vital action within the cells. In acute primary disease adequately treated, with no suppression of vitality either from incorrect treatment or lowered vitality, a full recovery can be expected.

Secondary effects are found in lowered vitality, a lowered tissue response, an overwhelming infection, emotional disease e.g.. depression/anxiety.

Treat the cause not the symptom is an aim of treatment. Symptoms point us in the correct direction for healing purposes. Removal of the cause is often enough to allow the tissue to heal and the blood impurities to clear. Short fasts and the liberal use of the cold shower [hydrotherapy] will stimulate the vitality within the patient. **T lymphocytes** have been shown to increase within the blood of people using regular hydrotherapy. Remove the cause and the disease will clear. The removal of the cause may not always be sufficient as some diseases create organ damage and secondary consequences that require further herbal medication and dietary adjustment. Where damage occurs in joint injury it should be remembered that joints don't forgive injuries and osteoarthritis can develop years after the initial damage. Infection and inflammatory causes could damage an area of tissue, upon healing it becomes scarred e.g. pleurisy, pneumonia.

The vital force working through the tissues is always trying to heal and bring about healthy cell function. It will always do its best for the tissue to encourage healing and removal of impurities.

Predisposing and exciting aetiology of disease.
Predisposing causes of disease operate prior to the development of actual symptoms. The predisposition of the body encourages the disease progression together with its effects upon the tissues.
Local predisposing aetiology are deficient nutrition, sclerotic arteries, previous disease, tissue degeneration and enervation [deficient nerve supply]. *These local influences favour congestion rather than inflammation.*

Exciting aetiology brings into sharp focus the predisposition of the tissue towards disease. Aetiology includes extreme cold or heat, renal colic, infections, paralysis. Each has a tendency to disease before the exciting cause comes along e.g. Colic will have stones or some obstruction present, infection always supervenes upon unhealthy tissue, paralysis may occur from an embolus itself due to atherosclerosis.

Temperaments [See typology Chapter 10].
Among individuals are found certain temperaments. These are the **sanguine, nervous, bilious and lymphatic**. For full diagnostic interpretation of the patient, typology and temperaments are analysed.

In the **sanguine** temperament the circulation is active. Predisposed to heart troubles. Tendency to an excess of blood. Auburn or red hair. Such types are

Pathology

predisposed to high fever and haemorrhages. Haemorrhoids and contracted spasmodic sphincters create constipation and rectal trouble. They are the cheerful, hopeful, gregarious, excessive, impulsive and active types. Vital excitement is aroused early and usually with a rapid return to health.
Require large doses of medicine - *Crataegus*.

Nervous Genito urinary disorders may occur with catarrhal conditions, leucorrhoea, infections e.g. thrush. Disorders of the spleen. melancholic temperament has a disposition to being emotional, excitable, introspective, sensitive, solitary and thoughtful. They have rapid changes of feelings and are sensitive. Panic and neurasthenia are this type neurosis. Large frontal lobes. Neuralgic pain and depression are typical. Tend to have a low vitality.
Require small to medium doses of medicine - *Ginkgo, Rosmarinus.*

Bilious
Lung disturbances with mucus congestion. Predispose to hepatic and stomach disorders. Renal disorders and gynaecological problems. Chronic rheumatism and arthritis, tuberculosis, artherosclerosis and degeneration of cartilage. Easily angered, impatient, irritable, impetuous, spiteful temperament. Tenacious wiry types with strong resistance to disease.
Require large doses of medicine – *Taraxacum.*

Lymphatic
They incline towards oedema, tuberculosis, anaemia and fatty degenerations. Gastro intestinal catarrh is common. Females are prone to gynaecological disorders. Large obese body, phlegmatic with a fair complexion. Temperament personality types are accepting, apathetic, dreamy, indifferent, lethargic, relaxed, sluggish and dull. Tend to have low resistance to disease aetiology and succumb easily to acute illness. Convalesce slowly towards health.
Require high doses of promptly acting medicine - *Chamomilla, Fucus, Scutellaria, Vitex.*

Combinations of the temperaments can be diverse, the most common being the nervous with sanguine or bilious types.

Diagnosis depends upon taking the dominant characteristics of that temperament and balancing with the environmental tendencies. Next determine the temperament and individuality, the constitution and character of the individual. The temperaments tend to change with advancing years e.g. menopause of male and female.
Thurston says that any continuous and persistent influence that alters cellular function will affect the functional capability of tissues and organs. Functional

changes within the tissues including cerebral neurones will tend to change the psychological and emotional makeup of that temperament.

Chronic conditions

By weakening the bodies reactionary power against one disease its power over all diseases are weakened. **Chronic disease** is encouraged by the incorrect kind of feeding habits. **Cell function** to be effective must have an adequate supply of nutrients in assimilable form. Lack of available nutrients causes the cell to malfunction; it is mineral elements that keep the cell healthy. **Drainage** of cellular waste needs to be cleared away by the lymph.

A lack of mineral elements for the cell creates disease resulting in intracellular fluid toxins. Interstitial fluid becomes clogged with impurities. Venules and lymphatics struggle to move the toxins away. As the condition progresses symptoms can emerge. Not until **compensation** has taken place in the tissue and **failed** that symptoms arise. Few symptoms suggest a chronic condition has progressed or depleted vital force [vasodepression] is present. Vasodepression means there is not enough vital energy to remove the cellular impurities.

Nerve current is disturbed in any toxic or chronic disorder. Blood impurity and cellular toxins impinge upon the nerve cells distorting their function, resulting in interrupted and/or depleted nerve transmission. Nerve fibres signal danger from disease aetiology. Any reduction of nerve transmission means the tissues may not be warned of impending danger and cellular action cannot be improved for its own needs. Chronic disease means that tissue cells are unable to arouse themselves to an **acute eliminative effort** in the form of an inflammatory response or elimination phase.

Deficiencies of alkaline substances create an accumulation of waste in the tissue. Minerals needed to heal and cleanse acidity and toxins from the tissues are of an alkaline nature; these neutralise acidic substances. Sodium phosphate is the best mineral to remove metabolic acid.

Chronic disease frequently occurs because of inadequate organ elimination. The secernants; intestine, skin, liver and kidneys have become sluggish and atrophied. Eventually these organs become hypotrophic and less able to perform their eliminative function correctly. Where the organ is in a weakened state, inadequate elimination causes blood impurity and creates further disease aggravations. Building up the organs of elimination [tone and trophic state] is a prior requisite to promoting elimination of toxins.

Pathology

Tissue changes

Priest explains 'organic deterioration follows two well defined courses:

1. hardening and shrinking = ischaemia, increased waste toxins, fibroid and mineral degeneration, dry gangrene, cirrhosis and sclerosis. [Contraction atrophy]

2. softening and dilation = overhydration, congestion and stasis, fatty and fluid degeneration – wet gangrene and liquefaction. [Relaxation atrophy]

The over contracted and the over relaxed conditions both lead to atrophy of tissue. Priest says' it is important to determine the cause which gives rise to the end condition as over contraction or over relaxation both give rise to atrophy of tissue'. Cook says 'pathological changes ensue from reduction or occlusion of neuro-vascular control' [384].

Gangrene means death of tissue. Dry gangrene usually involves a limb, there is a clear line of demarcation between the healthy and gangrenous tissue.
Wet or moist gangrene can affect an organ or limb. Both types of gangrene are due to gradual arterial occlusion and less commonly venous occlusion. Infection complicates the gangrenous condition.

Changes without destruction

Hypertrophy - an increase in the size of the tissues due to an increase in cell size. Physiological as in heart enlargement from continued exercise. The breast during lactation. Pathological from venous backpressure, chronic congestion e.g. prostate enlargement. Replacement as hepatic enlargement following damage.

Hyperplasia - an increase in the number of cells.

Atrophy - a decrease in the number or size of a cell, tissue or organ. Atrophy generally advances slowly and may be unaccompanied by pain. Muscle is especially liable to atrophy this is due to an insufficient supply of nutrients. Constitutional disease e.g. TB, chronic intestinal disorders or malnutrition cause atrophy due to the poor assimilation of nutrients. Persistent vasoconstriction impedes blood flow to the tissues it is especially common within the gastro intestinal tract. Lack of arterial blood perfusion to an organ creates atrophy.

Induration – creates a hardened area of tissue and can occur from inflammation, hyperaemia or infiltration from a neoplasm.

Changes with degeneration
Fibrotic tissue
A frequent accompaniment to disease conditions where atrophy encourages structural change, which is known as retrograde change within the tissue e.g. fibrosis. Fibrous tissue is of an inferior quality and tends to shrink as time goes on further impeding the circulation to the tissue concerned. Further a reduced amount of nutrients are available for the health of the cells. It is not impossible for tissues to recover and essential fatty acids have been known to improve myelin nerve sheath damage. Ol Oenothera Sig 500mg twice daily given long term for myelin degeneration.

Fatty degeneration
Arteriosclerosis is a common accompaniment of increasing age. Sclerosis is a disorder of the arteries and arterioles which causes obstruction to the circulation when sclerotic plaques build up within the arteries these are composed of calcium and cholesterol and constrict the lumen of the artery reducing blood supply and tissue nutrition. The liver plays an important role in the pathogenesis of arteriosclerotic disease. Deficient secretion and excretion of cholesterol in the bile salts accumulate within the blood.
Thyroid and pancreatic disturbances cause hypercholesterolaemia.

Changes with destruction
Liquefaction
In the processes of **decay** tissues commonly pass into some form of organic breakdown known as liquefaction. The decomposition begins in a few cells that break down into a liquid form. Their contents are injurious to the adjacent cells. In this way liquefaction may advance to neighbouring parts to successively destroy those cells. Fluid forms may appear as pus exuding from the tissues e.g. abscesses, furunculosis, ulcers.

Tissue decay depends upon the vigour or feebleness of vital action in the surrounding parts. The decay will not begin until capillary circulation has been obstructed and will advance as this obstruction extends.

Suppuration
Suppuration of the skin or mucous membrane has its origins in the blood. It may heal once the blood impurities are cleared and the capillary circulation restored. Or it may extend some distance along the affected tissue e.g. ulcerative colitis. Localised ulcerations can be observed on the cervix, tongue, skin, eye, tongue, mouth etc. Pain, irritation and hyperaemia accompany suppurative conditions. Ulcerative damage can cause scarring.

Pathology

Organ parenchyma
Organ parenchyma can become subject to suppurative processes. An **abscess** formation results in fever and throbbing of the part. If the vital effort is vigorous enough exuded lymph will dilute the impurities and help protect the adjacent structures. An abscess may be acute when concurrent with sharp vital action and a tendency to early discharge. When the vital action is feeble a chronic abscess can **infiltrate** surrounding tissues and be absorbed strong vasotonic alterative are required.

Suppuration is a condition of **hyperaemia with stasis** and is irritating to the nervous system. **Absorption** of pus occurs when vital action is too feeble to establish consolidation of the toxins. Other parts may become implicated and destroyed by the pus that frequently contain **infection**. The impurities and infection absorbed into the lymph and blood stream create a condition of **pyaemia**. Powerful vasotonics are required such as *Baptisia, Commiphora, Echinacea, Hydrastis, Iris, Phytolacca, Sassafras, Smilax, Uncaria and Zanthoxylum* against infective processes and pyaemia.

Hyperaemia may also be seen when cold hands or feet indicate inflammation of the heart or brain.

Changes with new growths [neoplasms]
1 Cysts
2 Fatty tumours e.g. lipoma
3 Fibroid
4 Glandular tumours
5 Malignant tumours

All new growths are the result of inadequate circulation and deficient cellular drainage. These factors cause retention of accumulated cellular toxic waste. The tissue fluid, lymph and blood cannot be adequately cleansed so adding to the problem of cellular encumbrance. The other problem is the lack of blood from vasoconstriction. Venous return and adequate lymph drainage is dependent upon respiration and muscular action. Use vasotonic remedies to detoxify the tissues to help shrink the tumours. Medicines for neoplasms see Chapter 31.

Different modes of dying
Death begins either at one's head, heart or lungs. These three points may be reached by disease advancing through a multitude of channels. The symptoms will exhibit the advance of disease upon the organs.
Death beginning at the head - cerebral arteriosclerosis it is seen in the iris and is called an arcus senilis.

Herbal Medicine - Keys

Death beginning in the lungs - disease from chronic bronchitis and emphysema with eventual basal lobe atelectasis.

Death beginning in the heart - disease brought on from valve defects, sclerotic conditions, hypertension and eventually heart failure.

Aetiology of disease

Typically the medical profession look for infection as the main cause of most disease. Bechamp has another point of view, his research reflects on the microzyma as the living entity upon which all life exists. The microzyma is always present in the blood and every tissue. Variations in the tissue and hence the types of microzyma determine the microzymas functional purpose.

Germ theory of disease

Drawing upon the works of Koch and Bechamp it is argued that infection is due to several factors operating simultaneously. [85]

Koch a German scientist formulated his postulates [laws]. There are five requirements for an organism as the causative agent of a disease

1.   micro-organisms must be present in every case of the disease
2.   are not found with any other disease
3.   ability to be recultured in a pure culture
4.   when inoculated in pure culture, it must produce the disease
5.   must be recoverable and grown again in pure culture.

Pasteur [1822-1895] invented nothing whatsoever. He had no medical training and he falsified, perverted and plagiarised the works of Bechamp. Pasteur proclaimed 'life is a germ and a germ is life.' Although many knew that Pasteur's claims were false they did not dare oppose him because Pasteur had made friends with the emperor Napoleon. Pasteur enriched himself at the expense of others.

Antoine Bechamp [1816-1908] was a scientist who worked at the Institute in Paris at the same time as Pasteur. It was not until Pasteur was dying that he made the important announcement that the 'soil was more important than the germ.' Today we encounter the orthodox treatment of infection using antibiotics. This is proving to be dangerous because of the growth of antibiotic resistant superbugs for example MRSI. The opposing principle is to use natural treatment, clear the infection and cleanse the tissues so that infection is much less likely to gain a hold in the future.

Pathology

Micro-organisms inhabit diseased tissue. People can become infected because they are ill and not healthy. Popular germ theorists tell us infection comes from the air. It was Bechamp who proved their existence. Germs of the air he said occur from dead or decayed tissue from vegetable, animal or mineral matter. The germs of the air are microzymas or bacteria set free when the substance was broken down [death]. In the case of chalk rocks the microzymas could live in a dormant state forever. Microzymas were the living remains of the animal, or plant forms that had been the constructive cellular elements of a living being.

'Nothing is the prey of death: all things are the prey of life – Bechamp'.

Bechamp researched and wrote *The blood and its 3rd anatomical element* amongst other books together with a score of research papers. In this book he describes microzymas, infection and the concept of the soil [the tissues]. Once the body has become weakened then micro-organisms gain a hold and are carried around the body. The *Competes Rendes* records indicate that Bechamp was always ahead of Pasteur. It was Pasteur who was seen as the favourite at the institute.

Henry Bastian wrote two books *The evolution of life* in 1872 and *Evolution and the origin of life* 1874.

Rene Dubos was a microbiologist. He stated micro-organisms exist within the body and become pathocausatives under certain conditions of disease. Micro-organisms can exist in a body without disease. He observed microbes changing form. Take a throat swab and it's possible to find diphtheria organisms present with no actual diphtheria disease.

Bechamp draws from other researchers of the day as he explains the principles of ferments. He took up the study of ferments and established that moulds changed sugars and caused them to ferment. He was the first to distinguish the difference between organised [living ferments] and the soluble ferment. Moulds seen under the microscope are formed by a collection of **molecular granulations** which Bechamp named **microzymas** [from Greek meaning 'small ferment']. He also showed that **granulations** under certain conditions **evolved** into bacteria and change their shape, this was proved by Loehnis and Smith [136]. The name microbe was applied to bacteria and is better known than that of microzyma. Microzymas are of immense longevity and are indestructible. Microzymas are necessary for cell life, repair and growth. Bechamp denied spontaneous generation while Pasteur continued to argue it. Mould accompanied fermentation and contained living organisms and could not be spontaneously generated but must be an outgrowth of some living organism carried in the air. Bechamp proved that each micro-organism might vary its fermentative effect in conformity with that medium in which it finds itself.

Lister derived his knowledge from Pasteur on antisepsis. Lister's patients died in great numbers and it came to be a gruesome joke to say that 'the operation was successful but the patient died.'

Bechamp's work on fermentation is the phenomena of nutrition, assimilation, dissimulation and excretion. The microzymas function as anatomical elements. They are the physiological and chemical elements of the transformations that take place during the process of nutrition, digestion and assimilation. The basic anatomical element is the microzymian molecular granulation known as a [**Russell body**]. These are *molecular granulations present within all living cells.* **Virchow** believed the cell itself has microzymas as anatomical elements. The microzymas of the bacteria undergo evolution that essentially are ferments. In a condition of disease the microzymas that have become morbid determine special changes that lead to disorganisation within the tissues, destruction of the cell and evolution [infection]. The cells are therefore changed, altered and destroyed by the disease processes. The microzyma can only be changed and never destroyed. The microzymas of the blood become the bacteria of disease.

Berthelot's experiments displayed the **decomposition of protein that provoked fermentation**. Both animal and vegetable substances contain all the products necessary to cause them to alter spontaneously.

> **'each granulation is a spherical mass of albuminoid matter**
> **having a microzyma for its centre'** [Bechamp]

The blood is composed of the red and white blood cells and microzymian molecular granulations. 'The microzymas are living elements that I have proved to be living by their function as ferments' says Bechamp. The microzymian molecular granulations become the first to be effected by changes within the blood proteins. 'The microzymas change into the fungus, virus or bacterial particles by evolution and return to microzymian form by an inverse phenomenon of evolution'. What happens when tissues alter? Chemical changes [**fermentation**] create change of form or function in the resulting microzymas. In certain conditions microzymas do not become bacteria. It is evident that the spontaneous chemical alterations within the blood are the result of fermentation or putrefaction. Fermentation is a process of nutrition that is of digestion, followed by absorption, assimilation, excretion and elimination. Microzymas act physiologically as ferments, effect the chemical transformation of the proximate principles and thereby changes which end in disorganisation of tissues and cells.

Pathology

Bechamp say's microzymas are living beings of a special order. The blood contains the microzymian molecular granulations; microzymas are the molecular granulations.

Microzymas are seen under the microscope and are known as Russell bodies [large cell wall deficient bacteria] which are immunoglobulins [proteins].

Microzymas are the cell granules observed by many cytologists. **Henle** in 1841 suggested that the microzymas are cell units or bioplasts. These are capable of assimilation, growth and division. They are to be regarded as elementary units of structure, standing between the cell and the ultimate units of living matter.

Bechamp say's 'microzymas are chemically and physiologically figured ferments', producers of zymases, which are called soluble ferments. 'Microzymas are autonomous anatomical elements.' 'There are many species of microzymas'. They are different in each bodily organ. 'For one can only distinguish a microzyma and consequently a bacterium by the origin and function of the microzyma.' 'Microzymas are organised, living individual ferments.' Bacteria by an inverse process can be reduced to the microzyma. Microzyma - virus - fungus - bacterium is the order of mutation and back again as health improves. The virus stage may produce few symptoms. Bechamp said that bacteria were not due to external invasion [current knowledge also confirms infection can occur from outside the body to alter the host microzymas]. It is when the tissue becomes affected by the invasion of a pathogen that the microzymas become altered. Germs carried by the air are not essential for infective processes to begin. The microzymas in their bacterial stage are sufficient to assure by putrefaction the circulation of toxins. Cellular death occurs from rupture of the cell membrane. However the microzyma does not die. Microzymas are present in pus, vaccines, infections etc. but are altered by the process. Hence the introduction of vaccines into a body can only bring about deterioration of health and subsequent alteration of the hosts microzymas to an unhealthy condition.

'Microzymas have been constituted physiologically imperishable'
Bechamp

The microzyma is at the beginning and at the end of every living organisation. It is the fundamental anatomical element whereby the cells, tissues, organs and the whole organism are constituted living. The microzyma becomes by nutrition that which it needs to become so as to accommodate itself to each new condition of existence. 'Microzymas remain morphologically similar to themselves.' They function in each cell and organ, naturally chemically and physiologically for themselves while preserving their individuality; at the same time that by co-ordination they function for the benefit of the microzymian molecular granulations of the cells, organs and systems taken altogether, whose physiological condition of health is preserved by them. Microzymas are organised ferments under certain circumstances they become bacteria at others cell builders.

Virchow's view was that the cell was the unit of life. Bechamp disagreed saying it is [the cell] built up by the cell granules within it. These **cell granules are the microzymas and the rod like groups we now know are chromosomes**

Pidoux concisely expressed **'Diseases are born of us and in us'.**
If the microzyma is physiologically imperishable what is the death of the living whole? It is the absolute disharmonisation of the functions of the microzymas explains Bechamp. The cell protoplasm always contains microzymas. The microzyma is capable of multiplying of becoming diseased and of communicating disease. In the condition of disease the microzymas do not act harmoniously and fermentation is disturbed the microzymas have either changed their function or are placed in an abnormal situation by some modification of the medium [a change within the tissues].

Microzymas direct the life of the cell [Bechamp]

The concept of infection
In Physiomedicalism tissue health is seen in terms of the following:
a] an infective organism is the product of unhealthy tissues
b] cellular, tissue, lymph and blood impurities create the necessary environment for infections
c] the ability to neutralise toxins from micro-organisms together with the micro-organism
d] once this has been achieved the tissues return to normal

Treatment aims to restore the tissues to their healthy condition. Physiomedicalism regards the body as being in an unhealthy condition in the presence of such an unhealthy tissues. It is necessary to take steps to limit the infecting organism and to inhibit its development or control its activity. It takes time to clear the blood and tissues of impurities. Hence the need to limit the pathogenic organism until the tissues can be detoxified and cleansed.

McDonagh in *Nature of Disease* stated that Escherichia coli is a primary form of bacteria. Transmutation from the E. Coli form into other types of bacterial micro-organism can occur.
The following précis explains the nature of infection from a number of viewpoints.

Pathology

Cantwell in *The Cancer Microbe* while researching scleroderma and cancer say's: acid fast mycobacteria are closely related to fungi. Acid fast mycobacteria cause TB and leprosy. There are different forms of the infecting organism found on microscopical examination.

Edgar Cayce in *Handbook for Health* explains that all healing is the changing of the vibrations from within – the attuning of the divine within the living tissues of a body to creative energies. **Disease is disturbance of vibration.** [Homeopaths give a potentised remedy, which is a vibration of the original diluted drug]. He further says 'microbes can originate in diseased cells and altered tissue.

Roy Allen in *The Microscopy of Micro-organisms associated with Neoplasms*, stresses that the cancer microbe is pleomorphic, indicating it has more than one appearance. The microbe can be rod-shaped or a coccus [round] shaped. The microbes live inside and outside cancer cells.

Virginia Livingston in *Cancer - a new breakthrough* and *The Conquest of Cancer*, was able in her research to **induce bacteria to develop from viral particles.** She discovered that the cancer microbe [*Progenitor cryptocides*] secretes a hormone called the choriogonadotropic hormone [HGC]. HGC protects the microbe from destruction. A newly fertilised embryo is also thus protected because sperm carry HGC.

Wuerthele-Caspe, Alexander-Jackson **and Anderson** [91] described 'these organisms, which appear primarily as small acid fast granules in young cultures and tend to become non-acid-fast in the larger forms present in old cultures. They may exhibit a number of types, such as: [a] minute filterable granules beyond the limits of visibility of the light microscope; [b] larger granules approximately the size of ordinary cocci, readily seen with the light microscope: [c] still larger round globoidal forms; [d] rod like forms with irregular staining and [e] occasionally globoidal forms which appear to undergo polar budding'.
Microbes can vary considerably in their appearance [morphology] depending upon the culture and laboratory media used. It all depends on what they are fed. Bacteria are pleomorphic; they regularly change their shape and size enabling them to pass through a filter. It follows the correct stain must be used in order to see the pleomorphic microbes.

McTaggart in march 2002 quoting from two papers [260] says that epidemiologists believe that *Bordetella pertussus* has mutated – changing its DNA fingerprint and the genetic coating of its outer coat of surface protein. Genetic changes have also been noted by scientists in the Netherlands, Poland and Finland. Vaccines are given to prime the immune system to recognise and attack the virus. However newer forms of virus are not recognised by the immune system. Pertussus vaccine given today may not protect against the newer forms of virus infection. Clinical evidence shows the disease is changing in character – lack of the characteristic whoop cough. Some 30% of individuals with an irritable or persistent cough have been shown to be infected with pertussus [260].

In 1908 **Hans Much** wrote about TB granules. These granules can enlarge to the size of cocci or rods or they can degenerate into coccobacilli [corynebacteria]. These TB granules initiated the tubercular infection by attacking the cell. In 1928 **HC Sweany** proposed that granular forms of TB could cause Hodgkin's disease. This was backed up by **Mellon & Fisher** [92] and **Beinhauer & Mellon** [93] also declared mutant TB microbes caused Hodgkin's disease. Acid and non acid-fast microbes were described that looked like staphylococci, corynebacteria and fungi. In 1931 **Armengol** a scientist from Barcelona grew pleomorphic TB microbes that had the appearance of fungi. TB bacteria do not die easily they survive by transforming into pleomorphic forms. **Eleanor Alexander Jackson** [94] managed to culture the virus of leprosy these were similar to cell wall deficient forms.

Lida Mattman and colleagues have seen cell wall changes in the TB microbe [95]. The cell wall is deficient in these forms, they can be as large as a red blood cell. The cell wall deficient microbe is always present in cancer. However its forms are variable: staphylococci, rods, large globoid and yeast-like forms, acid fast granules, fungus like forms and large body forms these are known as Russell bodies.

William Russell [1852-1940]. A pathologist at Edinburgh University identified microbes in cancer slides from tumours. Variable in shape and size, these were intracellular and extracellular. Microbes mutate according to natural phenomenon. Antibiotics cause mutation of microbes.

Wilheim Reich [96] found T-bacilli [cancer microbes] in cancerous conditions. Later on he would also find these T-bacilli in the blood and excreta of healthy people. Reich concluded

'the disposition to cancer is therefore determined by the biological resistance of the blood and the tissues to putrefaction' [Reich]

Aymes argues in '*Magic Bullets*' that the increasing use of antibiotics are causing more drug resistant infections. Drug resistant pneumonia and tuberculosis are becoming commonplace. Infections are mutating, this further supports Bechamp's view of infection mutations [350].

Pathology

Further work by **Enderline** [confirmed by Haefelu] calls the microzymas 'Endobyons'. His research on red blood cells explains the phenomenon. Endobyons are tiny particles in the membrane of red blood cells. They have a protective action against fungi and bacteria. They regulate their own growth and are part of the immune system. He found that good forms of microfungi e.g.. aspergillus are guardians of health and guard blood viscosity. A lack of endobyons generates an accelerated growth of fungi. When fungi grow they also attack leukocytes this is due to the size and number of them. Leukocytes suffer a reduction in their numbers and this causes a weakened immune system.

Acidic blood and a deficiency of nutrients disturb the endobyons and produce an increase of fungal growth. Fungi grow on the red blood cell, are aggressive and may be hidden and in a latent state. Alfatoxins [moulds] are excreted by fungi. Red blood cells put acids into their outer membrane [a homeostatic mechanism in order to keep the blood at pH 7.4]. Excess acid causes vacuoles and changes in the membrane. As the red blood cells travel through the capillaries they become flattened. Acids make red blood cells thicker and harder making them get stuck in the capillaries.
Acidosis is found in myocardial weakness and infarction. Bodily processes, antibiotics, radiation, steroids and sulphonamides create acidosis. Sugar, refined carbohydrates, fermenting juices, alcohol, excess animal protein, mercury have all been implicated as causes of acidity. Nitrates and pesticides in water. Stress, anxiety and negative thinking also contribute.

Endobyons can be changed back to their healthful state - they cannot be killed only changed in nature and function for as long as the tissue is unhealthy.
Treatment - adjust the tissue health by cleansing and detoxifying.
Enderline's treatment for fungi is as follows
- Essential oils with antifungal properties e.g. Szygium, Thymus.
- Cinnamomum bark
- Diet - avoid dairy products, animal proteins and sugar.
- Use antioxidants:
- Selenium rich food e.g. Soya, coconut, sesame seeds, herring, tuna, cows and pigs kidney, wheatgerm, Brazil nuts and pistachios.
  Vitamin C, E, betacarotine, Co enzyme Q10.

Yeasts and fungi
Fungal pathogens are becoming much more prevalent in systemic infections because there is a larger immunocomprised patient population, this includes patients with Carcinoma, Aids and transplants explains Dr Robert T. Wheeler.

Essential fatty acids, immunity and viral infections

Sufficient essential fatty acids on the cell membrane support reduction in the ability of the virus to replicate. Horrobin states there is evidence of a close relationship between fatty acid metabolism and the ability to respond to viral infections. [102]. EFA's are required to enable interferon to exert its antiviral effects. Viral infections induce abnormalities in EFA metabolism. EFA's have been useful in treating atopic eczema and post viral fatigue syndrome. EFA's enhance Interferon as it plays a part in resisting viral infections. Linoleic acid is required for the normal structure of all cell membranes. Other nutrients are required for the normal metabolism of linoleic acid - Vitamin C, Biotin, Vitamin B6, nicotinic acid, magnesium, iron and zinc.

Vitamin C and zinc deficiency lead to a depressed immune response.

It can be seen from the extensive works of Bechamp and other researchers that the concept of infection from outside the body is false in most cases of disease excepting those cases where an external infection overwhelms and depletes the vital force.

Primary requirements of the cell

Three cellular needs are defined without which cellular death occurs.

Innervation – sufficient vital force to maintain vital activity of the mitochondria together with an adequate nerve and blood supply.

Nutrition – provides for suitable food and fluids. This must include adequate vitamins, minerals and trace elements for optimum functioning.

Drainage – elimination of waste material. Drainage of the cell, tissue fluid and filtering of the blood.

The primary cause of disease

Lindlahr states **the primary cause of disease** is due to:

1] Lowered vitality
2] Abnormal composition of the blood and lymph
3] The accumulation of morbid waste [impurities] and toxins in the system.

A lowered state of vitality frequently occurs from long standing emotional and stress disorders.

Constitutional causes include **miasms** [miasma] from Cancer, Rabies, Psora, Tuberculosis, Gonorrhoea and Syphilis. Radiation miasm is gaining prominence. **G. Vithoulkas** states 'If the vital force is significantly weakened in the parents the child's **electrodynamic field** [electromagnetic field] can be weakened at the moment of conception.' Tuberculosis has its origins in a lack of sufficient nutrients to sustain health and found in the malnourished. Venereal disease has accumulated from the 1840's when around thirty thousand prostitutes in the London area alone serviced one million men yearly, quite a legacy for the current population. Miasmas create a weakened body and reproduce in the offspring a structural inherited weakness [**hypotrophic weakness**]. Miasma can create chronic inflammatory processes in the blood and lymph leading to congestion of the lymphatic drainage and circulation. Arthritis can be a legacy of a miasm. Each miasm emanates from a taint transmitted from generation to generation. Sometimes the miasm can skip a generation.

Aetiological causes for the degeneration of the cell
Deterioration of the vital fluids within the blood and lymph occur from denatured refined food. Refined food clogs the lymphatics and capillaries leading to inflammatory processes and infective conditions of the blood and lymph. Impurities in the system result from an excess intake of non-supportive foodstuffs and inadequate elimination. Inadequate trace element, vitamin and mineral intake deplete health and cause disease. Synthetic drugs used long term can lead to an impregnation of the drug picture onto the tissues, this leads to miasmic effects especially those with the gonorrhoeal [sycosis] miasm. Synthetic drugs add to the encumbrance along with vaccines and food additives, often absorbed into tissues from a very early age. Miasms tend to block or reduce the efficacy of the remedy. Residues can be cleared using vasotonic alteratives.
Acute disease is consistent in its cause, purpose and development - even when an infection is present it shows the need to detoxify and cleanse the tissues of encumbrance.

It is necessary to bear in mind that the healthy body has a healthy immune system. **Lindlahr** states that waste toxins and impurities give the micro-organisms of disease the opportunity to multiply. The infection is a **secondary** cause of disease. An infection thrives and multiplies in a weakened body. Unhealthy tissue allows infection to overpower the immune processes. The immune system resides in the blood-WBC's, spleen and bone marrow. These areas rely on a clean blood condition to work effectively. Elimination of blood impurity occurs via the eliminative secernants - liver, bowel, kidneys and skin.

Treatment aims to remove impurities within the tissue cells and blood in order to restore health. Hepatic and intestinal treatment must always be considered along with vasotonic alteratives in acute disease.

Herbal Medicine - Keys

Inflammation

Inflammation is a natural response to injury and should never be suppressed. Many medicines of a herbal nature do allay excess inflammation when required. Inflammation may be acute, sub acute or chronic and is always tissue supportive. During inflammation the blood rushes to the area of irritation. The blood vessels dilate and increase in size. Distended blood vessels allow the migration of WBC's to engulf invading organisms and neutralise infection or toxins. Impurities, toxins and poisons are neutralised by the cellular defences resulting in infection debris called pus. Bodily inflammation is often continuous until the infection or other disease process has taken its course. The tissue changes brought about during inflammation create disturbances within cellular function. Symptoms change as a result of tissue cell impurities from disease processes. Symptoms can become low grade and ineffectual in removing the disease aetiology. When inflammation becomes excessive or uncontrolled we may see delayed healing or chronic inflammatory action. Specifically the prostaglandins and the leukotrines regulate a large part of the inflammatory process. Both prostaglandins and leukotrines are pro- and anti-inflammatory having a homeostatic mechanism inducing or allaying inflammation as decided by the cell. A direct result of inflammation is an increase in free radicle activity. Retained secretions are frequently found to be an irritation factor that provides the stimulus to inflammation.

Inflammation has five cardinal symptoms:

redness, heat, pain, swelling and loss of function.

Acute inflammation is treated using relaxing remedies to vasomotor function e.g. *Asclepias, Lobelia or Nepeta.* Encumbrance, that is toxin build up within the tissue, becomes worse with the congestive phase. Congestion calls for stimulation to vital activity, hydrotherapy - cold water, cold compress.

Chronic inflammation or congestion require more stimulation to vital force for example *Capsicum, Cochleria, Myrica Ocimum, Zanthoxylum, Zingiber.*

There are five stages in the inflammatory process each stage must be allowed to run its course in order to clear the causative obstructive condition and to heal the tissue in the final resolution phase.

Inflammation can lead to irritation of the tissues with resulting **congestion**.

Stasis results from suppression of the vital effort, either from lack of vitality, drug suppression or forceful disease circumstances. An excessive level of inflammation may be soothed and allayed through the use of astringent, relaxant or demulcent medicines. Anti-inflammatory remedies that allay inflammation should not be used in chronic inflammatory disorders when more stimulation is required.

Pathology

According to Lindlahr there are five stages of **inflammation** these are:
Incubation, Aggravation, Destruction,
Abatement [absorption], **Resolution** [reconstruction]
Incubation is the time between the exposure [to infection] and its development. Cell debris along with toxins and micro-organisms accumulate in an area. The vital force reacts to the obstruction by means of the inflammatory response. Before inflammation can arise there needs to be some exciting cause for example obstruction of blood supply, infection, encumbrance [toxins], or blood impurity may create the necessary changes at cell level to excite an inflammatory reaction. Tissue reactivity at this stage is a necessary requirement to maintain health.

Aggravation is natures battle whereby the fight between micro-organisms and bodily defences gain the momentum accompanied by fever and inflammation. Fever is at its highest during this period of greatest vital activity.

Destruction
Disintegration of tissue occurs at this stage. Due to the accumulation of pus formation, some elimination must take place to rid the body of harmful toxins.

Abatement
The stage in which absorption of the toxins takes place and the exudate is eliminated from the tissue. The temperature abates along with the pulse and respiratory rate. Pain subsides and the redness consequent upon inflammation reduces. Oedema is reabsorbed.

Resolution [reconstruction]
Once the obstructions and accumulations of toxins have been removed during the period of abatement, reconstruction may then take place. Full recovery cannot take place if the inflammation has been suppressed during the stages of incubation or aggravation. When the inflammation has progressed through the five stages of acute activity the vital force has been given the chance to rebuild the tissue cells in the trophic restorative way.

The resolution phase supports the reconstruction of the tissues, regenerating the cells for the trophorestorative process. The trophic rebuilding will take place at a much faster rate because the area requiring to be healed has been cleared of toxins and impurities. It is suggested that Vitamin C. Sig 1g TDS/PRN be given in acute inflammatory disease.

Inflammation is an active hyperaemia
As inflammation proceeds the blood vessels become dilated, along with variation in the blood current. Capillary dilation, in an inflammatory state, increases the

arterial blood to the area. The area of inflammation may be small e.g. inflamed pustule or large as in hepatitis. **Equalising the circulation relieves active hyperaemia**. Equalising the circulation is achieved through diaphoresis this helps to clear the internal congested blood and relieve the hyperaemia. Remedies should be relaxant – *Asclepias, Eupatorium perfoliatum, Lobelia, Nepeta, Sambucus.*

Congestion is passive hyperaemia.
During inflammatory action blood vessels dilate, this continues for a time until the capillaries and venules become weary creating a relaxed state this is called **passive hyperaemia**. The blood still present in large quantities becomes congested, as the venules are unable to carry it away fast enough. Blood tends to become sticky and clot in a congested area, thrombus formation is possible. If the blood slows further then **stasis** of blood becomes evident. Blood colour becomes darker, cyanosis and oedema occurs in the tissue.
Relaxed tissue in venous engorgement is deep red or a pale colour.
Deep blue from venous stasis.
With venous stasis the tissues are full, oedematous and flabby e.g. haemorrhoids, varicose veins, menorrhagia.

Passive hyperaemia is also relieved by equalising the circulation, using stimulating astringent tonics. Catharsis and diaphoresis will also help to clear the internal congested blood and relieve hyperaemia.
A small frequent pulse indicates a change towards **stasis**. Stasis is reduced capillary flow with consequent obstruction – stimulate using diffusive stimulants

Pain during the inflammatory response
Pain is due to swelling of the blood vessels and extravascular spaces causing effusion of blood from the dilated vessels, with consequent pressure upon the sensory nerves.
Sympathetic pain as referred from the area may also occur.

Disturbances of function during inflammation
The functions of inflamed organs and tissues are always disturbed, as are the adjacent parts. Tissue of the same class can also become affected through reflex action. Secretions are always modified as to quantity and composition when the organs forming them are inflamed.

Pulse during inflammation or fever
Where the **pulse is firm** relaxants are indicated. If the **pulse becomes softer** it may indicate approaching congestion when stimulation is required. Mild **tonics**

are then required to balance the secernant activity. An irritable pulse could require relaxing nervines.

Treatment in acute inflammatory disease

1] Relieve inner congestion and consequent pain of affected parts. Achieved through relaxation to relieve the tension and capillary excitement. Relax the sensory nerve to ease the capillary tension.

2] Keep the temperature below the danger point by promoting heat radiation through the skin use diaphoretics/antipyretics.

3] Increase the activity of the organs of elimination to remove toxins and impurities [direct organ relaxation/stimulation]. Secernants may require relaxation and thus encourage the elimination of impurities [*Galium*-renal, *Cassia*-intestine, *Leptandra* or *Eupatorium perfoliatum* - liver, *Sambucus* or *Nepeta* - skin/secernants, *Mentha* species-antispasmodic, *Cochleria* – mucous membranes, *Lobelia*-primary relaxant. **Early congestion** in an illness requires full stimulation to vital force with *Capsicum, Myrica, Composition essence.*

4] Enervation of the nerves in that they tire easily, requires stimulation to the nerve tissue. *Cinchona* is a central and peripheral nerve stimulant and sustainer for cases of nerve exhaustion or *Cola, Ginkgo, Panax, Paullinia.* Recovery from congestion is slow and calls for mild tonics suited to the case e.g.. *Acorus, Agrimonia, Angelica, Centarium, Geum, Lavandula, Mentha species, Ocimum basilicum.*

5] Solid food is not required during an acute inflammatory condition. Fluids in the form of herbal infusions as required see crisis.

6] Proteolytic enzymes may be used in the treatment of inflammation and accompanying pain.
Bromelain from pineapple
Papain and chymopapain from papaya
Fungal protease from aspergillus oryzae fungi
Trypsin, chymotrypsin and pancreatin from pig and cow sources [Pig is higher than cow].

7] A very light diet is to be used during convalescence - baked apple, brown rice, cous cous, semolina, arrowroot, slippery elm food [Ulmus], vegetable soups, fruit juices - diluted.

Inoculation with Vaccines
Immunology [See also **infection** above].
Russell bodies [large cell wall deficient bacteria] are immunoglobulins [proteins].
It is these bodies that mutate to become fungi, viruses and bacteria. Microbes mutate according to natural phenomenon e.g.. flu virus. Microbes are affected by antibiotics and vaccines such also cause mutation of the microbes. Mutation of the genetic material can be switched backward and forwards.

Rosenow argued that certain serums used in their experiments had an affinity with the heart valves. He found that certain micro-organisms in the serums attacked the heart valves and joints.

The 1918 flu epidemic was caused by the mutation in vaccines used to prevent typhoid in the armies of Europe. When the typhoid had mutated to a paratyphoid infection.

In 1881 the Hungarian government said of the anthrax vaccine that 'pneumonia, catarrhal fever etc. have exclusively struck down the animals subjected to the inoculation.' It follows from this that the Pasteur inoculation tended to accelerate the action of certain diseases and to hasten the mortal issue of other grave affections'.

In 1888 at Odessa, Russia - 4564 sheep were inoculated against anthrax and 3696 of them died from that 'preventative' vaccine. Pasteur was forced in a similar incident to compensate many owners in France for animals killed by his vaccines. Kinnerman in 1929, a state epidemiologist believed that active immunisation may actually increase the virulence of diphtheria bacilli. He stated that **immunised carriers pass organisms of the more virulent type to non-immunised children, with the result that the fatality rate is increasing each year among non immunised children who contract diphtheria.**

Vaccines are dangerous and disrupt the normal functioning of many cells including the T cells of the immune system. Vaccines can provoke degenerative diseases such as cancer and aids.

Animal and human cells harbour all sorts of viruses. Animal tissue is used in cell culture lines. It is possible for a vaccine to become contaminated with viral particles and to be passed on to the recipient. At one time aborted foetus was used to grow cell lines for vaccines.
Some vaccines use mercury as a preservative. Injected vaccines containing mercury may cause CNS developmental anomalies.

Pathology

Millions of African people are infected with the Aids virus. This is most likely to be due to contaminated vaccines. During the years 1960-1977 WHO administered 24 million doses of vaccine worldwide. The Times newspaper reported in May 1987 the story – 'Smallpox vaccine triggered aids virus'. There have been 18 million aids deaths. HIV virus tricks the immune system and affects the white blood cells. Plague [smallpox] and aids virus both target the immune system. Steve Chrohn an American gay man, although his friends died, never contracted aids. In vitro cells were inoculated with the virus-no subsequent infection with the virus was found this proves something is blocking the virus to Steves cells [178].

Microzymas are the actual builders of body cells and our well being depends upon them. Microzymas are present in pus, vaccines, infections etc. but are altered by the disease process. Hence the introduction of vaccines into a body can bring about deterioration of health and prior alteration of the hosts microzymas to an unhealthy condition.

Bubonic plague also known as the black death killed over 25 million people. In 1347 the plague infection was brought in by ships to Sicily. It was carried by fleas on rats. The infection swept through Europe and by 1348 established itself in England. Typical symptoms were fever, black boils on the neck, groin and axilla. If the infection reached the lungs it was called pneumonic plague. In medieval England some 75% of the populus died in that locality. There was a tremendous fear that if you contracted the infection you would die – it was a death sentence with a high mortality. Plague infections went on for 300 years, however there were some survivors in London and elsewhere.

Dr Steven O Brien, a scientist at the National Institute of Health, Washington researched his theory on why some people contracted the infection and lived. There are documented areas of people who survived. One such area was in the village of Eem in Derbyshire. Eem village was quarantined, food was brought by carriage and left outside the village. In September 1666 one year after the plague visited Eem, there were survivors. How many survived? – according to parish registers of 1665-1725 which provided evidence of births, marriages and deaths it appears half the village populus survived. It was wondered whether the disease was anthrax as symptoms are similar, according to inventories of the period no evidence of animal loss was reported so Anthrax was ruled out. Perhaps crowded towns and cities, poverty or bad housing aggravated the problem – these factors were considered irrelevant. Death affected all equally. At Eem some people never got sick. Elizabeth Hancock contracted no plague, however in August 1666 her youngest son became affected. Within one week she had buried six children and her husband. In spite of all this Elizabeth never contracted the plague. Marshall Howe was in charge of burying corpses – he survived the plague. There was something different about those people who survived. Genetic resistance to the plague baccilus was considered a factor. Answers were to be found in the descendents genes. DNA was checked and a CCR5 gene was found in those survivors. The gene had mutated. Delta 32 mutation confers resistance, this meant that individuals with the delta 32 gene would survive.

Margaret Blackwell was in 1665 a survivor of the plague, a descendant in 2002 is Joan Blackwell. Dr Ric Tidwell researched specific action on host cells. He found the plague bacteria in blood could outwit the immune system. The bacterium highjacks the white blood cell and hitches a ride to the lymph nodes and once there it destroys the immune system. Delta 32 gene is present in 14% of descendents. Worldwide searches have been made and no delta 32 genes have been found in Africa or South America. Delta 32 is unusual in that it is found in previously infected areas and the location matches the infection in Europe with the bacteria. Analysis of the worldwide database shows that 700 years ago the gene was around. The rogue gene was passed onto survivors and protected them from plague. Survivors passed down the blood line. [See also AIDS/178].

Link between plague, typhus and smallpox

Writing about the history of epidemics in Britain, **Creighton** suggests that typhus fever and smallpox replaced plague. Later on measles insignificant before the middle of the 17th century began to replace smallpox. Observe a measles lesion of the skin, it looks remarkably like a smallpox lesion but much smaller. Distribution affects the same areas. Interestingly in 1847 typhus killed 30,320 people, this was half of all recorded deaths at this time. Typhus was treated with Plantago. An inhalation, wash and infusion was used before entering houses and to limit the infective process using Artemesia absinthium, Calendula, Mentha piperita, Salvia and Ruta, Ilex aquifoleum [177].

Genetic aspects

Glen Dettman of Australia explains that the AIDS retrovirus contains an enzyme called reverse transcriptase that allows the virus to reproduce itself backward by transferring RNA into DNA. This transfer can occur in both directions.

Vaccines weaken the immune system

In 1994 an article in the BMJ read 'it was well known among immunologists that auto immune diseases such as asthma, eczema and diabetes are the price we pay for eradicating infectious diseases'.

The immune system develops and with each new infection encountered an immunity is established. Access to infectious disease is essential for the immune system to develop. Before an individual develops immunity infectious disease would kill because there is no natural immunity. Infections tend to strengthen our immune system.

Pathology

Vaccines offer a partial immunity but only a temporary immunity. Vaccines are made from a bacteria or virus that has been manipulated in a tissue culture. Within the vaccine some bacteria or their proteins are killed or denatured by heat, some are live. They elicit an antibody response within the host. Because vaccines create subtle changes to an infection, the antibody response within the cell is no longer able to initiate the full-blown disease symptom complex. The vaccine tricks the immune system into an artificial immunity. The artificial immunity eventually wears off. Hence the need for booster jabs. It is not known how long the effect of the vaccine will last. Vaccines can produce a change in the effects of the original disease. Altered response can change the symptoms of a future infection. Once the vaccine particles are put into the body they are given free access to the blood, major organs and tissues resulting in an antibody reaction without an inflammatory response. Vaccines stay within the tissues and create further disease. With no inflammatory response the body cannot remove the vaccine. Susceptibility to other infections occurs in such immunocompromised individuals.

Vaccines can interfere and suppress the immune response. It is difficult for tissues to mount a vigorous response to a vaccine. The response to vaccination are chronic symptoms. Once the vaccine is in the blood it affects the intracellular elements because they are immunosuppressive. The circulating antibody of the viral or bacterial vaccine is intended to keep the virus within the cell and thus prevent any inflammatory response.

This can create atypical disease but only recognised if looked for. Latent 'time bomb' effects can occur when the immune system becomes compromised by another infection, stress, depression or another autoimmune disease is 'diagnosed.' More and more autoimmune diseases are being diagnosed vaccines are at the root of some of these illnesses.

Coulter writes in Vaccination, social violence and Criminality where he tells of cases of chronic sleep disturbances, night terrors, autistic behaviour etc. associated with vaccinations. Sociopathic tendencies are also reported; these he states follow vaccination with DPT/MMR.
The Times newspaper stated that the Urabe strain vaccine used against mumps and banned in Britain since 1992 causes viral meningitis.

Centre for disease control and prevention, Atlanta has identified 34 major adverse reactions to MMR and DPT including asthma, blood disorders, infectious diseases, diabetes, polio, meningitis and hearing loss. Most significant was the increased rate of seizures. Within three days of receiving the jab the rate rose to three times the national average. Reactions to the DPT were immediate. The worst reactions to MMR occurred within 8 to 14 days [100].

Dr Ken Aitken believes the MMR vaccine could be causing a new form of autism. 2000 families claim, since 1998, that their children have been damaged by the MMR vaccine.

Hepatitis B
Associated with a hepatitis jab is multiple sclerosis.

Measles
Poor nutrition and overcrowding predispose people to measles. Death from measles is uncommon with only one death per 10.000 cases. Measles can protect against future allergic reactions. Inhaled measles infection undergoes incubation within the lymph tissues of the tonsils, nasopharynx, and regional lymphatics. Symptoms indicate antibodies within the blood. This situation remains the same for all infections of this nature. The spleen and thymus glands are involved, as is the entire immune system. Symptoms increase with the peak of the disease. The illness is the effort of the vital force to clear and protect the body and clear the virus from the blood. The virus is eliminated from the body exactly the way it entered in the first place via the lungs. The skin lesions represent a vicarious elimination as the virus is expelled.

The MMR vaccination is preserved with mercury - a known neurotoxic agent. The MMR vaccine contains three live viruses and are capable of establishing long term illness explains Dr Wakefield. The MMR vaccine has been associated with inflammatory bowel disease. Viral proteins have been found in the lymph glands. The virus has been isolated in 95% of autistic children. There are now 1 in 32 children that is around half a million children in the UK with autism [168]. There are 1000 cases [January 2002] seeking redress through the courts against the vaccine manufacturers

It is considered by some writers that plague was replaced by typhus and smallpox itself mutating to a measles infection.

MMR vaccination link
1998 showed the biggest decline in vaccine uptake. Dr Andrew Wakefield of the Royal Free Hospital, London, published a study in 1998. The study showed an increased rate of inflammatory bowel disease. Such as bloating, diarrhoea and pain. Autistic behavioural problems were found to co exist with GI symptoms. The parents of most of these children said symptoms started soon after their MMR jab. Inflammatory bowel disease could allow proteins found in wheat and

milk to pass through the gut wall and into the blood to be carried to the brain. Vaccine encephalitis [brain damage] could be a result.

According to department of health figures, deaths from measles had decreased by 95% before the first vaccine was introduced in 1968. The decline was steady, indicating that the disease was dying out naturally. Deaths from measles had reduced from 1145 in 1941 to 100 in 1967. Improved sanitation from the early 1900s and improved diet contributed in the main to the reduction of the disease.

Polio

The disease has been redefined in name and called aseptic or viral meningitis. Most cases of polio are harmless. Enterovirus [polio] is found in the gut of healthy individuals. Millions of young people become infected by polioviruses yet suffer no harm from the infection. Infection can occur without producing the symptoms of disease. Sometimes the infection causes a sore throat, fever, aching limbs and vomiting. Infection induces viraemia and intense inflammation. If the virus enters the CNS - neck stiffness, joint pain, and paralysis of the limbs or respiratory muscles ensue. Polio causes eventual cranial nerve damage. Non paralytic polio often manifests as pyrexia. Some 90/95% of polio cases remain asymptomatic. Recovery is complete in non paralytic cases. 80% of paralytic cases improve within 6 months with ongoing improvements. There is a mortality of 4% which rises to 10% in adults with the bulbar variety. Respiratory failure occurs from paralysis of the respiratory muscles.

For every million people vaccinated 2 will have serious complications e.g. encephalitis [186].

Polio has been associated with Guillian barre syndrome [GBS], which causes varying levels of paralysis. Cases of GBS, studied in China were found to be infected with a variation of polio. Polio vaccine can lead to a mutation of the virus. Viral mutation would create a different type of disease but with a similar symptom picture. In Brazil the poliovirus has been isolated in patients suffering from GBS. Polio vaccine can cause a sore at the vaccination site, fever, headaches, extensive rashes and insomnia. Patients with lowered immunity can develop explosive infections. Immunocompromised patients with HIV, Aids, heart transplant patients or cancer should remain vaccinated.

Pertussus

Pertussus vaccine is probably the most common cause of recurrent childhood pyrexia. Pertussus vaccine introduced into the blood can drive the infection into deep body tissues where it will become a pathocausative.

Rubella

Determined by an upper respiratory infection with pyrexia. The rash of raised papules appears on the face, behind the ears and trunk. Primary risks are for pregnant mothers who on contracting the disease can pass the virus to their unborn. Following vaccination, immunity to rubella falls away at around 11 years of age [137]. Infection with a natural strain of rubella at a younger age would give immunity to a female and thus prevent the later infection or transmission at childbearing age. Rubella contracted in childhood gives life long immunity. Rubella infection of a foetus causes defective vision and hearing, heart disorders and autism.

Tetanus

Clostridium tetani a spore forming bacteria causes tetanus. Infection follows an insufficiently cleaned puncture wound. Because tetanus requires oxygen to reproduce treatment should allow the wound to drain naturally and thereby support elimination of the infection. Before the vaccine was introduced tetanus was largely in decline due to improved hygiene and wound management. During world war two only 12 cases of tetanus were reported [70].

Naturopathic & Herbal medication for infectious diseases-measles, polio etc.

If the following is carried out no residual paralysis [polio] or prolonged illness will develop.

1] Rest and fresh air. Keep the feet warm.

2] Fasting depending upon the case. Avoid food at the first sign of pyrexia or pain. Continue to avoid food until the pyrexia has eased. Once the pyrexia has subsided and the temperature is normal feeding may be resumed.

For the first day water is freely given [to dilute toxins]. Fruit juices – especially lemon juice every half to one hour. Whole fruit [on the second day after the fever has broken] with grains, beans and nuts given for seven days. Avoid all food until the temperature is normal.

3] Enemas if necessary to clear the lower bowel –
Chamomilla, Eupatorium perfoliatum, Nepeta cataria.

4] High doses of vitamin C, 3g daily.
Vitamin C helps reverse the toxic effects of vaccination.

5] Herbal medication - Thuja immediately action after vaccination.

Pathology

6] Diaphoretics.

7] Fomentation/poultice.

Medicines for infectious disease. [See also Chapter 36].
Achillea, Allium, Aloe, Baptisia, Berberis, Calendula, Chamomilla, Capsicum, Cinnamomum, Commiphora, Echinacea, Eupatorium perforatum, Hydrastis, Juniperus, Lavandula [wash], Lobelia, Nepeta, Petroselinim, Phytolacca, Sambucus, Scrophularia, Scutellaria, Thymus, Urtica. Astringents. Grapefruit seed extract [279].

Summary
Most orthodox pathology books cite the cause of most disease is due to an infection. In physiomedical herbalism tissue health is paramount, toxaemia from any cause [often from leaky gut or retained secretions from any cause] will give rise to unhealthy blood and tissue fluids, this encourages infections to become established. Healthy tissues withstand infections to a greater of lesser degree. When overwhelmed by infection herbal medicines can control the infective organism and limit its activity. A change in the physiology of the tissues creates the environment, which aids the infective process.
Certain temperaments and bodily typology [types of build] create tendencies to disease processes: these are called predispositions towards disease. Tissue physiology changes as age advances and disease processes gain hold.
Bechamp's work shows us the cause of disease lies within the blood and to detoxify and cleanse the blood enables all tissues to benefit from the cleansing process. Every cell requires nutrition and the elimination of toxins for adequate metabolic processes. Disturbance of either process encumbers the cell and leads to its demise. Inflammation is purely protective to tissues but it may be necessary to limit the inflammatory process always supporting the eliminatory efforts of the organism towards health.

Vaccinations should not be used. When immunisation is required suitable protection from infection is obtained through good living methods. Where overwhelming infections predominate, medication - vasotonic alteratives are available to neutralise the infecting organism and promote elimination. Inadequate elimination [with consequent infections] is always found when chronic disease is present.

7
Principles of physiology

What this Chapter is about
Physiomedicalism uses three basic principles to establish variations in function of bodily tissues. These three principles have special meaning to the physiomedicalist:

Stimulate, Contract, Relax.

Stimulate is the word used in relation to the vital force, where stimulate is an expression to encourage vital activity. It is the vital force that heals the disorder and by stimulating this force you are increasing the life power in the tissues. Direct the vital force using **stimulants** to focus and increase functional action and activity to an under functioning part or organ area.

Contract also means **astringe**, in this text - the terms are synonymous. Once the tissues are contracted, a tightening of the tissues takes place.

Relax is the term used to describe a slackening or loosening of the tissue also known as laxity or atony.

Cook gives his interpretation of the principals of contraction and relaxation 'Regularity in periods of alternate labour and rest is characteristic of all vital action'.
The period of labour or activity is one of contraction in which the muscle fibres are shortened while the period of inactivity [rest] is one of relaxation. Alternate contraction and relaxation is the means of function in muscle organs [11].

Contraction produces action while **relaxation** allows rest in all of the muscles, along with organs that contain muscle fibre e.g. stomach, intestine, heart and gall bladder. It is natural to associate the bodily effect with the function of the tissue. Observe action within the tissue during contraction balanced with rest during the relaxation phase.

Greer stated 'although there are many forms of disease the degree of interference to the vital force affects the symptoms and the parts affected.' Changes within the tissues, the tissues become either too relaxed or to contracted. **Relaxed tissue** is unable to gain normal tone. **Contracted tissue** is unable to relax sufficiently. Both abnormal tissue states [those of contraction or relaxation] are unable to maintain normal physiological function [p112]

Principles of Physiology

Nerve activity is determined by the irritability and conductivity of impulses.
Excess tension in the nerves creates:
excitement, sensitivity, irritability, wakefulness, active delirium
Excess relaxation of nerves creates:
depression induces lethargy, dementia, enervation, and passive delirium.

Irritability with weakness whereby sensitivity is increased while motor strength is reduced. Often found in the panic attack and neurasthenic [asthenic] patient.

Peripheral nerves react to arterial excitability with reduced venous drainage by:
[a] in the contracted state – muscular spasms and cramps.
[b] a relaxed state - loss of skeletal muscular action via the motor nerves results in problems with balance, standing or walking.

- Balance of calcium and magnesium, potassium and sodium will also require to be checked as they all affect nerve function.

Autonomic activity
Noradrenaline is methylated via its synthetic pathway to adrenaline. Each step is controlled by enzymes. Noradrenaline is found in the adrenal medulla and postganglionic sympathetic nerve fibres. Noradrenaline is an alpha receptor stimulating drug and is released at postganglionic sympathetic nerve end plates. Noradrenaline pools in the nerve terminals ready for activity. It increases blood pressure through vasoconstrictor action causing vasoconstriction of the skin, splanchnic and coronary blood vessels, pupil dilation and gut relaxation. This activity demonstrates the vasoconstrictor action upon the blood vessels.

Complimentary action
Bodily tissues must have a period of rest in order to recuperate otherwise the tissues will become full of metabolites as Cook tells us:
'The duration of an effort in any organ may have a considerable range but relaxation must come or the part will suffer from not receiving [in rest] a supply of nutriment equal to its waste'.

Cook also says 'the earliest departure of the tissues from under the full control of the vital force will be in a lack of ability either to relax or to contract some of the tissues as readily as in the healthy state. The balance of complimentary action is lost and either the tendency to contractility increases while the power of relaxation diminishes or laxity of the structures becomes more marked as the power to effect their contraction diminishes. These departures from the normal condition may be slight and gradual or distinct and rapid but as the change is in either direction the loss of vital control is manifest in the other and the longer the disturbance the greater the disposition to remain in an abnormal state. This loss of equilibrium constitutes a primary element in most diseases.'

Organ composition
Each organ has **four classes of tissue**
- parenchyma
- fibrous tissue
- arterial and venous blood vessels including lymphatics
- sensory and motor nerves

'Each of these classes of tissue may depart from health in either one of the two directions that constitute the primary elements of disease. As the tissues depart more and more widely from the normal standard the life power can use them less and less perfectly but still using them the imperfect execution of the functions will correspond in character with the particular nature of each deviation'.

[Cook p51]

Contraction and relaxation excess's interfere with the action of the different parts and create abnormal functional changes within those parts.

Physiomedicalism is tailored to an individuals needs while the herbalist treats 'to preserve organ reserve [because ageing equals loss of organ reserve] and to modulate intercellular messengers' - **Jeff Bland** 1999. Zinc is considered important in the role of modifying gene expression by intercellular means.

Tissue conditions
Altered conditions of the tissues occur in two directions this will result in:

1 Increased tension is usually associated with a tendency to increased activity
2 Undue relaxation is accompanied by a diminished effort

The **functional state** of the organ is influenced by the vasomotor system. The vasomotor system is the arterial blood supply together with its nerve activity. The function is influenced either by contracting or relaxing the tissue. Secretions will be duly increased by relaxation or decreased by contraction through the vasomotor blood supply.

Each change in a tissue, by embarrassing the normal discharge of the function pertaining to the organ involved, will cause aberrations in that function. As the function in its entirety depends upon the harmonious action of all the tissues entering into that organ, the diseased change in each of these tissues will create a functional disturbance. A diagnosis in terms of the tissue state and the level of physiological disturbance will give a true picture of the condition to be treated.

Contracted [tense] conditions
Arterial capillaries
Arterial capillaries of the skin under a moderate degree of tension induce a more active flow of blood. Considerable tension induces an accumulation of blood towards and in the part causing redness and oedema from distension of the capillaries - inflammation [See inflammation/active hyperaemia Chapter 6].

Veins
Increased tension of the veins impedes the return of blood and causes oedema and redness. A partial venous hue is seen over the skin surface.

The above condition within the veins is the essential basis for **Congestion** that may exist in any part or organ.

Relaxed conditions
Suderiferous [sweat] glands reduce heat and eliminate toxins. Where they are relaxed perspiration is increased and warm.

Relaxed glands and circulation increase perspiration that is cold while the skin surface is shrunken and flaccid. Flaccid skin moves blood from the skin towards the heart. This increases the requirement for increased heart action. A heart weakness may be aggravated by the extra recession of blood upon it.

Secretory organs
All the secretory organs are similarly disturbed in function when their tissues are affected by relaxation [laxity]. Laxity is at the basis of many chronic conditions. It is characterised by lack of tone in the parts. The vital chi force does not have sufficient control to produce the alternate contractions and relaxation required for correct function of the part. Hence congestion within the tissue of an organ will encourage an accumulation of waste and toxins that will be eliminated or accumulate in the tissues.

Secretions accumulating in the blood render the blood impure.

Substances retained by one organ will be carried by the blood to an exit from the body often through a mucous membrane this is called a **vicarious elimination** and becomes nature's support system to eliminate the toxins.

Examples of vicarious elimination are numerous as when bile is eliminated through the skin and mucous membranes in biliary disorders e.g. jaundice. Retained biliary pigment can affect the eyesight, which becomes blurred and floaters may be seen in the aqueous.

Herbal Medicine - Keys

Urobilinogen will give a yellow or green coating to the tongue. Urobilinogen affects the nervous system it can cause depression, irritability and melancholy.

Accumulated renal secretions urea and uric acid can give rise to smelly feet, rheumatic pain, catarrh and coughs.

Intestinal reabsorption of toxins find their way out through the breath that becomes offensive or an acne skin disturbance with comedones and pustules. Sweat glands try to eject urea that may render the perspiration offensive.

All the above are secondary consequences of vicarious elimination that is a purely protective function of the system. Unfortunately some treat the secondary effect without going back to the primary unhealthy organ function, which must be, if any permanent cure be possible, to heal the organ weakness in the primary cause of the disease process. Quicker return to health is obtained if the eliminatory function of intestine, liver, kidneys and skin are balanced.

Stomach disorders
Stomach glands
Laxity of the stomach **glands** creates deficient secretion of hydrochloric acid with resulting indigestion.
Mucous membrane
Tension of the **mucous membrane** creates thirst and stomach sensitivity.
Stomach capillaries
Stomach **capillary tension** causes engorgement of blood and deficient secretion, a tender gastric surface and heartburn.
Nerve supply
Undue **nerve tension** can produce vomiting with little nausea. If the nerve tension extends to the muscular walls of the stomach, nausea, retching or painful spasms with little vomiting may occur.

Similar effects occur in other organs of secretion.
In many cases of disease more than one secretion is disturbed. As when liver or gall bladder disorders provoke disturbance within the stomach, intestine or skin. The vital effects of retained secretions in the **acute stage** display through the nervous system as irritation and pain. **Chronic** disease indicates depressed vital function and consequent aberrations within the body. Symptoms become low grade and can give much distress as when the 'arthritis' sufferer complains about pain in the joints however the primary cause of disease may lie within the kidneys.

Principles of Physiology

Changes within the blood vessels

Venous obstruction causes distension of the capillaries and veins. Cyanosis and right heart trouble will give a bluish appearance to the lips and ears, coldness of the skin surface and dyspnoea. Effusion of serum may take place from obstruction of the veins with resulting oedema of the feet and ankles. Common presentations of venous obstruction occur in portal hypertension with backpressure affecting the liver. Consequences are vague digestive disease, splenomegaly, and evidence of a collateral circulation, oesophageal or gastric varices. Anaemia and ascites could also occur. Venous feebleness make the organs described inefficient in their task. Thrombus may form due to the venous insufficiency.

- Uterine disease may result from pelvic venous congestion. Obstructions within the veins lead to menorrhagia with clotting and pain. Lumbar lordosis and tilted pelvis may obstruct the venous return.

Vasomotor system

The vasomotor system is the controlling device of the body. **The vasomotor system consists of the autonomic nervous system and the circulatory system. It is the system that maintains the level of blood volume and the control of blood volume, through vaso-contraction and vaso-relaxation of the blood vessels; decreasing or increasing the amount of blood required in any given area. The autonomic nervous system controls and regulates the bodily functions through the vasomotor system.**

- The circular muscle fibres of the blood vessel walls are also part of the vasomotor system.
- The digestive, secretory and excretory paths are similarly controlled by the amount of blood in the area at any one time. The vasomotor control exerts its function over the systemic processes. Organ secretions are reduced or increased by vasomotor control. The mechanism operates by simple reflex arc nerve impulse to make the vasomotors relax or contract and affect the secretions of the gland on receiving impulses.
- The trophic state of the viscera is affected by the amount of blood available to feed the viscera and restore trophicity.

Medicines correct visceral function are specific and act through the local autonomic ganglia and reflex nerve arc to the vasomotor function enhancing end organ functional activity.

Factors that influence the vasomotor function

Circulatory control mechanism.

Thurston tells us 'the vasomotor system, working through the digestive, secretory and excretory organs absolutely controls the waste and repair of every tissue cell, tissue, and structure of the body'.

The vasomotor system co-ordinates the functional work of every organ excluding the voluntary muscular system [which is under the control of the will].

The vasomotor control of bodily organs is affected by the local nerve supply to that organ. We call the nerve supply the innervation of the nerve plexus.

The complete means of vasomotor control is achieved by and through the **circulatory system and the autonomic nervous system.**
The essential nature of the vasomotor function is primarily circulatory and secondarily motor [13]. The function and trophic state of organs are dependent upon the vasomotor function.
Other factors are mentioned below.

Vasomotor control is affected by a number of complex mechanisms. These are pressoreflexes, chemo reflexes, medulla influence and higher brain centre mechanisms and the local control of arteries. Some local effects induce blood flow through the arteries these will be discussed later.

The **physiological mechanisms** consist of many parts -
A] Factors include the level of oxygen required by the tissues and levels of carbon dioxide in the blood.
B] The level of nitric oxide within the blood.
C] Local and general ganglionic nerve fibres to the end organ.
D] Nerve centres within the organ itself.

A change in the arterial blood pressure or in the levels of oxygen or carbon dioxide content set vasomotor control mechanisms into operation. Arterial blood pressure changes initiate a vasomotor pressoreflex. A change in arterial oxygen or carbon dioxide content acts in two ways to bring about a change in arteriole diameter - by stimulating chemoreceptors and thereby initiating a vasomotor chemo reflex and by stimulating the medulla's vasomotor centres directly and thereby initiating the medullary ischaemic reflex.

Factors, which increase arterial blood pressure locally or generally, stimulate aortic and carotid baroreceptors. This leads to stimulation of the cardio inhibitory centres and inhibition of **vasoconstrictor centres**. More impulses per second go out to the heart over parasympathetic vagal fibres and fewer over sympathetic fibres to the blood vessels of the skin and abdominal viscera. As a result the heartbeat slows the arterioles and venules of blood reservoirs dilate. **Sympathetic** vasoconstrictor impulses predominate in the homeostatic balance of the circulation. Inhibition of these impulses is considered the major mechanism of vasodilation.

The main **blood reservoirs** are the venous plexuses and sinuses in the skin and abdominal organs [liver and spleen]. The venous networks serve to act as blood reservoirs for the storage of blood.

Reduction in **arterial blood pressure** causes the aortic and carotid baroreceptors to send more impulses to the medulla's vasoconstrictor centres thereby stimulating them. These centres send more impulses via the sympathetic fibres to smooth muscle in arterioles, venules and veins of the blood reservoirs, causing their constriction. This squeezes more blood out of them, and increases the venous return. This extra blood is eventually redistributed to the skeletal muscles and the heart because their arterioles become dilated due to locally produced substances. The vasoconstrictor pressoreflex and the local vasodilation mechanism serve to shift blood from reservoirs to structures that need it more. It is a valuable mechanism during exercise.

Vasomotor chemo reflexes.
Chemo reflexes located in the aortic and carotid bodies are particularly sensitive to a deficiency of blood oxygen [hypoxia] and excess blood carbon dioxide [hypercapnia] and to decreased blood pH. When one or more of these conditions stimulates the chemoreceptors, their fibres transmit more impulses to the medulla's vasoconstrictor centres; vasoconstriction of arterioles and venous reservoirs soon follows. This is an emergency device when severe hypoxia or hypercapnia endangers survival.

Local action from some factor decreases the level of oxygen, which stimulates the vasoconstrictor centres. More impulses are sent over the sympathetic fibres to the vessels of skin and abdominal viscera, which causes a reflex vasoconstriction.

Vasodilation and blood flow through the blood vessel results from the chemical nitric oxide produced in the vessel endothelium. Nitric oxide is derived from argenine. Nitric oxide is an enzyme and present in brain, immune system and endothelial blood vessel wall. Animal fats can prevent the diffusion of endothelial nitric oxide to the vessel smooth muscle by inactivating the nitric oxide via the oxidative mechanism. Reduced perfusion of blood to the tissue creates cellular changes and eventual hypotrophicity. Excessive doses of the amino acid argenine and nitric oxide are toxic [71-74].

The medullary ischaemic reflex.
When medulla ischaemia occurs its neurons suffer from oxygen deficiency and carbon dioxide excess. Hypercapnia intensely stimulates the vasoconstrictor centres to bring about marked arteriole and venous constriction.

Vasomotor control by the higher brain centres.
Impulses from centres in the cerebral cortex and hypothalamus are transmitted to the vasomotor centres in the medulla and thereby help to control vasoconstriction and vasodilation. Sensory fibres that terminate in synapses with neurons in vasomotor centres conduct impulses from chemoreceptors and baroreceptors. From the centres sympathetic neurons relay impulses to smooth muscle in blood vessels. **More impulses cause vessels to constrict. Fewer impulses cause them to dilate.** A hormonal flush is an example of a vasomotor flush.

Local control.
Norephinephrine, histamine, lactic acid and other substances act as stimuli to activate the local vasomotor mechanisms.

Vertebral subluxation
Impulses travel over the spinal reflex arc through sensory nerves to glandular tissue. Interrupted impulses at the spinal level affect organ areas. Adjustment or manipulation of those constricted vertebrae can bring relief.

Vasomotor control is affected by nerve balance/imbalance. The balance of nerve action affects the:

1] Trophic state of the viscera.
2] Secretory organ activity.
3] The functional state of plain muscle fibres of hollow viscera [contraction and relaxation].
4] Regulation of the ANS divisions: sympathetic and parasympathetic.

Visceral functional control
Tone and trophic state of the tissue and organ systems require to be evaluated against the background of typology [see Ch 10].
An organ may be either over-contracted or over-relaxed and this is the *functional state.* **Apart from this the cells and tissues are in a certain state of** *nutrition* **and conditions of** *hypertrophy* **and** *hypotrophy* **[atrophy] indicate the**

Principles of Physiology

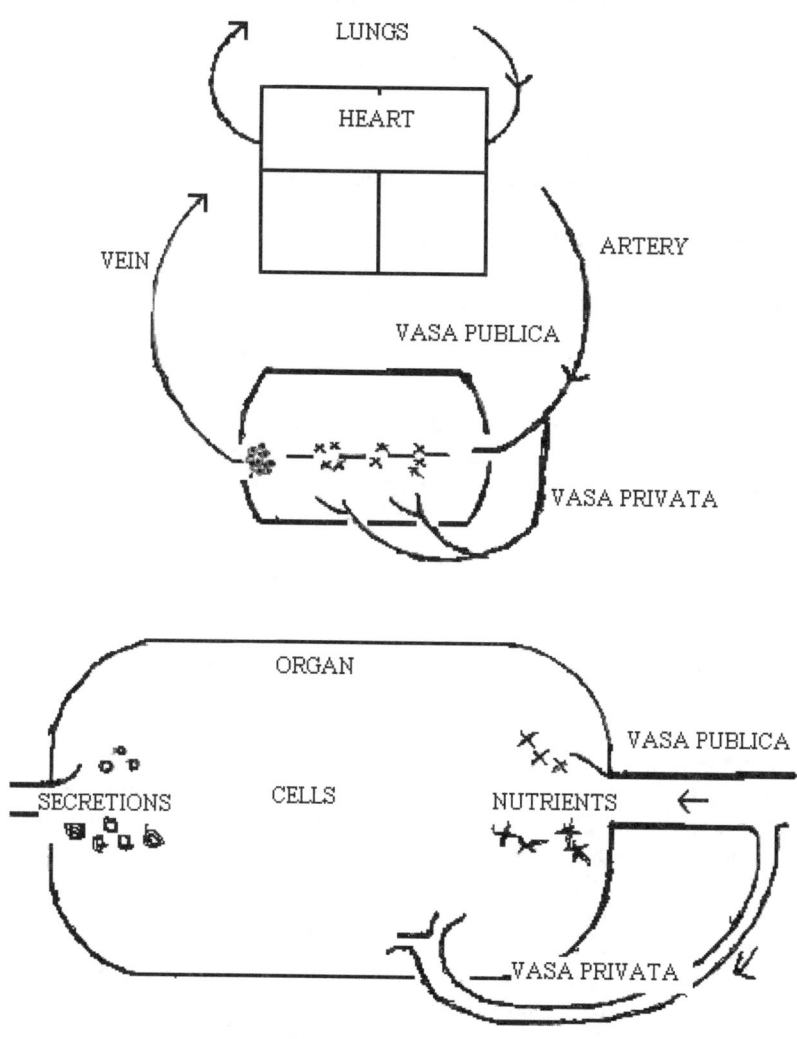

Visceral functional control, continued
condition of these cells and tissues. The trophic state depends upon the blood supply to the cells of the organ as quite distinct from the blood supply to the cells of the organ for its functional purposes. Remedies to improve the function [functional tonic] of the heart/kidney/liver differ from the remedy that looks after the trophic state [trophorestorative].

A nerve centre within the organ controls the trophic state.

The vasomotor system contains the nerve ganglion and blood vessels.

Kaspar Blond explains the term *Vasa publica* and *Vasa privata* of the vasomotor system.
**'*Vasa publica* Ganglionic fibres that control the lumen of the artery; the functional blood supply, through its plain muscle fibres is provided by vasomotor regulation and controls the blood going through the organ.
The functional state of the local ganglionic nerve centre with its fibres activates organ activity through the plain muscle fibres controlling the arterial blood supply'.**
***Vaso privata* blood supply is the blood supply to the organ for nutrition and waste removal. *Vasa privata* is the ganglionic nerve centre that controls the trophic state of the organ, i.e. its general health, and the blood supply to the organ.**

> **Over contracted** states of the vasomotors - vaso compression
> **Over relaxed** states of the vasomotors - vaso dilation

Both are affected by the local blood flow activated by the nerve plexus for the organ.

Viscero motor supply
The viscero motor supply regulates the **activity of the hollow muscular viscera**. The plain muscle activity at the organ end is effected by its own unique viscero nerve activity. The autonomic activity governs the amount of impulses activating the end organs. Stress often upsets the balance of the nerve impulses to the end organs with organ activity detrimentally challenged. The viscero motor nerves are activated through the muscle longitudinal and circular muscle fibres. The muscles are fed from their respective sources within the autonomic nervous system. Branches from the vertebra run to all the organ areas. Parasympathetic fibres activate the longitudinal muscle fibres. The sympathetic fibres activate circular muscle fibres. It is the aim of herbal treatment to restore a balance of autonomic nerve function to the supplying nerve and the end organ.

Principles of Physiology

So far as the secretions are concerned the **vasomotor supply** is involved. The vasomotor supply determines the amount of blood [+ or -] passing through the parenchyma.

Increased vasomotor relaxation = more blood supply - **increased secretion**
Vasomotor contraction = decreased blood supply - **decreased secretion**

Vasomotor - supplying glandular structures
- over contraction - small thick secretion
- over relaxation - profuse watery secretion

Stomach
Viscero motor - muscle layers [longitudinal and circular fibres] –
over contraction = colic
Secretory - surface vessels subject to astringents and stimulants

Secretions are affected by vasomotor control:
When the vasomotors are contracted [vasocompression] they decrease the secretions
Relaxed vasomotors [vasodilation] increase the secretions.

Thurston explains the ganglionic and local organ nerve supply will vary in its own **tonicity and trophicity.**
The trophic state of the ganglionic centre - vasotrophesy.
The peripheral mechanism - vasoatony.
Vasoatony and vasotrophesy effect the trophic state of the ganglionic nerve centres or peripheral vasomotor system.

Thurston's classification of disease syndromes.
Vasoexaggeration when there is an undue acceleration of vasomotor function. Found in acute conditions and pyrexia. Pyrexia is where all the functional activities are excited into action. Check the BMI, CVI and body temperature as these effect both vaso exaggeration and vaso depression.

Vasodepression is a condition of subnormal vasomotor functional activity. A deficiency in the reserve vitality of the cell. Found in reduced function of an organ or tissue area. **Lack of normal tone** and loss of tonicity of the cells making up the tissues. A lack of functional reserve energy. It is found in depression following acute illness. The asthenic constitution typically reflects vasodepression.
Vasocompression means **contraction** and vasospasm [spasm] of the extravascular spaces as well as the blood vessels. Irritation of the local ganglionic nerve fibres. All **contracted** [spastic] conditions are under this heading.

Vasodilation is a condition of excess **relaxation** of blood vessels and extravascular spaces that leads to passive congestion and ultimately stasis. All conditions of excess **relaxation** fall under this heading.

Vasoatony is a condition of loss of tone resulting in atony. Atony of the involuntary muscles and mucous membranes of the organ. Because of loss of reserve energy within the cell. Vasoatony is a trophic deterioration of the organ involved and will require stimulation to the vasomotor function and local circulation.

Vasotrophesy occurs when the neurons are enervated from inefficient or obstructed vasomotor function - this is the basis of degeneration of the CNS. All hypotrophic conditions are of a degenerative nature. Vasotrophesy is the trophic degeneration of the ganglionic nerve centres. Neurological degeneration falls under this heading.

Thurston says medicines used to treat conditions are referred to as vasostimulants, vasodilators, vasocompressors, vasotonics [Vasotonic alterative] and trophorestoratives.

Vaso stimulants: *Capsicum, Zanthoxylum*, and *Cochleria*.

Vaso dilators: *Chamaemelum nobile, Viburnum species, Lobelia*.

Vaso compressors: *Myrica, Zingiber* and astringents.

Vaso tonics [eliminative and restorative Vasotonic alteratives]:

> *Alpinia, Agrimonia, Berberis Sp.*

Trophorestoratives:

> *Avena, Bacopa, Crataegus, Dioscorea, Hydrastis, Phytolacca, Verbena.*

Summary

An adequate circulation must be present for essential organ activity. Decreased blood volume encourages hypotrophic states to manifest. The organ declines in health because insufficient blood is available to carry nutrients to tissue and waste from it. Trophorestoratives are used which improve the quality of organ health. Vasocontractants [astringents] tighten up the blood vessels. Vasorelaxants [including relaxing diaphoretics] loosen or dilate the blood vessels.

8
Contraction and Relaxation of Tissue

What this Chapter is about

Tissues contract or relax depending upon the activity required at any one moment. This action is common to all tissues. Nerve tissue is excited by neurotransmitters. Bringing the tissue balance toward normality from the over tense [contracted] state or from relaxed [sluggish, atonic state] is the object of medication. Toxic removal will commence once the tissue has improved tone. The following gives an appreciation of the different types of tissue under consideration together with the effects.

Lindlahr says 'There are two forces at work in the human organism, the one tensing and contracting the other relaxing and expanding. Normal function or health results from equilibrium between the two. This equilibrium between the contending forces we call the positive condition of health, departure from it in either direction, the negative condition of disease'.

Two tissue states exist these are known as relaxed and contracted tissue states. The effect upon the system is that:

- **Relaxed states produce a diminished effort**
- **Contracted states increase activity until excessive contraction**
  produces stasis

Basic formula of therapeutic application

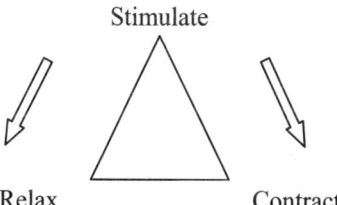

The functional state of tissue is affected by the condition of either
Over contraction - **hypertonia** and over [excess] relaxation - **hypotonia**

Treatment aims to restore this equilibrium of balance within the individual so that there is sufficient tension to produce action e.g. respiration, digestion, elimination and a relaxation phase for the cellular and organ rest periods.

Issues concerning contraction and relaxation of tissue in organs, nerves, circulation and secretions follows.

J. H. Greer. M.D. Physician in chief at Harvard Medical Institute.

Greer contributed his book - *Physician in the House* in 1897.

He says protoplasm has pulsating motion he observed this pulsation using a microscope. 'The protoplasm involuntarily and alternately contracts and relaxes with perfect rhythm. Diffusion of particles across the cell membrane allows the expulsion of waste and absorption of nutrients into and out of the cell.

Although there are almost innumerable forms of disease, manifested by a great variety of signs or symptoms these vary according to the degree of interference to the action of the vital force and according to the parts affected.

General departures from the normal conditions [of health] are:

[a] The tissues may become too relaxed or loose and thus be unable to regain their natural tone. In the alternate relaxation and contraction of the tissues there would be evidence of a lack of power to contract sufficiently.

[b] The tissues may become too contracted or tense and be unable to relax sufficiently [to carry on the normal rate of alternate contraction and relaxation].

[c] The tissues may have become damaged.

[d] There may be accumulations of waste material.

[e] There may be an improper environment that will interfere with the control of the vital force over the tissues. Especially excessive heat, cold or moisture.

Greer's formula was:
- Tone and stimulate relaxed conditions.
- Relax tense and contracted conditions.
- Remove accumulations, obstructions and toxins.
- Provide proper environments.
- Equalise the circulation as between the upper and lower circuits, and between the inner and outer circuits.
- Ensure normal excretory function [14].

Contraction and Relaxation of Tissue

Too much Relaxation

Cook gives insight into the tissue conditions of relaxation and contraction. Taking relaxation first, observation of the tissue with the relevant effects relaxation produces.

Muscle

'When muscular fibres are relaxed they perform their motions inadequately - the degree of motor loss corresponding to the degree of muscular laxity until complete relaxation leaves the part helpless. The effect of such a state upon the organs of locomotion is at once apparent. It is seen in the feebleness of the convalescent who totters as he tries to walk even if he can walk at all. In the helplessness of the paralytic whose fibres are too enervated and flaccid to make any contractile responses to vitality. Atony of the intestinal muscles induces constipation by not being able to keep up the natural peristaltic motion and simultaneous laxity of the abdominal muscles permits a pendulous abdomen and very persistent costiveness.'

Organs

Laxity in the tissues of the stomach will disable it from digesting food and also from secreting gastric juice, indigestion is the result. A similar condition of the liver will disable it from secreting bile and leave the secretion of bile to accumulate in the blood while its absence in the intestinal canal impairs chylification and deprives the intestines of their natural stimulus'.

Secretions

'All the Secretory organs are similarly disturbed in function when their tissues become partially disabled through too great laxity and this condition is one of the greatest mischief's in most chronic conditions and lies at the root of many acute diseases. It is characterised everywhere as a lack of tone in the parts, the vital power not having over them the control necessary to produce alternate contractions hence organ torpor with the accumulations of injurious toxins into the blood are provocative of disease'.

Circulation

'The same condition arises in the circulatory system - gives a weak and inefficient pulse and a limited blood supply to the whole body or to so much of it as may suffer enfeeblement of its vessels'.

'Some disturbances begin in the larger vessels and travel to or from the heart. In the vast majority of cases the trouble **starts in the capillaries** and then extends to the larger vessels then the heart'.

Capillary walls are capable of marked **contractions** and **dilations**. When they contract persistently – as under the influence of a retained secretion or other irritating substance or from any local excitement on the vessel nerve loops an impediment is produced which sends a reverse back current of blood to be met with a stronger onward wave. Problems occur when the onward wave is unable to remove the obstruction. A local accumulation of blood takes place in the capillaries. The amount depending upon the degree of localised obstruction. Insufficient arterial action produces further back pressure of blood towards the larger vessels and eventually the heart will become effected. An increased arterial action excites higher capillary tension and local excitement. During the state of **capillary tension** the part will exhibit a change of function. When contraction is excessive there will be a diminution of function in that part. In essence there will be a **decrease in secretions** in secretory organs e.g. pancreas, liver, gall bladder, stomach or kidneys. Once the tension subsides the secretions are renewed to normal.

Pain may be felt as a result of secretory organ tension.

'Capillaries may become relaxed in their venous or arterial portions. Disturbed functional action follows in the form of torpor of the area concerned'. Organ torpor produces a flaccid [relaxed] state of the organ and pallor of the part arising from deficiency of blood.

Nerves
'The nerve tissues either in whole or part sink into a corresponding loss of function when enervated by relaxation - the sensations in that part are diminished.

When it is remembered how closely the nervous system represents life itself all effects of torpor in the discharge of functions are to especial relaxation in the nerves of that part.
It is more practical to consider the several classes of tissue separately, that the effect of their too great relaxation may be more clearly appreciated' [11].

Over [excess] contraction - **hypertonia** and
over [excess] relaxation - **hypotonia**.

Too much tension
Tension within the tissues. Observation of the tissue with the relevant effect's contraction [tension] produces.

'As the vital power loses its ability to relax any part at will, the tension or contractility increases and with this increase are presented various disturbances in the functions quite unlike those pertaining to increased relaxation'.

Contraction and Relaxation of Tissue

Muscles

'In the muscular structures is observed an inclination to rigidity - exhibited through a wide range according to the degree of irritability of the parts. Sometimes this is seen in the motor nerves in the form of light jerking and spasmodic action and the extreme degree is met as tetanus or epilepsy. Spasmodic excitement in any muscular part is due to contraction'.

Organs

'Intestinal contractions are the basis of colic, IBS, in the tenesmus of dysentery. Asthma, physiological recurring uterine contractions during labour and the similar contractions observed in certain cases of dysmenorrhoea' [11].

Mucous Membranes

Tension of the mucous membrane causes an accumulation of mucus.

Circulation

'Exalted contractility of the circulatory system manifests in the pulse becoming more rigid and excited, labouring more rapidly and with less distinctive softening of its walls between the pulsations. In the nervous system it is seen in elevated sensibility - a part becoming peculiarly impressible to trifling influences or the entire nervous system exhibits a similar extreme and unnatural irritability'. Venous obstructions within organs become impediments to the circulation with the liver and gall bladder on the venous side, with kidneys and skin on the arterial side. Disordered secernants cause localised circulatory obstructions to the capillary circulation. Treatment of the heart, arteries, arterioles, capillaries and veins as necessary equalises the circulation. Diffusives are used to arouse local circulation e.g. *Zingiber, Nepeta, Achillea.*

Nerves

'Close associations exist between the nerves and the blood vessels, from the great vital centres to the minute ramifications throughout the body. So that the results of contractile excitement in one place can be felt in another area'; for example contraction of the neck muscles may give rise to migraine.

'The nerve distribution in a gland determines its degree of tension and activity both by stimulating its local circulation and increasing its glandular function. Increase of function cannot be dissociated from local nerve and circulatory excitement. The **Secretory action being dependent on the circulation**' [11].

Nerve & Muscle

'Undue contractility in a part may not always be associated with increased activity there are important and significant exceptions'.

'Extreme tension of the motor nerves creates rigidity of the parts and may become so great as to prevent any motion. This departure of the tissues has reached its greatest limit, the vital power cannot put into operation any degree of that alternating relaxation on which motion depends. The same condition is observed in other purely tonic spasms of the muscular structures - as in strangury, the spasms of tetanus, laryngismus stridulus and the spastic contractions that sometimes arise in parturition. These are usually uncertain in their duration, sooner or later giving way to some degree of relaxation while the condition lasts; the true function of the part is almost wholly inactive'. [11]

Secretory organs
'The same fact is observable in other organs. In the liver great excitement may induce such high tension that during the continuance of this state the bile is not secreted at all, or cannot escape from the fibrous or contracted tubuli. Tension of the skin prevents an escape of perspiration and causes an accumulation of heat'.

Secretions
'In a similar manner a secretion long suppressed by over tension in the part may at last find sudden exit by the rigidity yielding - as when pent up bile is discharged rapidly following long continued contraction and perspiration or mucous secretion pours out by a similar variation in the condition of their respective secernants'.

'When observed in the Secretory organs this inclination to tension is often exhibited in an increase of function. More bile is secreted by the liver, more urine by the kidneys, more perspiration by the skin, more menstrual blood' - these occur in the early stages of disease with congestion and stasis following on *e.g. Connect a hose pipe to the water supply, turn on the tap. Then gently put your foot on the hosepipe. Initially the pressure of water will increase - contraction. As more pressure is applied to the hosepipe, the pressure of water slows down - greater contraction. Eventually the water will stop flowing; the water will be held back by the pressure on the hosepipe – obstruction causing congestion & eventual stasis.*

Contraction & Relaxation
'These are conditions that cannot be maintained indefinitely, for even the longest period of tension must come to an end to be followed by at least a fair degree of relaxation, according to the alternating laws of nature. Contraction being a vital act its extreme manifestation under the influence of provoking causes may continue so long as the suppressed function does not prove directly threatening to life. When it has continued to this point, endangered vitality can no longer maintain the contraction, even under a

Contraction and Relaxation of Tissue

persistent provocation. Hence, spastic contractions yield at the moment of imminent danger, as when spasms of the glottis give way just short of actual suffocation'.

The foregoing text has been quoted in full from Cook. This is necessary so that a full insight can be gained into the tissue states of contraction and relaxation.

With contraction or rigidity of the tissues, as you find in tetanus, muscle cramp and wakefulness, medicines will include those of a relaxing nature. If a relaxed condition is found such as diarrhoea, leucorrhoea or varicose veins, these would require a stimulating or stimulating tonic. In the case of menopausal night sweats, paralysis or irritability occur a tonic nervine is required.

Over contraction - **hypertonia** and over [excess] relaxation - **hypotonia**

Relaxation of the tissues
Tissue becomes relaxed as a secondary consequence of poor and inadequate nutrition. The basic tissue state reflects physiological disturbance and give rise to the symptom complex.

Cook says:
[a] 'While excessive contraction will often yield when its continuance begins to endanger life, extreme relaxation cannot similarly take such a rebound towards contraction'.
[b] 'Even moderate over-relaxation can be removed only by slow processes of repair and gradual increase of nervation. With extreme relaxation, progress is slow if possible at all. Extreme torpidity of the stomach or liver may recover only part of its tone only after years of patient care and application'.
[c] 'Long continued and very great tension may result in extreme laxity when the reaction ultimately occurs; thus feeble and ineffective uterine contractions may follow a spell of tonic spasm. Obstinate constipation may follow a period of diarrhoea'.
[d] 'Conditions of over-relaxation, following over contraction are far less serious than when a similar or less degree of laxity was the primary form of disease'.

'The further the tissues have receded in either direction from the normal, the greater the disease and the more distinct the agitation in the function of the affected part. The change in the direction of relaxation leaves the vital power with less control over the structures than a change in the opposite direction'.

Herbal Medicine - Keys

'Tension with functional excitement, exalted sensitivity, increased arterial action and accelerated secretions, is more favourable than relaxation with diminished functional capacity. It is easier to relax the tissues than to astringe [tone] them. Relaxed conditions create less functional activity within the tissues with reduced capacity to heal'.

Contraction [hypertonia] and relaxation [hypotonia] reflect the functional state existing at any one time within the tissues. Physiomedical principals accept the need to balance the tissues so that neither over contraction or over relaxation occurs. **McDonagh** describes the pulsating motion of the blood proteins. Over contraction or over relaxation of immunoglobulins [blood protein] will have effects upon cell nutrition as less able to utilise the amino acids. Blood Vasotonic alteratives are the medicines used.

The therapeutic formula has been advanced upon and now includes sedate as another therapeutic advantage to treatment.

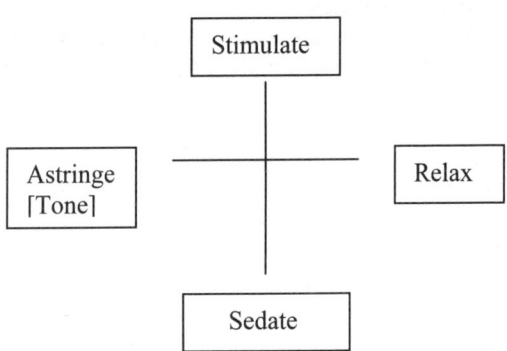

Evaluation of the case involves:

1] Secretory and excretory organ deficit of the eliminative organs. Every secreting organ in an abnormal condition presents some degree of obstruction to the circulation.

2] circulatory system balance

3] nervous system balance

4] endocrine level

Disease among the secretory organs involves some of the tissues comprising that organ or system suffering either tension or relaxation. Remedies are employed either as stimulants, e.g. *Zingiber* with tonics or relaxants as indicated.

Each organ is treated using medicines that support its natural function and activity

Contraction and Relaxation of Tissue

Medication is directed towards
a] secretions
b] excretions
c] local circulation
d] sensory nerves

The cell is regulated by the:
Blood and tissue fluid
Endocrine glands [hormones]
Nerve innervation

Function and trophic state of organs are dependent upon CNS and ANS functions. These nerve functions effect the vasomotor control of blood to the viscera. [See Chapter 7].

Tonicity and trophicity
Assess the patient in terms of their level of tonicity and level of trophicity. Tone is altered to the atonic form, from the over relaxed or over contracted state. Trophicity is either hypotrophic or hypertrophic. Either of the four states listed will depend upon the typology and effect the tone or trophic state locally or generally.

Summary
Careful reading and analysis of the above tissue conditions will enable you to assess the tissue state. Treatment will follow from the tissue condition diagnosed. It may be that the patient under your care has a number of different conditions at one and the same time. The kidneys may be relaxed, the duodenum over contracted, nervous system excitable, toxic encumbrance with catarrh as the focus. Always treat the eliminative organ secernants and balance the nervous system as excess nervous anxiety will deplete the patient and delay recovery. The requirement is often for a compound prescription - particularly in chronic cases.

9
Symptomatology

What this Chapter is about
Symptoms guide you to the cause of health problems. Take a careful case history and perform an examination. Check the iris of the eye for further analysis. All the systems and organ areas are easily seen in the iris. Further blood, urine and tissue analysis is available if required. Analyse the findings to make a diagnosis in terms of the physiological state.

Symptoms may indeed be the result of an extra effort by the vital force to rebalance the body. The symptoms that occur are always variable. Sometimes symptoms are excessive and at others hardly noticeable. Freedom from symptoms does not necessarily constitute health. Health is a variable and symptoms are a positive action by the vital force to some harmful [inimical] influence. Lack of symptoms could be interpreted as reduced vitality. In the absence of symptoms with a disease encroachment upon the cells and tissues such disease is dangerous because steps cannot be undertaken to heal, if vitality has not been aroused for a protective action. Symptoms are evidence of action to eliminate any pathological influence.

Disease occurs from some cellular disturbance. Once the cell function is disturbed the tissues produce symptoms. Symptoms guide you to indicate the sequence of the disease effects. Symptoms are not the disease. It is not the symptom that requires treatment but the cause of the symptom. Once the cause of the symptom is removed the symptom clears.
Symptoms fluctuate in accordance with the amount of vital force available and the cycle of a condition. Symptoms are produced by the Vital force and will reflect the level of vitality within the patient.

Posture [*decubitus*]
The patient during an exacerbation of illness frequently adopts certain postures.
- Restlessness occurs from fever, nervous debility.
- Lying recumbent [reclining] suggests lung or abdominal disorders.
- Knees drawn up suggest abdominal disorders – peritonitis, colic, gallstones, perforating ulcers, flatus.
- Lying on one side indicates lung, heart or liver disease.
- Prone position - pain, flatus, colic, gall stones.
- Sitting upright occurs in respiratory disease e.g. asthma, bronchitis, TB, pneumothorax, valvular heart disease.

Symptomatology

Symptom variability

Symptoms are rarely continuous in the course of a disease. Generally the vital efforts abate considerably after a time but not entirely until the disease condition has been resolved. Vital efforts return vigorously and subside when obstructions have been removed. Examples of obstructions are:

[1] invasive from infections
[2] congestive
[3] poor circulation
[4] enervation.

Fluctuations of symptoms are in accordance with physiological laws.

Three levels of vital energy are observed within the tissue:

Exacerbation: An exacerbation is a period of excited activity.
Intermission: Symptoms calm during an intermission [lull].
Remission [Abatement] - a remission can last months or years.

Changes take place once in 24 hours. The duration of an exacerbation may occupy nearly the whole of the 24 hours. This period of excited activity gets shorter as the system approaches health. The intermission becomes more distinct and prolonged as health returns.

Continuous symptoms with no tendency to abate indicate a continuous condition. Exacerbations and intermissions are feebly marked in chronic conditions [11].

Relapse

During convalescence even minor causes like overeating, undue excitement, emotional traumas, over exertion and insufficient rest could all create a relapse of the condition. Skin conditions, infections, rheumatic and inflammatory disease can all relapse. A relapsing fever is the result of accumulated toxins a common finding from pyrexia in the asthenic patient. Scarlet fever suffers no relapses however it can leave rheumatic or aortic valve disease. [See also typology].

Disease stages

In the clinical history as disease progresses there are changes marked by alterations in the symptoms and level of vital action. Where inflammation is present it has an incubation stage then an aggravation stage, common to all inflammatory action.

Disease commonly displays three stages.

* Invasion
* Reaction
* Termination

Herbal Medicine - Keys

Invasion is when the causes of disease gain their hold upon the tissues.

Reaction when the vital power springs into resistive action, arousing all the energies to overcome abnormal conditions present. At this stage occur the **exacerbations and remissions**. During the reaction such eliminative symptoms as effusions, exudations, eruptions and symptoms as are customary to the condition present.

Termination of the condition gives way to improvement, death a modified course of the disease or a secondary form of it. Modified disease is found if suppressive drug treatment has been used. Disease may become chronic with acute episodes occurring when the vital force gains sufficient energy for another reaction.

Chronic inflammatory action

Chronic inflammatory activity is common and found in arthritis, bronchitis, dermatitis, colitis, prostatitis, etc. Chronic symptoms suggest the need to allay an excess of inflammatory action within the tissue concerned. This is achieved by using medicines that stimulate the vital force to increased action and encourage elimination of toxins that cause irritation and inflammation in the tissues. However, the picture is more complex than just elimination of toxins whatever kind they are. Infections must be cleared and neutralised first before any deep tissue cleansing can be undertaken. It is not sufficient to merely stop an inflammatory response. Remove the encumbrances that give rise to inflammation then the symptoms will ease. The elderly patient with arthritis who moves about very little, eats a poor diet and is suffering from chronic anxiety may not have the vital reserve to get better. Medicine alone cannot be expected to cure the patient where other lifestyle measures are required to support the patient. Inflammatory and other chronic symptoms such as pain and discomfort need a number of supportive measures to improve health. Inherited weaknesses in an individual are genetic but can also acquired from bad living habits. Toxic accumulations from vaccines, suppression from drugs; preservatives, colourings, flavourings and sweeteners in foods, all provoke disease. A lot of improvement can be made in the patient's condition and level of symptoms if dietary changes are made. Fewer symptoms suggest a better control of the tissues by the vital force. Just removing salt from the diet can encourage the removal of fluid.

Summary

Symptoms reflect the vital force in action within the tissues. It is the aim of the medical herbalist to support the systems and cleanse the tissues of impurities. In most cases it will be found that impurities are at the root of the disturbance. Nerve irritability is often provoked because there is a toxic focus affecting the nerve.

Symptomatology

Don't be too quick to think it's all anxiety when nerve disturbance is found; it may be a toxic problem. Sciatica is caused by acidity of the blood, itself the result of chronic renal inactivity from a basis of anxiety and long standing nerve depletion from hypotrophicity. Structural disturbances and poor posture with ligamentous laxity may also play their part in the sciatica. Observe the patient. Typology enables you to form a clear, reasoned approach to the individual.

10
Diagnosis

What this Chapter is about
Diagnosis of the patient is based on each individual and not confined to a disease label. The more in-depth a case history, obtained, sometimes over a few visits, the more likely it is to find the root causes to the problem. Most cases of recurring illness are due to inherent [genetic] weakness. Acute conditions reflect the effort of the body trying to heal itself. Healing should be encouraged with herbal medicine and not suppressed with synthetic drugs.

Diagnostic concepts and principles
'The human organism possesses the highest possible degree of inherent immunity from disease causations [infectious and contagious] when its cells are kept free from toxins. Abstinence from stimulants and narcotics alone do not insure natural or physiological immunity from pathocausatives. One can so overwork the digestive apparatus, overwhelm the excretory organs and blockade the whole system with a surplus of putrefaction, even with wholesome food substances taken in unreasonable quantities and at unreasonable times as to render one's health an easy prey to contagion says Thurston.

How to diagnose the patient
Physiomedicalism provides a systematic diagnosis of the tissue state and level of physiological disturbance within the body. **Disease consists of a change in the structures of the body, due to an altered condition of the tissues. Symptoms are a reflection of physiological disturbance within the tissue [12].**

Symptoms occur when tissue becomes diseased and affects the vital force as it tries to heal and organise tissue recovery towards health.
The absence of acute symptoms is unlikely to give us a clear picture of health. Symptoms may not be clearly indicative of a disease state. Symptoms or lack of them are part of the picture of health or disease. Symptoms generally follow 1, 2 or 3 below and reflect the crises of Naturopathy.

[1] **Compensatory** and perhaps tolerant to the disease causation [hypertrophy].
[2] **Resolvent** towards a positive vital state in which the symptoms are produced by the vital force in action.
Clearing of the pathophysiology – pyrexia [a healing crisis].
[3] **Degenerative** as when the vital force is no longer able to clear the disease and heal the tissues [a disease crisis]. The symptoms are indicative of steadily encroaching disease upon a negative state of vitality [chronic catarrh].

96

Diagnosis

Diagnosis & assessment

Diagnosis is made not on a named disease entity but to a specific tissue condition assessed upon the features of the individual patient. Diagnosis demands that each person is seen as an individual, with their mental, emotional and physical aspects revealed in their true light.

Diagnosis can thus never be hypothetical but must be based upon a correct interpretation of the findings at that moment in time.

A full patient's history includes the following:

- Main complaint
- Past health
- Family health
- Mental/emotional aspect [ones thoughts and feelings]
- Drug treatments
- Review of all the body systems - at this moment in time.
- Identification of individuals typology
- Physical examination: a minimum of radial pulse, blood pressure, heart, abdominal and renal examinations.
- Urine test
- A diet diary of at least one week [not a pre-menstrual week as the diet can change on that week], with all foods, snacks and drinks taken.

Family health has relevance as the tendency to disease conditions, since these can be passed through the generations to become pathocausatives.

Wooster Beach arrived at a diagnosis of physiological function by observing - facies, tongue, pulse, examination of urine and faeces and an assessment of pain, temperature, thermotaxis, skin function and nerve sensibility.

Review the assessment plan for the patient:

1] Restore balance of function to the organs of elimination.

The tongue reflects conditions of the gastro intestinal tract. Moist coating on the tongue implies an open state of the secretions, dry - deficient secretions. Fissures suggest chronic disease. Colour of the coating - brown coat - infection and congested condition of the intestinal mucus layer, yellow or green a biliary disorder. [See also Chapter EENT - tongue].

2] Improve circulatory function - thermotaxis, peripheral circulatory function.

Thermotaxis: are there any parts of the body excessively hot or cold, this will determine if there is too much blood in one area or another. Extremes of heat and cold will be self-evident: pyrexia or hypothermia.

Vasomotor function - Pulse and blood pressure. Assess typology.

The pulse determines the extent of vital force/vitality in the body and the level of vital resistance within the tissues to further resist disease conditions. The radial pulse will easily show conditions of the blood vessel walls, whether tense or relaxed, obstructed through hardening, etc.

3] Balance nervous system

4] Organ weakness using trophorestoratives.

5] Deal with encumbrance [within the capacity of the organism to detoxify]. Toxic conditions past and present. Secretions, excretions, effusions - an indirect way to assess hydration.

6] Restore the blood to a healthful condition by clearing infection, removing acid wastes and controlling cholesterol impact within the arteries.

7] Balance the endocrine function.

Pathocausative influences of disease
Thurston describes the levels at which the cell is affected together with the causative phenomena – these are:
The pathocausative influences.
'All influences upon the cell or tissue that are inimical to cellular function'.
 • Causative phenomena.
'Cellular reaction within the tissues that may not be sufficient to occasion functional departures of the tissue or organs'.
 • Functional consequences.
'All abnormal functional actions of the organs or systems that are the consequence of pathocausative invasions and causative phenomena'.
 • Secondary results.
These are the secondary results from the above. The diseased tissue states and disturbed functions result from primary disease and the functional consequences.

A localised disturbance of the tissue may not produce a symptom. **Thurston** refers to the symptoms and functional aberrations:
'The primary causative conditions may advance no further than a circumscribed area within an organ and may not be sufficient to affect its function so that its work may go on practically uninterrupted'.

A persistent disease encroachment upon the tissues will eventually give rise to symptoms and is a pathocausative influence.

Diagnosis

When extra functional activity is required then a level of symptoms arises from the backlog of congested toxins. Toxins that have not cleared, often over a long period of time.

Pathocausatives will eventually effect cellular function. At the cell level, the vital force springs into action to eject the unwanted influence. If this is achieved no symptoms are observed. Once the adaptation mechanisms are overwhelmed then functional symptoms are produced. Causative phenomena affect the severity of symptoms. The more a cell or series of cells are disturbed, the greater the response required by the body. A cellular reaction ensues to rid the cell and tissue of a pathocausative influence. Where the unwanted influence remains and cell damage persists, pathology will ensue.

Organ weakness from any cause can delay recovery if the organ is weak from any cause. Organ weakness or incapacity from a recent illness induces further pathology. Treatment aims to heal the organs and remove the pathocausative influences.

Typology

Typology [somatotype] guides the herbalist towards the characteristics of the individual patient. Observe also the temperaments in your diagnosis [See Ch 6]. Kretchsmer says each person has certain characteristics built within their own body framework this will be explained.

Body typology determines whether the individual has a tendency or particular predisposition to illness. While there are variables within any typology the three basic types remain as a standard upon which to hang other references. Typology provides us with a grounding of physical evidence, which is a clear help in diagnosis. An understanding of typology will enable the herbalist to consider possible problems to which the patient might be predisposed to, even before they have been mentioned. It is such knowledge that constitutes the real background of interpretation of the later history and examination. Normal depends upon the normal level for that type and the presence of those same tendencies in a different type would be quite abnormal. There is no sharp dividing line between normal and abnormal typology. **The physiological becomes the functional-pathological and ultimately the organic-pathological.**

The makeup of the body, it's typology and how it responds in health and disease is significant in the prognosis. Certain physical tendencies towards disease are apparent with typology. Each body type has its own characteristics of physical disease and personality. For each of the three types there are differences in skeletal and visceral structure and from these differences flow certain typical predispositions. Typology indicates the mental, emotional and physical makeup of the types.

Thurston considered typology important in diagnosis and also to assess the prognosis and the quantitative level of medication. Thurston says 'humoral types give the constitutional reaction and include the relative proportion of this reaction'.

Constitutional reactions depend upon the following:
1] Vitality - the degree expressed and the amount available
2] Will - the quality of purpose and direction
3] Sensation - with particular influence upon subjective values
4] Thermotaxis – the level of combustion and metabolism
5] Hydration – water and electrolyte balance

The quality of the vital reaction is determined by the typology
[Priest]

It remains to show the various bodily types - they are named:

asthenic - ectomorph
athletic - mesomorph
pyknic - endomorph

Asthenic – ectomorph - cerebrotonia
Skin surface is derived from ectoderm. Asthenic types tend to have a large skin surface area compared to body mass. Asthenic types are deficient in their strength.

Skeletal - They have fragile body features and a prominent hyoid cartilage [Adams apple]. Asthenics have long thin bones, long limbs, weak muscular development and weak connective tissue. They are flat chested. Compensation occurs in skeletal muscle from hypoplasia of muscle cells.
The long, lean extremities produce a bowing effect due to that extension. The arms hyper-extend. There is ligamentous hypotonia and sacroiliac weakness which can create chronic backache. There is either a narrow pelvis with *genu varum* [bowlegs] or wide pelvis with *genu valgum* [knock knees]. Scoliosis and spondylosis can occur. There is a tendency to contraction of muscular tissue.

Cardio-pulmonary-renal-vascular [CPRV] – There is a reduced cross section of the thorax and low position of the ribs, which can lead to asthenic respiratory conditions: bronchitis, pneumonia, pleurisy, TB. Poor costal expansion and

Diagnosis

hypotonic diaphragm can lead to – hypotension, anaemia and peripheral circulatory insufficiency.

Gastro intestinal – A long narrow abdomen with weak supporting tissue within the gastrointestinal tract can lead to atony of the stomach. Visceral tone is often poor leading to intra abdominal visceroptosis. Transverse colon prolapse may become a feature. Tendency to duodenal ulceration. Bowel disorders from poor tone, shorter bowel and slow motility – irritable states e.g. irritable bowel syndrome, internal ulcerations. Other tendencies are gall bladder disease, dehydration, pelvic organ displacement, uterine retroversion.

Hyperglandular activity can lead to nervous and mental disorders.

The asthenic is the weakest of the three types and often shows excessive kinetic energy [they have difficulty relaxing].

Personality characteristics – On the behavioural level – cerebrotonia, sensitivity, sensory exposure to the outside world, inhibited and reserved, anxiety, nervous exhaustion and reactive depression. Autonomic instability. Hyper-irritability of the nervous system. Weakness and a tendency to passive delirium. Tendency to like privacy and seeks solitude in times of stress. Unpredictable attitudes and feelings. Attentive with rapid reactions. Sympatheticotonia - continuous adrenal activation produces the anxiety. Asthenics function under stress. Schizophrenia – extremely shy and introverted.

Re-educate the patient in their breathing habits. This will encourage circulatory improvement and help to decongest the liver, spleen and reduce spasm of the abdominal contents. Asthenics always need relaxing and *Humulus, Valeriana* or *Pulsatilla* are valuable nervines. The asthenic requires nervine relaxants with emphasis upon trophorestoration which is very difficult in the asthenic because they always live on their nerves. Relaxation of nerves supports the process of vasorelaxation and rehydration.
Calcium disturbance predominates with poor absorption and ability to use the calcium as needed. Calcium is required. Gentle tonic and bitter medicines are used for the ectomorph.

In the asthenic constitution: the trophic tendency is hypotonic and hypotrophic.
Cook says of the asthenic constitution 'support the nervous system and overall strength of febrile reaction, avoid over stimulating and rely more upon nervine tonics and trophorestoratives than upon stimulants'.
Astrologically affected by Saturn and Mars.

Athletic –mesomorph - somatotonia - sthenic

Muscle is derived from mesoderm.

Skeletal - coarse boned type. There is predominance of somatic structures of the body – bone, muscle and connective tissue. Athletic manifest as the strongest of the three groups, usually with heavy muscular development and consequent muscular strength. They can suffer from structural damage from a tendency to overstrain. There is a tendency to suffer from strains of joints and ligaments, fractures and hernia. Low back pain can occur from torn ligaments. Athletic types are also known as sthenic. There is a tendency to hyperpituitarism with disturbance of bone metabolism, arthritis, etc.

CPRV- athletic types push themselves to their limit. The over demanding lifestyle causes stress to the cardio vascular system leading to arteriosclerosis and nephritis. Cardiac function always needs supporting with: *Crataegus/Convallaria/Leonurus/Sarothamnus/Selenicerus.*

The three somatotypes

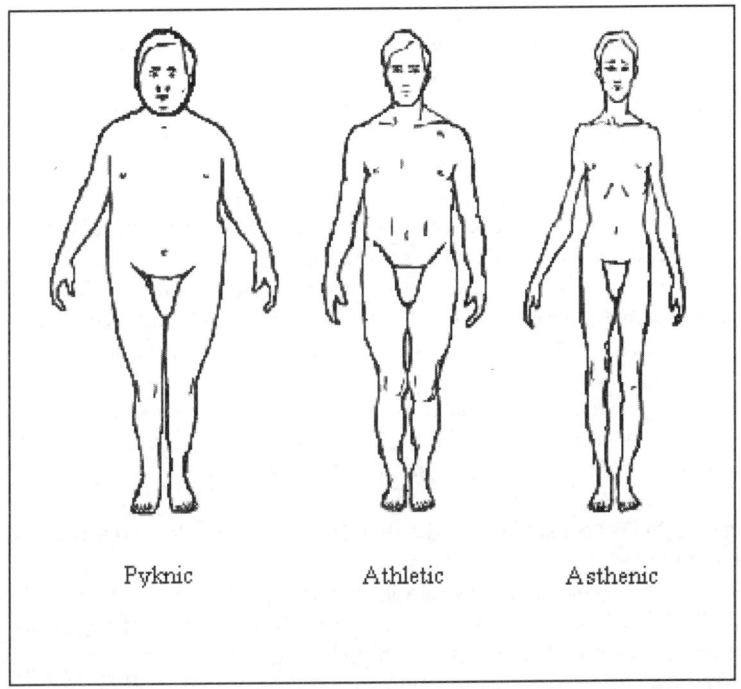

Pyknic   Athletic   Asthenic

Diagnosis

Personality characteristics – behavioural level is somatotonia with schizophrenic tendencies. Excitable with a tendency towards active delirium. Self assertive, direct, active and courageous. These are dominant types who like to take risks. They can be competitive and aggressive, which makes them insensitive, with lack of sympathy and tact. In times of stress they need action.
In the athletic constitution: the trophic tendency is hypertonic and hypertrophic.
Nervine remedies are chiefly relaxant.
Affected by Mars and Jupiter.

Pyknic – endomorph - viscerotonia - hypersthenic
Viscera are derived from endoderm and are well developed.
Pyknic types have large, soft, body cavities, short arms, fingers and neck. They tend to be fat with rounded body cavities and well-developed viscera.

Skeletal - medium boned types. Tendency to neuromuscular hypertension. lumbar lordosis, visceroptosis and spondylosis.

CPRV - emphysema and low tidal capacity. Circulatory disturbances include hypertension, vascular trouble, e.g. CVA, venous and lymphatic stasis; passive hyperaemia, varicosities, uterine fibroids.

Gastro intestinal - abdominal breathing. Abdominal ptosis, longer bowel, developing lumbar lordosis resulting in congested leg veins. Tendency to solar plexus tension. Tends to produce diaphragmatic rigidity, costal hyperelevation, affecting pancreatic function [diabetes]. It can produce congestive stasis of the liver and gall bladder with rheumatic tendencies from biliary retention. Rapid alimentary motility.

Glandular disorders of the hypothyroid type. Pyknic types with a gross accumulation of fat produce ptosis and lumbar lordosis.

Personality characteristics – behavioural level is viscerotonia an extrovert personality and a tendency to manic depression. Even tempered in the main and need others in times of stress.
They have greater autonomic stability as compared with the asthenic.
They tend to be relaxed, enjoy comfort and are sociable, jovial and tolerant. Love food and the companionship of other people. Parasympatheticotonia manifests as anger. *Chamomilla* is a preferred remedy.
Magnesium is required.

In the pyknic constitution: the trophic tendency is hypertonic and hypertrophic.

Cook says 'prevent congestion and encourage adequate perspiration'[75-79].

The pyknic constitution requires renal and thyroactive medicines.

Affected by the Moon and Jupiter.

Evaluation

In the evaluation of the individual patient, it is a prime necessity to establish which body type that you are dealing with. Normalisation of health can only be possible in as much as it brings the patient back to what is considered 'normal' for that type of constitution. Every person is subject to his or her own typology and it is a determining factor in any prognosis.

How long will it take to get better?
Acute and chronic cases

It is usually possible to achieve faster results in acute cases [a healing crisis], when there is an abundance of vital force for healing at this time. Treatment can include fasting or mono diets.

It takes longer in chronic cases when we encounter a disease crisis, often because there is a deficiency of vital force to utilise in the healing process. A minimum of a wholefood diet is required in treatment for chronic cases organic foods are best. Medicine will be required for months or years depending upon the syndrome being treated.

Curing a patient

Improving the patient's constitution will enhance their physical health. It may not be possible to cure the patient, always remembering that the cure is dependent upon the typology and level of trophic weakness together with encumbrance of the tissue.

Children usually heal more quickly than adults in the main. This is mainly because children do not carry as much emotional trauma as adults. In some ways we are slaves to our emotional desires. Negative emotions deplete vitality. Providing we can produce for the patient an increase in vitality together with an improvement in their quality of life – we have a cure [See Prognosis].

What to do when symptoms get worse?

Check the following.
- Is the patient taking the medication as prescribed?
- Has the prescription been changed? Is it too strong, too stimulating? Encourage the vital force don't force it to perform.
- Is any other medication being taken?

Diagnosis

- Have any synthetic drugs been abruptly changed or stopped?
- Has the diet changed?
- Has there been a fast?
- Is there a healing crisis or disease crisis?
- Check biorhythms and stress levels.
- Only if necessary reduce or change the prescription.

How long to continue with the prescription?

Once all the symptoms are settled, it may be possible to reduce the level of medication to once or twice daily but only if you are sure the tissue being treated has gained sufficient strength to warrant the reduction in medication level.

Summary of treatment aims.

Medicinal substances must produce increased integrity within the human body to restore balance and eliminate obstructive conditions. Pathocausatives including synthetic drugs decrease vital integrity by suppressing and obstructing vital action.

Medicines are given to support the elimination of toxins, renew cellular action and stimulate the vital force to heal.

11
Trophorestoration

What this chapter is about.
The vital life force guides, repairs and heals the organism. The life processes are constant and allow cell renewal to take place - life is a constant renewal of cells. The trophic level of tissue nutrition is determined by a large extent upon the patient's typology. Improvement or decline results from the ability to respond to disease provocation. Typology shows the weak areas that could become disordered when disease presents. The tendency to disease is thus reflected by the typology. Treatment aims to restore organ balance and is required before any deep tissue cleansing takes place. Thurston furthered Cook's work by introducing the normalisation of organismic balance by means of vasomotor regulation. Thurston maintained each organ has a vasomotor area. He classified the tissue changes in terms of various aberrations.

Tissue types

Tonicity - over contracted states [hypertonic]
            - over relaxed/flaccid states [hypotonic]

Hypertonic -
[hypertrophic] - pyknic types - vaso constriction, spasm, sclerosis, overhydration, reduced secretory activity, fatty infiltration.

Hypotonic -
[hypotrophic] - asthenic types - vasorelaxation, atony, dehydration, stasis.

Trophicity - atony [Hypotrophic] - dehydration and sclerosis [asthenic response]

            - hypertrophy [spasm] - over hydration [anasarca] & fatty infiltration
                                                        [pyknic response]

[Priest 1985]

The sympathetic nervous system affects the hormones as regulators of the systems e.g. adaptation syndromes.
Sympathetic adrenal syndromes [sympatheticotonia] affect vasomotor function this in turn determines the organ function and organ trophicity

Trophorestoration

Muscular structures - over contracted states exhibit in the following as:

- Heart - spasm [angina, MI, eventual infarction]
- Intestines - colic/constipation
- Bladder - strangury
- Stomach - achlorhydria from over contraction of the muscle layer
- Blood vessels - hypertension
- Ureters - colic, spasm
- Urethra - colic and obstruction
- Oesophagus - stricture
- Bronchi - asthma
- Secretory organs - contraction
- Liver - more bile [initially only]
- Kidneys - more urine [initially only]
- Skin - more perspiration [initially only]

Muscle – over relaxed/atonic muscle induces:

- Intestines - atonic constipation
- Bladder - incontinence, if the sphincter is involved inability to void fully

Organ insufficiencies/deficiencies/trophorestoration
Trophicity

An insufficiency of nutrients creates tissue disorders, the vital force being unable to keep the tone of the tissue in a healthy condition. The trophic centre, a part of the CNS, controls trophicity. The trophic influence of the bodily organs, systems and central nervous system is effected through the vasomotor function. The trophic influence refers to the local nutrition of each cell within the body. Conditions that create malnutrition will starve the part and degeneration is the result: the cause is always due to obstruction to the vasomotor function. The obstruction can be a local or generalised problem. Kollath explains trophicity, as does Thurston when mention is made of trophic conditions. Hypotrophicity means a general reduction in vasomotor functional activities. The autonomic nervous system is necessary to the nutrition, growth and maintenance. Bodily tendencies towards disease can be found in organ weakness known as trophic weakness.

Trophic disturbance occurs from:
[1] genetic weakness of the individual
[2] inadequate circulation of blood with corresponding nutritional disturbance to the tissues
[3] damage from acute disorders, e.g. serious infections
[4] poor nutritional status can produce trophic weakness and prevent full recovery

Trophic weakness indicates poor tone of the parenchyma, laxity and loss of tone within the tissues.

Trophic weakness is caused by a hypotrophic disturbance, which affects:
[1] nutrition
[2] cell nourishment and
[3] cellular drainage.

Over relaxed or over contracted states reflect the functional condition of the organ tissue.

The level of trophic function of an organ limits functional adjustment of that organ. Functional action is variable in all organs, at times more active than others depending upon the amount of over relaxation or over contraction of the tissue. The tone of the tissues will affect the functional action of that tissue. Whether the tone is one of atony or loss of tone or increased tone, its total trophic state is compromised. Limitation of function depletes the trophic state leading to hypotrophia.

Hypertrophic

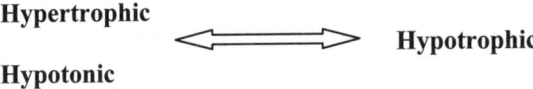 **Hypotrophic**

Hypotonic

Hypotrophia can occur from **hypotonic** or **hypertonic** states of the tissue.

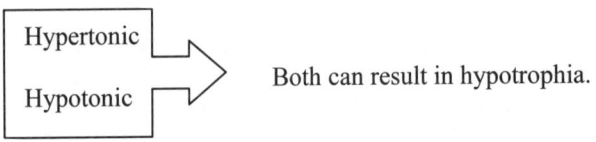 Both can result in hypotrophia.

Hypertonic
Hypertonic conditions are contracted or spasmodic conditions.
Hypertonic effects are due to inadequate tissue nutrition from prolonged vasocontraction [vasoconstriction].

Priest argues that hypotrophia can be arrived at by way of hypertonia and hypotonia.

Hypotonic
Hypotonic [atonic] conditions are relaxed or flaccid conditions.

Trophorestoration

Hypotonic effects occur from prolonged vasorelaxation. Vasorelaxation causes inadequate removal of fluid from the tissues, extra fluid encourages the circulation to slow with eventual stasis of the body fluids typically found in the hypotrophic and hypotonic state.

Hypertrophy can be a compensatory mechanism as in the heart in athletes. Hypertrophia of the muscles in an asthenic is due to compensation for a hypotrophic CNS or hypotrophic connective tissue. Remedies to treat the hypotrophic state are called trophorestoratives they invigorate the tissue.

<u>Representation of trophic volume within an organ.</u>

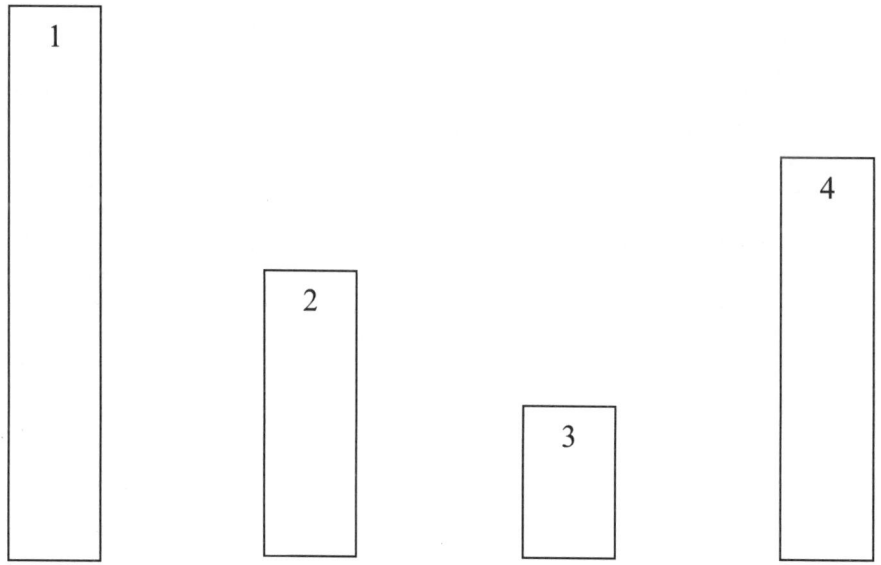

One - shows the ideal level of trophicity for any organ. This is the best possible level of trophic response.

Two - shows the amount of response available when the organ has a reduced trophic level, this is a variable.

Three - indicates organ utilisation used on a day to day basis.

Four - as demands increase [any illness] on the organ, more activity is required for the organ to function effectively. Problems emerge when the organ capacity is only at 2 and the demands outstrip the response this pushes the organ into failure.

Blood vessel anomalies

Hypertrophy is the result of **active or passive hyperaemia** – inflammation or congestion.

Active hyperaemia results from an over stimulated arterial function. Passive hyperaemia from over relaxed capillary/venous function.

Acute disease is often the result of a local active hyperaemia, it occurs from inflammation.

Chronic conditions of the abdominal organs are associated with arterial excitement and venous obstructions. An effusion of tissue fluid into the tissues causes fluid build up from poor venous return. Reduced capillary function encourages reduced organ action – the area is usually cold and pale. [See also Chapter 14 on hypertrophy].

Summary

Cellular health depends upon an adequate level of nutrients. The tissue supports the ability of the cell to absorb the nutrients. Capillary blood and activity carry those nutrients. The amount of blood in the vessel is dependent upon the local capillary action. Nerve action upon the larger arterioles and arteries is affected by general nerve activity [innervation]. Nerve irritability may be detrimental to cellular activity. Trophic response in a cell, tissue or organ reflects all the activity spoken about so far together with the typology and predispositions of the individual. Careful assessment of trophic state is of paramount importance in organ restoration. Trophic condition assessment is not always used with other types of empirical herbalism, opportunities for much more effective treatment could thus be lost. Trophorestoration builds up the organ tissue that supports all other organs in turn.

12
Prognosis

What this Chapter is about
Prognosis means the probable cause and outcome [the effect] of a disease [Blakistons medical dictionary]. Herbalists are frequently asked by patients, 'How long will it take to get better?' This question can only be answered if a thorough analysis is made of the symptoms and history together with an examination of the patient. The symptoms presented by the patient are an expression of the vital force in action within the tissues of the body. The vital force expresses itself in conditions of health and disease through functional effects. Functional effect refers to the level of activity in the cell, tissue and organ. Disease conditions pervert the functions of the vital force within the tissues. Function becomes disturbed in various ways depending upon the tissue affected and the causative factors.

Prognosis is viewed in the light of Physiomedicalism.
This approach focuses on three main factors these are:

1] The main focus of any disease causation is a lack of vital force at the cellular level.
2] An holistic approach is required. Without an holistic approach one falls into empirical diagnosis and symptomatic treatment.
3] Typology is a systematic way of assessing bodily physique and gives indications toward certain types of condition which the patient could be predisposed.
To explain these a little deeper

1] Vital force in prognosis
The Vital force is a term often used in medicine to explain the level of cellular activity. The life force is always seeking to create its best advantage in healing disease conditions.

The Vital force is eliminative, restorative and reconstructive
Thurston 1900

The vital force is a directive energy within the cell. Cellular vital force is always healing and supporting to the cell and tissues. For adequate cellular health every cell must have a supply of nutrients and eliminate its waste in order to remain healthy. Imperfect elimination of cellular waste creates an encumbrance within the cell. Encumbrances are inadequately eliminated wastes and toxins. Cellular impurities are then likely to find their way into the blood. Detrimental

111

consequences follow the build up of impurities e.g. infections. Infection gains a hold within a cell or tissue under such an encumbrance.

When the tissues are in a healthy state and eliminating adequately, waste toxins and blood impurities are detoxified by the liver and eliminated by the skin, bowel and kidneys - these eliminative organs are called secernants.

In order to evaluate the effects of disease encroachment it is necessary to **assess the level of vital force** within the tissue.

[a] Assessment is made of the pulse and blood pressure which are indicators of vital energy within the tissue. A flaccid radial pulse suggests relaxed tissue; this can produce a low blood pressure and may be indicative of hypoglycaemia or an asthenic state.

[b] The tongue will show the quality of the secretions and excretions of the eliminative secernants [See EENT].

[c] Skeletal structure gives evidence of the typology of the patient, known as one's somatotype].

Dr William Cook says:

Feeble, irregular symptoms or symptom cessation are unfavourable because they indicate a diminished vital response.

> [Science & Practice of medicine. Cook 1879]

Strong vital symptoms are always a good thing for the patient. However symptoms have often been suppressed before we see the patient. When symptoms have been suppressed are feeble or irregular, stimulate vital action. The suppression of the disease must stop in order for the health to return.

Cook further says:

Vital efforts in resistance to disease produce aberrations of function under abnormal conditions of the structures [tissues]. [Cook. p46]

2] Holistic approach in prognosis

'And while this [empirical approach] **may occasionally be successful it can assign no relation between cause and effect and can inspire no confidence as to future results'** [Cook]

An empirical approach to medicine and the treatment of the individual at best may occasionally give temporary relief of the symptoms. Fixed herbal prescriptions are useless for accurate treatment of the patient. Each patient must be assessed individually.

Prognosis

3] Typology – somatotypes.

Typology pertains to the framework of the body, that is, bodily physique.
There are three main bodily types and these are explained in Chapter 10.

Prognosis

Prognosis will determine the cause and effects of a disease. Two things are
required to produce disease conditions.

Firstly, the predisposition of the body and secondly the application of the exciting cause

[Cook p128]

Once disease is established in the tissue, the function of that tissue will change
according to the nature of the predisposing or exciting cause.

Exciting aetiology

Infection, inflammation, congestion, trauma or thermal effects are examples of
exciting aetiology of disease. In some cases, a thermal effect, from a chill could
be enough to induce hypothermia in an elderly patient. It is the predisposition of
the body that is generally more important than the exciting cause. Unless the body
is overwhelmed by an exciting cause of acute disease e.g. chill, meningitis,
pneumonia, etc.

Predisposing aetiology

Predisposing causes towards bodily malfunction occur from a genetic or familial
tendency. **Constitutional disease** includes one's inheritance, the trophic level of
the cells and organs and the effects of environmental factors e.g. diet, living
habits. Constitutional factors include genetic disease e.g. breast carcinoma,
prostate carcinoma, familial disease, e.g. diabetes.

Iridologists agree that disease tendencies have a genetic background and these
can be observed in the iris of the eye [80-82].

Where there is a trophic weakness treatment aims are:
1] Improve circulation to the end tissue/organ.
2] Tonics/astringents to the parenchyma.
3] Hydrotherapy and nutritional support.

Factors to be assessed in prognosis:
1] the vitality level - dependent upon the patient's individual personality
   [e.g. levels of anxiety/depression, and there is a psychoimmunological effect].
2] vital force and how its influences are felt through the tissues. Check the
   a] pulse - rate, rhythm and tone as indicators of vital energy
   b] tongue – it's shape, coating, movement

3] typology – bodily shape

4] past health as it <u>can affect one's future health</u>:

Rheumatic fever, scarlet fever, tuberculosis, pneumonia, diabetes, whooping cough, operations, cancer, glandular fever, aphthous ulcers, chronic inflammatory conditions, meningitis – these can all affect future health

5] vaccinations can be detrimental to health - see pathology

6] the amount of encumbrance within the tissues

7] indications from iris analysis [iridology] will indicate trophic weaknesses, encumbrance, nerve weakness among other things

8] genetic makeup of the organs, where a disease state may present as a trophic weakness.

9] environmental toxins, e.g. from:

pesticides/antibiotics/colourings/flavourings/preservatives/artificial sweeteners/GM foods [genetically modified/engineered]

10] nutritional and dietary factors

The patient may eat sufficient food yet still be undernourished and deficient in adequate nutrition to tissue cells.

* At this juncture it is plausible to question whether herbal medicines can affect the genetic makeup of cells in any way. Some examples found in the pharmacopoeia are: Astragalus membranaceus – inhibits cell RNA metabolism and prolongs the life span of some human lung diploid cell strains. Boswellia serrata inhibits the synthesis of DNA, RNA and protein in human leukaemia cells. Inhibits topoisomerase 1 and 2 enzyme by interacting with binding sites on the DNA molecule.

Law of cure

Healing occurs in the following sequence.

- **From the head downward**
- **In the reverse order from which disease arrived in the first place**
- **From within outwards - most important organs are healed first**

From the above we see how healing takes place. Healing is under control of the vital force. Healing starts at the head. When the patient says 'I feel well, I feel better' this is proof that healing is progressing satisfactorily, the prescription is continued in these cases. The prescription may be changed if the patient is moving towards a healing crisis. Disease conditions present the longest will be the last to clear. More recently acquired conditions clear first. Important organs are healed in turn by the vital force.

Prognosis

Crisis
There are two types of crisis. One crisis tends towards healing and the other crisis towards disease. Some symptoms are similar, however they are operating under different circumstances [see Chapter 16].

Getting the patient better
The herbalist needs to know three things to get the patient better.
1] how long it will take a patient to get better, whether this is months or years.
2] approximately how long it will take to start the healing process. There should be some improvement in the patient's condition within four weeks.
3] whether it is at all possible to get the patient cured, depending upon the individual typology [trophic response, blood condition/cleansing - 3 years].

A conversation with Wilfred Morley FNIMH some years ago produced the following 'What happens when the patient comes off the medicine I asked?'
Morley laughed and said, 'you never take the patient off the medicine.' What he meant by this was that patients with chronic conditions would be required to continue with the prescription in order to remove encumbrance and build up the trophic level of tissue integrity. Continued herbal therapy must also try to offset various other influences from disease aetiology whether they are of a constitutional or typological nature.

Five factors are considered in the prognosis and depend upon patient compliance to effect a return to health.

1] the herbal medicine must be correctly prescribed for the syndrome being treated
2] patient psychological state of mind - clearing of those negative emotions involved in the disease process. For instance: backache from feeling unsupported. Sleeplessness from worry. Hay's book gives detailed information on the causes and effects of mento-emotional disease [83]. Habit of a negative pattern is a barrier to healing.
3] a nourishing wholefood and organic diet where this is possible
4] lifestyle changes if required, such as posture alignment, physical exercise, breathing exercises, counselling.
5] reduction of any environmental pollutant where this is a factor in the disease condition

An accurate prescription for the patient is based upon treating the primary disease state and not the symptoms. Make sure the patient takes all their medicine at the prescribed times.

Curing a patient [See Chapter 10].

Conclusions
Reduction in the level of vital force available for healing encourages the diseased condition to persist. Presented to us in the patient is a collection of symptoms that should be interpreted against the background of typology.
Herbal medicine will rebalance the cellular vital energy and attempt to bring about a restoration of normal function. Always understanding that medicine is subject to the trophic weaknesses in the tissues. Trophic weakness may not allow full recovery.

Summary
Using physiomedical prognosis we are able to accurately assess and treat an individual using herbal medicine and diet together with lifestyle changes where appropriate.

As herbalists we are always trying to bring about
an improvement in the patients quality of life.

13
How herbal medicines work

What this Chapter is about
Medicines have active constituents that bring about physiological changes within the tissues. Herbal medicine has one object says Cook:

to restore the disordered body to a state of health

Medication will be effective only if it co-operates with the vital force against disease conditions - it is the vital force that heals. We must therefore render assistance to the vital force. 'A drug in itself affects nothing by its mere chemical influence, it is the vital power which the drug calls forth that is the true healer' [11]. True medicine acts in harmony with the vital force.

Dr. Elizabeth Williamson of the London School of Pharmacy argues:
'that in view of the prevalence of synergistic activity within a herb the search for isolated plant constituents might be pointless' [330].

Remedial impressions are made upon the tissues
When the tissue disorder has been healed the vital force will regain more control over those tissues. In disease states the tissues are sluggish in their functional activity. Sluggish function results from imperfect vital effort.
Functional activity and bodily symptoms in health or disease are constantly changing. The changes are always towards health; the vital force will always attempt to heal the tissues. Remedial action with herbal medicine must aim to improve the function of the tissue structure.

Lyle says of the action of remedies; '**to find out how the herbs work observe the remedy in action by itself**'. Observe the vital force to see if there is a favourable or unfavourable response to the medicine. Herbal medicines act specifically to effect the tissue structures and the function of that tissue.

The **length of remedy activity** is often short and therefore the stimulus to vitality has to be **repeated frequently**. Herbal medicines will act together in a compound prescription. Their action is synergistic and each enhances the therapeutic efficacy of the others without any inhibition of their own isolated activity. It is often a necessity to cleanse and detoxify the blood and tissues when an alterative is used, more correctly known as a **Vasotonic alterative** these are immune system scouts and work as cellular detoxifiers.
Alteratives improve the cleanliness and quality of the blood. Reabsorb the inflammatory products of disease. Modify disordered processes of nutrition

together with the elimination of toxins. Alteratives will mobilise stored toxins within the tissues. A funnel effect is found when using alteratives therefore detoxing and cleansing of the blood and tissues should be carefully undertaken. They are used in combination with renal, hepatic or intestinal remedies.

Physiomedical treatment is applied to encourage the vital force to remove the original damaging influence and provide a healing influence to the tissues. Where a reactive effort by the body has occurred as a result of disease processes, it must be remembered that the organ systems only have power to heal within their capacity and require support.

Synthetic Drugs

Orthodox medicine uses drugs to control bodily actions and symptoms. It has been said that the drug replaces the disease it is meant to cure with another disease. Perhaps a more manageable disease for the patient to live with. This is not an encouraging prospect for the patient. Herbal medicines work with the vital force to heal an unbalanced condition and help to return the tissues towards health.

Herbal and drug interactions will always need to be checked during the history taking because many patients are taking synthetic drugs when they come for treatment. Some synthetic drugs can be stopped immediately. While others e.g.. Steroids must be reduced slowly if they have been taken over a long period of time. Always ensure the patient has herbal medication cover before reducing their drugs. In the case of cardiac drugs, anticoagulants and steroids, extra care is necessary when withdrawing the drugs. It must be remembered that some drugs are keeping the patient alive and cannot be stopped - Thyroxine is one example. While the writer prefers herbal medication to synthetic drugs the above information must be taken into consideration when treating patients. Some patients are so delicate and in a poor state of health that without their synthetic drugs they would deteriorate.

Combining herbal medicines

Medicines will influence an organ and tissue: Lobelia will effect muscle and nerve tissue, Asclepias affects the mucous and serous membranes, Hydrastis influences the skin and mucous membranes, Capsicum lends influence wherever required. Some medicines will expend their influence on two or more organs. With proper combining of the remedy an effect can be produced to make the remedy affect either organ or tissue.

Althea heals mucous membranes in the lungs, stomach, bladder and bowels. The principal remedy would be added to carry the remedies and influence the organ required, e.g. use Barosma with Althea for renal problems. Use Inula with Althea for the lungs, etc.

How Herbal Medicines work

As the tissues become more healthy, changes to or less medication are required by the vital force. Healthy tissues respond with greater vigour to remedy application. Those medicines of a more gentle nature will then be used to treat the patient while keeping the more powerful remedies for other cases.

At the start of treatment use small doses of medicines. Watch the vital force in action within the tissues, through the symptoms and signs. Medicines of a weaker variety are preferable to the more potent in the early stages of treatment in chronic disease, e.g. Cassia [senna] is preferable to Aloes in sensitive cases.

Herbal constituents

The pharmacopoeia describes the active constituents of each medicine, with explanations of how the drug component works upon a certain set of tissues.

We are not merely concerned with the active constituents as Dr Gilani, Pakistan University medical college says:

A pure compound is not always a true representative of the plant

Kerry Bone says: Phytopharmacology - more research should be undertaken on herbs as whole herbs, not just to find the active constituent. Science is an imperfect tool that relies a great deal on in vitro and animal experiments. Digestive and other processes lead to the change of plant constituents to different effects within the human body

Active compounds in plants

Acetylcholine

Acetylcholine is:

Inhibitory to the CVS - decrease's heart rate, dilates the blood vessels. Excites and stimulates other organs - respiratory airways, GIT, bladder, uterus.

Laxative plants contain acetylcholine.

Acids

Organic acids are derived from aldehydes when these are combined with oxygen. Acids are nutritive as they contain sugars, mineral salts and vitamins. Diuretic, laxative and sialogogue. Salicylic acid allays inflammation and is anti rheumatic Medicines e.g. Filipendula, Salix alba.

Alkaloids

Synthesized from amino acids. They influence the CNS receptor pathways.

Raise or lower the blood pressure via the CNS, Affect respiration and circulation as either excitants or depressants, Stimulate the ANS – Analgesic, Anaesthetic, Antispasmodic, Mydriatic.

Alkaloidal activity - HIV inhibitor alkaloids, benzophenanthridine alkaloids - fagaronine chloride, nitidine chloride, columbamine iodide and protoberberine alkaloids, the isoquinoline alkaloid 0-methylpsychotrine sulphate and the iridoid fulvoplumierin [J of nat prod. 1991 54 [1] 143-54].

Alkaloid medicines e.g. Atropa [atropine], Berberis vulgaris, Cola [caffeine], Chelidonium, Colchicum [colchicine], Cinchona quinine, Fumaria, Galega, Leonurus, Opium [morphine], Scoparium, Rauwolfia, Symphytum, Strychnos nux vomica, Viscum.

Anthracenosides

These are aperients/laxatives/purgatives. Purgatives are potent remedies e.g. Aloe, Cassia [senna], Rhamnus purshiana, Rheum.

Antimicrobials

Under this heading are grouped anti infectives:

antiviral [virucidal], antibacterial [bacteriocide], antifungal [fungicide].

Medicines

Allium Inhibits bacteria, fungi, virus, and parasites. Indicated for infections cholera, dysentery and typhoid.

Aloe succus is Antimicrobial.

Arctium is a blood detoxifier. It has been shown to inhibit staphylococcus. Polyacetelines are antibacterial and active against bacterial and fungal infections.

Baptisia

Cetraria

Chamomilla - Volatile oil contains chamazulene, bisabolol and umbelliferone. Bactericidal effects upon staphylococcus, salmonella. Antimicrobial, fungicidal.

Cinnamomum - Essential oil is antibacterial and antifungal. Inhibits staphylococcus, E-coli, typhoid bacillus.

Echinacea

Eucalyptus

Eucalyptus - Antiseptic action via the volatile oils.

Honey - raw, unrefined and organic honey is antiseptic.

Hydrastis - Alkaloid action of berberine is active against diarrhoeal infections.

Causative organisms inhibited are E-coli, guardia, klebsella, paratyphoid, shigella, salmonella, vibrio cholerae [34].

Myrica - Flavonoid: myricitin is bactericidal.

Piper cubebs - Antibacterial and antiviral.

Potentilla - Anti typhoid remedy having clear antimicrobial action.

Quercus - Antimicrobial.

Szygium [cloves] - The volatile oil from which is found eugenol is a powerful antiseptic against bacteria, fungi and viruses.

Bitter compounds

Bitters stimulate glandular activity and secretions. A bitter taken before a meal is a strong aperitif. Bitters are tonic to the stomach and gastro intestinal system, they aid appetite and digestion. Bitters stimulate bile flow and pancreatic secretion. Some are diuretic.

How Herbal Medicines work

Medicines e.g. Artemisia species, Carduus, Erythrea, Gentiana, Humulus, Lactuca, Menyanthes, Peumus, Taraxacum.

Coumarins

Coumarins smell of vanilla. They are antibacterial and anticoagulant.
Medicines e.g. Amni visnaga, Asperula odorata, Avena, Galium, Melilotus, Parsnip.

Essential [volatile] oils

Essential oils are aromatic, volatile compounds. Several actions are attributed to these compounds they are:
antiparasitic, antiseptic, carminative, facilitate digestion, diuretic, emmenagogue, expectorant, intestinal disinfectants, stomachic, spasmolytic
Medicines e.g. Cinnamomum, Juniperus, Lavandula, Mentha species, Melissa, Thymus, Zingiber plus dozens of others.

Flavonoid glycosides

Glycosides selectively affect one organ or another. Glycosides when hydrolysed separate into two parts. One is a sugar [glucose or fructose] and the other the aglycone component. Each aglycone combines with an enzyme to create an active affect on to the target organ. Aglycones are non sugar components. Aglycone structures are anthraquinones, phenols, tannins and triterpenoids. Glycosides are poorly absorbed from the ileum.

Allay inflammation, antiviral – herpes simplex, influenza, polio, antiallergic, antineoplastic – skin cancer, hepatoma, ovarian cancer [230 p159], inhibit mitosis, cell surface receptor blocker against cancer cells, collagen supportive by strengthening capillaries to aid the inhibition of cancer cells, TGF is transforming growth factor and is a cytokene, inhibits hyluronidase enzyme, inhibit toxic damage to cells, diuretic, spasmolytic, remove excess copper from the tissues, flavonoids and vitamin C have synergistic activity, strengthens fragile capillaries, hepatoprotective, bind type two oestrogen binding sites, analgesic, anticholesterolaemic, venous tonic.

Flavonoid groups also called bioflavonoids [vitamin P] – Flavones and Flavonols – quercetin. Flavonoids are yellow pigments found in plants. Quercetin is antioxidant and allays inflammation. Conditions benefiting from quercetin are arthritis, asthma, cataract, dermatitis, diabetes, dysentery, gout, heart disease, psoriasis and urticaria. Dosage around 600mg daily, catechins [green tea], proanthocyanidin oligomers, Anthocyanins and anthochlors.

Isoflavonoids – genistein [Soya, Trifolium are plant molecules that possess oestrogenic activity. Isoflavones modulate the sex hormones. Around 60g of soy a day is helpful to balance the hormones. An endocrine modulating effect is found at the level of the hypothalamic, pituitary, gonadal axis. Increases time between menses. May also help in the reduction in prostate disorders.

Herbal Medicine - Keys

Sources - chickpeas, lentils, soya,

Medicines Capsella, Citrus, Crataegus, Convallaria, Euphorbia, Equisetum, Fagopyrum, Helianthus, Medicago, Ruta, Sambucus, Trifolium, Tussilago, Viola tricolor.

Limonine

Limonene effective in pancreatic and colorectal cancer. Limonene is found in the essential oils of citrus fruits, lemongrass, and other herbs.

Mucilage - glucide

Mucilage is produced by plants during metabolism and then stored. Mucilage calms peristalsis and is antidiarrhoeal. Large doses cause food to swell and thus aid its elimination from the intestine – laxative action. Mucilage acts by reflex from the gut. Mucilage is protective, reduces irritation and allows healing over raw surfaces. It is useful in ulcers both internal and external. Polysaccharides in these demulcent medicines are antiseptic. Mucilage is vulnerary and haemostatic.

Medicines e.g. Agropyron, Althea, Borago, Ispagula, Plantago, Symphytum, Tussilago, Ulmus.

Ispaghula causes relaxation of the intestine at high doses. The relaxant activity dominates in the plant.

Oestrogenic compounds

Interact at oestrogen binding sites. Lignans and isoflavones are sub groups of oestrogenic precursors.

Medicines e.g. Arctium, Linum, Podophyllum, Silybum, Soya, Schizandra and Trifolium.

Phenols

Phenolic acid esters are simple phenols. Salicylic acid, gallic acid, caffeic acid and rosmarinic acid are examples.

Activity - febrifuge, sudorific, affects thermo regulatory centres and peripheral blood vessels. Are antibacterial and antifungal. Tumour inhibitors.

Medicines e.g.

Calluna, Filipendula, Rhamnus purshiana, Salix alba, Uva ursi, Vaccinum.

Polysaccharides

Polysaccharides are simple sugars. They have immunostimulating properties.

Medicines e.g. Astragalus, Coriolus versicolor, Eleutherococcus, Ganoderma, Lentinus edoides, Panax, Poria cocos.

Resins

Resins are antiseptic and soluble in alcohol.

Medicines e.g. Commiphora, Guaiacum, Zingiber.

Saponosides - saponins

Sapogenin from plants contain glycosidal saponins. Saponins increase the bioavailability of non-water soluble plant compounds.

Saponins are Antispasmodic, Antiphlogistic, Expectorant, Diuretic [weak], Antineoplastic - inhibit metastasis, Anticholesterolaemic – inhibit cholesterol absorption, Adaptogenic, Allay inflammation, Alderosterone effects that increase the amount of available and circulating hydrocortisone to the tissues.

Steroidal saponins

Medicines e.g. Caulophyllum [caulosapogenin], Chamaelirium, Dioscorea [diosgenin], Saponaria officinalis, Scrophularia, Smilax, Trigonella [diosgenin], Tribulus terrestris, Trillium [trillarin].

Triterpenoid saponins

Medicines e.g. Aesculus, Angelica sinensis, Astragalus membranaceus, Glycyrrhiza [glycyrrhetinic acid], Panax, Paeonia lactiflora, Rehmania glutinosa, Schizandra chinensis.

Tannins are water-soluble polyphenols and sugars. Tannins can associate with proteins to form polymers. Only small amounts of tannin are absorbed from the gut. Two main groups exist condensed tannins and hydrolysable tannins. Tannins bind with protein. They are all antiseptic and anti fungal. Tannins are anti neoplastic and inhibit HIV by inhibiting the cytopathic effects of HIV and HSV. Tannins are free radical scavengers. Tannins inhibit enzymes – lipoxygenase, lipid peroxidation, cycloxygenase and histamine release. Inhibit ascorbic acid peroxidation. Inhibit adrenaline-induced lipolysis. Tannin sub-group - Anthocyanidins, Gallic acid phenols [red wine].

Astringent and possess a local inflammatory allaying action. Vasoconstrictors.

Medicines e.g. Agrimonia, Ajuga reptans, Alchemilla vulg, Banana, Euphrasia, Hamamelis, Polygonum, Potentilla, Quercus, Scolopendrium, Stachys.

Terpenes – composed of three groups – monoterpenes – limonene, triterpenes – asiatic acid, boswelic acid and sesquiterpenes – parthenolide.

Medicines e.g. Boswellia, Centella, Commiphora.

Sesquiterpenes

Some sesquiterpenes are found within the essential oils of plants.

Medicines e.g. Tanacetum parthenium has a sesquiterpene lactone named Parthenolide. Artemesia annua – artemisinin.

Volatile oils – see essential oils.

Summary

Medicines are specific to tissue conditions, not a disease name. Treat the tissues, found upon examination to be unhealthy, using medicines with the ability to restore the tissues to health. Prescriptions will require to be modified as time progresses, the patient will require varying herbs to stimulate the vital force and relax or tone the tissues. Knowledge of the available constituents supports the use of the medication to activate healing of the cell and tissue fluid.

14
What is disease?

What this Chapter is about
Disease is a condition of the tissues whereby the vital force working through the tissues is unable to heal them effectively. Weak tissues provoke further disease because cellular activity is less robust in eliminating disease causes.

Disease is a departure from health, the consequence of which means that physiology is interrupted leading to discomfort inconvenience or suffering.

Disease consists in the organic changes themselves not the deranged processes that proclaim them explains Cook.

The cure of disease depends upon the knowledge and application of correct principles and these must be worked out in every case.

Symptoms announce that the structures are not under the full control of the vital force. Robust symptoms indicate the vital force is vigorous and trying to heal the tissues. Disease conditions are favourable when the level of functional activity falls below the normal standard. Restore the tissues to their normal condition and the disturbed functions will normalise [11].

There is no fixed standard for health in the body; any deviation from health could be called disease. A chief characteristic of a living body is not a fixed state but variation by self-adjustment, to a wide range of circumstances. Taking into account self-adjustments, it is not practical to mark a line separating healthy, from those which may as reasonably be called diseased [13].
Cook says 'The external signs of disease are shown in the functional aberrations upon which we must sometimes rely and occasionally come long after diseased conditions in the tissue cells have been fully established. For immediately the tissue cells are invaded to any extent, even locally, a warning pain, ache or distress is produced - **this is where ease ceases and disease commences.'**
The vital force may quickly resist and the excretory organs totally eliminate the disease aetiology, so that the illness is transient and the individual continues in an even balance physically and mentally. No indefinite line can be drawn between health and disease.
The change in functional action produces symptoms that are not the disease but an expression of the abnormal conditions of the tissues.

What is Disease ?

All recoveries take place by virtue of the Vis medicatrix nature – the healing power of nature. Vital efforts never destroy life but when disease gains a hold in the body the vital actions decrease in vigour.

Thurston's definition of disease

'Disease is an enforced resistive, eliminative and constructive extra functional intrinsic activity, general or local, because of invasion, exhaustion or destruction of living matter and tissue cells, by extrinsic inimical substances, forces, influences or environments. These are sufficient to disturb or destroy the physiological harmony between assimilation and dissimulation' [13].

Disease is made up of symptoms and called a **syndrome**. Disease is what we see occurring from a secondary result of tissue invasion. The vital force is the producer of symptoms. Extra functional action by the vital force occurs once the tissues are invaded. The level of symptom reaction is due to the disparity between the invasion of the tissue and the response by the vital force to the invasion. The integrity of the cell function is a factor in disease response; that is the response by the vital force. The cell tries to limit any pathological influence and will do so, within its own capacity to adapt and neutralise the offending problem. Symptoms will not arise until the cells require an extra level of action. Because the capacity of the organ to heal itself has become exceeded, due to the inimical influence overwhelming it, extra functional activity is required. More energy is required by the vital force to heal and consequently more symptoms emerge.

The ability of the cell to withstand disease influences depends upon its own structure. The cell is affected by intrinsic and extrinsic disturbance and cell structure will be weakened intrinsically. Effects that occur within the cell: encumbrance, toxicity, impurity, exhaustion; in fact any negative effect will weaken the cell and allow disease conditions to become established. Extrinsic effects, factors from outside the cell, will also weaken it for example excesses of heat or cold.

Disease is a tissue state

Disease consists of cellular changes affecting the tissues locally or generally. This will produce changes in the function of those tissues.

Disease - signs & symptoms

The signs of disease the herbalist may observe within the patient, during the consultation, may have occurred a long time after the disease conditions have become established in the tissues. The symptoms arising from bodily disorder arise as the ability of the organ systems to heal becomes reduced. This reduction arises as the organ systems become unable to adjust to the need for extra functional action required for healing. When an organ cannot bring about enough energy to heal the disorder and its capacity to heal is exceeded symptoms will then be experienced.

Bodily adjustment is influenced by cellular function. Disordered cellular function is **functional - symptom free** or can be **extra functional - producing symptoms**. Nutrition and drainage of the cell is a vital effort. During any cellular process the cell can become disordered and still maintain its functions, local environments may become disturbed and give rise to extra functional cellular activity - producing symptoms.

Inflammation, fever and pain are not diseases; they are physiological manifestations occurring within the tissues and indicate the level of vital resistance that is present. The vital force attempts to overcome disease by putting into activity physiological [extra functional] processes for the removal of encumbrances.

End result - functional consequences
Following any cell reaction, that has not been sufficiently cleared or neutralised by the vital force ensures symptoms may result. Tissue damage can lead to an unresolved condition. Unresolved conditions encourage pathology with further symptom complexes. Pathology can arise from damage that has occurred to bodily organs as a result of the disease process. [See Chapter 15].

Periodicity [law of sevens]
Lindlahr says 'crises often develop with marked regularity and in well-defined periodicity'. Periodicity is the timing of an exacerbation. The law of sevens suggest that aggravation of symptoms in a healing crisis [acute or chronic]. The law of sevens suggest that alteration of symptoms will occur, as a reaction, change or crisis during the course of the condition. A change in the symptoms may be towards healing or disease depending upon the type of crisis. A reaction by the body to a disease process is brought about by the vital force. Critical discharges typically occur every seven days e.g. abscesses, glandular swellings, haemorrhages, skin eruptions. The health level of the patient and their level of vitality influence the process of the crisis.

The seventh day is often marked by symptom changes. Further symptoms occur during a healing or disease crisis, depending upon the patient's level of vitality. The level of vitality will determine the severity of symptoms.

It should be remembered that:

vital efforts never destroy but always support life

What is Disease ?

Chronic disease

Chronic disease in the patient is similar to acute disease regarding periodicity. A crisis may develop on the seventh day, week or month following commencement of the illness. The patient must be healthy enough to produce an acute eliminative effort [a crisis]. An exacerbation of symptoms requires vital energy, produced by the vital force.

Acute disease

Acute disease is an effort by the body to rid itself of unhealthy conditions within the tissues. Accomplished by and through the vital force all acute reactions represent increased cellular activity. The vital force cannot act correctly in a body that has encumbrance within the tissues. Impurities need to be eliminated. When the vital force tries to clear impurities, acute reactions may develop depending upon the amount and level of energy within the tissues. Acute symptoms reflect a healing crisis taking place in the tissues. Typical acute symptoms are eliminative in effect and include catarrh and sinusitis, boils, abscesses and certain forms of diarrhoea.

Encumbrance is dangerous as it can pollute the cell and causes its death. Encumbrance will add to the cellular burden this makes cellular activity decline over time.

The vital force will never do anything that is not an attempt to heal and cleanse the tissues. Vital force can be depleted through the ingestion of too much food.

In acute disease it is advisable to fast for at least a day. **Short fasts are very stimulating to the vital force.** Fasting rests the digestion making vital energy able to concentrate upon the healing process rather than digestion. Even when healthy, if the body is given too much, or the wrong kind of food it can precipitate illness and become a pathocausative [a cause of disease].

Lindlahr states: 'acute disease is the result of a healing effort of nature. It is natures attempt to establish health'.

Fever, pain and inflammation are not disease, merely the bodily reaction to a condition of encumbrance. Any remedy that is anti-inflammatory may be suppressive to the vital force. Suppressed disease causes the blood become full of impurities these are tolerated within the tissues where depleted vital force is encountered. Stimulation to vital force will again attempt to remove the impurities. Depleted vital force can lead to a selection of low-grade symptoms. We use the word chronic in these cases.

Building up the vital force takes time and the patient needs to understand that acute reactions need to be treated correctly without suppression. Suppression of disease is much more likely to bring about serious pathology. The tissue requires a healing crisis to become healthy again.

Inflammation

Thurston states 'Inflammation is an exaggerated state of vasomotor functional activities because of invasion or destruction of living matter and tissue cells involving a more or less circumscribed area' [13].

Inflammation is a helpful and healing effect by the body as it limits unwanted influences.

Inflammation is the reaction by the tissues to some form of injury or invasion. It is characterised by the clinical signs of: heat, pain, redness and swelling. Vasomotor relaxation can result in inflammation.

Congestion

Thurston states 'Congestion is an inability of the vasomotor function to maintain the normal balance between assimilation and elimination, locally or generally, because of functional obstruction, vital depression, or lesion of the tissue units of the vasomotor apparatus' [13].

Congestion may occur anywhere in the tissues. It results from a reduced level of vasomotor function: a reduced level of blood or nerve supply resulting in congestion.

Congestion can occur in the cell, lymphatics, circulation and organ areas, in any part of the body that has a circulation and nerve supply. Congestion is the disturbance between the normal balance of nutrition and waste.

Congestion is caused by an obstruction to the circulation/vasomotor function, from:

- Damage [injury] to motor nerves
- Degeneration of motor nerves [trophic degeneration]
- Vital depression from nerve weakness
- Spinal problems causing pressure and disturbance

In the last example it may be necessary to manipulate or adjust the spine to improve the condition.

Congested conditions require stimulation to the vasomotor circulatory function.

Irritation

Thurston states 'Exaggerated local and reflex impressions of peripheral sensory nerves arising from long continued inefficient inflammatory action' [13].

Irritation arises from the chronic inability of the tissue involved to heal. Long standing inflammation will create this irritable state.

What is Disease ?

Pain

Thurston states 'Exaggerated functional action upon sensory nerve centres due to violent disturbance or destruction of tissues' [13].
Pain is the physiological response to some form of abnormal tissue state. It is a reflection of an abnormal condition within the tissues.
In health there is no pain. Pain is not the disease but is a response to an abnormal tissue condition. Pain is a requirement of life. It gives warning to a disease state. It is an indication of an abnormal process occurring within the tissues and has a protective function. Remove the causes of that pain and the pain subsides.
Pain may in some instances be a prayer for nutrition of the tissue cell.
Pain can become a pathocausative due to an irritative nerve effect. Some remedies can remove the irritation of the nerve to encourage healing e.g. *Hypericum, Scutellaria, Lobelia,* and *Viburnum opulus.*
The sympathetic nervous system affects the hormones as regulators of the systems e.g. adaptation syndromes.
Sympathetic adrenal syndromes [sympatheticotonia] affect vasomotor function this in turn determines the organ function and organ trophicity

Vertical and horizontal assessments

A **horizontal assessment** is made using the past history, typology [which reflects the vitality level] and the long-term objective to arrive at a prognosis. Iridology can provide confirmation of the horizontal diagnosis for assessment purposes. The patient is more suited to long-term assessment of future health when they are treated.
A **vertical assessment** of the patient is arrived at through blood tests, pulse diagnosis and acute level of symptoms.
Iridology reveals organ areas and level of health of these areas – the lighter areas suggest sub acute or acute tissue activity.
Disease encroachment frequently reflects the trophic weakness of a specific organ area.

Summary
Bodily and organ system and cellular relationships

The actual amount of renewal within an organ is dependent upon the organism as a whole because **the cell is dependent upon the organism and the organism upon the cell.** We need to consider the system of cellular function as it reflects upon the overall structure of the body. Structure reflects the function of the organism; the two coexist. When disease arises function becomes disturbed. Disturbed function eventually affects the structure of an organ area. Poor elimination of toxins and retained secretions have detrimental consequences and affect tissue regeneration. **Function affects the structure and structure affects the function.** [See also trophic Chapter 11].

15
What is health?

What this Chapter is about
Thurston gives his **definition of health**.

'Health is a state of the whole organism, or any part of the vital body, in which there is sufficient vital vigour in the tissue cells, and functional activity in tissues and structures, to maintain physiological co-ordination between assimilation and dissimulation, nutrition and waste, of the normal body elements, with sufficient potential vitality for all reasonable extrinsic body work and intrinsic resistive, eliminative and constructive functional action'.

The moment diseased conditions of tissue cells cover sufficient area to derange functional work of the organs and systems; the potential **reserve vitality** is required for extra functional work. It resists and eliminates the disease causes and repairs any damage that may have resulted from the invasion. During the temporary engagement of the reserve vital energy the individual is incapacitated for physical or mental labour, because of a withdrawal of vital energy for interior resistive, eliminative and reconstructive functional work. This reserve vitality is inseparable from ordinary kinetic energy. Therefore any definition of health must necessarily include both the energy levels of potential and kinetic vitality. Potential energy is a resting level of vitality, whereas the kinetic level is energy producing action and motion, it is another conversion stage.

Vital energy determines the level of tissue activity. Depleted vitality encourages the development of diseases as it depletes the vital force. Depleted vitality will result from chronic anxiety and stress. Depression also depresses vitality. Organ disturbance can occur from tension and lack of relaxation. When rest and relaxation are withheld the organism will use reserve vitality to keep things going. The depleted vital force at a low level can no longer afford protection from infections whether they be intracellular, extracellular or contagion from an overwhelming infection. Rest is required to enhance the vital force and the vitality levels. It is unwise to keep going when ill as rest will be very beneficial for the tissue cells. An acute crisis will support the renewal of cellular renewal, repair and trophorestoration but only if there is sufficient rest and suitable food.
Never feed a diseased body to excess - this will merely make the disease longer lasting or reduce the functional activity of the healing capacity of tissue cells.

At this point it is useful to identify the difference between fitness and health. One can be fit but not healthy. Healthy but not fit. There have been a number of athletes who have died of cancer they were fit but not healthy. Identification of health is made from the history, examination, laboratory testing and an Iridology analysis, such analyses can produce a certain measurement of ones level of health.

Summary

Health is a balance of function as determined by Thurston. The World Health Organisation in the year 2000 agrees with Thurston's statement.

16
Naturopathy

What this Chapter is about
Naturopathy is a system of healing using natural methods of treatment and is
patient orientated medicine.
Naturopathy has **six** pillars of function for the enhancement of life processes.
These are **fasting, hydrotherapy, diet, light, air and exercise.** For current
purposes we shall look at the effects healing treatments have upon the tissues.
When a treatment is given certain effects should be the result. Effects are shown
as **symptom change or amelioration.** New symptoms may emerge which could
form part of an old disease, this is known as a **healing crisis.** Reduction of vital
symptoms as manifested through the living tissue, as a decline of vital response, is
found in a **disease crisis** [See also Chapter 4].

Crisis
There are two types of crisis, one tends towards healing and the other crisis
towards disease. Some symptoms can be similar to both crises however they are
operating under different circumstances.
Crisis is defined as: a decisive change in the tissues due to a healing or a disease
crisis. A crisis is an attempt to re-establish the secretions and excretions that have
become more or less suppressed during acute or chronic illness.

Healing crises and chronic ailments depend upon the following conditions:
healing will be towards either a resolution of the condition or further disease
conditions. Acute robust symptoms are favourable. Decline in the function of an
organ or its vital capacity would prolong the disease, this often happens in chronic
disease states, where vitality is slowly drained away. The patient must possess
sufficient vital energy for a healing reaction to occur. Treatment aims to build up
tissue vitality so that the tissue is supportive to any healing crisis. A short term
[24 hour] fast is supportive and beneficial to the vital force. The vital force
becomes energised in a crisis. Strong vitality and adequate elimination creates
robust symptoms.
Patients approaching a healing crisis usually have more vital energy and
symptoms may abate. This is known as 'calm before the storm' or there may be
an exacerbation of symptoms that herald the onset of a healing crisis. A fever
suggests a healing crisis. The symptoms reflect the vital force resisting disease
conditions. A healing crisis can occur when the body is attempting to clear some
obstructive condition. A healing crisis helps the body to recover from disease and
is always supporting the body towards health. An acute flare up of eczema under

Naturopathy

treatment can reflect a healing crisis. A healing crisis shows the herbalist a positive state is emerging within the tissues. It occurs as the tissues try to heal and clear the causes of disease. It is a restorative effort by the tissues towards health. Symptoms are to be seen as a *positive vital state* in the cells and tissues of the body.

Acute tissue reactivity during a crisis can be safely controlled with vasotonic alteratives [antimicrobial] and organ support together with antiseptic and nervine herbs. It is preferable to use the herbal infusion in an acute condition. Herbal medicine and hydrotherapy are valuable to promote healing as opposed to suppression of the reaction by using synthetic drugs. If acute reactions are suppressed the constructive healing crisis may be changed into a destructive **disease crisis**.

Secernants

The secernants [eliminative organs] are required to carry away toxins and must be healthy in order to achieve their eliminatory work.

Secernant organ weakness delays recovery and prolongs the illness. Weak secernant activity can prevent full healing from taking place. In certain disorders secernant organs can be obstructed and at other times one or more of them will be freely eliminating while the others are inactive. Cook says 'such failures in eliminating the secretory toxins and impurities constitute the essential cause of numerous conditions'.

When suppressed elimination occurs within the tissues it will intensify a local condition because further impurities are being added to the already existing toxic load. Blood impurity and lymph congestion can result in encumbrance of the tissue this delays recovery. The re-establishment of the secretions is an aim of treatment.

Re-establishment of the secretions from the liver, bowel, or skin during a crisis is called a **critical discharge.** Critical discharges are an excess of such evacuations being due partly to the relaxation following a considerable degree of tension and partly to the amount of unelimimated impurities that had accumulated during the obstruction of the secernants. Critical discharges are sometimes presented in the form of haemorrhages, eruptions, glandular swellings, boils or abscesses. Such discharges have the tendency to appear at intervals of about seven days and are known as **critical days** [See law of sevens].

Healing crisis

To heal the tissues of disease causes the vital force must raise the level of vitality. An inflammatory effort by the tissues is nature's way to heal. However, the acute symptoms may have occurred before and been unable to heal the tissues which thereby pass into a chronic condition. Fasting, correct diet and herbal medicine enhance the vital force enabling healing of the diseased tissue. Getting better may not always be comfortable for the patient. The vital force provokes inflammatory processes. The inflammatory process is a completely natural process and is vital for the preservation of tissue. A healing crisis always results in an improved condition of the health of tissue. The vital force must remove disease encumbrance from the tissue. Encumbrance is a chronic accumulation of waste within the tissue. Typical symptoms of elimination are: colds, catarrh, some diarrhoeas, fever, certain skin rashes. The existing symptoms may become worse. New symptoms can appear in the crisis. These symptoms can belong to either a healing or disease crisis but they are operating under different circumstances.

As soon as any acute elimination starts it is best to stop eating, use fluids only until the acute episode has passed.

To determine the aetiology through evaluation by history of symptoms and examination of the patient to determine the aetiology. Diagnosis is confirmed from the above. During the healing crisis the patient will need a lot of encouragement to keep with the treatment. No one likes to feel ill and it is worth reminding the patient they are getting better.

Sometimes a healing crisis may not develop -- *Why doesn't the patient get better?* this can be due to:

1] low level of vital force

2] some nervous diseases like depression which can rob the nerve tissue of vitality and prevent healing

3] the tissue having been destroyed by a disease process

4] damage to a nerve supply or blood vessels could stop the healing process. As no nerve signal or adequate blood supply would be available to that locality for healing

5] damaged tissue, from trauma or infection, may be unable to respond and heal itself it would be liable to chronic degeneration with little or no healing able to take place

6] inherited weakness [trophic weakness] from birth, making an organ area more vulnerable to disease processes. Trophic organ weakness can also follow damage from infection, injury or obstruction to the circulation.

Disease crisis. A disease crisis is simply a different form of elimination by the body - a vicarious elimination. It arises from encumbrance of the tissues due to waste matter, toxins, impurities, etc. Where toxins or impurities are to be eliminated they will be ejected from any surface of the body. The body is self protective in this effort. Symptoms include the following; abscess formation, catarrhal elimination from any mucus surface, skin surface for example dandruff, fever during an infection, infection symptoms, ulcers created and discharging pus.

Naturopathy

Disease processes that are unable to heal effectively will create a disease crisis. The patient will always feel unwell in a disease crisis. Whereas the healing crisis patient feels well.

Inflammation is frequently found during a crisis and is common to both crises. [See the section on inflammation].

When conditions within the tissues become chronic the vital force is depleted. This reflects a disease crisis. Symptom fluctuation is but little marked in the chronic condition. Symptoms are the result of the *negative vital state* within the cells. Chronic long standing symptoms like acne, chronic bronchitis or arthritis all fall under the term disease crisis. When disease conditions encroach further upon the tissue, symptoms are of a chronic nature. Medicine that is stimulating to the vital force arouse vital integrity within the tissues and aid healing e.g. Stimulants - *Capsicum, Cochleria, Composition essence, Myrica, Zanthoxylum, Zingiber.*

How many crises would the patient have to go through to get better? It would depend upon the level of vitality. Chronic conditions require herbal treatment to raise the level of tissue strength to enable a crisis to develop.

Detoxification

A large number of diseases result from **auto intoxication** [self poisoning]. This auto intoxication begins in the intestine. Instead of toxin removal the tissues retain toxins that become reabsorbed into the blood causing further disease. The unhealthy intestine reabsorbs toxins in this way

Treatment aims to cleanse the intestine of toxins. One way to achieve this is through purging. Epsom salts [magnesium sulphate] has an irritant effect and a strong attraction for carbon. Epsom salts saturate the entire lining of the GI tract. By the process of osmosis, carbonaceous [organic] waste is removed from the blood as it passes close to the surface of the GI tract. Organic waste is thereby eliminated from the body.

Dosage: One heaped teaspoonful in 500 ml of warm water. Followed by herb tea if desired. Results are expected within 24 hours. One dose is sufficient at any time. Repeat if required 3/7 days later.

Suggested light diet to follow the elimination process.

Breakfast: fruit e.g. apricots, figs, prunes, grapefruit.

Lunch/dinner: vegetable protein – rice, soya, cous cous, green leafy vegetables, wholewheat bread/crisp bread, vegetable soup, fruit.

Fluids: herb teas, fruit juice, Chicory, No caff, Barleycup, Dandelion coffee.

Sebastian Kneipp

Kneipp [1821 - 1897] wrote several books on hydrotherapy they are worth reading as they contain references to the herbal therapy of disease conditions.

Herbs used in baths and sitz baths offer remedial benefit by dermal absorption. Essential oils from plants are readily available and can be added to the bath water.

Hydrotherapy

Hydrotherapy is the use of water to arouse bodily reactions for healing purposes. Hydrotherapy is described as the use of water, hot or cold, in any form, for the maintenance of health or the treatment of disease [388].

Disease states respond to the use of hydrotherapy to arouse the vital force and if required, an acute eliminative and healing effort to dispel disease. The application of hydrotherapy must be related to the level of the vital response. Warm, hot and cold water are used in the treatments. Sometimes a compress or a spray [shower] is beneficial.

Acute and chronic disease is treated using hydrotherapy

Cold water applications are used as sprays [showers] and compress [wraps, compress]. Bodily tissue function can be altered to improve tissue health. A healing crisis can be brought about with the use of hydrotherapy - to increase the temperature use a full body compress.

The temperament of the patient and their physique should be taken into account. Asthenic types often under react in pyrexia, their need is for a nervine trophorestorative in order to raise the temperature. Gentle treatment is often effective, using the spray for a short time, the patient will also find it refreshing and stimulating.

Whenever the treatment is finished it is best to pat the area dry. A different signal is created in the tissues if rubbing the area dry after the hydrotherapy. Rubbing the area dry will heat the skin and warm the area once again.

Cold water:

        1] stimulates the circulation
        2] supports the elimination of impurities and toxins
        3] regulates the temperature

Law of action and reaction

Therapeutic agents have primary, temporary and a secondary permanent effect.

In the case of heat above 37c [98.6 f] blood is drawn to the skin surface. The primary and immediate effect of hot water is to make the skin red and hot. The temporary effect of heat is to draw blood to the skin surface.

Secondary and lasting effects of water are that the blood temporarily recedes towards the interior of the body once the blood has receded towards the interior it needs stimulation to bring it back to the surface once again, cold water will achieve this effect.

Excessive cold is suppressive to the tissue's capillary circulation.

Naturopathy

Derivative effect of water
The application of water alters the blood volume within an area of the body. Organs can be influenced in this way. The prolonged use of cold water will drive blood out of an area [vasoconstriction]. Hot water draws blood into an area [vasodilatation]. Hot water foot baths draw blood from the head.

Spinal reflex effect of water
Water applied to the skin causes a reflex activity. Spinal reflex activity is stimulated to corresponding areas supplied by the dermatomes. The spinal reflex arc is the mechanism for this action. Intense hot or cold applications affect the skin and encourage altered blood flow to the tissues.

Reflex affects
Immersion of one hand or arm will increase the blood flow to the opposite arm.

Cold applications
  decrease acid production
  calm peristalsis
  increase tone in the stomach
  slow the heart
  contract the blood vessels

Hot applications
  increase acid production
  quicken peristalsis
  increase tone in a relaxed stomach
  decrease tone in a contracted stomach
  decrease intestinal blood flow
  relax muscles of the chest, abdomen and pelvis
  decrease the pulse rate
  dilate blood vessels
  increase menses

Cutaneous stimulation creates a reflex visceral reaction, particularly vasomotor [circulatory] reactions. Alternating hot and cold applications produce marked stimulation to the local circulation [388]. Vasomotor control of blood volume is altered by using water applications. The tone of visceral muscle can also be altered. Many visceral disorders are affected beneficially by the appropriate stimulation of the corresponding cutaneous area [36].

Several points are worth noting with hydrotherapy treatments.
Some side effects may occur with hydrotherapy. Headache is common and results from the release of toxic products into the blood.

Herbal Medicine - Keys

There are times when the treatment must be stopped - if there is discomfort, hypotension, dizziness, palpitations or shivering.

Bodily areas of treatment and effect

Applications create an effect upon organs by stimulation of the dermatomes, e.g.:

Knee/upper leg treatments have an effect upon
bladder
stomach
reproductive organs

Knee to ankle treatments affect
nose
throat
bladder
intestines
ovaries

Feet treatments affect the
head

Elbow to wrist treatments influence the
heart and lungs

Right shoulder treatments affect the
liver and gall bladder

Abdomen treatments
arthritis of the hip

T shaped compress for
congestion of the pelvis

Preparation of the patient.

If the patient is cold, never use cold water to start the treatment. Warm the patient first using warm or hot water. Follow with the cold application.

Cold water sends the blood to the core of the body. The blood returns with vigour bringing heat to the surface this is called the revulsive effect.

The patient needs to be suitably prepared they need a warm room, without draughts. Avoid treatments within an hour of meals.

Hydrotherapy effects

1] the temperature of the water, 2] the length of a treatment 3] the area treated.

Naturopathy

Cold water treatment is used to relieve an inflammatory condition as described above. Treatment must take into account the vitality of the patient. Cold can be a suppressant to the vital force and should be used with care in depleted patients. Cold water stimulates the skin and capillary circulation. Capillary action is vital to organ function. Local dermatomes receive impressions from the hydrotherapy and effect to deeper organs is produced. Inadequate organ function [vasodepression of gastro intestinal, genito urinary] is stimulated to improved action by cold applications. It will also control fever naturally without suppression providing the temperature is kept sufficiently high to resolve the inflammatory state and complete the healing process. A fever is a healing and cleansing process and needs to be supported and never suppressed.

Hot water
Hot water is not generally used during inflammation. Heat will bring more blood to the area and increase an overheated [inflamed] condition. There is already an excess of blood an inflamed area and cold applications are required to restore the balance of blood.
Hot applications are used for:
otitis media, spasm, abdominal colic, pain and asthma.

Affusion - spray
Affusions are more powerful than compress they are used in acute conditions and short-term. They can be used cold, hot or as a combination of cold/warm/hot. An affusion using hot then cold water creates a quick impression upon the tissues. Use hot water at 38c for 3 minutes followed by cold water for 20 seconds. Always finishing the treatment with cold water.

Face affusion
Used cold the face affusion brings more blood to the head. The face can be sprayed or use a circular motion with the jet of water moved around the face. The sinus area can be affected if the water is allowed to run over them.
Affusions are used for:
headache, tiredness, depression, catarrh, and sinus conditions.

Head bath
Cold water to the head and neck will stimulate the blood flow to the brain.

Limb treatments/water treading/dew walking
Water treading is also useful to warm the body up. This is treading in knee high water, alternately lifting the leg up high and placing down again. After the treatment pat dry and have a walk to warm the legs. One easy way to tread water is to use a bucket. Water treading and dew walking tones the legs and encourages

blood drainage from the feet. Where one limb is treated the other benefits, this is known as a consensual reaction.

Compress [wrap]

The effect of a compress is dependent upon the amount of moisture contained within it.

Cold wet compress and sprays, draw blood to the surface and open the skin glands, they aid perspiration and eliminate impurities.

Separate cold compresses are laid over an area of inflammation.

Heat is beneficial in some painful conditions. Warm water bottle wrapped in a tea towel can ease pain and needs to be followed by a cold application to prevent any congestion returning.

A compress is used to influence any part of the body, it may help a variety of conditions. During a fever a compress is used to reduce the temperature and encourage perspiration. Perspiration encourages detoxification. Methodically used, a compress can affect the dermatomes below the skin surface and thereby organ function is stimulated to improved function.

Two methods can be used when applying a hot or cold compress.

A hot compress up to 40c or a cold compress up to 18c. Method: a towel is wrung out in hot/cold water and applied to the area. It is left on until the patient notices the compress has become warm. Repeat the process. Tea towels are suitable for use as compress. Compress can be left on for 60 minutes renewing as required. The patient should be lying down during the treatment. The patient should rest after removal of the compress.

The hot compress is anodyne and may be used for painful conditions. Always follow a hot compress with a cold splash to prevent any congestion of blood. Compress can be repeated as often as required.

Compress

Squeeze all the water from a towel apply the cold, wet compress for up to 30 minutes it will increase vasodilation.

To increase fever the wrung out compress is applied for up to 2 hours.

Used for achy joints, throat congestion, fever, chronic conditions and sub acute states e.g. poor elimination of the skin, blood impurity, and immune depression.

Chest compress - cold

Applied cold from the axilla to cover the entire chest area. The compress is applied for up to 90 minutes. Used in all chest complaints where there is fever or inflammation.

Naturopathy

Chest compress - hot
Hot chest compress are contraindicated in fever. Applied until the compress heats – use for up to 30 minutes. Hot chest compress are used for bronchial conditions.
Cold leg compress
Cold leg compress are applied from knee to ankle and left in place until it becomes warm. The compress can be replaced up to three times in a treatment. Repeat use hourly as required. Remove before it gets too hot.
Used in: fainting, fever, headaches, gently allays inflammation, achy legs, bruising, depression, heat stroke, tension, induce sleep and calms the patient.

Compresses can be made to carry medications [soak the compress in an infusion and wring out or apply oils to the skin e.g. Symphytum for bruises, Avena in eczema, Chamomilla for cramps.
Raw onion crushed and put into muslin and held on the ear will bring relief from earache.

Cold wet compress/wet sheet treatment
Eye compress
Worn over the eyes it supports drainage from the eye and is used for tired eyes.

Neck compress
Compress applied to the neck can release spasm and congestion. Used in brachial neuritis and for throat conditions [See below].

Throat compress
The cold compress will reduce congestion of the blood vessels and lymphatics of the neck. The compress is renewed once it has heated up to be replaced with a further cold compress. The compress is covered with a dry cotton or wool covering.
Apply a cold compress for all ear, nose and throat problems e.g. tonsillitis, sore throat, mumps, catarrh, sinusitis.

Foot bath
Hot footbaths dilate blood vessels and lowers vascular tension.
Used in fever, pelvic congestion, haemorrhoids, prolapse, seminal emissions, hip arthritis, and varicose veins.

Wet sock treatment [natural fibre]
Put on socks wrung out in cold water. Used in insomnia to draw blood from the head and aid restful sleep. It is calming to the nervous system. Do not use where there are varicose veins as the socks would become too warm if left on overnight

and tend to aggravate the veins. If the feet become cold and do not get warm discontinue treatment, it may be that the patient has a circulatory deficit.

Ice compress

Ice compress should only be used in acute injury and in acute inflammatory disease with caution and for short periods only.

Hay sack/bean bag

Used as a small compress full of cut herb. Grain such as barley and known as a beanbag can also be used in the compress as grain holds heat. The sack is heated for a few minutes then applied to the area. The main advantage is in **holding the heat in the bag**. Less changing is required as one would have to do with a water compress. The bag may be left on for two hours. It can be used as a natural painkiller.

Used in arthritic conditions, backache and to the chest in bronchial trouble

Whole body pack
How to apply the whole body pack

After application of the pack the patient should become warm in a few minutes. If this is not the case the reaction is said to be bad and the whole treatment discontinued.

What happens in the cold compress to the body functions?

A cold compress will lower body temperature by increasing heat radiation. The compress draws heat from the internal congested areas to the skin surface relaxing the capillaries and promoting heat escape and temperature reduction. The compress can be left on for 90 minutes.

Prepare a double sheet that has been wrung out in cold water. Put two blankets then the sheet upon the bed. Lay the patient on the sheet. Then wrap the patient in the sheet. Cover the feet too. Next wrap the blankets around the patient. Give diaphoretic medicine to encourage a reaction.

Dry skin brushing

Wearing too many clothes depletes skin action. Synthetic nylon and it's derivatives encase the skin preventing the skin from 'breathing', skin tone is thus reduced. Continuous hot bathing further depletes the tone and reactivity of the skin. As the tone of the skin diminishes flaccidity increases. When the skin ages it becomes thinner. Ageing skin allows cellulite build up and produces thick, dry, leathery skin. Dry skin contains bacteria that can infect fissures and add to the total burden in any skin disease. Enlarged pores are seen with aged skin. Flaccidity of the skin occurs from loss of elastin due to reduction of collagen. Collagen can be improved with Ol Oenothera and Vitamin C. Cellulite forms from the deposition of fat around the cells. Movement of the skin with brushing mobilises these fats to be carried away by the lymph.

Skin brushing decreases muscle tension and relaxes the nervous system.

Skin brushing supports the body and encourages the removal of toxins. Brushing the skin encourages the stimulation of capillaries. The lymphatic vessels of the skin are stimulated to increased action. The movement of lymph is dependent upon the contraction of the skin tissues. The skin has sensory nerves that are stimulated by brushing. This in turn affects the lymph, capillaries and tone of the skin by stimulating smooth muscle. Venous blood flow is increased with skin brushing.

A loofah is used to dry skin brush. This brushing removes dead skin cells. Dry brushing can be used for hyper/hypotension. Using small strokes - start with the legs, then abdomen, bottom, chest and back, finishing on the face. Always work towards the heart when skin brushing. This exercise needs to be done gently to avoid scratching the skin.

Air and light baths

The skin is stimulated to healthier function using natural daylight and air. Wearing a swim suit use the natural air and daylight. Take in warm weather as exposure to cold will cause a chill.

Skin loses its tone and becomes shrivelled, dry [enervated] and atrophied in many individuals, it is therefore unable to eliminate toxins, etc. Too many clothes also obstruct the skin.

Poor skin function is observed in the iris as a scurf rim. It tells us the skin's circulation is defective and elimination of toxins has been reduced. This can lead to auto intoxication and will place a heavier burden upon the renal system.

Use the light and the air baths to help the capillary circulation to improve its function.

Correct breathing

Deep breathing controls the body and balances the nervous system. Control the breathing and you control the body and its emotions. Deep lower lobe expansion can be experienced by laying face down. The breath is allowed to find its own rhythm. As breathing continues you notice the abdomen pushing against the surface on which you are lying.

Another way to fill the lungs with air is to use the sitting position for breathing techniques; fill the lower lobes, then middle and upper lobes.

This type of breathing is known as a full yoga breath. Used as an exercise it calms both mind and body. Instant effects can be produced. Panic attacks can be eased with deep breathing.

Herbal Medicine - Keys

Balneum [Baths] [See also Chapter 26]
Baths are a total skin treatment. Their effects depend upon:

1] length of time in the water
2] temperature of the water
3] individual reaction

Baths are taken warm or cold
A warm bath opens the skin pores and increases peripheral blood. The skin becomes warmer and it takes on a glow. Peristalsis is also increased. Warm baths are relaxing to the nervous system. They increase blood alkalinity and ease pain. Mobility is increased. Some exercises are more easily performed in warm water.
The cold bath stimulates the sympathetic nervous system. Reduces peristalsis and tones the skin.
Baths can be used for **medication of the skin**. Infusions, decoctions, oils and aromatic waters can all be used. Oils can be added and by absorption through the skin, affect the body, either locally or generally. Ten drops of essential oil may be added to a bath if required. Choose either relaxant or stimulant effect for the oil. Chamomilla, Lavandula are relaxing. Syzygium is stimulating.

Baths are relaxing [warm water] or stimulating [cold water]
Both will have an effect upon the patient's state of mind

Types of bath
Three types are used in treatment with varying immersion times and temperatures

- warm - up to 20 minutes 36C - 38C
- cold - up to 30 seconds 12C - 18C
- warm alternating with cold - 5 minutes warm alternate 10 seconds cold.

Specific hydrotherapy
Arm bath alternating hot then cold.
Two bowls are used, the arms are put into the hot [38C] for 1 minute then transferred immediately into the cold for 15 seconds.
Used for the following:
Arthritis, Bronchitis, Blood pressure regulator, Depression, Eczema, Exhaustion, Hypotension, Tennis elbow, Tiredness.

Epsom salts
A powerful way to clear the skin and support detoxification. 100g epsom salts is added to a body temperature bath. Stay in the bath for up to 30 minutes. Follow

with a cold spray. After a bath containing epsom salts the patient is put to bed. Perspiration through the skin supports the eliminative detoxing process.

Hydrotherapy for children

Water treatments are contra indicated if the child is cold or shivering.

Warm to hot baths are used to increase the temperature and so aid the elimination of toxins. Warm baths aid restful sleep, relieve tension [hyperactivity] and difficulty in sleeping.

Footbaths are used to clear catarrh and colds on the chest.

Fever

'Fever is an exaggerated state of the vasomotor function, resulting from invasion of the tissue cells by inimical substances, forces or influences, and involving sufficient area of tissue cells to require extra functional action of the general vasomotor apparatus' [13].

Fever is a cleansing and healing effort by the body to rid itself of toxins in the tissues such as infection or waste impurities from metabolism.

The vital force cleanses and detoxifies the tissues during any fever condition. Fever is a natural action of the vital force. Many pathogenic microbes cannot be killed, except under very high temperatures. It is not the temperature during the fever that reduces any microbe by itself. The fever enables the blood capillaries to carry the pathogen to the skin for elimination.

Types of fever

Continued fever

Even course – rising and falling in the evening.

Remittent fever

Reduction of the fever for 1-7 hours then an exacerbation.

Intermittent fever

Cessation of symptoms, increased secretions, acute pyrexia, returning at intervals. Definite course.

Relapsing fever

Cessation of symptoms but a relapse after several days and may be repeated more than once.

All fevers are in accordance with the amount of vital resistive strength available

Typological bias in the treatment of fever

The athletic or sthenic reaction - when congestion is prevented by adequate surface perspiration.

Asthenic reaction - an inadequate pyrexia in most cases. Support the nervous system and encourage sufficient pyrexia. It is preferable to avoid strong stimulants and rely upon nervine tonics and trophorestoratives to elevate the fever.

Cook explains the treatment of fever according to the typology. 'The level of stimulation or relaxation must be adjusted according to the vital resistive strength'. A combination of relaxation and stimulation is required in acute disease. The relaxing influence is obtained from Sambucus, Nepeta. Stimulation with Achillea.

Fever treatment

The following regime is used for fevers of all kinds including the treatment of infectious diseases. Some fevers may require a less powerful treatment depending on the pathocausative condition.

Complete rest is required – physical, emotional and intellectual. A room that is well ventilated and warm with the exclusion of everyone except the carers is needed. Feet should be kept warm. Food should be avoided until fever, pain or convulsions have cleared. Filtered water can be given with a suitable diaphoretic.

Medicines for the skin, capillaries and nerves in the pyrexial state

Relaxants are employed to take the blood to the skin surface together with stimulating herbs. Nepeta or Asclepias as relaxants with Zingiber as a stimulating capillary remedy.

Relaxing nervines of the diffusive class - *Lobelia, Nepeta, Sambucus, Tilia, Eupatorium perforatum*. Lobelia has the advantage of possessing the power of relaxing arteries and capillaries and soothing peripheral nerves.

Suitable nervines are *Piscidia* [CNS], *Primula* [peripheral nerve], *Lactuca* [spinal], *Pulsatilla* [ENT and reproductive system], *Humulus* [CNS], *Dioscorea* [GIT], *Viscum* [GIT], and *Chamomilla* [both types for GIT].

Fasting - the digestive processes need to be engaged in the processes of elimination not digestive assimilation. Because fasting takes a lot of vital energy from the tissues it is preferable to build up the tissue strength before commencing the fast.

Acute disease and inflammatory processes call for a fast. In deficiency diseases and chronic disease states, intermittent fasting helps more than the consumpton of health foods [190 p15].

In acute disease the body gives off large amounts of morbid and toxic waste. The vital energies are concentrating on the cleansing and healing processes. Kuhne claimed that disease consists of an accumulation of waste and morbid matter in the body, the most efficient way to clear the tissues is to fast. In many cases of weakness, lowered vitality and low resistance the tendency towards encumbrance of the tissue increases. Toxins that are not eliminated would create autointoxication - where toxins produced from cellular processes are reabsorbed into the tissues. To keep the elimination active the secernants are stimulated to remove the toxins. Secernants - bowel, skin, liver and kidneys.

Extra functional elimination always creates new symptoms. It is quite natural for the tissues concerned to produce eliminative symptoms. Gastro intestinal symptoms include a coated tongue, nausea, sometimes vomiting and purging.
Nervous symptoms always accompany the elimination of toxins - fear, depression, hallucinations, irritability and irritation commonly surface when fasting. Emotional temperaments and sensitive/negative people need a lot of support with fasting. Lindlahr suggested great care with the asthenic types. More robust athletic types can fast more easily, they have less nervous fragility.
Fasting has been continued for up to 104 days with no apparent ill effects [190].

Ketosis
Starvation is not the aim of therapeutic fasting [190 p16].
Fasting is catabolic and breaks down toxins. When fasting, the body scours the system for fats and sugars. Fatty acids are broken down with the liberation of ketone bodies. *Sweet smelling breath* is found as acetone is excreted. It is usual to have ketosis with fasting. When ketosis is found the patient must take nourishing fluids. It may be necessary to use fruit juices or grated carrot or apple if the patient becomes unwell from hypoglycaemia.
Following the fast use non-citrus fruits, vegetables, millet, cous cous, bulgar wheat, sesame, brown rice and an allergen free diet. The diet must be built up very slowly using mashed foods for the first six hours or so. Gradual change towards a more normal diet can follow.

Summary
During disease the diet needs to be simple or there may need to be a fast. Where food is eaten it must be light and easily assimilated. Fruits, salads and vegetables together with juices are best for nourishment. Acute disease requires no food whatsoever, only water as thirst dictates.
Too much or the wrong kind of food will delay healing and it will not be properly assimilated.
Eating will interfere with the elimination of waste. When food is eaten the vital force is diverted from its work of combating disease to digestive processes, thus delaying recovery. A short fast on fluids for 24 hours will be very beneficial to the vital force. See also food regime.

17
Treatments for the systems

Each system contains information on medication, diagnostics, conditions and treatments. The lists of medicines at the start of each chapter reveal a quick reference guide as an aid to memory.
Refer to the Pharmacopoeia for detailed information on any particular medicine.

EYES, EARS, NOSE AND THROAT

Eye medications
For inflammation, bacterial, fungal or viral infections, soreness, ulcers, weakness of the ocular eye muscles, degenerative conditions of the eyes.

Adonis vernalis - local anaesthetic in iritis, iridocyclitis.
Allium - antimicrobial.
Aloe vera - allays inflammation, antimicrobial.
Artemesia abrotanum – conjunctivitis – poultice [228 p349].
Berberis vulgaris - antimicrobial.
Butea frondosa - inflammatory states.
Calendula - allays inflammation, antimicrobial.
Chamomilla - allays inflammation.
Chamaemelum nobile - conjunctivitis, meibomian cyst, use the collyr and
fomentation.
Chelidonium - conjunctivitis, inflammation, infective opthalmia.
Cimicifuga - cranial nerve remedy.
Cineraria - opacity.
Euphrasia - optic astringent tonic. Antiseptic.
Foeniculum - allays inflammation.
Hamamelis - astringent. Antiseptic.
Hydrastis - antiseptic, antimicrobial, antiviral, antibacterial, astringent and tonic.
Oenothera oleum – collyr gtt for dry eyes.
Pilocarpus jaborandi - reduces ocular pressure, conjunctivitis, glaucoma, iritis, detached retina, optic neuritis, retinal haemorrhage, iridocyclitis [iris & ciliary body], keratitis.
Piscidia - inflammatory or painful conditions of the eyes.
Pulsatilla - allays inflammation, nervous eye disorders, astringent, antiseptic.
Ricinus communis – soothing demulcent to the eye.
Rosa damascena aromatic water - a cooling astringent.
Rubus - optic astringent.
Ruta - ocular muscle tonic.
Salvia - antiseptic.

Eyes

Sambucus - inflammatory eye conditions, antiseptic.
Scutellaria - cranial nerve remedy.
Sempervivum – allays ophthalmic inflammation, astringent.
Solidago – antimicrobial.
Stellaria - collyr for eye inflammation, emollient, demulcent, discutient.
Thymus - visual disturbances - infection, inflammation use collyr.
Uva ursi – anti-infective, antimicrobial, mucous membrane astringent.
Vaccinum myrtillus - optic vasodilator, optic trophorestorative.

Miotic – dilates pupil
Areca, Atropa, Cannabis, Pilocarpine.
Mydriatic – constricts pupil
Coca, Datura, Duboisia myoporoides [192 p164], Gelsemium, Grindelia, Hyoscyamnus.

Formulary for ocular medicines – external use

Carrier for eye medications
Ocular lubricants
Althea, Aloe vera gel, Cetraria, Chondrus, Ricinus communis - will soothe the skin and eye.

Eye fomentation
Infuse the herb and apply as a fomentation. Aromatic waters or LE can be used.
Chamomilla, Euphrasia, Foeniculum, Quercus.

Eye drops
Always instil eye drops with the patient lying down. Get the patient to look up and hold head backwards. Instil the drops and close the eye for one minute. Cover with an eye pad if required.

Collyr applications. [Collyrium - Eye Lotion]
Eye preparations should be sterile. [See Sterilisation technique Chapter 34].

Collyr Aloe
Aloe vera succus. Dispense undiluted. Sig 5gtt directly into the eye.
Collyr Euphrasia
Tincturae Euphrasia Sig 10gtt et aqua Rosae in an eyebath.

Collyr Euphrasia et Hamamelis
LE Hamamelis 5ml LE Euphrasia 5ml Aqua rosae 30ml
Inflammatory and infected conditions of the eye. Sig 3-5gtt in an eyebath.

Herbal Medicine - Keys

Variation of the medicament for the condition presenting:
Althea, Calendula, Chamomilla, Foeniculum, Hydrastis or Rubus.

Collyr Ricini [Castor oil eye drops]
> Ol Ricini

Dispense 10ml Sig 1gtt PRN

Unguent pro oculis [Eye ointment] Euphrasia eye ointment.
> Paraffin molle   60g
> LE Euphrasia   5ml

Apply PRN. Variation of the medicament for the condition presenting.

Unguent Hydrastis Hydrastis eye ointment

Hydrastis [1:5] 2ml. Hydrous wool fat to 60g. Melt under a gentle heat add the tincture and mix.

Eye examination

Using a good light observe the face, eyes and lids. To examine the underside of the lid roll the lid over a cotton wool bud.

Diagnostic stains

Fluorescein – strips or drops, after examination of the eye drops use saline to wash out the eye.

Mydriatic. Atropine dilates the pupil – never used in glaucoma or raised intraocular pressure. Pilocarpus 1% counters the effect of atropine.

Irrigation of an eye

Normal saline/Aloe vera. Patient holds a dish next to their face and looks away while the collyr is run across the face to the eye. Running the collyr across the face and then on the eye helps the patient to get used to fluid on the face before it before it reaches the eye thus avoiding shock.

General treatment perspectives for eye conditions

Palming the eyes involves placing the palms of the hands over the eyes and applying gentle pressure for half a minute. The technique encourages more blood supply to the eyes. Massage of the occipital bones encourages relief of tension - Oleum Lavandula diluted is helpful when applied to the temporal or occipital bones and helps to relieve head pain.

Hydrotherapy - apply a cold compress for inflammatory conditions and to improve arterial blood supply and eye drainage.

Vitamins A and C support eye health.

Eyes

Cause of many eye troubles

Many eye troubles result from reflex disturbances in the body. Sometimes areas seemingly unconnected with the eye e.g. liver, renal or bladder disturbance. Any mucous membrane disorder could affect the eyes. Treatment is aimed at the cause of the condition.

The eyes reflect one's health and many common conditions are first seen in the eyes. Typical examples are; sclerotic changes, cholesterol pigments, conjunctival irritations, blepharitis, corneal changes, scleral abnormalities and thyroid disorders. The iris shows disorders of the body; alterations within the fibres of the iris, the amount of light or dark, pigments superimposed upon the iris, organ health etc., the subject is called Iridology.

Eye conditions

Bags or shadows under the eyes
Aetiology
Anxiety, Depression, Exhaustion, Hepatic disorders, Insomnia.

Blepharitis
Raw red lid margins and enlarged lid. Irritation but no pain.
Aetiology: Possible renal trouble, infection or mucous membrane disorders

Blurred vision
Aetiology
Blocked tear ducts
Acute conjunctivitis
Acute iritis – blurring, floating spots, pain in eyeball
Acute glaucoma
Degenerative conditions – atherosclerosis
Hepatic disorders.
ME
Thyrotoxicosis

Cataract
An opacity of the lens becoming milky white with a waterfall appearance.
Aetiology
Defective circulation to the eye and accumulation of impurities. Due to inadequate nutrition. Associated with sclerosis in the blood vessels. It may result from disorders of the kidney, liver or pancreas, X-rays or sunlight damage, steroid therapy, shampoos containing laurel sulphate.
Treatment
Use foods as listed under retina also vitamin B2, C, E. Zinc.

Herbal Medicine - Keys

Collyr made from Chelidonium fresh plant tincture or the expressed juice.
Cineraria maritima - smarts a bit [or Euphrasia] requires long term use.
Ruta is effective in cataract.

Conjunctivitis
Redness affects the conjunctiva. Usually bilateral. Eye feels hot and gritty with itching or irritation. Discharge is mucoid. Mildly photophobic. Variable discharge. A frequent cause is an allergic sensitivity or a lacrimal obstruction. Vision is not affected.

Aetiology
Blepharitis
Catarrh
Corneal exposure from lid deformity
Foreign body e.g. dust/chemicals
Hay fever/allergy
Infections/toxins due to: flu/bronchitis/pneumonia
Ingrowing eyelash - entropian
Keratitis
Opthalmia neonatorum [newborn] from gonococcus infection
Sub tarsal concretions, beneath lower lids
Symblepharon
Stye
Trachoma – a viral infection produces tiny warts, distorts the lids and scratches the cornea [see also lacrimal system].

Corneal/dendritic ulceration
Ulcer pain may be considerable. Vision may not be affected. Corneal opacities can occur in the late stages of severe disease.
Aetiology
Drugs, injury.
Treatment:
Injury to the cornea requires soothing demulcents/Aloe vera eyewash and trophorestoratives. Vitamin A and C.
Collyr: Aloe vera, Ulmus, Hydrastis.
Used in an eyebath and as a compress to the eyelids. Internal Px of the same.

Chalazion
An infection of meibomian gland
Treatment
Eye drops of an antiseptic nature e.g. Hydrastis/Echinacea/Euphrasia.
Cleanse the blood using vasotonic alteratives.

Eyes

Dermatitis of eyelids and face
Aetiology
Cosmetics may cause a dermatitis. Infection. Scratching.
Treatment
Remove the offending cosmetic [See under skin for treatments].

Diabetic retinopathy
Medicine
Ginkgo biloba, Vaccinium myrtillus, Vitis vinifera, Zanthoxylum.

Dry eyes
Aetiology
Associated with rheumatism - Sjogrens disease – deficient lacrymal secretion.
Menopause
Secretory disturbance of the pancreas.
Treatment
Collyr Aloe vera or Oenothera.

Foreign body not fixed to the lens or cornea
Treatment
Remove the foreign body by flicking out with a cotton wool bud using an aseptic technique.

Floaters
Transparent, grey or black floaters [black specks] in the vitreous fluid. They can occur singly or as multiple floaters.
Aetiology. Blood impurities from hepatic disturbances. Migraine
Treatment
Agrimonia, Artemesia vulgaris, Chionanthus, Cnicus, Echinacea, Erythraea, Filipendula, Leptandra, Taraxacum.

Glaucoma
Raised intraocular pressure due to blockage of the schlemm canal, the aqueous humour cannot be removed from the anterior chamber.
An important **cause of blindness.**
Often secondary to other diseases. Acute congested glaucoma is due to obstruction [blocked drains]. Sometimes due to inflammation or tumours. Anxiety raises intraocular pressure. On examination the eye feels stony hard to palpation. The eye is red/brown and there is severe pain often above the eye. Vomiting can occur. Shallow anterior chamber. Rainbow halos around lights, intermittent **blurring of vision which is severe.** Photophobia is frequently present. Corneal oedema. The pupil is oval, semi dilated and fixed. Intraocular pressure is raised.

Opthalmoscopy reveals: pale cupped optic disc.

Treatment

Acute condition - referral may be necessary. An notifiable disease.
Because of the chance of developing blindness glaucoma is a very risky condition to treat.

Medicine

Calendula, Cannabis, Capsicum, Equisetum, Fagopyrum, Pilocarpus jaborandi, Pilocarpus pinnatifoleus, Pilocarpus microphylus - from which is derived pilocarpine, as a treatment for glaucoma – it is cholinergic, increases salivation and produces diaphoresis [60]. Urtica. Vaccinum. Collyr Capsicum.

Hay fever/allergy

Medicine

Aloe vera, Euphrasia.
Ephedra will stop irritation of the mucous membranes [vasoconstrictor].

Hordeolum/styes

Aetiology

Blood impurity/lymphatic congestion. Rundown condition. Check secernants - it can occur from toxic intestinal reabsorption.

Treatment

Warm water bathing and epilate the eyelash [pull it out]. Bathe the eye with Calendula and Sambucus
Local antimicrobial as drops or preferably an ung of Baptisia, Echinacea, Hydrastis.

Hypermetropia see Refractive error

Injury

When stained a lesion may be seen. Pain is common. Vision is affected in corneal trauma. Lacrymation is increased. Photophobia is usual. Corneal or conjunctival foreign body may be present.

Iritis - acute form

Dull constant pain. Blurred vision due to exudate. Rainbow halos. Worsening of sight. Radiating pain.
Aetiology - Mild and relapsing associated with spondylitis. When more severe – gonorrhoea, syphilis or TB. Associated with chrohn's disease.

Medicine - Iritis

Achillea, Aloe, Chamomilla, Cimicifuga, Euphrasia, Hydrastis, Pulsatilla, Sambucus. Collyr - Aloe vera, Hydrastis.

Eyes

Ingrowing eyelash
Can occur from a scar as in entropian where the eyelid turns inwards. Sometimes a congenital condition.
Treatment
Epilate eyelash using an aseptic technique.

Itchy eyes - treat as catarrh or hay fever.

Keratitis
An acute inflammation of the cornea that may progress to a corneal ulcer. Often secondary to conjunctivitis. Little blurring of vision unless the ulcer is centrally placed. Persistent discomfort, grittyness and pain. Ulcers hard to see. Greyish patch of infiltrate.
Treatment as iritis

Lacrimal system
Dacrioadenitis – an inflammation of the lacrymal sac often with infection. A tender, swollen lacrimal gland. Oedema of the upper lid. Chronic cases show painless enlargement.
Bilateral causes - reticulosis, sarcoidosis, TB.
Treatment
Use antimicrobials - wash out the sac using Aloe vera collyr.

Lid - abnormalities
Congenital or genetic predisposition. Epicanthus – Asian faced appearance, overgrowth of eyelids.
Lid retraction
is present if a band of white sclera is visible above the iris when the eyes are looking straight ahead.
Aetiology
Usually due to thyrotoxicosis and associated with frequent blinking and lid lag – exothalmus [the upper lid seems to lag behind the eyeball when the patient looks downwards].
Space occupying lesion
Myopia – eye larger than normal

Macular degeneration – age related
Age related macular degeneration – affects the macula region of the retina. Commonest cause of blindness in England. It is due to the degeneration of the macula. It causes loss of central vision and makes peoples faces go blurred. The central words disappear from any sentence. The lens is frequently at risk from free radicle damage. Free radicles promote macular degeneration.

Opthalmoscopy reveals: atrophic patches, clumps of pigment, elevated macula - grey encircled with hard edged white exudates, splattered with superficial haemorrhages and punched out circular hole. It is genetically determined.

Treatment

Carotenoids are concentrated in the macula lutea. Carotenoids increase the density of the macular pigment. The most significant carotenoids are:
[1] Alpha carotine; carrots and pumpkins. [2] Beta carotine; apricots, carrots, cantaloupe, peaches, spinach. [3] Cryptozanthin; oranges, papaya, peaches, tangerines. [4] Leutein and Zeaxanthin; broccoli, celery, kale, peas, red pepper, spinach. [5] Lycopene; pink grapefruit, tomatoes, water melon [57]. Selenium. Vitamin C, E.

Medicine

Vaccinum myrtillus. [See also diabetic retinopathy].

Meibomian cyst see swelling

Myopia [see refractive error]

Neoplasms
Benign
Papilloma. Zanthelasma – a disturbance of fat metabolism. Globules of fat in the eyelid or surrounding tissue.

Treatment

Cleansing of the blood using vasotonic alteratives. Adequate liver and gall bladder excretion.

Malignant
Rodent ulcer
Treatment - Trifolium pratense. Allium.
Melanoma – lumpy swelling which is of a brown or black colour. Hard swelling with proptosis.

Night blindness
Aetiology
Vitamin A deficiency

Opthalmia neonatorum
A notifiable disease which occurs from a gonococcus infection.

Orbital cellulitis [See under nose section].

Eyes

Pain in the eye
Aetiology
Glaucoma. Migraine. Herpes zoster.

Pinquecula fatty deposits on the iris

Pupil size
Aetiology
Head injury, multiple sclerosis, neurosyphilis, tabes dorsalis, sarcoidosis

Ptosis
[Blepharoptosis] drooping of the upper lid.
Aetiology
Congenital either unilateral or bilateral.
Acquired - usually unilateral if due to [1] cranial nerve paralysis [2] paralysis of the cervical sympathetic.
Bilateral due to myopathy or bells palsy.

Pterygium
A triangular patch of mucous membrane growing on the conjunctiva.
Treatment
Hydrastis. Microdesmis puberula - fol and emulsion.

Puffy eyes
Aetiology
Catarrh
Foreign body
Inflammation
Renal disturbance

Red eyes
[See under conjunctivitis]

Refractive error
Hypermetropia - long sightedness causes the image to fall outside of the eyeball, the image does not converge and is due to diminished power of accommodation.
Rarely causes symptoms in adolescence.
Called presbiopia in those over 40
Myopia short sightedness causes the image to fall in front of the retina. Distance vision is lowered. Usually found in late childhood.

Retinitis

Aetiology

Retinal inflammation secondary to infective or systemic disease processes - diabetes. Parasitic toxoplasmosis infection from undercooked meat. Eclampsia.

Retinitis pigmentosa

Is a common condition. The peripheral retina is affected. There are peripheral deposits of black pigment.

Retinoblastoma

A highly malignant tumour.

Scleritis

For causes see conjunctivitis.

Sore white eye

Aetiology

1 Majority of pains in normal looking eyes without visual loss have no organic basis. Some are forms of stress headache.

2 Blepharo - conjunctivitis or iritis - inflammation is barely visible.

3 Glaucoma - mild

4 Acute retrobulbar neuritis – multiple sclerosis gives pain on movement of the eyeball, tenderness of the eyeball, blurring of central vision.

5 Sore white eye present on waking – neuralgia from sinusitis.

Squint/strabismus

Aetiology

Ocular muscle weakness

Treatment

Eye muscle exercises using the formula -x-

The eyes are put through movement in three planes that will strengthen all six pairs of ocular muscles in both eyes. [1] horizontal plane [2] imagine a large X in front of the eyes, next look at the upper top right then lower bottom left, repeat upper left and follow to lower right corner.

Ruta graveolens tones the ocular muscles.

Styes [See under hordeolum]

Swelling and deformities

Aetiology

External stye. Injury.

Sebaceous cyst – eyelid skin

158

Eyes

Meibomian cyst – pea size swelling
Papilloma – lid margin grow into long horns
Treatment
Constitutional - alterative and eliminative vasotonics.
Chamamelum nobile.

Symblepharon
Are adhesions between the eyeball and the eyelid. They can occur from irritants, sprays and burns.

Retinal problems
Detached retina
Aetiology
Injury. Possible implication with pancreatic disease
Treatment
Beneficial to treat the pancreas and liver/ gall bladder.
Vitamin A may help the retina along with
Carotenoid foods: carrots, peaches, apricots, broccoli, spinach, cantaloupe, celery, pumpkin, tomatoes, watermelon, pink grapefruit, red pepper, peas, kale, oranges, papaya, tangerines.
Medicine
Vaccinum myrtillus.

Retinal haemorrhage
Central retinal arterial changes. Opthalmology will reveal retinal changes.
Aetiology
Arteriosclerosis, Blood disorders, Hypertension.
Diabetes.
Treatment
Lycopus. Vaccinum. Plus constitutional treatment.

Trachoma
A common cause of blindness in poor countries. The infection Trichomonas is responsible. It is an infective condition. The infection sometimes returns.
Red, swollen, tear filled eyes, half shut with discharge that virtually glues the eyes together. Then the eyelids turn inward, making the lashes like sharp bristles. Corneal scarring occurs in untreated patients, this causes blindness.
Treatment
Allium and Echinacea ointment. Aloe gel.
Vasotonic alteratives. Berberis vulgaris. Hydrastis.

Herbal Medicine - Keys

Trauma
Black eye
Bony damage, oedema, haematoma, ecchymosis and discolouration. Often from injury.
Treatment
Use a cold compress frequently.

Ulcers [See under cornea].

Uveitis
An acute emergency.
History may include urethritis, infection, diabetes. Aching of the eye and severe photophobia. Considerable visual loss. Corneal redness and oedema. Pupil is contracted and irregular. Possible raised intraocular pressure. Treat as iritis.

Watering of the eyes
Aetiology
An uninflamed eye may water with a blocked tear duct.
Tears - depression/happiness/sensitivity.
Arc eyes: the eyes become sensitive to bright light - associated with use of welding torches.
Allergy, Conjunctivitis, Catarrh, Hay fever
Foreign body
Photosensitivity
Sticky discharge of infants

Worms in the retina
Aetiology
From ingestion of worm eggs
Treatment
Allium.

Ears

Ear treatments
Many of the remedies used for eye conditions apply to ear disorders.
Allium - antiviral, antifungal, antibacterial.
Cimicifuga - vasotonic alterative. Motor nerve antispasmodic and sedative.
Euphrasia - anticatarrhal. Aural astringent. Antiseptic.
Glechoma - anticatarrhal. Astringent. Antiseptic.
Piscidia - Inflammation or pain of otitis media.
Pulsatilla -
    anticatarrhal, stimulating and astringent to the mucous membranes. Nervine.
Sambucus - anticatarrhal. Antiseptic.
Solidago - anticatarrhal. Astringent. Antiseptic.
Verbascum - anticatarrhal.

Formulary for aural medications
Ear drops [guttae]
Use the otoscope first to examine the meatus.
The following may be used in guttae - diluted tincture, liquid extract or Oleum
[essential oils must be diluted].

- Guttae oils should be warmed first. Put the oil onto warm a teaspoon . Lie patient on the unaffected side then instil the drops into the ear.
- Guttae - to soften hard wax Ol Almond/Ol Olive/Ol Verbascum. Instil warm oil 3gtt into the ear.
- Guttae - for otitis media – dilute Tr Commiphora 2gtt and Tr Hydrastis 2 gtt with Oleum Almond 2ml. Lie the patient down for 5 minutes.
- Sig drops 5gtt into the ear.
- Guttae - antiseptic etc. Allium capsule oil can be instilled into the meatus.
- Guttae – deafness, otosclerosis, tinnitus.
- Various guttae can be used – Oleum Verbascum or Cimicifuga or this can be made by using LE Verbascum, LE Cimicifuga diluted with almond oil.

Pulsatilla can be used for inflamed conditions, infective conditions, deafness etc. With these above conditions the rule is a daily application over a long period of time. Keeping the sinuses clear always helps ear problems.

Poultice
Perforations, infections, hearing loss – put crushed material onto gauze. Bind into place over the ear. The following poultice can be applied to the ear - bulb of Allium sativa or onion, Chamomilla or Plantago.

Hearing tests for auditory loss
Use a watch, with the opposite ear closed this will give the range of hearing.
The Rinne test.
The vibrating tuning fork is held on the mastoid bone then in front of the ear. If the sound is louder on the bone than in front of the ear the rinne is said to be negative and the deafness is conductive. If the sound is better in front of the ear the rinne is positive and is either normal or there is perceptive deafness. Sound carries better in air.
Middle ear deafness - air conduction diminished or lost, bone conduction normal.
Auditory nerve damage - air and bone conduction diminished or lost.
Total deafness gives a negative rinne, [no ear sound]. Bone carries sound to the good ear.
Weber test.
Test with a watch first to find the poorest ear. The vibrating tuning fork is then held in the midline on the forehead. Sound is heard in the ear with conductive deafness. Sound is lateralised to the deaf ear.
Middle ear deafness - sound is heard better on deaf side.
Auditory nerve deafness - sound only heard on the healthy side.
The occlusion test.
The tuning fork is held on the mastoid bone. The ear is covered with the finger and the sound is louder. In conductive deafness there is no change.

Hearing disorders

Deafness [Also see under hearing loss].
Deafness has either a conductive or perceptive loss.
Aetiology:
Conductive deafness occurs in the outer ear, from the ear to the tympanic membrane.
Perceptive deafness has its causes in the inner ear. Perceptive deafness is due to a sensory neural deficit and is due to a cochlear or retrocochlear lesion.

Skin conditions associated with the ears
Basal cell carcinoma
An ulcer of the helix which has a history of long duration See Chap. - malignancy.

Erysipelas
Raised erythematous rash that spreads to involve the face.
Haemolytic streptococci are implicated. [See Chapter on dermatology].

Eczema
[See dermatology].

Ears

Furuncle
Painful. Enlarged lymph nodes adjacent to the pinna are painful. [See Ch 3 & 26].

Gouty tophy
Occur on the helix as fixed, hard white lumps. [See Chapter 3 & 26]

Herpes zoster [See Chapter 3 & 26].
A vesicular eruption confined to the distribution of the nerve. Often very painful.
Keratosis
Warty growth of the helix that may become malignant, they may be multiple.
[See Chapter 3 & 26].

Otitis externa/eczema
An itch is the main symptom. It may be aggravated by an ear discharge. Fungal infections give rise to irritation and pain. [See dermatology].

Squamous cell carcinoma or melanoma
An ulcer of the helix of short duration. [See Chapter 31].

Ulcers
Ulcers of the helix are often inflammatory and may have a secondary infection.
[See dermatology].

Hearing loss [See Chapter 3].
Aetiology
Outer ear - catarrh
Foreign body
Injury - perforated drum
Inner ear – drugs, neomycin
Tinnitus
Otosclerosis

Cholesteatoma
A white mass of epithelium within the middle ear may resemble a neoplasm. It can become infected and produce a painless foetid discharge.
Where pain, vertigo or headache occur they suggest intracranial complications or labyrinthritis.

Mastoiditis
Resulting from infective processes within the ear. Brain abscess is a serious complication. Promote elimination via the intestine.

Medicine - mastoiditis
Baptisia, Capsicum, Commiphora, Echinacea, Hydrastis, Phytolacca, Pulsatilla.
Vitamin C.
Inhalation of Eucalyptus, Menthol, Tea Tree, Thymol.

Meniers disease
Signs and symptoms - vertigo, tinnitus, deafness, nausea and vomiting.
Aetiology
Allergy
Anxiety – sometimes severe anxiety can aggravate the Meniers.
Drugs
Focal sepsis
Hypotension. Sodium retention.
Medicine
Antispasmodic tincture, Chamomilla, Cimicifuga, Crataegus, Ginkgo, Humulus, Passiflora, Stachys, Tanacetum parthenium, Valeriana, Viscum, Zanthoxylum. Magnesium.

Mucopurulent discharge [See Chapter 3].
Aetiology
Catarrh. Infection.

Nystagmus
Nystagmus is seen as rapid eye movements either slow or quick and occurring in rapid succession. The movement of the eyes is towards the involved labyrinth during the quick phase. Nystagmus occurs in abnormal balance. The semicircular canals of the labyrinth are disordered by the disease process.

Otitis media [See Chapter 3].
Of an acute nature, produces earache with conductive deafness and fever.
Aetiology
Catarrh, infection, enlarged tonsils or adenoids
Neoplasm.

Otosclerosis
Aetiology bilateral conductive deafness eventually.
Chronic mucus in the middle ear
Bone changes e.g. arthritis

Ears

Pain in the ear/earache [See Chapter 36].
Aetiology
Cold air, draughts, foreign body, impacted wax
Otitis media
Perforated drum
Yeast infections

Pre auricular sinus [See Chapter 3].
May produce a discharge and inflammation. Furuncle in this site strongly suggests an infected sinus.

Perichondritis [See Chapter 27].
Pain, red, swollen pinna with fever. Chronic cases can produce hoarseness. Nasal septum may collapse. Often associated with an infection of the knee cartilage.

Pinna lumps [See Chapter 27].
Aetiology
Uric acid, rheumatic disease.

Red Drum
Aetiology
May follow a head injury
Bleeding into middle ear from infection, otitis media.

Tinnitus
May follow any form of ear disease e.g. trauma, otitis, otosclerosis, wax. Nervous tension. Noise induced deafness. Meniers disease – deafness, headache, vertigo. Drugs – salicylates, quinine, antibiotics. Avitaminosis – B vitamins.
Anaemia, cardiac disease, vascular insufficiency [tinnitus not severe]. Renal affections. Fractured base of skull. Intracranial tumours. Syphilis.
History - localise the condition. Right ear or left ear? both ears? inside head? Is there any hearing loss?
Characteristics – continuous, pulsatile, clicking, whistling, ringing, hissing etc.
Associated symptoms – hearing disorders, vertigo, headache, visual symptoms.
Past health – past inflammatory disorders, ops, trauma, noise, drugs, metabolic disorders [thyroid], hypertension, and allergies. Enquire about psychiatric history.
Medicine
Capsicum, Cimicifuga, Crataegus, Echinacea, Equisetum, Ginkgo, Glechoma hederaca, Hydrastis, Primula veris, Salix alba, Scutellaria, Tanacetum parthenium, Tilia, Verbena, Viscum.

Herbal Medicine - Keys

Tumour

Glomus jugulare tumour. Red drum, no pain, slow growth, intracranial spread – fatal. Cholesteatoma. Neuroma.

Medicine

Echinacea, Galium, Iris, Phytolacca, Rumex, Thuja, Viola odorata.

Vertigo

Aetiology

Disorder of the labyrinth

Drugs

Epilepsy

Head injury. Post traumatic

Hyperventilation

Hypoglycaemia

Inflammatory - from an upper respiratory infection

Lesions in the cerebellum e.g. tumours. Nystagmus has no latent period or fatigue in cerebellar lesions where vertigo is sensitive to movements of the head.

Meniers disease

Migraine

Multiple sclerosis

Positional - positioning of the head, backwards, when lying down, bending backwards or to one side produces severe vertigo but clears after several seconds. Usually self limiting in its effects. Nystagmus may also be present.

Stress

Vesicles on the drum

Aetiology - often associated with glue ear.

Osteoma

White bony hard swelling deep within the meatus of the ear is common.

Nose

Nasal treatments
Many prescriptions will be aimed at the sinuses as they affect the nasal passages.

Anticatarrhal medicines
Allium, Baptisia, Berberis Vulgaris, Cochleria, Echinacea, Ephedra, Euphrasia, Commiphora, Glechoma, Phytolacca, Sambucus, Sticta, Solidago, Uva ursi, Also see the eye and ear sections for medicines.

Formulary for nasal drops and sprays
Nasal drops are known as Naristillae or Narist. For short.

Naristillae Ephedra Ephedra nasal drops
> Ephedra 5ml
> Aqua to 25ml

Administer using a dropper to each nostril. Sig 3gtt.
Indications - Profuse nasal catarrh or hay fever.

Nebulae Cinnamon compound Cinnamon nasal spray
> Tr Commiphora   7ml
> Tr Cinnamomum 7ml
> Aqua Camphora 3.5ml
> Aqua Rosae   300ml

Spray the nostrils as required
Used in nare ulceration and infective catarrh and colds.
Alternative remedies e.g. Ol Eucalyptus/Menthol can be used.

Nasal diagnosis
Nasal Blood supply - Ophthalmic artery
                                  - maxillary artery
                                  - littles area
Venous return - via the skull into the internal jugular artery

Nasal sinuses
diagnostic pressure points
> 1] Frontal sinus
> 2] Ethmoidal sinus
> 3] Maxillary sinus

Trans illumination techniques. A technique to observe the sinuses. With the room darkened, a bright light is held in the mouth. It is used to illuminate the sinus area. A dull maxillary sinus suggests sinus disease. Dental cysts illuminate brightly.

Nasal Conditions

Loss of the sense of smell

<u>Aetiology</u>

Catarrh. Pharyngitis. Viral infection. Injury.

Epistaxis

<u>Aetiology</u>

Trauma – blow
        foreign bodies
Hay fever, Atrophic rhinitis
Infection – common cold
Tumours
Hereditary telangiecstasis
Hypertension
Bleeding disorders e.g. Haemophilia, Leukaemia. Thrombocytopenia [low platelet count]
Anti coagulants
Jaundice – vitamin K deficiency, Scurvy
Enteric fevers e.g. typhoid

Mucocoele/pyocoele [See Chapter 3].

Collection of mucus within a sinus which causes swelling and pushes the eye forward and down [proptosis]. Examination looking down onto the head is necessary. Where erosion of the sinus occurs swelling will be seen over the frontal sinus. Progression to pyocoele may occur.

Orbital cellulitis

A localised infection with inflammation can occur with sinusitis, it may progress to an abscess with possible complications [brain abscess, meningitis]. The affected orbit could be very swollen. A rapidly growing neoplasm [rhabdomyosarcoma] may simulate a cellulitis. History of an infection would confirm the diagnosis. [See Chapter 3].

Nasal polyps

Polyps do not usually bleed. Pigmented, ulcerated or a bleeding polyp may be malignant.

Aetiology of polyps: Excessive mucus production from toxic encumbrance

<u>Treatment</u> - polyps

Cold water splash to the face.

<u>Medication</u>

Teucrium chamadrys orally and as snuff.

Thuja orally and as a paint.

Polyps continued
Snuff: Myrica, Quercus and Sanguinaria - powders.
                    Powdered Sanguinaria, use tiny amounts only.
Nebulae or Naristillae: Commiphora, Ephedra. Essential oleum diluted.

Sinusitis [See emergency herbal medicine]
Aetiology
Catarrh, fumes e.g. petrol, paint, infection, polyps.

Sneezing
Aetiology
Allergy, smoke, dust, colds, rhinitis, fever, foreign body.

Snoring
Aetiology
Alcohol, catarrh, depression, infection, obesity. Hay describes the inability to let go of old thoughts and feelings as a cause of snoring.
Treatment
of the cause. Garg. and inhalations.

Throat, tongue and mouth

Oropharynx medicines for periodontal gum disease and hygiene.

Acacia senegal - Oral plaque. Periodontal infections.
Allium – antiseptic, bacteriostatic in aphthous ulcers,
Aloe vera - protects mucous membranes. Sprayed or used as a mouthwash helps in pain and infection. Eases the ulcers by clearing infection and healing the ulcer.
Aloe and Echinacea - provide cover for Gingivitis, Stomatitis, Dental caries and Pyorrhoea
Althea – allays inflammation, protects mucous membranes.
Apple cider vinegar - astringent and antiseptic for all mouth, tongue and throat disorders.
Azadirachta indica - dental caries.
Baptisia – antiseptic.
Berberis vulgaris – antibacterial, antifungal. Oral inflammation.
Calendula – antiseptic, soothing and allays inflammation.
Chamomilla – antiseptic, allays inflammation, oral inflammation.
Chamaemelum nobile – as above.
Chondrus crispus – demulcent.
Collinsonia - congestion with redness or hoarseness.
Commiphora – antiseptic and disinfectant, stimulating to mucous membranes.
Coptis – astringent and to mucous membranes. Aphthous ulcers.
Echinacea – anti infective.
Galium - fresh juice painted on the tongue soothes inflammation and heals ulcers.
Geum urbanum – astringent.
Gnaphalum – astringent.
Hamamelis - oropharyngeal inflammation, gingivitis.
Hydrastis – mucous membrane astringent tonic, antiseptic, allays inflammation, mucous membrane trophorestorative.
Massularia acuminata [Randia acuminata] is antimicrobial against oral pathogens associated with orodontal infections - Bacteroides gingivalis, Bacteroides melaninogenicus, G. Gigivalis and G. Meelaninogenicus and Streptococcus.
Melaleuca – antifungal.
Mentha piperita - oral antiseptic, anaesthetic.
Myrica cerifera – astringent.
Olea europaea - contains calcium elenoate, a potent antimicrobial for toothache and mouth infections.
Pilocarpus - eases the pain of ulcers.
Piper methysticum - local anaesthetic
Piscidia – inflammation, infections or gum bleeding.

Tongue

Populus candicans – anti infective. Propolis tincture - swab the area with diluted Tr. 5 gtt. Mouth ulcers, soreness of the lips or mouth. Use the Collutoria.

Quercus - astringent.

Salvia - rubbing a leaf around the gums will help to prevent pyorrhoea. Syrupus Salvia gives relief in tonsillitis, gingivitis and aphthous ulcers. Fresh leaves clean and whiten the teeth.

Sanguinaria - stimulating. Oral plaque. Oral antibacterial – streptococci.

Styrax benzoin – antiseptic.

Symphytum – mucous membrane trophorestorative.

Szygium - toothache, oleum applied on cotton wool will ease the pain and is antiseptic.

Thymus - tonsillitis, aphthous ulcers - oral antiseptic and anaesthetic.

Trifolium - salivary gland congestion, pharyngitis.

Tsuga canadensis - aphthous ulcers, gingivitis, stomatitis.

Uncaria – anti viral - vesicular stomatitis.

Urtica – cleanser.

Vaccinum – aphthous ulcers, leucoplakia.

Formulary of preparations for mouth disorders

Gargarismata or garg. for short [Gargle].

Garg antiseptic [Antiseptic gargles]

- Apple cider vinegar 15ml and dilute with 30ml aqua.
- Baptisia 1ml dilute with 30ml aqua.
- Echinacea and Commiphora 0.5ml aa dilute with 30ml aqua.
- Aloe gel is suitable to use undiluted for the above conditions.

Use in catarrh, halitosis, aphthous ulcers, pharyngitis, and tonsillitis.

Sig 30 ml gargle [swallow if desired].

Garg halitosis

Carum 10g. Cinnamomum 15g. Myristica 5g. Szygium 5g. Ethanol 125ml Aqua 375ml. Sig Garg. 5gtt et aqua 50ml.

Collutoria 1 [Mouthwash]

Compound Thymus et Glycerine
Tr Thymus 10ml Glycerine 30ml aqua to 50ml
Sig 5ml et aqua for oral health.

Collutoria 2

Stryax 5gtt et aqua 100ml Sig Rinse oral cavity PRN.

Collutoria 3

Mouthwash of 5% zinc is antiplaque.

Herbal Medicine - Keys

Stomatitis prescription
Glycerine, Hydrastis and Commiphora.

Irritated or sore throat prescription
5ml lemon juice, 5ml glycerine, 5ml honey, dissolve in 300ml hot water.
Drink freely.

Nutritional therapy for mouth conditions
Vitamin A, C, beta carotine. Minerals - copper, zinc. Zinc stabilises the mucous membrane, inhibits plaque and mast cell histamine.

Tongue & Mouth Disorders
Test for taste and smell sensation can be done by making up some small bottles of strong solutions. Then ask the patient to confirm the taste and smell of the solutions.
For taste use sugar [sweet], saline solution [salt], vinegar [sour], gentian [bitter].
Smell sensation is tested with ammonia, cloves or peppermint oil.
Check for lack of salivation in patients ask the patient.

Tongue

The tongue is reflective of the alimentary tract

Taste
Loss of taste – colds and infections adversely affect the taste buds.
Metallic taste - hepatic/biliary disorders. Myalgic encephalomyelitis.

Atrophy
Aetiology
Atrophy may produce a **smooth** tongue in pernicious anaemia, iron deficiency anaemia, hypoglossal cranial nerve damage/disease, accompanied by burning sensations.

Burning or dryness of the tongue and mouth
Aetiology
Dryness of the tongue indicates deficient fluid intake. Dryness occurs with a tendency to deficient secretion [Cook].
Excessive dryness is found in internal inflammation. Without any related evidence of inflammation or lack of salivation it may occur as a manifestation of anxiety. Diabetes. Typhoid fever. Ulceration of the small intestines. [See also tongue soreness] Penicillin hypersensitivity induces burning sensations on the tongue.

Tongue

Ulcerations
Painful greyish or white ulcers in the mouth.
Aetiology
Aphthous ulcerations, Bechet's syndrome, Blood impurity, Diphtheria, Erythema multiform, Leukaemia,
Pemphigus, Secondary ulceration is common and infection by streptococci or staphylococci.
TB may produce painful inflamed ulcers of the tongue, lips and mouth.
Trauma from ill fitting dentures, Vitamin B2 deficiency.

Coatings on the tongue

Has the patient been eating anything coloured?
Black furry tongue
Aetiology
Fungal infection, diabetes, blood poisoning, mucous membrane disorders of the stomach/intestine.
Brown and dry
Aetiology
Found in many severe illnesses – local inflammation, stomach or liver disorders, acute intestinal obstruction, malabsorption, diabetes, typhoid fever, uraemia.
Brown like gingerbread
Aetiology
Found in malignant and bilious fever, typhus.
Brown like leather
Papillae are pointed, patchy or elevated – typhoid fever.
Creamy appearance [furry]
Aetiology
Aids - candida. Inflammation of the stomach, catarrh of the stomach.
Dull slate grey
Aetiology
Brown buccal pigmentation opposite molar teeth. Is a feature of adrenal disease.
Furring of the tongue [See black tongue]
Aetiology
Smoking. Mouth breathers.
Inadequate dietary fibre.
Green
Aetiology
Disorders of the biliary tract.
Grey
A dusky or grey coating may infer nervous weakness.

Majenta

<u>Aetiology</u>

Cheilosis – riboflavin deficiency [B2] there are superficial fissures at the angles of the mouth [angular stomatitis]. The tongue is majenta.

Fissures are subject to fungal infection.

Orange red

<u>Aetiology</u>

Arteritis nodosa, pernicious anaemia - treated with Vitamin B12 injections. Oral preparations of B12 will not work once the pernicious anaemia is present.

Pallor

<u>Aetiology</u>

Anaemia

Deficiency of blood to the tongue.

Purple

<u>Aetiology</u>

Lung or heart disease.

Red tongue

<u>Aetiology</u>

Allergy may cause erythema, swelling and ulceration of the tongue.

Atrophic glossitis [beefy tongue] See also smooth tongue/local itis.

Alcoholism, anaemia, gastritis, diabetes, intestinal haemorrhage, malabsorption, pellagra, pancreatic deficiency, steatorrhoea.

Red tip and edges

Inflammation of the stomach.

Scarlet tongue see inflammation

Strawberry colour

<u>Aetiology</u>

Scarlet fever.

Early stages - the tongue has a white coat and bright red papillae. After a few days the white coat disappears leaving a strawberry appearance – strawberry tongue.

Yellow tongue

Biliary disturbances.

White coating

<u>Aetiology</u>

Aids. Candida. Fever. Leucoplakia. Gastric derangements or Mucus congestion.

Dry tongue

<u>Aetiology</u>

Dehydration. Mouth breathing

Deficient secretion from the mucous membranes of the stomach or intestines.

Stomach nerve derangement. Diabetes. Intestinal ulceration.

Typhoid. Wasting diseases. Rheumatoid arthritis produces a dry mouth. Sjogrens disease.

Tongue

Shrunken tongue implies insufficiency of blood. Feeble heart action.

A moist tongue implies an open state of the secretions
Mucus coating
Dyspepsia, bad taste in the mouth,
Thick white coat
Catarrh. Malnutrition
Secondary syphilis – produces flat, superficial, white to grey mucous patches which bleed easily when scraped. Glazed appearance.

Enlarged tongue
Aetiology
Enlarged and swollen red tongue with a white fur suggests derangement of the stomach/intestine with effect on the brain. Chronic digestive insufficiency. Mercury poisoning. Tertiary syphilis
Vitamin C deficiency

Flabby tongue
Glandular disease. Delirium tremens.

Fissuring
The deeper the fissure the more chronic the disorder. Fissures are subject to fungal infection.
Aetiology
Stomach nerve disorder
Congenital fissuring of the tongue produces symmetrical furrows and normal papillae.
longitudinal fissure
Stomach or intestinal irritation.
transverse fissure
Renal irritation.

Geographic tongue
Aetiology
Hypotrophic gastro intestinal tract. Diabetes
Pyrexia

Papillae
Loss of filiform papillae of the tongue
Aetiology
Niacin deficiency [B5, nicotinic acid] this causes – chronic dyspepsia, glossitis, papillary atrophy, stomatitis, dematitis, diarrhoea, finally dementia.

Papillae unnaturally prominent and moist, bright red and clean.
Derangement of stomach nerves.
Movements of the tongue
Shakiness - virtually always suggests a nervous temperament
Deviation to one side – upper motor neurone lesion [stroke]
Thrusting or darting tongue suggests chorea.

Sore or painful tongue
Aetiology
Aphthous ulcers. Burns to the tongue
Erythema multiform from drugs, infections or systemic disorders
Vitamin deficiency. Collagen disease.

Staining of the gums and teeth occurs in fluorosis and tetracycline use. Fluorosis, once evident confirms poisoning of tissue, the teeth can have a mottled appearance. The mottling of the teeth is permanent.

Under surface of the tongue
An ulcer on the frenum may be due to coughing
Varicosities are found in some elderly patient

Mouth

Oral mucous membrane may be involved in allergic reactions, purpura, liver disease, telangiectasis and scleroderma, pemphigus, lichen planus, and vitamin deficiencies.
Cheek pigmentation occurs in addisons disease and small intestine polyps.
Addisons disease produces grey or blue pigmented spots.

Measles
Small bluish white spots surrounded by a red areola, known as Koplicks spots. [See Chapter 12]

Abscess
Collection of pus and infection from inadequately eliminated toxins. [See Ch 3].

Breath bad [See halitosis]

Candida
White plaques like milk curds can cover the entire oral cavity in severe cases.
If found as a symptom of aids this is a poor prognostic sign. [See Chapter 24].

Mouth

Diphtheria
Fever and toxaemia with white plaques that bleed on removal. [See Ch 24].

Fillings
Vitamin E, antioxidants, and selenium can reduce mercury toxins from fillings.

Gingivitis
Inflammation and soreness of the soft tissues and the gums with bleeding.
Swollen and necrotic in chronic mercury poisoning - see below.
Gingivitis can accompany pyorrhoea, diabetes, systemic disease, anaemia, leukaemia or vitamin C deficiency. Food impacted between the teeth. Oral sex can initiate gingivitis. Pregnancy.

Halitosis
Aetiology - inadequate intestinal elimination, infected intestine.
Treatment: Promote elimination via the intestine. [See under laxatives].
Medicine
Agrimonia, Allium, Artemesia, Baptisia, Cassia, Commiphora, Filipendula, Glycyrrhiza, Iris, Linum, Papaya, Petroselinum, Phytolacca, Salvia, Trigonella.

Herpes simplex and zoster
Attacks the tongue and mouth with very painful vesicular eruptions.

Leucoplakia
White plaques inside of the cheeks or tongue.
Aetiology
Aids – when found in association with aids – poor prognosis. Dental troubles.
Dietary irritations. When the tongue is involved it is characteristic of tertiary syphilis.
Medicine
Aloe, Calendula, Commiphora, Hydrastis, Salvia, Sempervivum, Vaccinum.
Vitamin A, C.

Lichen planus
Distribution – buccal mucous membranes, sacrum, wrists, legs.
Medicine – lichen planus
Capsicum with Commiphora as a small dose in oral lichen. Plus constitutional treatment.

Mumps
Enlarged parotid gland, high fever and loss of appetite. Orchitis follows mumps.

Medicine - mumps
Capsicum, Angelica archangelica, Baptisia, Calendula, Echinacea, Erythraea, Phytolacca, Pulsatilla, Scutellaria.
Use a cold compress to the throat.

Papilloma virus
Papilloma can develop on the vocal cords. Children complaining of hoarseness require to be checked as the papilloma can occlude the larynx.
Medicine
Capsicum, Commiphora.

Paralysis of the vocal cords
Aetiology
Nerve damage or tumour.

Periodontal gum disease
Parotitis, stomatitis, glossitis, gingivitis, loose teeth, receding gums, plaque, bleeding and tender or painful gums.
Treatment must be constitutional with advice upon diet along with frequent collutoria [mouthwashes].
Co-enzyme Q10 Sig up to 100mg daily. Maintenance dose: 15-30mg daily.
Vitamin C, B12, folic acid. Zinc.
Medicine
Anti infective and astringent.

Poisoning
Lead: deposits a black line along the gingival margins.
Poisoning with mercury, may cause severe swelling, redness, necrosis, erosions and ulcerations of the mouth, tongue and gums.

Pyorrhoea
Infective condition of the gums.

Salivary gland cancer
Ascorbic acid can influence the risk of salivary cancer. It inhibits the conversion of nitrate to nitrite and reduces the formation of cancer forming nitrosamines [22]

Sore throat
Infectious mononucleosis
Known as glandular fever. A sore throat is seen with a white membrane covering the tonsil.

Mouth

Stomatitis
Red, dry and sore mucous membranes.
Aggravated by dentures

Plaque
Folic acid binds toxins secreted by plaque.

Thirst
May be seen in mouth breathing, dehydration, diabetes, diarrhoea, fever, haemorrhage.

Toothache
Toothache: Oleum Szygium 2gtt applied on cotton wool will ease the pain. It is powerfully antiseptic.

Inflammation of the larynx
Laryngitis [See inflammation]
Acute or chronic laryngitis presents with hoarseness. The mucous membrane is hyperaemic. Vocal cords may swell and hypertrophy.

Laryngitis acute
Aetiology
Chill from cold. May follow upper or lower respiratory tract infection.
Overuse of the voice. Tobacco smoke.
Papilloma on the vocal cords. Myxoedema.

Loss of voice
Aetiology
See laryngitis
Acute nervous reactions - panic, shock.
Head injuries
Vascular troubles e.g. CVA.
Laryngeal nodes. Polyps. Carcinoma.
Pharyngitis - chronic
A hyperaemia of mucous membrane on the posterior wall of the oropharynx.
Persistent slight sore throat is a main symptom.

Quinsy
An abscess may form with tonsillitis. Symptoms can be severe with fever, pain in the throat and ear, dysphagia, and malaise.
If the quinsy bleeds, erosion of an artery is suspected.

Scleroma

A painless chronic inflammation of the upper respiratory tract in which a white plaque forms. Use the mirror to see behind the uvula for plaques.

Tonsillitis

Aetiology

Patients are often very ill with acute tonsillitis. Sore throat, pyrexia and dysphagia, hyperaemia and purulent discharge are common. Tonsillar lymph glands at the angle of the mandible are large and tender. Infection, often from a toxic intestine.

Treatment

Fast. Fluids only.

Cold compress to the neck – remove when warm. Vitamin C.

Garg Salvia. Garg Lemon juice. Garg Apple cider vinegar.

Collutoria – Salvia.

Medicine

Baptisia, Capsicum, Commiphora, Echinacea, Hamamelis, Hydrastis, Phytolacca, Salvia.

18
Respiratory system

Expectorant and carminative medicines
Mild expectorants which also exert a gentle carminative action upon the digestive system making them suitable for children and to counteract the nauseas effect of stronger expectorants:
Hyssopus
Pimpinella

Antiallergic and antihistamine medicines
Althea, Baptisia,
Chamaemelum nobile, Chamomilla recutita,
Echinacea, Euphrasia, Ephedra,
Ganoderma lucidem, Gnaphalum,
Hydrastis, Hyssopus,
Mentha piperita,
Paeonia lactiflora, Picrorrhiza kurroa, Pinellia ternata, Propolis, Pulsatilla,
Quercetin a flavonoid found in onions has a natural antihistamine effect,
Rehmannia glutinosa,
Salvia officinalis, Sambucus, Schizandra chinesis, Scutellaria baicalensis,
Stephania tetranda, Szygium, Tylophora indica, Uncaria tomentosa, Urtica,
Verbascum. Vitamin C has an antihistamine effect.

Bronchodilators
Angelica archangelica, Aspidosperma, Atropa,
Ephedra, Euphorbia,
Grindelia, Hyssopus, Lobelia inflata,
Passiflora, Pilosella, Symplocarpus,
Thymus, Trifolium.

Pulmonary and expectorant medicines
Drosera - demulcent, expectorant. Antiasthmatic.
Ephedra - antiallergic, bronchodilator.
Euphorbia – antispasmodic, expectorant. Sedative.
Grindelia - antispasmodic
Hyssopus - carminative and expectorant.
Inula - gently stimulating tonic expectorant. Diaphoretic and diuretic.
Lobelia inflata - relaxant
Marrubium - gently diffusive tonic expectorant. Diuretic. Bitter tonic.
Pimpinella - pectoral and carminative. Add to lung mixtures.
Prunus serotina - astringent, tonic pectoral. Sedative.
Pulsatilla - stimulating to mucous membranes, antiallergic.

Herbal Medicine - Keys

Sanguinaria - powerful stimulating expectorant with tonic properties.
Sticta pulmonaria - demulcent and astringent pectoral.
Tinospora – [Guduchi] antimicrobial and immunostimulant
Tussilago - demulcent, diffusive expectorant & tones the bronchi.
Urgenia – stimulating expectorant
Verbascum - demulcent, astringent and alterative to the lungs.

Fluids are essential in the treatment of respiratory and infective conditions.

Formulary of Inhalations, linctus and syrups

Inhalation of Menthol
Menthol crystals 3g. Tinctura Benzoin to 100ml.
Sig 5ml to 500ml aqua frig. Inhale the vapour.

Inhalation of Menthol & Eucalyptus
Menthol crystals 3g. Ol Eucalyptus 3ml Aqua to 100ml.
Sig 5ml to 500ml aqua frig. Inhale the vapour.

Linctus
Linctus Acacia
Acacia 6%, Syrup 74ml, Aqua Auranti 20ml.
Cough linctus Sig 15ml

Sedative linctus
Acacia 20%. LE Prunus Serotina 40ml. Syrupus to 100ml.
Sig 10ml PRN. Sedative and demulcent to irritable coughs. Remedy may be changed to Tussilago if desired.

Mucilage
Ulmus, Cetraria, Chondrus produce large amounts of mucilage for allaying irritable inflammatory conditions of the respiratory [and other] mucosal surfaces. Pour boiling water upon the required amount of remedy. After 10 minutes strain.
Add for stimulation of tissue and antimicrobial effects;
essential oleum e.g. Ol Cinnamomum, Melaleuca, Szygium or Salvia 1gtt.

Pastilles and lozenges
Obtain gelatine in fine powder. Melt on a water bath and incorporate the medicament as a suspension. Triturate [mix] if necessary. Lubricate moulds with almond oil then pour mixture into moulds to set. Each lozenge/pastille should weigh two grams. Sig Suck a lozenge PRN.

Respiratory System

Syrupus [Syrups]
Syrups are best for coughs due to the relaxing effect the syrup has on the respiratory mucous membranes.
To make a syrup: take Althea, Glycyrrhiza, Urtica, Prunus, Symphytum.
Simmer for 10 minutes. Strain and add 250g sugar, mix well and bottle.
Volatile herbs - Thymus, would require a sealed container. Menstrum brought to the boil and then the heat is turned off, the lid being untouched until the menstrum had cooled. Melt the sugar and add to the menstrum.

Respiratory conditions

Allergy
Aetiology
Hay fever
Food allergens can encourage hay fever attacks. The most common allergens are citrus fruit, chocolate, food colourings, dairy produce and wheat.
Dietary sodium can increase histamine sensitivity, cheese has sodium.
Medicine
Euphrasia, Ephedra, Pulsatilla, Sambucus, Urtica.
Prescription to relieve irritation.
LE Euphrasia, Drosera, Pulmonaria and Solidago - equal parts.

Asthma
Various medicines are used according to the conditions present:
Aspidosperma, Drosera, Ephedra, Euphorbia, Grindelia, Lobelia, Urgenia, Polygala senega, Sanguinaria, Symplocarpus.
Compound prescription - bronchial antispasmodic.
Tr Commiphora   7ml
LE Euphorbia   7ml
LE Grindelia   7ml
LE Lobelia   3ml
LE Symplocarpus 7ml   aqua to 250ml
Sig 10ml aqua cal.

Bronchitis acute/chronic/emphysema
Some suggested prescriptions.
Px1 Mentha pip, Symphytum, Marrubium, Tussilago, Glycyrrhiza, of each 15g
    add a pinch of Capsicum. Add 550ml of boiling water and infuse for 15
    minutes in a closed vessel.
    Sig 10 - 20ml in a wineglassful of hot water every 2 hours. Add essence
    Pimpinella 2gtt to each dose.
Px2 Marrubium, Hyssopus & Althea.
Px3 Tussilago1, Marrubium1, Pimpinella 1, Glycyrrhiza 1.

Px4 Acute Bronchitis; three day fast, follow with three day fruit diet. Epsom salts bath once a week. cold compress placed on chest as required.
Inula, Verbascum, Achillea - 30g of each.
Gently decoct in a closed vessel for ten minutes cool and strain.
Sig 30ml every 4 hours.

Cough mixture
Althea rad, Angelica, Chondrus crispus, Hyssopus, Marrubium, Mentha pip, Origanum, Sambucus, Symplocarpus, Thymus equal parts of each.
Decoct then add Chondrus separately. Add Glycyrrhiza last.
Sig 30ml PRN.

Carcinoma of the bronchus [lung cancer See Chapter 31].
Symptoms include: persistent chest infections, cough for more than three weeks, tiredness, haemoptysis, dyspnoea, loss of voice, chest pain, wt loss, facial and neck swelling.
Pre malignant cells could be detected by screening sputum from deep coughing.

Catarrh
Mist Nasal catarrh Mixture for nasal catarrh
Arctium, Iris, Phytolacca, Zanthoxylum, Dect. Sarsae. Co.
Colds
Herbal cold and cough medicine:
Infusium: Hyssopus, Marrubium, Tussilago aa equal parts. Sig 60ml TDS.

Vapour inhalation and vapour rub
An inhalation of volatile oil to clear the passages and remove catarrh.

Px Ol Camphor	2ml
Ol Eucalyptus	2ml
Ol Mentha piperita	1ml
Ol Pinus	2ml
Ol Thymus	2ml

Sig Put 5gtt into a bowl. Pour on 500ml boiling aqua. Lean over the bowl. Place a towel over the head and bowl - inhale the vapours.

Vick rub
Make a "vick" rub.
Two methods [1] by adding the essential oils to the infused oil of Helianthus or similar and rub onto the sinus area, chest and back.
[2] Paraffin molle can take 5 gtt essential oleum, then apply over the sinuses.

Respiratory System

Hay fever see allergies above.

Influenza
Influenza virus is spread through droplet contamination by coughing and sneezing.
Symptoms start suddenly with pyrexia, headache, sore throat, cough, aching limbs and back, and general weakness. Symptoms can be severe enough to require complete rest. Convalescence may take some weeks in order to enable a return to a normal level of energy.
Medicine
Sambucus or Achillea with Mentha and Composition essence.

Mist Influenza
Infusium - Mentha pip, Angelica archangelica and Melissa 10g aa.
For cold on the chest Marrubium is advised instead of Melissa.
Make the infusium @ 30g to 500ml
Sig 30ml QDS

Influenza formula [anti influenza to protect against influenza].
Achillea, Eupatorium perfoliatum, Marrubium, Mentha pip., Sambucus 12g aa.
Syzygium 10 cloves.
1 litre hot water leave, add pinch of Capsicum.
Sig 45ml with hot water and sweeten with honey.

Laryngitis
See EENT.

Mucovisidosis - cystic fibrosis
Pulmonary and anticatarrhal medicines [See above]
Chionanthus. Juniperus, Iris, Uva ursi.

Pertussus
Medicine
Allium, Hyssopus, Hieracium, Lobelia, Marrubium, Tussilago, Urgenia.

Mist pertussus [1]
Mentha pulegrum 10g, Hyssopus 10g, Angelica archangelica 10g.
Infuse 30g in boiling water. Strain and sweeten with honey if required.
Dose - babies 5ml QDS.
       - up to 5 years 10ml QDS.
       - adults 30ml 2 hourly.

Herbal Medicine - Keys

Mist pertussus [2]

LE	Drosera	3.5ml
LE	Hieracium	14ml
LE	Echinacea	7ml
LE	Trifolium	14ml
Tr	Lobelia acid	7ml
Infusion Thymus to		240ml
Syrupus simplex		240ml

Sig 10-15ml Aq cal frequently.

Syrup Pertussus [3]

LE Thymus	10ml
LE Trifolium	7ml
Tr Lobelia acid	3.5ml

Syrupus simplex to 100ml. Mix together.
Sig 5-15 ml PRN

Pneumonia/pleurisy [See Emergency conditions]
Inflammatory condition of the lungs and pleura often due to infection. Pleuritic pain can be severe. Pneumonia can accompany bronchial carcinoma and aids.
Example mixtures are given below:
Mixture 1
Mentha piperita, Sambucus, Thymus, Tussilago aa.
Mixture 2
LE Asclepias 10ml, LE Achillea 16ml, LE Bryonia alba 3.5ml,
LE Eupatorium perf. 5ml, LE Pulmonaria 3.5ml Aqua to 240ml
Sig 10-15ml frequently.
Mixture 3
Asclepias 0.5, Nepeta 1, Mentha pulegrum 1, Sambucus 1, Mentha pip. 0.5.

Sarcoidosis
Although a rare disease it closely resembles tuberculosis. Sarcoidosis can affect many different organs. The commonest site of clinical involvement is the lung. A honeycomb appearance of the lung results from infiltration.
Treat systemically using antitubercular medicines below.

Tuberculosis [See tropical diseases]

Yawning
Aetiology
Anxiety, circulatory disease, depression, drug effects, hepatic disease, tiredness, thyroid disorders.

19
Endocrine System

Some of the following medicines are obtained from radiational physics quoted from Lesourd and Turenne [Reference 1 p91-93].

Adrenal supportive medicines
Many renal remedies also act upon the adrenal glands.
Avena – nutritive to vasomotor neurones.
Borago - adrenal supportive.
Cimicifuga - small doses support adrenal function in exhausted states.
Cola – stimulating to adrenal function, nerve enervation.
Glycyrrhiza - adrenal supportive.
Ledum [labrador tea], indicated in fatigue and weakness from adrenal exhaustion.
Panax - adrenal cortex supportive.
Rehmannia – adrenal trophorestorative.
Salix nigra for the adrenals and especially when impotence/sexual dysfunction is found.
Schizandra - Stimulating nervine trophorestorative - CNS. Adaptogenic tonic.
Zanthoxylum - adrenal tonic.
Pantothenic acid and potassium support the adrenal glands.
Plus:
Achillea, Apium, Berberis aquifoleum, Asclepias, Chamaemelum nobile, Euonymous, Gentiana, Iris, Leonurus, Mentha viridis, Nepeta cataria, Mitchella, Rubus idaeus, Verbascum.

Ovary, prostate and testicular medicines
[See also Gynaecology/Genito urinary tract]
Artemesia species, Carduus, Chamaelirium luteum, Dioscorea, Mentha pulegium, Pulsatilla,
Salvia officinalis, Serenoa, Sumbul – musk root, given in small doses for anxiety, hypertensive states associated with testicular trouble, Turnera, Viburnum opulus, Zanthoxylum, Vitex.

Pancreatic supportive medicines
Agrimonia, Agropyron, Arctium, Caulophyllum, Cassia, Chionanthus, Comiphora molmol, Eupatorium purpureum, Fraxinus americana, Gentiana, Geranium maculatum, Hydrastis, Inula, Iris versicolor, Mentha pip/pulg., Phytolacca, Rosmarinus, Rumex, Ruta graveolens, Sambucus, Sassafras, Scutellaria, Seneco aureus, Solidago, Smilax, Sticta pulmonaria, Stachys, Taraxacum, Tussilago, Verbascum.

Herbal Medicine - Keys

Pineal gland supportive medicines
Achillea, Baptisia, Berberis V., Calendula, Centella, Chelone, Convallaria, Crataegus, Equisetum, Fucus, Guaiacum, Hydrangea, Iris, Morinda citrifolia, Panax, Sambucus, Selenicerus, Taraxacum, Trifolium, Turnera, Tussilago, Valeriana, Verbena, Viola odorata.

Parathyroid supportive medicines
Achillea, Agrimonia, Asclepias, Berberis V., Borago, Calendula, Chelidonium, Chimaphilla umbellata, Cnicus, Convallaria, Crataegus, Dioscorea, Echinacea, Eupatorium perf., Euphrasia, Galium, Grindelia, Hypericum, Lavandula, Leptandra, Lobelia, Myrica, Populus trem, Rubus idaeus, Salix nigra, Salvia officinalis, Selenicerus, Stachys, Tanacetum parthenium, Thuja, Uva ursi, Valeriana, Viburnum opulus, Viscum.

Pineal and thymus gland supportive medicines
Agrimonia, Agropyron, Arctium, Caulophyllum, Cassia, Commiphora molmol, Echinacea, Eupatorium purpureum, Fraxinus americana, Gentiana, Geranium maculatum, Glycyrrhiza, Hydrastis, Inula, Mentha pip/pulg., Morinda citrifolia [Noni] - [The fruit contains proxeronine this converts into xeronine and is required for tissue repair - medicinal activity includes - adaptogenic, allays inflammation, antimicrobial, analgesic and stimulant - regulates the pineal, thymus and thyroid glands]. Phytolacca, Rosmarinus, Rumex, Ruta graveolens, Sambucus, Sassafras, Scutellaria, Seneco aureus, Solidago, Smilax, Sticta pulmonaria, Stachys, Taraxacum, Trifolium, Tussilago, Turnera, Tussilago, Verbascum, Verbena, Viola odorata, Viscum.

Pituitary anterior and posterior supportive medicines
Achillea, Baptisia, Berberis Vulgaris, Borago, Calendula, Centella, Chelone, Convallaria, Crataegus, Dioscorea, Equisetum, Fucus, Glycyrrhiza, Guaiacum, Hydrangea, Iris, Juglans sp., Medicago, Panax, Sambucus, Selenicerus, Smilax, Taraxacum, Thuja, Trifolium, Turnera, Tussilago, Valeriana, Verbena, Viola odorata, Zanthoxylum.

Thyroid supportive medicines
Althea, Arnica, Carduus, Chamaemelum nobile, Chionanthus, Convallaria, Dioscorea, Equisetum, Euonymous, Eupatorium purp, Fraxinus americanum, Fucus, Galium, Geranium maculatum, Hamamelis. Juglans, Iris, Leptandra, Leonurus, Lycopus, Morinda citrifolia, Phytolacca, Ranunculus, Seneco aureus, Thuja, Thymus, Uva ursi, Viola odorata, Vitex.

Endocrine System

Dysharmony in the endocrine system

A drop in the production of metabolites by receptor tissue induces overproduction of hormone from the stimulated organ. Adrenal disturbances induce excessive pituitary activity, often to the point of exhaustion. Similarly excessive target tissue function cuts off the production of stimulatory hormone. Excessive amounts of circulating hormone, cause reduced activity and atrophy of the producing gland. When hormones are not broken down due to a diseased liver resulting in oestrogenic cells ceasing production.

Acromegaly a growth hormone disorder. Typically found in adults and occurs from excess growth hormone. Bones of the jaw, hands and skull are enlarged.

Adrenal disease - hypoadrenalism

The adrenal glands weigh around 5 grams, have high oxygen consumption and have the highest content of vitamin C in the body. The cortex secretes adrenal steroid hormones [cortisol, DHEA's and Aldosterone]. The medulla secretes adrenaline and catecholamines. Adrenal activity is concerned with energy production, muscle and joint function, bone health, immune system health, sleep, skin regeneration and thyroid function. Muscles and bones are affected by too high cortisol levels. Sleep is disturbed by high cortisol levels. Thyroid disturbance may be due to adrenal insufficiency.

Low cortisol production from sluggish adrenal function can result in chronic fatigue syndrome. Recurrent stress depletes adrenal gland function.

Aetiology

Autoimmune disease, TB, Meningococcal septicaemia, continued stress, malignancy, amyloid infiltration.

Symptomatology is often vague.

Debilitating fatigue following exercise ME., weight loss, anorexia, enlarged lymph nodes,

Disturbances of mood and sleep. Impotence/sexual dysfunction, diarrhoea, confusion, amenorrhoea, hair loss, myalgia, buccal pigmentation which is a dull slate grey colour opposite molar teeth.

The immune system is also affected giving rise to an overstimulated or depressed response e.g. exacerbation of allergic responses [34].

Adrenal disorder can occur from steroid treatment and is known as Cushing syndrome. A moon face is found in the patient from fluid retention. Symptoms as above also diabetes, osteoporosis, frontal balding in males, plethora, purple striae of the skin, poor wound healing and peripheral muscle wasting.

Diabetes mellitus

Diabetes is a disorder of carbohydrate metabolism and is characterised by hyperglycaemia it is due to deficiency of insulin. Complications affect the eye, blood vessels, kidneys and nervous system. There are two types of diabetes: primary and secondary. Primary diabetes has two main types. Those which are insulin dependent and those which are non insulin dependent.

Diabetes can present as an acute, sub acute or chronic condition.

Acute diabetes often presents with weight loss, polydipsia and polyuria. Ketoacidosis and acute infection could be a first presentation.

Sub acute diabetes symptoms include pruritus, candida infection, fatigue, parathesia in the limbs and visual refractive problems [often myopia].

In all of the above cases a urine sample containing glycosuria and ketonuria is diagnostic of diabetes.

Anaemia is found in patients who have dietary imbalance, sugar disturbances, hypoglycaemia and potential diabetes.

Secondary diabetes often complicates hepatic, gallbladder, duodenal and thyroid disorders.

Cirrhosis, pancreatitis, adrenal disorder, thyrotoxicosis, stress, infections and steroids may precipitate diabetes.

Chronic diabetes eventually produces complications - retinopathy, cranial nerve lesions and peripheral neuropathy, renal disease/abscess/glomular damage, pneumonia, genital infections, balanitis, arteriosclerosis and gangrene. Impotence/sexual dysfunction, muscle wasting and proteinuria occur from renal involvement.

Anti diabetic synthetic drugs commonly used **do not prevent the effects** of diabetes from occurring.

Glucose tolerance test for the detection of diabetes.

Analysis of the medical history. Pulse and blood presssure checks.

Biochemistry checks for blood glucose, fasting blood glucose [taken AM before food or drink], triglyceride level, LDL, HDL., and cholesterol levels. Body mass index – see below. [417].

Treatment

It is inadvisable to fast diabetics.

Vegetarian diet.

Fish oil can be used in insulin dependency.

Medicine

Pancreatic disorders – Chionanthus, Galega, Gymnema sylvestre, Iris, Momadica charantia, Ocimum sanctum, Pterocarpus marsupium, Taraxacum, Trigonella.

Nicotinamide [B3] deficiency means an inability to synthesize glucose correctly.

Vitamin B6 may be helpful in peripheral neuropathy.

Vitamin C

Vitamin E 200mg daily may help diabetic ulcers.

Endocrine System

Chromium helps regulate sugar control. Low chromium is found in atherosclerosis – an effect of diabetes. Chromium is found in whole grains, nuts, brewers yeast.

Hypoglycaemia

Hypoglycaemia is a low level of glucose in the blood with consequent cellular starvation. Low blood glucose affects the brain to bring about a wide variety of symptoms. The brain uses some 40% of available blood glucose. Symptoms usually arise two hours after eating or early in the morning. It is aggravated by eating refined carbohydrates. Insulin makes the glucose available to the cell. Glucose is used for cellular energy. It is stored as glycogen in the liver and muscles. When the blood sugar level falls, the adrenal glands produce adrenaline, which stimulate the liver cells to release glycogen this produces glucose for the blood and cells. Hypoglycaemia tires the adrenals leading to hypotrophicity. Adrenal insufficiency can raise its head during a fast and treatment is needed to direct the medication towards the adrenal glands. Adrenal supportives are always required in treatment. For hypoglycaemia it is advisable to enquire about adrenal symptoms - exhaustion, chronic tiredness and thyroid function.

Most symptoms affect the intellect and the emotions. Symptoms range in their severity - headache, forgetful, irritable, temper tantrums, poor concentration, anti social behaviour, fatigue, muscle cramps – anywhere.

Diplopia, sweating, loss of consciousness and fits are often presenting features.

Hypoglycaemia

An **acute attack** of hypoglycaemia is best met with a spoonful of raw honey to provide blood glucose. The absorption of honey is a quick acting remedy. Treatment aims to stabilise the blood sugar levels. Diabetes must be treated if present. All patients must avoid refined sugar.

The **glycaemic index** [GI] of foods. Carbohydrates release glucose at different rates after consumption. It is preferable to reduce high GI foods as they cause insulin resistance and disturb blood sugar levels. If taken use a mixture of high and low foods to balance up. That is a diet with complex carbohydrates eg wholemeal bread, oats, sesame, nuts, wholemeal pasta, beans, pulses. Protein foods support the absorption and carry the carbohydrates encouraging the normalisation of the blood sugar.

Taking glucose as 100 we have some examples:

Parsnips	97
Baguette	95
Carrots	92
Honey	87

Cornflakes	80
Watermelon	72
Potato	70
Wholemeal bread	69
Rice brown	68
Muesli	66
Raisins	64
Oats	49
Baked beans	48
Carrots	49
Grapes	46
Soya beans	15

Hypoglycaemic dietary regimes

Chronic cases must attend to any problem associated with obesity.
Frequent small carbohydrate meals with complete attention to the diet.
Breakfast – fruit stewed, cereal,
Lunch – salad, potato, fruit
Dinner – protein; fish, meat, poultry with vegetables
Snacks in between meals will support the blood sugar – fruit including dried fruit, grains, nuts, yoghurt, oats, seeds – sesame/sunflower, muesli.

Hydrotherapy

A cold spray for 3 minutes daily will stimulate the pancreas.
Eat regular meals with a small snack in between. Snacks can consist of yoghurt, fruit, nuts, seeds, wholewheat crackers or bread.

Medicine for hypoglycaemia, the pancreas e.g. Chionanthus, Iris, Peumus, Taraxacum.
Liver and gall bladder *support* are frequently indicated e.g. Berberis vulgaris, Chicorium, Cynara, Mentha piperita, Peumus, Silymarin, Taraxacum rad.
Nervines are used if there is present any constriction further down the GIT. Treat any anxiety or stress issues found within the patient.
Muscle spasm can obstruct the outflow of bile from the gall bladder. Relaxing smooth muscle spasm can help, e.g. Chamomilla, Dioscorea, Scutellaria, Viburnum opulus, Viburnum prunifoleum, Valeriana, Verbena.

Mammary glands

Assess hormonal levels and any possible toxic focus when abnormalities are found. See gynaecology .

Endocrine System

Menopause

Known as the change of life as indeed the body changes in all its aspects – hormonally, physically and emotionally.

The menopause is a change of life and needs to be treated as such. What are the issues coming up for you or your partner at this time?

Symptoms of hormonal change:

flushes, mood changes, fertility cycle change [bleeding anomalies].

Oestrogen receptor binding medicines

Cimicifuga, Curcumin, Dioscorea, Glycyrrhiza, Humulus, Lobelia, Medicago, Oenothera, Pueraria – [kudsu], Rumex, Salvia, Sanguinaria, Smilax, Thymus, Trifolium, Turmeric, Turnera, Yucca, Viscum, Vitex.

Soya, peas, flaxseed, rye, wheat, sea vegetables, citrus fruits, grapes.

Vitamins A, B2, B6 B12, C, E, Magnesium.

Treatment perspectives

- Organs which can attribute to possible hypoglycaemia: liver/gall bladder, pancreas.
- Hormonal imbalance.
- Diet.
- Operations – are the ovaries remaining?
- CNS/ANS stress/tension/depression. Adrenal effects

Obesity

Obesity is a common condition and is defined as an excess of adipose tissue. It is found in overeating and in less than 1% of hypothyroid or Cushings patients.

Various weight to height tables with corresponding body frames give the level of weight for that body type as found in Davidson's principles and practice of medicine.

Weight – consider the waist measurement to be half or less that of the height.

Body mass index

The body mass index more accurately reflects the presence of excess adipose tissue. BMI is calculated by dividing body weight by the square of your height in metres. Over 25 is considered overweight.

BMI categories

	BMI [kg/m2]
- Underweight	less then 18.5
- Normal	18.5-24.9
- Overweight	25.0-29.9
- Obese	30-34.9
- Morbidly obese	more then 35

Herbal Medicine - Keys

Waistline circumference
Reflecting the amount of adipose tissue in the abdomen. Excess adipose increases the risk of cardiovascular disease and diabetes.
For men - a girth over 90 centimetres [37 inches]
Women – over 80cm [32 inches].

Basal metabolic rate at rest
The breakdown of food is a metabolic process and this process creates heat in the cells. The metabolic rate is obtained as a figure at bodily rest. The formula gives the resting metabolic rate in calories. This formula as given by Budd is as follows:
Under 30 years multiply weight by 14.7 and add 500
Over 30 years multiply weight by 8.7 and add 830
The resulting figure is the resting metabolic rate. This figure gives the calorie intake requirement per day. The calorie requirement figure is multiplied by 1.4 for a sedentary occupation and will increase by around 500 calories for an active person doing regular exercise.

Management of obesity
Treat any underlying - bullaemia, cushings disease, depression, hormonal disturbances or hypothyroidism. Encourage exercise.
Treatments
Clear the colon using laxatives. Stimulate the metabolism using stimulants. Diuretics if there is oedema, this is more common in pyknic types.
Amorphophallus konjac yields glucomannan – aids weight loss, is anticholesterolaemic and hypoglycaemic. [192 p239]. Capsicum, Foeniculum, Fucus, Galium, Stellaria.

Osteoporosis [See musculoskeletal system]

Parathyroids
Hyperparathyroidism
Hypercalcaemia occurs from excess of parathyroid hormone.
Adenoma is found in 85% of cases. Pancreatitis has been implicated.
Symptoms include: malaise, depression, peptic ulcers, hypertension.
Medicine
Centella, Fucus, Galega, Iris, Trifolium, Zanthoxylum.

Hypoparathyroidism
Signs and symptoms
Tetany, cramps, neuromuscular irritability, anxiety. Trousseaus sign – sphyg cuff inflated for 3 minutes resulting in tetany – spasm of the arm muscles.

Endocrine System

Calcium regulation

Governed by the parathyroid hormone, glucocorticoids, androgens and oestrogens, growth hormone, thyroid hormones.
Calcitonin is a hormone produced by the thyroid. It inhibits the reabsorption of bone and increases the excretion of calcium and phosphate. Magnesium binds to calcium and supports a balance of both minerals.
Medicine
Aphanes, Apium, Avena, Cetraria, Chondrus crispus, Equisetum, Fucus, Plantago, Scutellaria, Symphytum, Urtica, Zingiber.

Pituitary gland

Growth hormone deficiency. Hyperprolactinaemia. Hypopituitarism.
Hyperprolactinaemia – features galactorrhoea.
Hypopituitarism – has around 25 causes ranging from infective e.g. meningitis, vascular, traumatic, functional e.g. anorexia and tumours. Patients may have fluctuating emotions.
Bromine foods: asparagus, carrots, celery, cucumber, garlic, lettuce, melon, millet, mushrooms, onions, parsnips, peaches, rye, tomato.

Ovaries see above and gynaecology

Thyroid gland

Thyroid disturbance can be assessed by observing the **basal temperature** in the morning before rising over several days. A persistently lower oral temperature than normal assumes low thyroid function. Basal body temperature is between 36.6-36.8. The thyroid weighs between 8-40g.
A skin test for iodine absorption. Apply some iodine to the thigh, around an egg size. If the patient is very deficient in iodine the patch will disappear by the next morning. The test is dependent upon how rapidly the patch fades. Repeat the test to confirm the result.
The thyroid gland affects metabolism and the rate at which foodstuffs are utilised. Thyroid imbalance is a prominent factor in sexual dysfunction. Neuroendocrine links are complex and regulate the sexual function. Seaweeds are useful in patients who are hypothyroid and have related sexual weakness and nervousness. Adrenal activity is also impaired or exhausted in many cases of disturbed thyroid function. The thyroid is involved in immune deficiency conditions e.g. SLE, RA, Diabetes and Sjogrens syndrome. Some 30% of young people develop thyroid disturbances as a result of whiplash injuries to the neck. Puberty, pregnancy, postnatal depression, anaesthetics, glandular fever, lowered metabolism, post viral syndrome, alzheimers disease all affect thyroid function. Physiomedically speaking if one endocrine gland becomes disordered others may also be affected.

Women are affected with thyroid disturbances by 8:1. Females become more depressed and weight increases. Depression is a finding among all sufferers.

Thyroid conditions
Hyperthyroidism
Aetiology
Often occurs from an infective process.
Nodules may precipitate the reaction.
Malignancy – thyroid
Pituitary tumours. Ovarian tumour. Autoimmune effects.
Signs and symptoms: exopthalmus, hyperkinesis, atrial fibrillation, palmar erythema, muscle wasting/myopathy, diplopia, gritty eyes, weight loss, irritability, increased appetite.

Treatment Thyroid disturbances from iodine deficiency use Fucus. It is unusual now to find iodine deficiency, salt contains iodine. Fucus will not help where the thyroid has been removed. No changes in TSH have been found using Melissa it will not create a hypothyroid condition.
Reduce brassica and soya. Eat raw cabbage. Seafoods, Watercress.
Selenium is essential for the production of thyroid hormones. Low selenium causes a haemostatic increase in TSH. Glandulars affect the thyroid function.

Medicine for Hyperthyroidism
Fucus, Lycopus, Leonurus, sedatives.
For the conversion of T4 to T3 copper, iron, selenium and zinc are required. For the production of T3 vitamin A is required.
Glandulars. Adrenal supportives. Carnitine, Iodine, Phenylananine,

Hypothyroidism
Aetiology within the immune system, from infection or iodine/TSH deficiency.
Symptoms include goitre, menorrhagia, mental and physical fatigue, dry hair, loss of hair, anaemia, cold intolerance, neck and shoulder pain, polymyalgia type symptoms as muscles become affected this leads to fatigue, depression is significant, dry skin, slow metabolism, constipation, intestinal spasm, candida, slow reflexes, carpal tunnel syndrome, heart failure. Adrenals also become affected as they produce steroids and oestrogens after the menopause. Patients tend to feel worse in the morning: wiped out feelings, somnambulence. Hyperinsulinism. Underweight may occur in some individuals. Miscarriage. Progesterone deficit and oestrogen dominance with some hypothyroids. 35% of the oestrogen is formed in the adrenals and in fatty tissue.

Endocrine System

<u>Treatment</u> for Hypothyroidism
Response to treatment is often very slow.
Optimise nutritional status with whole foods. Care if fasting the patient.
Hydrotherapy - Cold throat compress to the thyroid, Sitz baths.
Treat the thyroid and adrenals together – Carnitine, Chromium, Iodine,
Phenylananine, Selenium. Vanadium.
Glandulars. Seafoods. Watercress.
<u>Medicine for Hypothyroidism</u>
Avena, Capsicum, Cetraria, Chondrus, Fucus, Ginkgo, Iris, Panax, Petroselenium,
Phytolacca, Smilax.
Elderly patients may require a long term maintenance dose.

Thyroid function tests
Ranges
T3 - blood life is an unreliable indicator.
Total T4   60-150 nmol/l - indicates the amount of thyroxine.
Free T4   8.8-27 pmol/l treat if under 15.
TSH   0.3-5.5 miu/l - abnormalities suggest a low level of thyroid hormone. TSH
is released by the pituitary in response to low blood levels of hormone.
Total cholesterol will be raised if there is a thyroid disturbance.

20
Cardio Vascular system & Blood Disorders

<u>**Cardio vascular medicines**</u>

Cardiac tonic and trophorestoratives
Aegle marmelos [Beli] containing aurapten, heals myocardial cells. Indications -
Angina pectoris, arrhythmias, pericarditis, and palpitations [263, 1991, 57 [1] p43
Capsicum, Crataegus, Convallaria,
Quillaja saponaria Aortic valve disease/hypertrophy Sig 0.25ml [BPC p364].
Pulsatilla, Selenicerus, Terminalia arjuna,
Calcium channel blockers [depress myocardial activity and nerve conduction].

Sedatives [Beta blockers]
Humulus,
Pulsatilla, Rauwolfia, Scutellaria,
Veratrum album/viride, Viburnum opulus, Viscum.

Arterial and capillary bed stimulants
Achillea, Angelica archangelica, Asarum canadense,
Capsicum, Cochleria
Fagopyron esculentum
Sarothamnus, Selenicerus, Serpentaria - CI in hypertension.
Zanthoxylum, Zingiber

Vasodilators
Capillary vascular bed relaxant including relaxing diaphoretics [Beta blockers]
Asarum canadense, Asclepias
Corallorhiza, Crataegus
Leonurus, Lobelia
Melissa, Nepeta
Ruta, Sambucus, Tilia
Viburnum opulus, Zanthoxylum

Venous tonics
Aesculus,
Cayenne, Collinsonia, Crataegus,
Fagopyrum,
Hamamelis, Hydrastis, Myrica,
Ruscus aculeatus, Stachys,
Vaccinum, Vitis vinifera.
Vitamin E.

Cardio vascular system & Blood disorders

Cholesterolaemia
See chapter 3

Formulary for circulatory conditions

Syrupus Stillingia

Stillingia	20ml
Iris	10ml
Sambucus	20ml
Chimaphilla	10ml
Zanthoxylum	10ml
Syrupus	160ml

Sig 5ml TDS aq cal pc.
A powerful lymphatic and immune stimulant that favourably influences the blood.

Blood disorders
Blood purifying mixture [1]

Arctium	0.5 ml
Cassia	1 ml
Fumaria	0.5 ml
Galium	0.5 ml
Menyanthes	0.5 ml

Sig 3ml TDS.

Blood purifying mixture [2]

Arctium	0.5ml
Capsicum	5 gtt
Echinacea	0.5ml
Iris	1ml
Rumex	1ml
Trifolium	1ml
Mixture of Senna Co.	6ml

Sig 10ml BD, TDS.

Blood purifying mixture [3] [Stimulating alterative after Dr England].
Arctium
Berberis aquifolium
Iris
Rhamnus purshiana
Sanguinaria
Trifolium
Zanthoxylum

Herbal Medicine - Keys

Naturopathic treatments
Hydrotherapy
- The alteration of blood volume is well established using hydrotherapy principles. Arm baths to increase coronary perfusion.
- Foot baths to draw blood from the head.
- Abdominal compress to relax and relieve inner congestion.
- The temperature of the water is significant in all hydrotherapy treatments.

Fasting is beneficial for cardiac patients. It is a requirement that patients drink not less than 1400ml water each day in addition to the fast. In one study cardiac patients in severe cardiac failure were fasted. Many of these recovered in our clinic, even after they had been shown to be previously refractive to cardiac drugs [190 p17]. For specific hydrotherapy treatments see also Chapter 16.

Cardio vascular conditions
Anaemia
1. Aplastic Failure of the bone marrow to produce enough red blood cells.
2. Haemolytic Abnormal destruction of red blood cells.

Pernicious anaemia - Vitamin B12 deficiency and requires Vitamin B12 injections
Sickle cell anaemia - gene defective DNA
Thrombocytopenia – Gentiana, Smilax, Vitamin K.
Medicines
Arctium, Capsicum, Centella, Chionanthus, Cichorium, Cnicus, Echinacea, Equisetum, Fucus, Gentiana, Medicago, Melilotus – Mononucleosis,
Petroselinum, Picraena, Rumex - iron, Salvia, Smilax, Stellaria, Taraxacum rad, Trifolium, Urtica - iron, Zanthoxylum, Zingiber.
Several bitter tonics are available for prescription in anaemias.
Vitamin C. B12. Zinc. Molasses. Watercress.

Angina pectoris
Is caused by sclerosis or spasm. Treat the liver, pancreas, arterial and nervous system.
Medicines
Ballota, Capsicum, Crataegus, Leonurus, Sarothamnus, Terminalia arjuna, Tilia, Zanthoxylum.

Arteritis
Onset 50-70. Headache with burning or tenderness is mainly unilateral. Clinical features – blurring of vision, fever, sore joints and muscles. Fundi – cotton wool exudates, flame haemorrhage, distended retinal veins. Ischaemic optic neuritis can develop in 50% of untreated cases.

Cardio Vascular system & Blood Disorders

<u>Medicines</u>
Capsicum, Convallaria, Crataegus, Filipendula, Gelsemium, Ginkgo, Selenicerus, Tanacetum parthenium, Ruta, Urtica, Valeriana, Zanthoxylum.

Atherosclerosis cerebral [Arteriosclerosis]
Cerebral ischaemia resulting from sclerosis. Check for diabetes.
Stimulate the cerebral circulation.
<u>Medicines</u>
Allium, Armoracea, Capsicum, Centella, Cola, Ginkgo, Phytolacca, Stachys, Zanthoxylum, Zingiber.

Arrhythmia/palpitations/tachycardia
<u>Medicines</u>
Ballota, Capsicum, Convallaria, Crataegus, Cytissus, Gelsemium, Leonurus, Passiflora, Rauwolfia, Terminalia arjuna, Tilia, Valeriana, Zanthoxylum.
Reflex disturbance e.g. flatulence, indigestion, anxiety can also cause conduction defects.
<u>Medicines for reflex conditions</u>
Dioscorea, Melissa, Rosmarinus, Zingiber.

Cholesterolaemia [See also Chapter 3].
Cholesterol does not cause heart disease. Dr Joel M. Kauffman introduces a book by Dr Uffe Ravnskov MD PhD 'The Cholesterol Myths'. In which he quotes 'no study has ever proven that lowering the amount of cholesterol in the diet reduces the risk of heart disease.... Lowering cholesterol through drugs won't prevent arteries from hardening if homocysteine is high' quotes from his book - Kilmer McCulty MD [2000].
Coronary mortality is not lowered by lowering cholesterol. BMJ 1992, 305.
Studies have been ignored or misquoted J Clin Epi. 1995 48, 713-9.
Statins not due to cholesterol lowering. BMJ 1995 311, 1436.
Coronary heart disease. Stehbens, WE [2001]. Experimental & Molecular pathology, 70, 103-119 & 120. Article in CAM April 2003.

Endocarditis, myocarditis, pericarditis
<u>Medicines</u>
Convallaria, Crataegus, Cytissus, Echinacea, Selenicerus, Terminalia arjuna, Tilia.

Glandular fever
Presenting symptoms are fever, lymphadenopathy. Splenic enlargement is found in 50%. Liver enlargement found in 12%. Recovery can take a year

Herbal Medicine - Keys

Medicines for glandular fever
Achillea, Allium, Baptisia, Berberis aquifoleum, Capsicum, Collinsonia, Commiphora, Echinacea, Eucalyptus, Hydrastis, Iris, Phytolacca, Sambucus.

Heart failure/CCF
Medicines
Capsicum, Convallaria, Crataegus, Hydrastis, Terminalia arjuna.

Hypertension
Assess the need for a relaxing impression upon the heart, arteries and capillaries. Tonic action upon the veins is required in most cases, rarely do the veins require a relaxing impression. Are there obstructions within the sercernant eliminative organs giving rise to the hypertension? Renal disorders – check the urine.
Hypertension medicines
Achillea, Capsicum, Crataegus, Gelsemium, Humulus, Lobelia, Parietaria, Sambucus, Tilia, Valeriana, Veratrum, Viburnum opulus/prunifoleum, Viscum.

Hypokalaemia
Low potassium can result from inadequate intake, diarrhoea, dehydration, vomiting, starvation, diuretics, digitalis and laxative abuse. Cardiac effects produce - premature contractions, tachyarrhythmias and AV block.
Signs and symptoms Muscle cramps - tetany and weakness.
Treatment
Increase fluids. Grape juice. Bananas. IV infusion in severe cases.

Hypotension
A low blood pressure results from cardiac disorders, hypokalaemia, adrenal disturbance, hypoglycaemia, renal disturbances. Emotional disorders - chronic anxiety, fear or shock.
Treatment - tone and stimulate the organism.
Medicines
Angelica archangelica, Capsicum, Convallaria, Crataegus, Cytissus, Ephedra, Myrica, Panax, Rosmarinus, Stachys, Zanthoxylum, Zingiber.

Inadequate peripheral circulation/arterial/venous
See hypertension
Ischaemia
Stimulate the arterial circulation.

Oedema
Treat the heart, circulation and kidneys. The precise remedy depends upon the cause.

Cardio Vascular system & Blood Disorders

Palpitations
Medicines
Antispasmodic Tr, Arnica, Avena, Chamomilla, Crataegus, Lavandula, Leonurus, Lobelia, Lycopus, Melissa, Panax, Passiflora.

Paralysis
Medicine
Arnica, Capsicum, Centella, Cimicifuga, Ginkgo, Rosmarinus, Scutellaria, Strychnos, Urtica, Zanthoxylum, Zingiber.

Phlebitis
Use venous tonics above.

Polyarteritis nodosa
Arterial wall inflammation.
Treatment
Avoid salt. Increase fluids. Vitamin E.
Medicines
Allium, Apium, Centella, Chionanthus, Crataegus, Fagopyron, Filipendula, Scutellaria, Taraxacum, Tilia, Viscum, Zanthoxylum.

Purpura
Haemorrhage into the tissues causing skin discolouration.
Aetiology
Blood disorders, smoking, vitamin C deficiency.
Treat the liver.
Medicines
Aesculus, Crataegus, Fagopyron, Ginkgo, Vitamin C, E. Lotion – Arnica, Hamamelis.

Raynauds disease
Aetiology
Arterial spasm affecting mainly the limbs.
Treatment
Massage of the trapezial and deltoid muscles helps relieve neuromuscular tension.
Medicines for Raynauds
Angelica archangelica, Antispasmodic Tr., Capsicum, Crataegus, Ginkgo, Ruta, Scutellaria, Selenicerus, Tilia, Valeriana, Viburnum opulus, Viscum, Zanthoxylum.

Herbal Medicine - Keys

Stroke - cerebro vascular accident [See emergency medicine]

      Haemorrhage – cause - tearing of a diseased blood vessel often associated with hypertension.
Symptom onset – sudden
Unconsciousness – always present
"   depth – deep
Paralysis of the upper motor neuron – complete
Vital functions – often severely disturbed
Death – a common cause of sudden death
Prognosis – severe residual disability
      Thrombosis – cause clot forming in the diseased vessel.
Symptom onset - gradual
Unconsciousness - usually present
"   - not deep
Paralysis of the upper motor neuron - weakness
Vital functions - usually not affected
Death - less common
Prognosis - some disability
      Embolus – impacted clot from another diseased blood vessel
Symptom onset - extremely sudden
Unconsciousness - uncommon
"   present - not deep, often only dazing
Paralysis of the upper motor neuron – weakness
Vital functions - may not be affected
Death - uncommon
Prognosis - variable.

Thrombus
Blood clots formed in a diseased blood vessel initially cause reduction of blood to the end tissue. Eventually this will lead to hypotrophia. This is a condition of obstruction of the vasomotor supply.
Medicine
Direct stimulation to the circulatory vasomotor supply – Capsicum, Zanthoxylum, Zingiber
Anti coagulants.
Hepatic/gall bladder/ pancreatic remedies.

Varicose veins/ulcers
See venous tonics. Ulcers [See emergency herbal medicine – wounds]

21
Digestive System

Intestinal and hepatic medicines including bitters and aperitifs.
The two main mechanisms for the activity of bitters are [1] reflex effects from the bitter taste buds and [2] a direct effect on the stomach lining.

Aloe vera - resin is purgative and anthelmintic.
Berberis vulgaris - tonic laxative, cholagogue.
Cassia angustifloia/acutifolia - anthelmintic, laxative, tonic.
Chondrus crispus - demulcent and mild laxative.
Erigeron canadense [Canadian fleabane] – essential oil is parasiticide [246 p451].
Ficus carica - fresh and dried fig is a mild laxative.
Gelidium amansii [Agar] - bulk laxative.
Glycyrrhiza glabra - demulcent.
Ipomoea purga - purgative, contraindicated in inflammatory conditions of the GIT
Jateorrhiza – bitter tonic.
Linum catharticum - mildly tonic. Laxative.
Linum usitatissimum - demulcent and emollient.
Morus nigra and alba - mild astringent laxative.
Plantago psyllium - bulk purgative, demulcent and stimulant.
Polymnia uvedalia - tonic to the intestinal muscles and liver.
Prinos verticillatus [Black alder] affects the mucous membrane
Rhamnus frangula - stimulating tonic laxative.
Rhamnus purshiana - influences peristalsis.
Rheum officinale - aperient and stomachic.
Rheum palmatum - small doses ease diarrhoea. Large doses laxative.
Ricinus communis - mild and suitable for children.
Rumex crispus - laxative where skin and blood disorders predominate.
Tamarandus indica - mild alkaline laxative.

Gastrointestinal smooth muscle relaxants
Atropa belladonna
Chamaemelum nobile, Chamomilla recutita
Dioscorea villosa
Ferrula assafoetida
Humulus lupulus, Hyoscyamnus niger
Lavandula officinalis, Lobelia inflata
Melissa officinalis, Mentha species
Valeriana officinalis, Viburnum opulus, Viburnum prunifoleum
Zingiber officinalis.

Herbal Medicine - Keys

Formulary for gastro intestinal conditions
Compound herbal formulae

Emulsion Emulsio
Emulsions are used to evenly suspend an oil, powder, tincture or fluid extract. Basically oil and water are mixed together then an emulgent is added. The required medicament is put in last.
Emulsions can be used upon the skin to aid absorption of the medication.
Examples: Agar, Chondrus crispus, Gelatine, Quillaia and Tragacanth.
Internally used to suspend resinous medication [See Chapter 33/34 & Priest].

Emulsio Oleum Amydalae. Emulsion of Almond oil.
Oleum Almond 120 ml, Acacia pwd 30g, aqua 30ml.
Mix together, then gradually mix in a further 240 ml of aqua.
Sig 30/60ml. Action: Demulcent.

Enemas
Enemas are used to promote evacuation of intestinal contents and to allay inflammatory and irritable conditions.
Enemas can be used in **acute conditions** – colic, colitis, collapse, constipation, CVA, dysentery, meningitis, pain, typhoid, vomiting [when oral medications are ineffective as a feeding method]. **Chronic conditions** include - carcinoma, constipation, diverticulitis and pain.
Intestinal enemas
Althea, Coffee, Dioscorea, Ferrula, Lobelia, Myrica, Picraena, Ricinus, Rubus, Nepeta, Ulmus,

Enema Asafoetida [Ferrula]
    Tr Asafoetida 3ml
    Mucilage Ulmus to 100ml
Mix together the Tinctura and the Ulmus mucilage.
Sig Inject 100ml administered as an enema.
Administered for pain, spasm or flatulent distension of the bowel.

Enema Dioscorea
LE Dioscorea 5ml, Infusium Nepeta or Eupatorium perf. 20ml
Sig Inject 25ml as an enema. Administered for spasm or flatulent distension.

Enema Picraena
Decoction of Picreana 120ml, Mucilage of Ulmus 60ml
Sig Inject 60ml BD An anthelmintic which will destroy nematodes - threadworms and round worms. Administered at body heat as a retention enema.

Digestive system

Mixtures
Extract Rhamnus compound. Compound extract of Rhamnus.
LE Rhamnus p.   15ml
LE Euonymous   30ml
LE Glycyrrhiza   7ml
Essence Zingiber 30ml
Syrup Juglans   180ml
Dosage 5ml BD Hepatic and laxative prescription.

Constipation decoction
Achillea 30g, Bidens 30g, Zingiber 15g Aqua 1500ml
Decoct in a closed vessel and reduce to 1000ml. Add molasses to sweeten.
Sig 30-120 ml PRN.

Laxative Confection
Prunes, Dates, Raisins, Figs aa 120g finely chopped
Cassia acutifolia powder 30g. Sig Up to 30g

Confection of Senna
Cassia acutifolia   60g
Tamarind   60g
Prunes   45g
Figs   90g
Sugar   360g
Simmer all ingredients for an hour. Cool. Then add 2 gtt of oil of Anethum, Carum and Mentha. Sig 5-30ml PRN.

Haemorrhoids mixture
Ranunculus, Hamamelis, Collinsonia, Aesculus, Rhatany, Sanguinaria, Thuja, Pulsatilla, Cinchona, Glycyrrhiza, Honey.

Inflammatory conditions using a Linseed broth
25g of linseed and 550g water. Bring to the boil and then simmer for 5 minutes. Strain. Sig 60 ml TDS.

Combining medicines
Cathartics are usually followed with suitable intestinal tonics.
Capsicum may be added to prescriptions if there is a severe sluggish, inactive bowel inducing constipation.
Leptandra increases the secretion of bile, best combined with Zingiber, Euonymous or Taraxacum. Capsicum if necessary. Some stimulant will be necessary to eject the bile from the liver and gall bladder.

Herbal Medicine - Keys

Euonymous and Taraxacum will enable bile to be secreted and excreted.
Lobelia is added to cathartics in spasmodic bowel problems.
Zingiber will prevent griping when added to cathartics.
Zingiber is a stimulating diffusive remedy and tones the liver and intestine when used with either class of hepatic or laxative.

Development of the gastro intestinal tract

Consideration of pain syndromes need some anatomical evaluation. As the gastro intestinal tract develops it divides into three parts these are:

foregut - midgut - hindgut

Foregut develops into:
    1] lower oesophagus
    2] stomach
    3] upper duodenum
    4] liver
Midgut develops into:
    1] lower duodenum/pancreas
    2] jejunum
    3] ileum
    4] ileo coecal junction
    5] caecum and appendix
    6] ascending colon
    7] hepatic flexure
    8] transverse colon

Hindgut [smallest part of the GIT] develops into;
    1] descending colon
    2] sigmoid colon
    3] rectum, anal canal, anus

Pain in the **foregut** is pure visceral and supplied by the vagus nerve
Pain in the **midgut** is visceral referred, supplied by the splanchnic nerve
Pain in the **hindgut** is viscero-somatic, supplied by pelvic parasympathetic S 2.3.4. Pelvic plexus is mixed sympathetic/parasympathetic.

It follows from the above explanation of the gastro intestinal areas, that the **same medicine will affect a number of sites.** The vital force carries the remedy to the selected site of disorder. Suitable combinations of other medicines enhance the prescription.

Digestive system

Intestinal disorders and general systemic disturbances

Acute abdominal pain considerations
Aspects to be considered – Pain
Site at onset
Site at present
Severity, Duration, Type of pain
Aggravating factors
Relieving factors
Physical signs
Movement and distension
Tenderness
Rebound/Guarding/Rigidity
Murphy's
Swelling
Hernial orifices and scrotum
Auscultate for:
High pitched tinkling in small intestine obstruction.
Absent bowel sounds suggest peritoneal involvement, obstruction, ischaemia or strangulated bowel.

Conditions of the acute abdomen
Myocardial infarction - sudden pain, which may be upper abdominal.
Pneumonia/TB
Diabetes/Pancreatitis
Inflamed or Perforated viscus – cholecystitis [pain right upper abdomen], peptic ulcer [severe, continuous pain of sudden onset, in the upper abdomen, aggravated by inspiration. it may become generalised], appendix [Mc Burneys point], diverticulitis,
Bowel obstruction – strangulated bowel is usually found in the sigmoid colon, or gall stones obstructing the intestine. Large bowel obstructions also occur from adhesions, intra abdominal carcinoma, or volvulus [bowel twisting]. Intra abdominal cancer is more likely if; patient is over 50, with pain for over 48 hours. They have constipation, dysuria, distension and an intra abdominal mass.
Small bowel obstructions are often due to a hernia, colic, enteritis, constipation, acute diverticular disease, IBS. Small bowel obstruction gives - steady pain and rarely blood or mucus in the stool.
Malaria/Typhoid/Cholera
Ectopic pregnancy/ovarian cyst – diffuse lower abdominal pain, shoulder tip pain [particularly left], Vaginal examination reveals tenderness on movement of the cervix.

Salpingitis – unilateral abdominal pain, right sided rectal tenderness. Left sided tenderness is an indicator of fallopian tube or ovary disease. Tenderness on movement of the cervix is a more useful sign in ectopic pregnancy.

Fresh bleeding, a boggy uterus and an open cervix are seen in an incomplete abortion.

Cystitis, pyelonephritis, renal stone, renal tumour – loin pain, colic in stone with loin to groin pain [males over 30], frequency, dysuria, scalding [cystitis in young females], check for white cells in the urine. Absence of guarding and rebound tenderness. When pain, pallor and a distressed patient present, a stone is more common. Dysuria and pyrexia is more likely with infection.

Haematemesis

Aetiology

Foreign body. Injury

Peptic ulcer. Portal hypertension – oesophageal varices

Drugs - aspirin

Tumours

Bleeding disorders

Liver function

The liver is secretory and has vascular and metabolic functions. It performs biliary secretion [bile salts are reabsorbed in the small intestine and sent to the portal vein where bile acids are synthesized from cholesterol]. 1.5 litres of blood pass through the liver each minute. The liver synthesizes vitamin K, prothrombin and clotting factors, plasma protein and heparin. It stores glycogen, fats, iron and vitamins B12, A, D, E, K. Detoxification of toxins and drug inactivation. Hormonal and Immunological function. Metabolic functions [heat regulation].

Carbohydrate, protein and fat are metabolised. Proteins are deaminated to urea and desaturated fat.

Conjugation of bilirubin

Old red blood cells are broken down to iron and globin, these are stored. Haem part is converted to bilirubin and attached to plasma protein. The liver removes protein and makes bilirubin water soluble [haemobilirubin]. These pass via the biliary system to the small intestine where the action of bacteria forms urobiligen. Most is excreted in the faeces some is reabsorbed and excreted in the urine.

Acute liver disease [primary biliary cirrhosis]

Often associated with viral disturbances. Symptoms include fatigue, low grade fever, anorexia, nausea and abdominal pain.

Signs include pale stools and dark urine, enlarged liver, spider naevi on the skin and jaundice.

Digestive system

Chronic liver disease
Sometimes the chronic form is asymptomatic. Symptoms - hormonal imbalance [PMS], loss of libido, amenorrhoea, icterus, confusion, drowsiness,
Signs - enlarged liver, abdominal distension, portal hypertension [ascites], spider naevi,

Cirrhosis
Cirrhosis has many causes that include alcoholism, viral disease gall bladder and liver disease. *Bright red palms* [acute and chronic form], portal hypertension, jaundice, fatigue, anorexia, nausea, abdominal discomfort, weakness, gynaecomastia, dupetrens contracture in some cases.
Icterus, hepatic and splenic hepatomegaly. Fatty cysts on the skin. Finger clubbing.

Hepatic carcinoma
Secondary carcinoma follows from metastases of the breast, lung, stomach or bowel.

Hepatitis
Hepatitis both A and B are acute illnesses. Transmission is via the oral faecal route, also by saliva, urine, intradermal injection or blood recipient. Children and young adults tend to be affected. Incubation is between 15 – 50 days. The virus is isolated from the faeces. Often infectious before the patient feels ill.
Symptoms:
anorexia, malaise, nausea, jaundice, pruritus, pyrexia. Dark urine and pale stool, depression, hepatic tenderness, palpable liver. Raised serum bilirubin.

Hepatomegaly
Classically an enlarged liver is found in:
1] smooth – hepatitis, allergy, cardiovascular disease,
2] small – cirrhosis
3] knobbly - cancer
Enlargement may also be due to hydatid cyst, metabolic disorders – fatty liver - lymphomas, leukaemia, venous congestion and hepatic vein occlusion.

Hepatomegaly can be a reliable clinical indicator of induced food disease - *intolerance, allergy or sensitivity* to a food may occur. The liver plays a significant role in the establishment of an allergy is evident from its role in protein metabolism. It has been shown that anaphylaxis does not occur when the liver has been excluded. Enlargement of the liver occurs when an intolerance to a substance was ingested. The average size of the liver is proximal to the rib cage. Liver size increases by up to 8cm distally measured in the mid clavicular line in induced food disease.

There occurs a relationship between hepatic enlargement and the following conditions: acute respiratory infections, restlessness and colic in infants, vomiting, diarrhoea, eczema, sleep disturbances, lack of concentration, hyperactivity, abdominal pain, pain in the legs, poor appetite, malaise, desire for sweet foods or liquids.

Jaundice

Jaundice occurs from

1] Blood disorders which may be haemolytic or congenital.

2] Within the liver from some infective process, damaged liver cells or cancer.

3] Or from external obstruction - impacted gall stones, cancer of the pancreas.

> 1] Haemolytic – no jaundice/slight jaundice
> 2] Hepatic – jaundice, stool normal, urine dark
> 3] Obstructive – jaundice, dark urine, stool pale

Icterus will present once the bile is greater then 3mg/100ml.

Enquire about holidays abroad, blood transfusions, surgery, shellfish allergy, leptospirosis, drugs and alcohol intake.

Courvoisers law

A distended gall bladder in the presence of jaundice is due to some other cause [generally to carcinoma of the head of the pancreas]. This is explained by the fact that gall stones eventually cause fibrosis of the gall bladder. The gall bladder is unable to contract to remove any stones with jaundice being the result. Irregularity of the gall bladder suggests stones or a tumour.

Gall bladder disorders

Cholangitis produces pain over the liver, jaundice and chills.

Cholelithiasis - stones or gravel are mainly composed of cholesterol. If the stones become stuck in the bile duct then colic is present. Dark urine and light stool are characteristic of obstruction in the gall bladder. Common findings with patients who have gall stones is chronic flatulence, indigestion and heartburn. Pain radiating to under the right scapula is common.

Dietary requirements for stones, hepatic and gall bladder disorders.

Reduce caffeine, sugar and alcohol.

Decrease or avoid saturated fats, sugar and red meat. Butter contains short chain buturic acids, which break down easily, and is better absorbed than margarines. Lecithin breaks down into choline, it is found in egg yolk and pulses.

Increase water soluble fibre: fruit and vegetables. Vegetables increase bile excretion. Eat a high fibre diet containing oats, flaxseed, green leafy vegetables and beans. Eat vegetable based proteins – grains [barley, oats, millet, rye, cous cous, brown rice]. Soya, tofu, yoghurt, wheat germ and spirulina. Methionine is an essential amino acid and once ingested the liver attacks sulphur this stimulates liver function. It is lipotrophic and protects the liver.

Amino acid methionine containing sulphur is found in:
 live yoghurt, cottage cheese, cheese, cream cheese, peaches, pears, pineapple, brassica, cabbage and artichoke.

Apples, beetroot, dandelion, grapefruit, lemon, parsley and watercress tea stimulate the bile flow.

Antioxidant foods, especially those containing vitamin C and E together with Selenium these help to prevent free radicle damage to liver cells.

Increase the fluid intake.

<u>Hydrotherapy</u>

Hot and alternating with cold compress over the liver. Spray may be alternated if this is more convenient.

Direct manual drainage to the liver using the liver pump.

Method: One hand is placed over the liver the other placed posterior, move forwards and back, using firm pressure on the upward and the downward movement. [Like doing a bi manual examination of the kidneys].

<u>Hepatic and gall bladder medication</u>
<u>Treatment</u>
Rest the digestive system and reduce carbohydrates.

<u>Loss of digestive tone</u> from hepatic or gall bladder disturbance is treated with Chionanthus and Filipendula.

<u>Cholagogue/choleretic</u>
Berberis vulgaris, Centaurium, Chelidonium, Cnicus, Cynarus, Dioscorea, Euonymous, Fumaria, Iris, Leptandra, Myrica, Peumus, Rhamnus sp, Silybum, Taraxacum, Viburnum opulus.

<u>Liver vasotonic alterative</u>
Equal parts of LE Phytolacca and LE Chionanthus.
Sig 2.5ml TDS

<u>Hepatic disorders general</u>
Leptandra is a relaxant, Berberis vulgaris is tonic, Berberis aq., is tonic but weaker than Berberis vulg.

Hepatic/stomach or pancreatic disorders - Euonymous with Filipendula and Chionanthus.

<u>Medicines for hepatic cirrhosis</u>
Acorus, Agrimonia, Artemesia sp., Berberis sp., Chelone, Dioscorea, Euonymous, Hydrastis, Iris, Leptandra, Menyanthes, Peumus, Rumex, Silybum, Stachys, Taraxacum, Zanthoxylum, Zingiber.

Herbal Medicine - Keys

Medicines for hepatic abscess
Artemesia sp., Baptisia, Berberis vulgaris, Calendula, Chionanthus, Dioscorea, Echinacea, Iris, Leptandra, Peumus.

Medicines for hepatitis - acute and chronic
Allium, Artemesia sp, Agrimonia, Arctium, Berberis sp., Chelone, Cinnamomum, Foeniculum, Glycyrrhiza, Hydrastis, Iris, Leptandra, Menyanthes, Peumus, Phyllanthus amarus, Rheum palmatum, Rumex, Silybum, Taraxacum, Stachys.

Gall stone treatment - Olive oil and lemon juice
1 pint of pure olive oil and the juice from 8 lemons.
Eat nothing after the midday meal, drink fluids as required. In the evening drink 500ml of olive oil [virgin] and the juice of eight lemons. This is taken in divided doses.
Follow on with grapefruit juice for up to three days if desired or a very gentle diet with no animal fats, use fruit juices, herb teas, cottage cheese, salad, jacket potatoes, vegetables, rice, and fruit.

The oral cavity and tongue reflect gastro intestinal conditions [See also EENT].

Anorexia and bullaemia are often associated with poor self image of the individual.
Treatment - Psychotherapy
Medicines
Marsdenia bark, Acorus, Gentiana. Nervine trophorestoratives e.g. Avena.
Zinc sulphate 15mg daily.

Colitis
Colitis can be quite incapacitating for the sufferer. Acute colitis requires bedrest and emotional rest. Relief from the pain and discomfort is an urgent matter. Severe haemorrhage can occur.
Medicines
Acacia, Agrimonia, Dioscorea, Geum, Glycyrrhiza, Humulus, Hyoscyamnus, Lobelia, Myrica, Potentilla, Symphytum, Zingiber.

Dyspepsia
Aetiology from the stomach e.g. ulcers, nervousness affecting stomach function. Flatulence, flatus. Constipation.

Flatulence
Aetiology
Commonly found if eating too fast or eating too many varied foods at one sitting.

Digestive system

Carcinoma of the stomach, ulcers, intestinal hurry [IBS].
Treatment for flatulence, dyspepsia or pain.

Tincturae Carminative
Carum, Cinnamomum, Elettaria, Zingiber aa equal parts of bruised sem.

Gastritis – Acidity – Hyperchlordria

Alkalies given to reduce the acidity of the stomach do not normalise but tend to deplete the functional efficiency of the stomach. Protein foods also tea, coffee and alcohol are acid forming. Antacids are calcium based they are best avoided. Filipendula given when required for conditions of hyperchlorhydria supports normalisation of function. Filipendula normalises an excess or deficiency of acid within the stomach. Mentha piperita is also used for its stimulating effect upon the stomach - they are amphoteric stomach medicines.

Stomach activity is closely linked to liver, gall bladder and pancreas function. Disorders in one organ will eventually produce disturbed functional effects upon other organ areas. Duodenal ulcers can be silent and the patient may have treated themselves with antacids for years however not treating the cause, merely the symptom. Duodenal ulceration can create [once healed] a constriction in the duodenum, if the constriction affects the ampulla this can impair the flow of bile. The gall bladder and eventually the liver respond by becoming inflamed then congested. Cholelithiasis, cholecystitis, jaundice or cirrhosis may follow.

Treatment for these conditions depends upon the tissues and the causative factors that preceded the disturbed function.

Stomach medicines - Agrimonia, Althea, Cetraria, Elettaria, Filipendula, Mentha piperita/spicata, Symphytum, Zingiber. Demulcents and astringents.

Hyper/hypochlorhydria antacids – Agrimonia, Artemesia absinthium, Chamomilla, Carum carvi, Centarium, Filipendula, Gentiana, Jateorrhiza, Melissa, Menyanthes, Taraxacum rad, Dec. Jam. Sarsae Co. [Compound decoction of Jamacian Sarsparilla].

Ulcers - peptic and duodenal

Ulcers can occur as a result of food intolerance. Helicobacter pyloris is a bacterium that affects around 40% of the British population. At least 95% of duodenal ulcer patients are infected.

Treatment
Clear the lower bowel with an enema every third day.

Medicines these all inhibit the growth of H. pylori –
Acidophyllus, Allium, Berberis sp., Calendula, Cinnamomum, Coptis species, Corydalis ambigua, Hydrastis, Magnolia officinalis, Phytolacca, Rheum palmatum, Thymus, Uva ursi. Grapefruit seed extract. Manuka honey - [Leptospermum scoparium].

Herbal Medicine - Keys

Dietary adjustment

Restrict food in acute cases. Severe cases may have food pureed until symptoms settle.

Papaya is a nutritive food healing to ulcers. Symphytum tea, carrot juice, cabbage juice, slippery elm gruel, rice milk, oat milk, soya milk. As improvement occurs give carrot, celery or cabbage juice.

Baked apples, steamed vegetables, baked potatoes, avocado pear, banana.

Increasing fibre and starch – oats, cous cous.

Prescription - Filipendula with a combination e.g. Agrimonia, Geranium maculatum, Mentha piperita plus Phytolacca.

Medicines

Acorus, Althea, Avena, Calendula, Chamomilla, Centaurium, Cetraria, Chondrus, Cinnamomum, Filipendula, Foeniculum, Geranium maculatum, Glycyrrhiza, Hydrastis, Mentha piperita, Symphytum, Thymus, Trigonella, Ulmus.

Vitamins A & E, Zinc. Along with relaxation techniques.

Where gall bladder disturbances are found with pain or deficient bile flow - use Taraxacum rad.

Hiatus hernia

Mainly found in the over 50 age group. The stomach herniates through the diaphragm and a portion or in severe cases the whole stomach can move into the chest. Reflux of stomach contents can be very disturbing for the patient. Some tension is often found in these cases with tension holding points in the stomach [undigested ideas for some].

Treatment

Eat dry. Eat small meals. Don't mix to many foods at one meal. Chew all foods well. Improve the posture – sit up straight. Don't rush meals. Exercises like sit ups and leg raising could prove helpful, yoga.

Medicines

Relaxed conditions of the stomach [atonic] astringents for the muscle wall: Acorus, Agrimonia, Erythraea, Filipendula, Gentiana, Herniaria glabra-Sig 3g, Hydrastis, Mentha species. Demulcents: Symphytum, Althea, Ulmus.

Halitosis

Occurs from putrefaction [infection] in the gastro intestinal tract. Which may lead to mouth ulcers. Anxiety can encourage the condition.

Treatment

Clear the intestine. Allium, Artemesia species, Baptisia, Berberis species, Calendula, Cassia acutfolia, Echinacea, Phytolacca.

Digestive system

Hernia
A hernia is the protrusion of an organ, or part of an organ through the walls of a cavity within which it is normally contained.
Strangulation occurs when oedema and resultant congestion interferes with the blood supply. The venous return is affected initially and later as pressure at the neck of the sac increases, the arterial supply is cut off gangrene may ensue.

Nausea
Assess the cause of the nausea. Aetiology – overeating, nervous vomiting, stomach – gastritis, gall bladder - cholecystitis/lithiasis, or pancreas disorders - pancreatitis. Infection, intestinal obstruction or carcinoma of any organ.
Medicines – antiemetics.
Ballota, Chamomilla, Capsicum, Cinnamomum, Filipendula, Geum urbanum, Glycyrrhiza, lobelia, Melissa, Mentha piperita, Menyanthes, Zingiber.

Oesophagus
Assess the cause of the primary symptom of dysphagia. It could be due to tonsillitis, anxiety causing spasm, stomach disorders – hiatus hernia, carcinoma or oesophageal pouches.
Medicines
Inflammation - Althea, Cetraria, Chondrus, Glycyrrhiza, Hydrastis, Symphytum.
Spasm - Chamomilla, Chamaemelum nobile, Dioscorea, Humulus, Lobelia, Viburnum opulus.
Stricture [exclude carcinoma] – Althea, Cetraria, Chondrus, Glycyrrhiza, Psyllium

Vomiting
A common symptom in many disorders. When nausea is present look for an abdominal cause. It is useful to divide vomiting into digestive and non digestive aetiology. Assess the frequency, quality and amount of vomit. Observe the vomit.
In a robust constitution: vomiting can clear the stomach condition immediately. Less viable types take longer for a reaction. Vomiting clears usually within 48 hours in cases of food poisoning. Small intestinal troubles - vomiting tends to occur later on.
Longer bouts of vomiting suggest severe infection e.g. botulism which is fatal.
Food poisoning is common and can be precipitated by ingestion of some poison or pathogenic bacteria e.g. salmonella.
Other causes of vomiting include carcinoma of the stomach, gall bladder disease, gall stones, appendicitis. Non digestive aetiology includes migraine, renal disorders, anorexia and bullaemia.
Persistent vomiting is most likely from acute pancreatitis.

Herbal Medicine - Keys

Emesis treatment
Physiomedicalists using the graduated emesis treatment - whereby the emetic is given and the contents of vomit examined - this gives reliable indications as to the condition of the separate tissues of the stomach e.g. excessive mucus - relaxed mucous membrane.
Treatment for vomiting depends upon the cause – see nausea.

Pancreatic disorders
Insulin production
Secretory enzyme function

    starches – amylase
    fats   – lipase, phospholipase
    proteins – proteases

Pancreatitis
Acute abdominal pain, nausea and vomiting. The intestinal muscle may produce spasm with ileus. Shock symptoms may occur with pain together with hypoglycaemia. Chronic cases produce pain and often diabetes. May follow alcoholic poisoning, impacted gall stones, chronic hepatic disorders, ulcers and carcinoma.
Medicine
Chionanthus is considered a sovereign remedy for pancreatic disorders.
Pancreatic carcinoma
Jaundice that gradually deepens, weight loss, steatorrhoea. Pain referred to the back. Diabetes and thrombus formation.

Spleen disorders
Medicines
Acorus, Allium, Astragalus, Berberis vulgaris, Chionanthus, Cichorium, Cinchona, Echinacea, Grindelia, Hydrastis, Myrica, Phytolacca, Scolopendrum, Tamarindus, Taraxacum, Thuja, Urtica, Vinca rosea.

Pathophysiology of gastro intestinal dysfunction
A] Impaired digestion - increased intestinal permeability
B] Intestinal endotoxaemia
C] Dysbiosis
D] Intestinal inflammation - malabsorption
E] Oxidative stress - impaired hepatic detoxification
F] Intestinal permeability defects - impairment of GI immune function.

Digestive system

Treatment aims to
1] Remove intestinal toxins
2] Eliminate intestinal pathogens
3] Reduce oxidative damage
4] Re-establish normal flora
5] Rebuild the intestinal mucosa
6] Improve digestion

Many systemic diseases are derived from toxins in the bowel - gut dysbiosis.
The treatment of systemic diseases is by elimination and detoxification. Digestion and absorption of foodstuffs play an important role. The intestine absorbs foodstuffs. It can also reabsorb toxins this is called **autointoxication**. The intestinal mucosa is not impermeable to intact protein molecules being absorbed. Not all proteins are broken down into macromolecules [37, 38]. There are around 400 different species of micro-organisms in the gastro intestinal tract. Beneficial organisms provide natural anti infective support and are immune stimulating.
Pathogenic effects of micro-organism -- carcinoma is often determined by the interaction of food in the body. Exotoxins, found inside a micro-organism and endotoxins, secreted from a micro-organism are pathogenic.
The microflora of the intestine also affects the way pathogens behave.

Conditions affected by the intestinal microflora:
Allergic reactions to dairy produce/eggs/wheat – these are the most common
[see allergy].
Candida
Diabetes, Pancreatitis
E. Coli has insulin like effects and can bind to insulin [E. Coli toxins] and initiate metabolic processes so disturbing the blood glucose balance.
Meningitis
Myasthenia gravis
Psoriasis
SLE and dematomyositis
Thyroid disease
Ulcerative colitis [See also Chapter 32].
Treatment
Fermented milk in the form of live yoghurt e.g. acidophyllus is known as probiotic. Probiotics assist the immune system. Healthy bacteria are enhanced which break down fibre and resistant starches. Gut bacteria help manufacture some B vitamins and vitamin K.

Herbal Medicine - Keys

Malabsorption
Lactose intolerance
A deficiency of the enzyme lactase causes an intolerance to milk products. Low levels of lactase enzyme in the duodenum are the cause of the intolerance.
Aetiology - flatulence, bloating, abdominal cramps and diarrhoea.
Treat by avoiding dairy produce and give lactase enzyme.
Soya beans in the form of milk, yoghurt and tofu can help patients with lactose intolerance, soya does not contain lactose.

Gluten enteropathy
May be found as an allergic reaction. Symptoms include diarrhoea, weight loss, pain and aphthous ulcers.
Treatment: Gluten found in wheat, oats, barley and rye *must be avoided.* Strengthen the intestinal mucous membrane.
Medicines
Agrimonia, Aloe, Berberis species, Calendula, Chamomilla, Capsicum, Collinsonia, Dioscorea, Hydrastis, Medicago, Melissa, Rubus, Smilax, Trigonella, Ulmus, Zanthoxylum, Zingiber.

Colic
Medicines
Acorus, Angelica archangelica, Artemesia absinthium, Capsicum, Carum, Chamaemelum nobile, Dioscorea, Elettaria, Geum urbanum, Levisticum, Mentha piperita, Nepeta, Pimpinella, Potentilla, Stachys, Valeriana, Viburnum Sp, Zingiber.

Diarrhoea [Gastro enteritis]
Aetiology
Inflammatory diseases – IBS, colitis with pain, diarrhoea and mucus. Infection, malabsorption, diabetes and thyrotoxicosis.
Infective conditions of the intestine – salmonella, typhoid, paratyphoid, dysentery – amoebic, shigella, giardiasis, campylobacter.
Allergic or intolerance to foods.
Artificial sweeteners, excess of vitamin C, lactase deficiency, antibiotics, laxatives, digoxin.
Diarrhoea may be part of a healing crisis. If there are other crisis symptoms then the use of astringents to stop diarrhoea is inadvisable.
Treatment
Live yoghurt - acidophyllus bacteria, will help to recolonise the intestine with 'good bacteria.'
Astringent medication to gently allay the diarrhoea.

Digestive system

Medicines - diarrhoea
Agrimonia, Allium, Aloe, Althea, Atropa, Baptisia, Chamomilla, Cinnamomum, Commiphora, Filipendula, Hydrastis, Trigonella, Valeriana, Ulmus.

Meleana

Aetiology – infections, enteritis, diverticulitis, ulcerative colitis, chrohn's disease, dysentery, haemorrhoids, malignancy - colon or rectal carcinoma [diarrhoea alternating with constipation, virtually always bleeding], over relaxed intestinal mucous membrane.

Signs and symptoms in acute haemorrhage - Low blood pressure, pallor, rapid thready pulse, cold clammy skin, restlessness. A rectal examination is required in all cases.

Treatment

Nourishing fluids.

Depending on the diagnosis and severity of the case a short fast may be indicated for around three days. Use a restricted diet of fruit or vegetable juices freshly made, this will balance the electrolytes, e.g. carrot juice alternating with apple juice. Grape juice for the potassium salts. Ulmus gruel is soothing for inflamed surfaces along with Symphytum to aid healing. Soups, grated apple or carrot, soya yoghurt can be used. Rest for the intestine is imperative in severe cases.

Once improvement occurs stewed apple, brown rice, cous cous, potato with a single type of vegetable. Following on with protein – tofu, beans [which must be mashed initially]. A rotation type diet may follow using bland foods, lamb and pears to start with. Gradually introducing one food at a time – after about two weeks.

Wheat, dairy items and oats may be introduced later and checks made for any sensitivity reactions to these products. Protein, wheat and dairy produce are the commonest allergens. By removing food that cause irritable states of the mucosa an allergy is removed. Vitamin C and beta carotine are healing to the mucous membrane. Lactobacillus acidophyllus is antiseptic, antiviral and antifungal to the intestinal contents.

Hydrotherapy

Cold compress or sprays are good to relieve the internal congestion and any nerve spasm affecting the intestinal vasomotor nerves.

Medicine

Specific medication depends upon the cause.

Over relaxed mucous membrane of the bowel can give rise to loose stools. Astringency is then required to tone the membrane – Hamamelis is gentle and useful for all age groups as it cleanses and astringes without griping.

Herbal Medicine - Keys

Constipation

Because impurities and toxins are reabsorbed from the intestine a focus of general poisoning [autointoxication] can be set up. Clearing the constipation is of paramount importance. Bile salts are reabsorbed with constipation, hence patients can feel ill and very toxic if the situation progresses. Depression can occur with bile salt reabsorption.

Treatment

Three ingredients are required for the relief of simple constipation.

[1] fibre [2] fluids [3] movement/exercise. Fibre - nuts, prunes, figs, raisins, fruit, green vegetables.

Where these are insufficient medication is required.

Bulk laxatives given with plenty of fluids - Ispagula, oat bran.

More stimulating remedies are Aloe, which require to be combined with an antispasmodic to prevent griping - Anethum, Foeniculum, Zingiber.

Relax the bowel wall in simple constipation, is often all that is required - Cassia angustifolia.

More stimulating medication in severe cases – Aloes, Rhamnus etc.

Contracted bowel needs relaxant and antispasmodic nervines – Chamomilla, Viburnum opulus, Viburnum prunifoleum.

Cholagogues are required if bile is insufficient and the stool pale.

Candida – thrush [See also gynaecology].

Candida is a yeast. It lives naturally in our bodies. Once the body becomes compromised, candida proliferates and causes all sorts of symptoms. It thrives in an alkaline environment. Candida results from long term dietary inadequacy. Poor elimination of toxic waste [auto toxaemia] and often emotional disturbances.

Oral candida requires an alkaline medium for it's improvement. The small intestine is acid therefore candida is unable to develop here.

When candida becomes established it secretes toxins [exorphins] into the blood. Candida can affect any mucus surface; vagina, uterus, fallopian tubes, intestine, bladder, kidneys etc. Symptoms are numerous from nervous irritability to colitis.

Treatments

Avoidance of sugar in all forms. Initially avoid fruit because of the fructose.

Give vitamin A, C, and zinc.

Detoxification of the intestine can be aided by a short fast. Restore the healthy micro-organisms with live yoghurt. Supplement with caprylic acid, lactobacillus and acidophyllus organisms.

Medicines

Intestinal cleansers and mucous membrane remedies.

Allium helps stop the invasion. Baptisia, Berberis species, Calendula, Hydrastis, Iris, Tabebuia.

Digestive system

Crohn's disease, Ulcerative colitis, Colitis, Diverticulitis, Irritable Bowel Syndrome, Megacolon, Anal fissure.

Crampy pain, flatulence, mucus with the stool, sometimes blood. It may be associated with colitis, ulcerative colitis, food intolerance, parasites [tropical diseases], candida, stress or drugs.

<u>Symptoms</u> are varied and many with these conditions.

Bloating, diarrhoea, pain, weight loss, bleeding, anaemia, fistula in ano are common findings. Palpable mass in diverticulitis, rebound tenderness and iliac fossa tenderness. A rectal examination is necessary. These conditions can be very severe and require in patient treatment. Chronic diarrhoea or blood loss will be very debilitating to a patient.

<u>Treatment</u>

Acute cases require bedrest, nervine medication, antispasmodics, demulcents, antimicrobials. Restricted food intake, pureed foods, fluids.

Check the transit time with charcoal tablets, beetroot or sweet corn. Maximum of 36 hours, over this time suggests constipation. Under the time diarrhoea.

Check for allergic reactions in these conditions.

Encourage regular habits of defaecation. A high fibre diet - No bran. Fluids. Gentle exercise

A short fast is followed by a diet that must be started with juices of carrot, apple, cabbage, watercress. Follow on with - brown rice, cous cous, oats, cooked apple, tofu, fish, yoghurt and banana.

<u>Demulcent medicines</u>

Althea, Glycyrrhiza, Plantago, Psyllium, Symphytum, Ulmus.

<u>Astringents</u> – Acorus, Agrimonia, Geranium maculatum – is best in haemorrhage, Hamamelis is gentle, Hydrastis, Plantago, Polygonum, Potentilla.

<u>Anti microbial agents</u>

Echinacea or Phytolacca are indicated for the mucosa and tissue fluids.

Allium, Berberis species, Hydrastis, Juglans regia, Quassia.

<u>Antispasmodics</u> [For flatulence, spasm, pain, IBS].

Artemisia absinthium, Chamomilla, Carum carvi, Filipendula, Foeniculum vulgare, Humulus and Mentha piperita.

<u>Supplement</u> with Vitamin A & C.

Carcinoma of the ascending colon

Notoriously silent

Anaemia – [lassitude, weakness and dyspnoea] in 20% of patients.

Systemic disturbances present for a considerable time before any change takes place in the bowel.

Abdominal pain - right side – steady deep ache/episodes of colic/dull nagging pain or soreness aggravated by turning or walking.

Loss of weight.

Vomiting in 33% of patients.
Altered bowel habit – constipation or diarrhoea.
Lump present – ascending colon – fixed tumour in 65% of cases.
Eating a meal provokes pain, borambygmi, nausea, anorexia.

Carcinoma of the descending colon
70% of cases have colicky abdominal pain, unrelated to meals.
Colon is very muscular, therefore symptoms tend to result from obstruction.
Acute on chronic obstruction.
Constipation that tends to get worse despite increasing doses of laxatives.
Constipation followed by diarrhoea – 60% of cases.
Alteration of bowel habit – sudden with increasing difficulty in defaecation.
Lump present, fixed tumour in 25% of cases.
Distention
Blood – small amount, mixed with faeces, appears dark to fresh in 10% of cases.
Feeling of fullness or mild cramps progresses to griping and true colic, relieved by passing flatus or evacuating.
Never any meleana in the left colon.

Carcinoma of the sigmoid colon
Alteration in bowel habit – constipation more frequent but the history is only of a few days or weeks.
Abdominal pain – colicky, dull ache over the lower abdomen, below umbilicus.
Lump present
Tenesmus – feeling a need for evacuation which may result in tenesmus accompanied by the passage of mucus and blood, especially in the early morning.
Bladder symptoms.

Carcinoma of the rectum
Commonly interfere with defaecation in 80% of cases
Changes in the sensation of defaecation – alteration in the size, shape and regularity of the stool.
Common – visible bleeding – mixed or unmixed.
Feeling of fullness, urgency to defaecate on standing. After the passage of a stool – usually only a small amount or the patient may pass – pus, mucus or flatus. There may be a harassing sense of incomplete evacuation, bowel irritability or tenesmus.
Change in bowel habit in 80% of cases in recent months.
Rectum painless – unless deep invasion occurs then there is dull perineal pain, may be referred to the low back or thighs.
Mucoid diarrhoea
Ribbon like stool

Digestive system

Urinary symptoms can occur
Constipation is unusual
Weight loss and lassitude is uncommon
Tumour is usually hard not tender
Rectal carcinoma reveals two characteristic features – induration and elevation, either an indurated disc or proturberant ulcerated growth. 75-90% can be palpated.

Summary
Changed bowel habits, rectal bleeding, abdominal pain, weight loss, anorexia and vomiting occur in carcinoma of the large intestine.
O/E
Rectum is normally smooth in health. Neoplasm – large bowel palpable in 75%+ of cases.
Diagnosis can be made in 98% of cases with a history and physical examination.
D/D
Appendix abscess
Colitis, Diverticulitis – long history, ileus, pyrexia, abdo tender.
Ulcerative colitis – unformed faeces
Crohn's disease, Intestinal TB
Endometriosis.

<u>Ano rectal disease</u> [See also p399]
Suppositories offer a soothing preparation to Anorectal disorders.
Local medicaments for use in suppositories
Belladonna extract, Conium extract, Hamamelis extract, Lobelia extract, Rubus, Solanum dulcamara.

Soothing haemorrhoidal preparations
Anodyne for painful conditions – anal abscess/fissure/fistula, vomiting, colic, diverticulitis, colitis, proctitis, haemorrhoids, cystitis, anxiety.

<u>Examination</u>
Check the following – history, weight loss, abdominal pain, bleeding, change in bowel function.

Peri anal irritation
      With a rash - eczema, abrasions, pruritus
      Colitis
      Coeliac disease
      Diarrhoea, Megacolon
      Fissure

Herbal Medicine - Keys

Commonly causing discomfort/irritation:
Abscess, Infection
Allergy
Proctalgia/Proctitis
Rectal prolapse
Spinal lesion/coccyx fracture
Ulcer
Threadworms

Fissure in ano
Anal ulcer in the long axis of the lower anal canal with spasm of muscles and pain.
Symptoms of a fissure: sharp agonising pain starting during defaecation overwhelming in intensity, lasting an hour or more. Ceases suddenly. Stools frequently streaked with blood. Slight discharge.
O/E Sentinel skin tag. Tightly closed puckered anus.
Medicines
Althea, Chamomilla, Geranium maculatum, Polygonum, Rhamnus frangula, Scrophularia, Symphytum, Trigonella, Ulmus.
Antimicrobials
Achillea, Calendula, Echinacea, Glechoma, Phytolacca, Trigonella.
External
Atropa, Calendula, Stellaria, Symphytum.
Allium suppositories or capsules can be inserted at night.
Injection of Althea, Calendula, Cetraria, Chondrus or Ulmus.

Anorectal abscess and fistula
Aetiology
Faulty intestinal elimination, carcinoma, haemorrhoids, IBS, tuberculosis, ulcerative colitis.
Signs and symptoms:
Faecal incontinence, rectal prolapse, haemorrhoids – bleeding/prolapse,
pilonidal dimples, protruding polyps, Imporforate anus – birth.
Anal and peri anal abscess – may have pain and fever before the abscess is palpable.
O/E PR – tender, boggy swelling, palpable in rectal wall.
Pregnancy could create a swelling in the rectal wall.

Fistula in ano – principle symptom is a persistent sero-purulent discharge that irritates the skin. External opening within 3.75cm of the anus. History for years. Tends to be chronic. O/E Nodule palpable in the wall of the anal canal.
Treatment as above - fissure.

Digestive system

Proctalgia/Proctitis/Pruritus

Anal itching can be very distressing. Tends to occur in nervous patients, infected skin, haemorrhoids and intestinal disorders e.g. colitis etc.

Treatment

Hydrotherapy - Cool the area with cold water splashes to the anus.

Chamomilla, Dioscorea, Lobelia, Mentha piperita, Viburnum sp., Stellaria or Calendula crem

Rectal prolapse

Astringe the area. Reduce when necessary use warm water and push the rectum back. Always use a cold sitz bath after warm water.

Medicine

Aletris, Capsella, Composition essence, Geranium maculatum, Polygonum, Quercus.

Haemorrhoids

Distended haemorhoidal veins which may prolapse at the rectum. Excess venous pressure results from an increase in portal pressure because veins drain into the portal veins. Chronic coughing, heavy lifting/straining, venous congestion from straining at stool, constipation, low fibre diet and pregnancy.

Treatments

Clear the bowel using a high fibre diet. An enema may be required in severe cases to clear the rectum.

Reduction of the haemorrhoid will give relief from pain and haemorrhage.

Hydrotherapy – cold water spray directly onto the area.

Sitz bath. Warm water will help to reduce the haemorrhoid, follow with cold water for one minute. Soothes the pain of haemorrhoids. Improvise with a bowl of warm water to reduce the haemorrhoid and sit in it, follow on with cold water to astringe the plexus.

Medicines

Achillea, Aesculus, Chamomilla, Chelone, Collinsonia, Dioscorea, Geranium maculatum, Hamamelis, Hypericum, Iris, Juglans, Plantago sp, Polygonum, Potentilla, Quercus, Rhamnus purshiana, Scrophularia, Symphytum, Urtica, Verbascum.

External

Ung Ranunculus, Sempervivum, Symphytum or Stellaria - eases pain and itching. Aloe, Hamamelis, Stellaria or Vitamin E suppositories – insert after bowels opened.

Intestinal obstruction

Symptoms – pain, distension, vomiting, absolute constipation.

Acute obstruction – small bowel. Chronic obstruction – large bowel

Herbal Medicine - Keys

<u>Aetiology of acute obstruction</u>
Adhesions. Volvulus. Paralytic ileus
Intussusception - red current jelly stool in child e.g. 9 months
Foreign bodies - gall stones
                      - mass of undigested material
Congenital – atresia and stenosis
<u>Treatment</u>
Antispasmodics via rectum e.g. Enema of Nepeta cataria and Dioscorea.

Physiological changes in acute intestinal obstruction
1. Pain – intermittent at first, colicky in type. Later the pain becomes continuous and is more persistent.
2. Vomiting – stomach contents
                     bile stained fluid
                     faecal vomit due to reverse peristalsis
3. Shock and dehydration - pale anxious patient with sunken eyes
     Continued vomiting leads to loss of fluid and electrolytes notably NaCl and P.
4. Abdominal distension – distended bowel allows absorption into circulation of toxins and bacteria from decomposing elements.
5. Constipation – absolute constipation, absence of flatus

Pruritis [See anal conditions].

Worms Helminthic infections
Nematodes – Roundworm [Ascaris] and Hookworm [Necator].
Threadworm [Strongyloides].
Cestodes – Tapeworm from beef, fish or pork, rats or hydatid disease.
<u>Medicines</u>
Allium, Artemesia vulgaris, Capsicum, Cassia, Chenopodium, Convallaria, Gentiana, Helleborus niger, Humulus, Myroxylon balsamum, Oleum Ricinus, Ruta, Spigelia, Tanacetum vulgare, Ulmus.
Pomegranite bark decoction, Pumpkin seeds.

22
Genito Urinary System

Genito urinary medicines - Diuretics

Diuretics [1] Increase the flow of urine. [2] Remove waste impurities from the blood and tissue fluid. [3] Promote the absorption of an effusion in oedematous conditions. They produce their effects in two ways. The first by increasing renal blood flow through the glomerulus and secondly by inhibiting the reabsorption of sodium by the renal tubule. All herbal diuretics promote diuresis. The skin enhances eliminatory processes by removing fluid and impurities from the tissues.

Medicines increasing renal blood flow

Crataegus, Convallaria, Sarothamnus, Urgenia, Zanthoxylum, Zingiber.

Medicines increasing glomerular filtration are:

Nervine relaxants also have diuretic activity.
Agrimonia - astringent diuretic
Agropyron - demulcent diuretic
Alchemilla [aphanes] arvensis – astringent and demulcent
Apium – antiseptic, uric acid solvent, diuretic
Arctium sem - antiseptic diuretic
Barosma - stimulant diuretic
Capsella - genito urinary tonic/astringent.
Curcubita [pumpkin seed] – prostatic enlargement, intestinal parasites. [192 p449]
Daucus - stimulant and deobstruent diuretic
Equisetum - astringent tonic
Eryngium - astringent diuretic
Eupatorium purpureum - relaxing diuretic
Galium - relaxing and diffusive diuretic
Hydrangea – demulcent diuretic and antilithic
Juniperus - stimulating diuretic
Parietaria - demulcent diuretic
Petroselinum - diuretic tonic
Plantago - astringent diuretic, antihaemorrhagic
Rhus - genito urinary tonic
Solidago - antiseptic tonic, diuretic
Tinospora cordifolia – indicated in impotence/sexual dysfunction and spermatorrhoea
Uva ursi - astringent and antiseptic
Zea - demulcent diuretic

Herbal Medicine - Keys

Diaphoretics - Sudorific [See also Chapter 26]
Included here are diaphoretics as they influence skin and renal function. Diaphoretics play an important role in pyrexia and capillary treatment, particularly in chronic conditions. Diaphoretics encourage blood to the skin surface and reduce blood congestion within the kidneys. Capillaries tend to become obstructed as age advances and the use of diaphoretics enables a better flow of blood to the tissues.
Diaphoretics influence the [1] sweat glands of the skin, [2] the peripheral nerve endings, [3] superficial capillaries and the [4] central nerve component - medulla and spinal cord.

Diaphoretic medicines
Achillea - stimulating diaphoretic
Aristolochia - stimulating diaphoretic
Asclepias - relaxing diaphoretic
Capsicum - general stimulant in tardy reactions
Chamomelum nobile – relaxing diaphoretic. Increases dermal blood flow
Eupatorium perfoliatum – relaxing diaphoretic
Hyssopus – dermal and circulatory diffusive. Mild diaphoretic
Lobelia – relaxant to all structures - best given with positive vital reaction
Mentha viridis – mild diaphoretic activity in pyrexia
Nepeta cataria – relaxing diaphoretic with antispasmodic activity
Pilocarpus – deficient secretions. Stimulating diaphoretic
Salvia officinalis – relaxing diaphoretic
Sambucus – relaxing diaphoretic
Thymus – relaxing diaphoretic. Antispasmodic. Antiseptic.

Examination of the genito urinary tract
Always examine a specimen of urine passed first thing in the morning before food or drink and test the sample within four hours.
Renal examination is carried out by direct palpation. Hand held at the level of the 12th rib posteriorly. Supported with the opposite hand at the same level anteriorly. The examining hands are brought into contact with the kidney angle on asking the patient to hold an inspiratory breath for a few seconds. The bladder can be delineated by percussion, if there is urine to be voided. Prostate examination is via the rectum, using a glove and gel. Always clean the patient afterwards. Scrotal examination see testicle.

Sodium foods help prevent the body fluids from becoming too acid or too alkaline. Sodium chloride [common salt is hygroscopic] and encourages fluid to be held in the tissues.

Genito Urinary System

Adequate daily fluid intake

Adequate water consumption is essential for renal health. Skimping on fluid intake can cause passage of more concentrated urine which encourages the risk of kidney stones and infections. 1500 ml per day is considered a minimum fluid requirement when genito urinary or infective conditions are present.

Excess protein intake has been associated with an increase in calcium loss in the body, through enhanced urinary excretion of calcium. The **decrease in calcium** absorption occurring with **increased protein** intake is related to the acid produced from protein metabolism. Around half of this increase in calcium loss is attributed to the breakdown of sulphur containing amino acids with a resulting acid imbalance. The remainder is due to the increased renal filtration.

Urinary Conditions

Cystitis and recurrent infections

In health the urine is sterile. When infection is present it often occurs from outside the body. The bladder surface and prostatic fluid have natural antimicrobial effects. E. Coli infection if found in the urine, has been transferred from the anus.

Treatment

In the female patient with cystitis keep the area of the vulva clean and allow the shower water to spray down and not upwards. Always use a spray after a bath.

Increase fluids

Cranberry juice reduces the ability of infection to stick to the bladder wall.

The diet should contain large quantities of juices. Use a juice fast for 3 to 7 days. Followed by salads with vegetarian proteins. Grapes for potassium content.

Medicines

Diffusive demulcent diuretics and antimicrobials for cystitis.

Agropyron, Allium, Althea, Barosma, Hydrastis, Uva ursi.

Uva ursi - Infusium for cystitis - Sig 30ml TDS.

External use

Ol Tea tree diluted and added to the bath water

Enuresis

Is the patient drinking late into the evening? Check the prostate. Typically frayed nerves from a background of chronic fear, insecurity or anxiety aggravate enuresis, it often starts in childhood. Tonic and antispasmodic nervines help.

Urinary astringents

Agrimonia, Althea, Bidens tripartita, Capsella, Curcubita pepo, Equisetum, Geranium maculatum, Lycopodium clavatum, Marsdenia, Pulsatilla, Rhus aromatica, Rubus, Scutellaria, Valeriana, Verbascum, Verbena, Vinca, Zea.

Herbal Medicine - Keys

Epididymitis
Medicines
Agropyron, Capsicum, Echinacea, Pulsatilla, Salix nigra, Serenoa, Zea.

Genital herpes [See gynae section].

Glomerulonephritis - acute
Aetiology
Infection - [E. coli, pseudomonas, Streptococcus], tonsillitis and inflammation can cause damage to the glomerulus, leakage of blood and protein into the urine occurs. Salt and water retention leads to severe oedema.

Pyelitis and pyelonephritis – infections, calculi, diabetes, synthetic drugs, pregnancy.
Treatment for Glomerulonephritis Pyelitis and Pyelonephritis
Diet must be low protein, salt free. Fluids. Bedrest. Steaming – hot steam room. Laxatives to prevent toxic reabsorption. Cold hip bath.
Medication using diaphoretics and cholagogues.
Medicines
Achillea, Agrimonia, Agropyron, Althea, Baptisia, Barosma, Calendula, Capsicum, Daucus, Echinacea, Galium, Hydrangea, Parietaria, Peumus, Plantago, Sambucus, Solidago, Taraxacum, Uva ursi, Zea, Zingiber.
General prescription for kidney disorders.
15g Uva ursi 5g Juniperus 15g Barosma 15g Agropyron. Simmer gently for 15 minutes in one litre of water. Sig 30 ml TDS. Uses - antilithic, bladder and renal weakness. Rheumatism. Flatulence.

Gravel see renal calculus

Haematuria
Aetiology
Blood in the urine – calculi, infection, tumours.
Treatment
Astringent diuretic for the haemorrhage.

Hernia
Areas are checked by asking the patient to cough while the examiners hand is placed over the site of possible herniation [umbilicus, inguinal].
Treatment
Astringents and poultices – Agrimonia, Herniaria glabra Sig 3g., Tinospora cordifolia.

Genito Urinary System

Hydrocoele
An increase in the amount of scrotal fluid.
<u>Treatment</u>
Aspiration using a syringe. Diuretics.

Hydronephrosis
Renal oedema with dilation of the kidney. Often occurs from back pressure from an impacted calculus, chronic infection, tumours or enlarged prostate.

Impotency & Nymphomania - Sexual dysfunctions
Impotency is common to males who may have had several sexual partners. Impotency can occur from the initiation of the sex drive when it is more likely to have a physical problem. Sex drive decreases from the age of 30 years onwards. Mento emotional disturbance create an excess sympatheticotonia to the pelvis - excitability of the pelvic nerves. Fears arrest adrenal hormones and put the body into flight or fight mechanism. These influences constrict vasomotor blood vessels and nerve plexuses resulting in sympatheticotonia.

Men can suffer from the damaging effects of arguments and hostility, these emotions create atmospheres which can deplete the sex drive. Sensitivity of the man or woman can also be a problem.

In the history find out from the patient: Do you like the person that you are with – their mind, body etc?

Past health conditions which have a bearing - common in diabetics, arthritis of the spine, chorea, multiple sclerosis, rheumatic fever, chronic anxiety, depression.

Nymphomania [addicted to sex] of either sex encourages a greater need for excessive sex and creates overindulgence. Aetiology - anxiety, depression, fears, insecurity, poor self image, it can encourage masturbation excesses as an attempt to relax the body and mind. Cure relies upon psychotherapy for the fragile personality and nervine tonics, antispasmodics and/or hormonal balancers.

<u>Management</u>
Relax, reduce worry and stress. Avoid becoming too busy with life. Exercise.

Psychotherapy: sort out any problems in the relationship; anxieties or hostilities, worries and fears. Two thirds of couples attending *therapy sessions* reported an improved and enhanced sexual life with their partners. Impotency where it was a problem improved by the same amount [66%] in this group.

It is important to spend regular time to be together. Respect for your partners needs and kindness towards them count for a lot.

Regular sessions of physical touching, caressing and sharing both mentally and emotionally sharing problems by talking and listening. Trading complaints can be helpful. There should be no sex until full sexual desire is rekindled.

Go to bed together around three times a week. Commonly partners do not go to bed together.

Herbal Medicine - Keys

Medications - impotence/sexual dysfunction
Acorus - a general tonic is beneficial
Avena - tonic trophorestorative with Serenoa and Cola if there is depression.
Chamaelirium luteum – CNS tonic
Cola - central nervous system stimulant
Eleutherococcus - tonic
Humulus – sedative to sexual drive. Avoid in impotence/sexual dysfunction.
Jasminum officinale – aphrodisiac.
Liriosma ovata - spinal nerve tonic
Panax - tonic when much stress is a cause
Pausinystalia - Yohimbe is used as a vasodilator to the penis.
Pulsatilla - in sensitivity of the nerves, it reduces nerve irritability
Salix nigra – sexual sedative - avoid in impotence/sexual dysfunction.
Schizandra – adaptogenic tonic.
Scutellaria - nervine antispasmodic
Serenoa – prostate tonic
Tinospora cordifolia – [Guduchi].
Turnera - insufficiency and inadequate erections, it strengthens the genitalia.
Valeriana – relaxant nervine.
Vitex - lack of virility, hormonal.
Withania – adaptogenic.
Zizzyphus – tonic nervine.
Medicines also include - Byrsocarpus coccineus, Funtumia elastica - stem and twig latex, Microdesmis puberula, Microglossa pyrifolia, Neubouldia laevis.
Aromatherapy – Lavandula, Patchouli, Rosmarinus, Ylang ylang with a base oil for massage or diluted essential oil in an atomiser. Massage each other and become intimate again.
Bach flower remedies
Larch, for lack of confidence and fear of failure. Walnut for over sensitivity.
Treatment - long term – Scutellaria, Valeriana, Viscum for nervous subjects.
Tablet of Cola, Turnera and Pulsatilla – Sig 1/2 TDS. Tablets provide a slower absorption to enable a gentle trophic effect within nerve tissue.

Incontinence
Medicines
Ephedra, Equisetum, Geranium maculatum, Passiflora, Uva ursi.

Infertility [See sterility]

Nephrotic syndrome
Moth eaten glomerular damage. Leads to heavy protein losses in the urine and thus reduction in plasma proteins.

Genito Urinary System

Treatment - nephrotic syndrome
Restrict fluids. Keep an intake and output chart of fluid consumed. Avoid salt.
Diet – protein not in excess of 60g daily.
Medicine
Astringent, tonic diuretics – Agrimonia, Capsella, [See renal failure below].

Oedema
Oedema persisting through the night is likely to be of renal origin. Oedema building up through the day and clearing through the night is likely to be of cardiac origin.

Orchitis
Inflammation of the testicles with pain.
Treatment
Cool the area with a cold or ice compress if retainable. Ice compress, applied for 30 seconds PRN.
Medicines
Echinacea, Galium, Pulsatilla, Salix nigra, Smilax.

Prostate disturbances
Falling levels of testosterone appears to encourage the prostate to enlarge. Enlargement is common to men over 60. Frequency and incontinence follow after a period of time. Cholesterol metabolites accumulate in the prostate and initiate cancer. Dioxins encourage prostate enlargement. Chemical oestrogens are naturally present in plastic and leach out into the food contained within, these can affect the prostate.

Diagram of the prostate gland

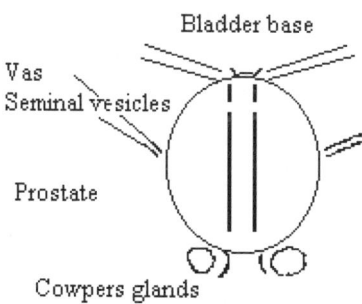

Unbroken lines palpated in health, plus dotted lines in disease

Prostatic calculi
Simulates the irregular hardness of carcinoma 'like beads in a bag'.

Acute prostatitis
Acute prostatitis - may cause retention of urine. PR examination reveals oedematous and a tender hot prostate gland.

Chronic Prostatitis
PR examination - reveals the gland can be enlarged or normal. Nodular enlargement with boggy areas. Tenderness is slight or absent.

Benign adenomatous enlargement
PR examination - increase in prostate size. Smooth, convex, elastic but may be firm enlargement. Usually middle lobe enlargement.

Carcinoma of the prostate
PR examination – posterior part of the gland near the surface is recognised as a rounded area of induration, as it enlarges the nodule acquires stony hardness. Later the vertical median groove between the lateral lobes becomes obliterated. Enlargement towards the seminal vesicles, like horns of a bull is characteristic. Due to the involvement of the lymphatics mobility reduces. Extension is in a backwards direction. Stony hard irregular mass interrupts the normal contour of the gland.

Treatment
Hydrotherapy includes hot/cold contrast immersions for the pelvis. Hot immersion for three minutes and cold immersion for one minute. Always finish with cold. Spray the perineum with cold water from the shower.
Exercise improves venous return and arterial output.

Medicines
Drainage of blood from the pelvis to relieve prostate congestion – Collinsonia. Myrica.
Acute prostatitis [usually abacterial] – immerse the pelvis in warm water for five minutes. Complete with cold effusion.
Prostate hypertrophy – Agrimonia, Aphanes, Capsella, Equisetum, Eryngium, Hydrangea, Serenoa, Solidago, Tussilago, Urtica, Zea. Oleum Borago. Oleum Linum.
Zinc picolinate will inhibit 5 alpha reductase.

Pyelonephritis/Pyelitis [See glomerulonephritis]

Renal failure – acute
Aetiology
Severe hypotension, shock, septicaemia, renal disease.
Oliguric phase – reduced urinary output with possible anuria.
Diuretic phase follows as improvement occurs.

Genito Urinary System

Treatment See glomerulonephritis.
Diet – low protein around 20g. Restricted fluids to 600ml in 24 hours.
Patients are often extremely ill.

Chronic renal failure

Chronic renal failure increases acidosis when potassium ions accumulate, this can cause disorders of heart rhythm.
Treatment See glomerulonephritis.
Restrict the amount of potassium in the diet.
Restrict sodium.
Dietary and fluid restriction.

Renal calculus

Calculi are formed mainly from calcium where there is an increase in renal excretion of calcium. Calcium oxalate and phosphate form crystals which create gravel and stones.
The condition is related to a diet of refined carbohydrates, low fibre and high animal saturated fats.
Vitamin and mineral treatment.
Vitamin B6 and magnesium working together help prevent renal calculi. Magnesium helps excrete calcium stones. Vitamin B6 increase the excretion of oxalates. Vitamin K prevents the crystallisation of calcium oxalate. A small amount of citrates found in the urine is normal. Calculi formation makes the citrates bind with the calcium and then the citrate is no longer available for oxalate elimination. Citrates prevent seeding of oxalates. A Low citrate can result from diarrhoea and UTI. **Sodium citrate and magnesium citrate can prevent calculi. Calcium citrate is better absorbed than calcium carbonate.**
Treatment
Adequate fluid intake is essential. Many renal medicines will break down calculi.
Agropyron, Alchemilla arvensis, Althea, Atropa, Collinsonia, Daucus, Eryngium, Eupatorium purpureum, Galium, Hydrangea, Parietaria, Zea.
Prescription for Renal calculus
Zea 30g, Althea 30g, Collinsonia 15g, Ess Mentha virida 20 Gtt. Aq ad 240ml. Sig 15 ml TDS.

Renal colic

Medicines
Use relaxing diuretics and demulcents.
Anodynes of an antispasmodic nature. [See emergency herbal medicine].

Retention of urine [See emergency herbal medicine]

Herbal Medicine - Keys

Sterility
Medicine
Avena, Capsicum, Centella, Cornus officinalis, Panax, Selenicerus, Turnera, Vitex, Zanthoxylum. Vitamin B complex, Vitamin E. Zinc.

Testicular problems
The examination of the testes is performed in two stages:
A] Observe the testes for size and shape. It is common to have one testicle slightly larger or which hangs slightly lower than the other.
B] Feel for any changes. Hold the scrotum in the palms of your hands so that you can examine each testicle in turn using the middle fingers under the testicle and the thumb on both hands. Place your index and middle fingers under the testicle and your thumb on top. You should be able to feel a firm, smooth tube running upwards from the epididymis - this is the spermatic cord. Feel the testicle itself by gently rolling it between the thumb and fingers. Note it's size, weight and consistency - it should be smooth, with no lumps or swellings. Both testicles should feel the same. The Left testicle always hangs lower than the right.

Swellings are found in:
Neoplasm [hard, eventually immovable enlargement]
Syphilis
Epididymitis. Is there a history of surgery causing infection?
Epididymo orchitis is a non translucent disorder. The cord thickens and the testes are hot.
Epididymis enlarged and nodular usually follows mumps.
Hydrocoele [watery soft enlargement]
Spermatocoele
Varicocoele [nearly always on the left].

Testicular cancer
Around 1600 men a year develop testicular cancer and accounts for around 2% of all neoplasms in males. It is the most common male cancer in the 20-35 year age group. Some 10% of men with testicular cancer had crypto-orchidism [undescended testes as children]. Any changes in testicle shape or size should be examined. A feeling of heaviness or a dull ache in the lower abdomen could be warning signs. [416]

Uraemia
Often the result of failing kidneys.
Treatment as renal failure

Genito Urinary System

Urethral stricture
May follow an infection. Scarring of the urethra can occur.
Medicine for urethral stricture
Althea, Atropa, Daucus, Echinacea, Equisetum, Eryngium, Eupatorium purpureum, Thuja, Zea.

Urethritis
Infection either ascending from E coli, or sexually transmitted disease.
Treatment
Irrigation via a catheter with urinary antiseptic medication from list below.
Medicine
Achillea, Agropyron, Althea, Apium, Barosma, Betula alba/pendula, Calluna, Echinacea, Equisetum, Eryngium, Eupatorium purpureum, Galium aparine, Piper methysticum, Serenoa, Uva ursi, Zea.

Varicocoele
Medicine
Venous tonics. Cold spray.

23
Urine analysis

Urine collection
For a correct interpretation of urinary constituents, the urine must be collected in the morning before food or drink are taken. Urine voided must be tested within four hours.
For microscopical analysis of the urine the area should be washed and a mid stream specimen obtained. A minimum of six hours concentration of urine in the bladder is required for a specimen test.
Mid stream specimen. The patient voids a little urine, stops, then voids into the specimen jar, stops once again and completes micturition. The mid part of the urine is used for analysis. Preservation of urine is with 1% boric acid.

Dipstix are used for the interpretation of abnormalities in the urine. The following can be found, if present, and indicate the need for further investigation: bilirubin, ketones, nitrite, pH, blood, protein, specific gravity [Sp.G.], glucose, leucocytes, urobilinogen.
It may be necessary to check three specimens of urine on different days for complete analysis of urinary constituents.

Centrifuge the urine and **microscopical** analysis can reveal:
amorphous deposits, bacteria/parasites, casts, crystals, epithelial cells, foreign substances, fragments of tumour growths, gravel/calculi, prostatic threads, RBC's. WBC's, sperm and yeasts.

Kova slide
Fill a capillary tube with bleach to clean both tube and slide. Put on the stage and leave to settle. Use 10x for focus and 40x for fine detail. Mid stream specimen will avoid contamination. The Kova slide has counting chambers.
Count the number of: RBC's and WBC's.

Observe for [a] Squamous cells and

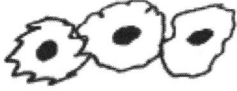

[b] Tubal epithelial cells

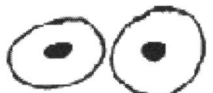

Genito Urinary System

Rolled up epithelial cells - cylindrical or elongated are found where bacteria, crystals or yeast exist.
Squamous cells and epithelial cells are not significant unless there are a lot of them.

Urinary abnormalities

Bacteria – seen as red shapes or spheres under microscopical examination. Bacteria are moving or non moving. Spheres are clusters or chains. [See also infection below].

Bile or B vitamins show a yellow discolouration of the sample.
Test - Shake a specimen – bile shows a frothy appearance.

Calcium elimination or infection produce high alkalinity.

Casts – bodies formed in the tubule of the nephron. Cylindrical mould shape. Proteinuria generally accompanies casts.
- found in some high fevers where the membranes become damaged.
- nephritis e.g. glomerulonephritis – basement membrane damage.
- strenuous exercise
- emotional stress [long standing]

Waxy and fatty casts
       tubular, inflammation, degeneration
       chronic renal disease of the collecting tubules
Pseudo casts are found in associated proteinuria, inflammatory disease of the renal pelvis or ureter, hydronephrosis. Pseudo casts have tapered ends.

Pseudo casts

Cloudy – albumin
       urates
Found in cystitis, inflammation and dehydration.

Conditions creating infections

Candida, Trichomonas, immuno compromised babies, diabetes, damaged urinary tract from catheters, descending UTI, antibiotics.
WBC's are seen in these conditions.

Crystals
1. Calcium oxalate
2. Urate
3. Phosphate

Epithelial cell casts – are always present but such may be abnormally high. Epithelial cell casts are found in disease of the tubule, severe tubular damage [a cement loss]. Unlikely to see cells unless 100x is used.

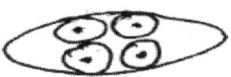 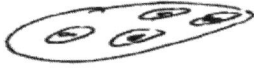

these degenerate to a coarse granular cast

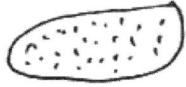

if the degeneration continues it produces a fine granular cast and these have a grainy appearance and are colourless, grey or pale.

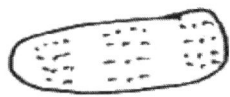

Fishy smell to urine – acetone [renal failure], ketones [diabetes, starvation], nitrogen [infection].

Frothy specimen – albumin [where 1% albumin can elevate Sp.G. by 3 points].

Fungus bulbs – puff balls

Hyaline cast – consists of protein and a mucoid substance. Semi transparent, no detail.
Detecting hyaline cast may not indicate pathology.
Found in:
acidity, extreme exercise, multiple myeloma, polyarteritis nodosa, proteinuria, severe parenchymal disease.

Genito Urinary System

Hyaline cast diagram

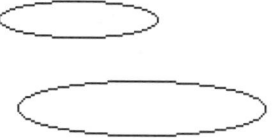

Infection [See conditions above]
90% of infections ascend from the bladder.
Descending infection occurs from: calculi, leptospirosis, TB, tumour, typhoid.

Ketones
Normally only 3-15mg of ketones are excreted in a day.
The quantity is increased in:
fasting, starvation, impaired carbohydrate metabolism [diabetes], pregnancy, ether anaesthesia and some types of alkalosis. Excess fat metabolism will induce a ketonuria. The acidosis accompanying ketosis will cause increased ammonia in the breath.

Nitrite
Nitrite is found in infections of the urinary system.
Ascorbic acid inhibits the conversion of nitrate to nitrite and reduces the formation of cancer forming nitrosamines [22].

Pseudo casts see casts

pH – preferable level is acid at 5

Phosphates
Turbid urine indicates **phosphates**.
Alkaline, cloudy - suspect phosphate crystals if dipstix show no protein.
Test
2% dilute acetic acid clears phosphates.

Protein [Albuminuria]
The presence of urinary protein requires investigation. Albumin can be detected by heating the urine, preferably after centrifuging to remove the sediment, then adding dilute acetic acid. A white cloud after addition of the acid indicates that protein is present. Normally not more than 30 – 200mg of protein are excreted daily in the urine.

Herbal Medicine - Keys

Albuminuria
Aetiology
[1] transient albuminuria could be due to: severe anxiety, pyrexia, strenuous activity, exposure to severe cold. In a few cases albuminuria may be found in the last few weeks of pregnancy.

[2] organic albuminuria [pre renal] operating before the kidney is reached.
Drugs causing toxic effects upon the kidneys. Heavy metals like mercury, arsenic and bismuth can poison the tubules.
Anaemia. Blood diseases.
Dehydration from pyloric obstruction.
Intestinal obstruction. Severe diarrhoea.
Intra abdominal pressure as in ascites and intra abdominal tumours.
Diabetic coma.
Addisons disease.
Heart disease with passive congestion of the kidneys.
Impairment of the renal circulation.
Pyrexia.

[3] Renal albuminuria [post renal] may arise in the renal pelvis, ureters, bladder, prostate or urethra. Mixture of vaginal or prostatic secretions may give a false positive.
Renal albuminuria can be found in all forms of renal disease whether from degenerative, inflammatory or destructive aetiology.
Glomerular proteinuria occurs with increased passage of proteins. Tubular proteinuria from impaired reabsorption of protein.
Acute glomerulonephritis occurs from damage to the glomeruli.
Nephrosis produces a marked proteinuria accompanied by oedema and low concentrations of serum albumin.
Nephrosclerosis, a vascular form of renal disease is related to arterial hypertension. The proteinuria observed increases with the increasing severity of the renal lesion. Although less is found than in glomerulonephritis.
In patients with lesions of the ureters or bladder blood may be added after the urine has left the tubules, in such cases we have haematuria.

Pus in urine
Aetiology: abacterial cystitis, acute infection, collagen disease, cystitis, renal tumour.

Red blood cells – if specimen stands – smoky, ground glass appearance. Normal urine will have some RBC's [5mm to C]

Genito Urinary System

Three forms of RBC's. [Dont confuse with yeasts]
1] Biconcave discs. Smaller than white cells.
  High Sp.G. in the urine and the RBC's become biconcave.
2] Crenated
3] Ghost [rare] have a larger nuclei

RBC's are found in:
- Benign familial haematuria,
- Glomerulonephritis, renal infarction, urinary tract infections,
- Calculi, collagen disease, SABE, strenuous exercise – transient,
- Vascular disease, capillary necrosis, endocarditis.
- Malignancy in 10% of patients over 40

Test: Cool the urine in a fridge.
Brick red colour suggests red blood cells.
Bleeding into the nephron gives a red colour.
Red blood cell casts are rarely seen.
Usually disintegrate into granular casts.

Semen
Normal sperm count gives a volume of between 3-5ml. pH is 7.4.
Count 60 - 200 million per ml.
Motility of 90% after 45 minutes. Around 65% after 3 hours.
Abnormal forms up to 20%

Sodium prevents the body fluids from becoming too acid or too alkaline.

Smoky urine – on standing or may suggest haemorrhage.

Specific gravity – normal level is between 1015 -1020

Tubular necrosis – red cell casts may be found in pyelonephritis, infection or partial obstruction.

Tissue necrosis – casts are found.
Aetiology - decrease in urinary flow, acid pH., obstruction.

Herbal Medicine - Keys

Urate crystals [uric acid crystals] give a brick red colour – acid pH, turbid urine, rheumatic complaints.

White blood cells – large numbers suggest invading organisms.
WBC's found in suppurative conditions. Large numbers of pus cells are seen in infections and inflammatory conditions. Scanty white cells observed may indicate ingested infection.
WBC casts are cigar shaped casts. Red cells are seen inside the cast. White cells are formed in the tubules.

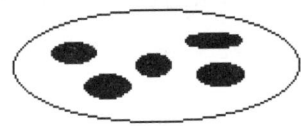

During pregnancy it is normal to have a large number of WBC's
White cell casts occur in:
Inflammatory and infection aetiology - drug/chemical intoxication, cystitis, glomerulonephritis, nephrotic syndrome, chronic pylonephritis, prostatitis, urethritis, intrinsic renal disease, suppurative disease.

WBC's qualitative count
2 million in 24 hours. 0-5 per mm3 [textbook normal].
Female   20 per mm3
Male   10 per mm3
           20 - 50 possible contamination with vaginal discharge
           50 – 100 significant.

Yeasts may be oral or budding
Put one drop of saline on a slide with a swab of the infection, cover slip and observe.

Oral   Budding

Trichomonas vaginalis
Present with four flagella and move with a wobbling/rotating movement. Once removed from the body for analysis it must be observed within five minutes or the trichomonas will die.

24
Immune system

Immune medicines

Vasotonic alteratives are immunoactive remedies. Activity involves
- the neutralising of toxins,
- inhibition of micro-organisms
- removal of cellular impurities together with blood cleansing.

Most organ medicines possess alterative activity. [See also Chapter 29].

Immunostimulants and blood cleansing medicines - vasotonic alteratives.

Allium sativa
Arctium lappa
Baptisia tinctoria
Calendula officinalis
Catharanthus rosea
Chimaphilla umbellata
Commiphora molmol
Daphne mezerium
Dicentra canadensis
Echinacea species
Fucus vesiculosis
Guaiacum officinale
Iris versicolor
Ligustrum porteri
Menispermum canadensis
Panax ginseng
Phytolacca decandra
Plantago major
Polygonum multiflorum
Polymnia uvedalia
Polypodium vulgare
Porea cocos
Rehmannia glutinosa
Rumex crispus
Salvia miltiorrhiza
Sanicula europaea
Sassafras officinalis
Scrophularia nodosa
Smilax officinalis
Stachys betonica
Stillingia sylvatica

Tabebuia impetiginosa
Thymus species
Trifolium pratense
Uncaria tomentosa
Veronica beccabunga
Veronica officinalis
Viola odorata

Remedies for the immune system

Vitamin C, D, E. }
Manganese   } all will increase oxygenation of the tissues
Selenium   }
Low levels of the above are found in toxic and allergic complaints.
T cell function is improved with zinc - use zinc citrate.

Immunology

Natural immunity is present at birth and is actively supported by breast milk feeding.
Acquired immunity means the cells have responded to an antigen. The cells keep this response as a memory for the future, in order to protect against adverse circumstances.
Natural immunity is provided by the skin. Perspiration is bactericidal. Mucous membranes secrete lysozyme which is antimicrobial. Extracellular fluids neutralise toxins, promote phagocytosis, provide antibodies and activate compliment.
Phagocytes – both macrophages and neutrophils destroy abnormalities within the blood. Phagocytes are found in the bone marrow, spleen, lymph nodes and the blood circulation.

Acquired immunity

Cell mediated immunity and humoral immunity are both acquired. Humoral immunity involves antibodies and compliment. Compliment within the plasma binds to antigen-antibody complexes.

Immune responses

Cellular immunity involves the activation of:
T cells
Cytokines
Lymphokines - activate macrophages and increase leucocytes.
Interleukins – affect prostaglandins, bone reabsorption, IgA synthesis.
Interferons – are proteins which are released by cells when infected by a virus.
Interferons once released interfere with virus replication.

Immune System

And from cellular responses there are effects of transmitting influences to the blood. All of the following transmit their influences to the blood for good or baneful effect.

Nervous system   }   Blood
GUT   }
GIT   }
Muscular/skeletal system   }

Treatment always goes back to the beginning with these cases.
1 Firstly look for secernant organ malfunction. Treat any eliminative organ insufficiency first. It is important to clear the eliminative organ before any deep cleansing takes place. Otherwise a crisis may develop which could be very difficult to control [See Chapter 11].
2 Next attend to the condition of the blood and lymph [including the immune malfunction]. There is about three times more lymph than blood. Cleansing the blood and lymph can take about three years of continuous treatment.
3 Nerve treatment is frequently required to settle an overactive immune system response.

Organism response to an allergen occurs from:
- Humoral antibody production
- Cell mediated response.

Humeral response involves **antigen – antibody reactions**, immunoglobulins and compliment. **Immunoglobulins** are glycoproteins. The main immunoglobulins within the body are IgA, IgD, IgE, IgG, IgM. Around 20% of IgA is found in the serum and secretions of the intestine. IgE is found in allergic reactions. IgG is mainly evidenced by antibody formation during an immune response. Compliment is a plasma protein. Compliment binds to antigen – antibody complexes. Compliment facilitates the elimination of micro-organisms.

Immune tolerance.
Immature immune cells are recognised as foreign and attacked by the T and B cells. **Autoimmunity** means a loss of immune tolerance. This occurs and the body produces antibodies to itself. The antibodies then become a damaging influence to an organ [thyroid] or system [SLE] and many sites can become affected.

Cells involved in the immune response
Lymphocytes involved in the immune response are T and B lymphocytes. T cells switch off activity whereas lack of T cells activates the problem. B lymphycytes produce antibodies that neutralise infectious organisms [antigen]. B lymphocytes

recognise virus infections. T lymphocytes are involved with cell mediated immunity, this includes T helper cells, T suppresser cells and others. T lymphocytes orchestrate and produce interferons. Null cells possess receptors for IgG antibodies. Killer cells are coated with antibodies and are cytotoxic. Mast cells release histamine and are involved in hypersensitivity reactions.

Basophils and eosinophils are respectively blood and mucus borne. Stem cells are found in the bone and lymph tissue. Some cells carry antigens.

Allergy, sensitivity and toxicity

Allergy and sensitivity to foods often have a basis in a toxic problem found within the cell or tissue fluids an overload of toxins find their way into the blood. Symptoms are found when toxins have sensitised the immune response to danger within the cell or blood stream.

Hypersensitivity reactions

Hypersensitivity reactions involve an increased response by the immune system to an antigen or a damaging effect that can affect any area.

Reactions:

1] anaphylactic - where shock may predominate

{antibody immunoglobulin reaction.

2] immune mediated cytotoxic cell membrane {   "

3] cell mediated   {   "

4] stimulated antibody reaction   {   "

5] antibody reaction

6] antibody dependent cell mediated cytotoxicity

Summary of above different hypersensitivity reactions [1 – 6]

1]   Immediate reaction. Antigen – foods, dust mite, drugs, parasites, pollen.
     Histology reaction – oedema, vasodilation, mast cell degranulation, oesinophils.
     Condition produced – allergic rhinitis, anaphalaxis, asthma [extrinsic], eczema [atopic].

2]   Cytotoxic. Antigen – cellular surface or tissue bound.
     Histology – damage to the target cells.
     Condition produced – addisonism, haemolytic anaemia, pernicious anaemia, transfusion reactions, myasthenia gravis.

3]   Immune complex. Antigen – bacteria, fungi, parasites.
     Histology – acute inflammatory reactions, neutrophils, vasculitis.
     Condition produced – glomerulonephritis, persistent infections, RA, environmental antigens from farmers lung e.g. mould.

4]   Delayed reaction. Antigen - cell or tissue bound.
     Histology - perivascular inflammation, mononuclear cells and fibrin.

Condition produced – contact dermatitis, insect bites, leprosy, pulmonary Tuberculosis.

5] Stimulating. Antigen - cell surface.

Histology – hypertrophy.

Condition produced – neonatal hyperthyroidosm, hyperthyroidism.

6] Antibody dependent cell mediated cytotoxicity. Antigen – antibody complex upon the cellular surface of target cells.

Histology – damage to target cells.

Condition produced – autoimmune tumour rejection.

Allergic phenomena and aetiology of allergy

The immune system signals an alarm bell to ring when allergy is present. It is rare to find only one allergen. Where one allergen is present, remove the allergen and the patient is cured. Multiple allergies are often found and suggest the need to detoxify the blood and clear the liver as a primary site of protein metabolism. The unique position of the liver in the splanchnic drainage system clearly illustrates its physiological function of detoxification. According to Heitner [128], the gastro intestinal tract is the source for the clinical syndrome of allergic reactions to **cows milk** [dairy produce]. The intestinal canal is equipped with various immunological mechanisms. Secretory IgA plays an important role in the immune response. Patients lacking IgA often have excessive absorption of numerous dietary antigens that result in immune complex formation. Immune complexes are transported to the liver. Hepatic drainage becomes obstructed in allergy and results in liver tumefaction [swelling] [61].

Alan Baklayan, a Naturopath, discovered a link betweeen ascarid infestation, Geotrichum candidum yeast infection in dairy allergy. Recommended treatment is [1] avoidance of dairy produce, [2] removal of worm infestation and [3] treatment of any yeast infection [415].

Some causes of allergy

- Blood changes/toxicity and blood impurity/allergies
- Eliminative organ disorders
- Hormonal changes - post pregnancy, PMS
- Malnourished – low Vitamin C, zinc
- Spinal nerve loop irritation [simple reflex arc] - irritated nerve supply
- Stress/depression - fatigues the immune system.

Allergic responses

Allergic responses are fixed or mobile. A mobile response can become altered with HRT and the contraceptive pill, enquire about this in the history.

Mobile responses:

a] The amount of food can effect the level of allergic response. You will want a response in the patient once they commence treatment. Check the patients symptoms to assess the response of a diet or fast.

b] Tolerance cut off. A small amount of allergen may produce no allergic response.

c] On/off response either all or nothing with symptom reaction. Either very allergic with symptoms or no reaction.

d] Foods containing histamine could provoke a reaction e.g. mackerel.

e] Lectins can trigger a histamine type response [a false food response].

Allergic reactions in an individual
Tendency to feel worse if they don't have the product.
Feel better if they keep on with it. This is due to tolerance to the product.

Treating allergies and food sensitivities
Immediate treatment
A short **fast** then introduce one food at a time. Bananas contain serotonin and may cause allergy. If there is no reaction within 24 hours [max 48] there is no allergy.
Removing one food from the diet at a time is another way to treat.

Long term
It should be remembered that over exercising can deplete the immune system.
Find out the patient's intake of food and drink, by using a diet diary to cover 7 days. Avoid the premenstrual week in women, holidays etc. The diet diary should give the patients full intake and amount of foodstuffs and include drinks. Adjustment of the diet, if required, can then be made. [See Ch 28]. Observe for allergies in foods, some examples are:
dairy produce, yeast, egg, red meat, gluten grains, cane sugar.
Foods producing less response are: rice, lamb, sunflower/pumpkin seeds, pork.

Detoxification is achieved through one or more of the following:
- avoidance of the allergen
- restricted food intake – remove the item for 14 days
- dietary changes
- fasting
- Detoxification can reduce the chemical overload in the body. This will support immune function.

Treatments to help detoxification of the tissues.
- Vitamin C   } all will increase oxygenation of the tissues
- Manganese   }   "
- Selenium   }   "
Low levels of the above are found in toxic and allergic complaints.

- T cell function is improved with zinc. Use Zinc citrate at around 15mg daily. Zinc sulphate has a purgative quality.
- Calcium carbonate is poorly absorbed. Calcium gluconate – better absorption.
- [See also cholesterolaemia Chapter 3]

General factors in immunity
Chemical sensitivity
Occurs from a build up of toxic chemicals in the system e.g. lead, mercury etc. Hyperactivity in children maybe, tartrazine or sunset yellow [colouring], induced, their zinc could be low.

Antioxidants and free radicles
Antioxidants are protective enzymes. They protect against free radicle damage.
Free radicles are oxygen molecules in a highly reactive unstable form and are found in the atmosphere, in food and within our own bodies. They are formed as a by product of normal cellular activity but can cause other cells to behave abnormally. Research implicates these molecules in a range of illnesses – including heart disease, cancer and aging. Free radicles are produced by many things e.g. pollution, chemicals, smoking. They only live for a few seconds. Free radicles damage chromosomes and fatty acids in the cell membrane. Other changes are triggered by peroxidation [rancidity]. Resulting in the cell membrane losing its ability to protect the cell. Free radicles attack the enzymes and proteins resulting in skin loss of elasticity, the skin ages and becomes wrinkled. The aging process is stimulated by this process. Cell damage creates aging, senility, and all chronic disease. It follows that free radicle damage is found in all illnesses.
Protection with enzymes made from our own cells together with nutrients from the diet, help neutralise free radicles. Antioxidants are nutritionally dependent and require copper, magnesium, selenium and zinc to perform correctly. Ubiquinone, Beta carotine, Vitamins A, B complex, C, and E are also antioxidants. Urea and bilirubin produced by the kidneys and blood are also antioxidants.

Pesticides
Pesticides are responsible for T and B cell reduction in the body.
Cadmium toxicity [cadmium is found in plastic] has adverse effects on host resistance to bacterial and viral infections.
Vitamin B6, Petroselinum and Allium help chelation [reduction] of cadmium.

Pulse test – used to detect allergies.
Take the pulse at rest. Give the patient, to hold in the mouth, the allergic product. When the reaction is positive [an allergy or sensitivity], an increase in the pulse is

measured. Pulse increases by around 10 over one minute. It may take 24 hours to produce a response. Avoiding the product will usually settle the reaction. Acute and severe IgE reactions may occur with allergies e.g. anaphalactic shock, asthma, urticaria.

Transit time

The time it takes for food to pass through the gastro intestinal tract. It may take up to 24 hours to process the food eaten. To test transit time ingest charcoal tablets taken after food, usually six tablets as a single dose. Charcoal colours the stool and is a useful indicator of the transit time for food passing through the git. Longer or shorter transit times will raise suspicion of absorption problems.

Main symptoms of food intolerance
Headache, Migraine, Fatigue, Depression/Anxiety, Hyperactivity
Recurrent mouth ulcers
Aching muscles, joint pain, rheumatoid arthritis.
Nausea/vomiting, Stomach/duodenal ulcers, Bloating/flatulence, Diarrhoea, Constipation
IBS, Chrohn's disease Oedema.
Eczema
50% of patients are allergic to eggs/dairy produce/wheat/citrus fruit/sugar.
One of more may produce a reaction.
Migraine
Oranges/cheese/sherry/chianti can produce pain. Oranges affect the liver.
Hepatomegaly [See above]
Children respond to allergens and often the effect is produced through mucous membrane sensitivity e.g. pharyngitis, headache, rhinitis, abdominal pain, otitis media, respiratory infections.

Glaser research
Children fed a diet free of cows milk, wheat, eggs and chicken, up to 10 months of age, were found to have less allergy.

Weight trouble
Could be caused by food sensitivity. Avoid certain foods and thereby lose weight if the patient is food sensitive. Increase fluids to encourage weight loss.

Conditions with an autoimmune basis

Adrenal glands
Addisons disease is a hypotrophic adrenal condition.

Immune System

AIDS Acquired immune deficiency syndrome.

The virus of AIDS is a retrovirus. A virus can only replicate itself inside of the cell. Groups of molecules – antigens on the outside of the cell are recognised by the antigen and by their own cells they are therefore not destroyed. CD4 antigen acts as a receptor to the virus. The virus attaches to the surface and is taken into the cell. The virus can only affect certain cells. The aids virus kills cells it lives in. Not all cases that have the virus get aids. Initially a small part of the lymph system is affected. Some cells die off as a result and toxins kill more cells. Failure of the response of B lymphocytes to a new antigen allow the virus to spread. Interferons are not produced in aids patients. Reduced alpha levels and raised levels of an abnormal acid labile interferon occur. Reduced interleukin 2 levels and elevated B – 2 microglobulin are found. Antibody +ve patients may not be infectious initially until the immune system becomes more damaged. Deterioration is greater in depressed patients.

Inactivating the virus. The virus will die outside of the body and can be destroyed with soap and hot water. Heat will destroy the virus at 560 degrees for 30 minutes.

New forms of the virus

Reports in 2002 indicate new superviruses. One reason for this is the supposed protection available through drug treatment. Synthetic drugs only control the virus when taken. Once the drugs are stopped the virus reappears. People are reinfecting each other with the new virus. HIV mutates faster than any other known virus and once mutation has taken place it becomes a synthetic drug resistant form.

Classification - [group 1] acute infection
[group 2] asymptomatic infection/lymph nodes
[group 3] persistent generalised/lymphadenopathy.

Some cases have an abrupt and sudden onset of watery diarrhoea. An incubation period of 11-28 days. Followed by pyrexia. After two days – clinical glandular fever, sore throats, rashes, headaches, night sweats, diarrhoea, fatigue, painful ulcers of the mouth, genitals or anus in some cases. The illness lasts between 5-44 days, the average just under 14 days. Majority of patients have no initial symptoms. Patients are lymphopenic – a progressive depletion of neutrophils along with thrombocytopenia.

Symptomatology - fatigue, weight loss, anorexia, lymphadenopathy, thrush, herpes, leucoplakia, meningitis, respiratory catarrhal symptoms, pneumonia, genitourinary symptoms inflammatory in nature e.g. herpes, leucorrhoea, gonorrhoea, warts. Patients with skin symptoms have GIT symptoms.

Herbal Medicine - Keys

Neurological complications – brain infections, malignancy, ischaemia, haemorrhage [due to thrombocytopenia], metabolic arteritis, meningitis, peripheral neuropathy, dementia.

Prognostic markers [poor prognosis] are oral candida, herpes zoster and leucoplakia. A single blood test confirms the diagnosis - Differential lymphocyte count: T cell sub sets and look for T4 + T8 cells. Condition requires to be present for about six months before the virus can be isolated.

Lymph nodes reveal follicular hyperplasia and is typical of viral infection.

Treatment

Strategy is to inhibit the virus.

Support the immune system.

Help positive psychoneuro immunological effects [slow deep breathing, Yoga, Tai chi, positive thinking].

Diet - Wholefood, omitting sugar and refined foods

Vitamin C, beta carotine,

Constitutional treatment

Precise treatment is constitutional.

Allium, Astragalus, Berberis, Buxus sempervirens [Boxwood], Echinacea. Glycyrrhiza, Hypericum, Lomatum, Siphonochilus aethiopicus [African ginger] and Sutherlandia frutescens.

The following have been tested and found to be active in inhibiting the virus.

Aphrosa villosa [60%], Breynia angustifolia [57%], Bridelia retusa [45%], Coptis chinensis [94%], Drypetes roxburghii [45%], Duabanga sonneratiodes [94%], Gardenia coronaria [51%], Harrisonia perforata [68%], Lithospermum erythrorhizon [60%], Paranephelium longifoliatum [45%], Schrebera swietenoides [53%], Securinga leucopyrus [68%], Terminalia catappa [97%], Terminalia alata [90%], Turpinia cochinchinensis (45%), [Figures in brackets are % aids virus inhibition values at 200 ug/mol] [278, 1991, 54, [1], p143-54].

Candida

Candida can produce in excess of 25 different symptoms. Candida colonises in the intestine, infection overgrowth is due to toxins and blood impurities [See also gynaecology].

Haemochromatosis

An excess deposition of iron into organs leading to fibrosis and organ failure. Features gonadal atrophy, loss of libido, lethargy, bronze skin, diabetes.

Hepatitis

Hepatitis A and B are acute illnesses. Transmission is via the oral-faecal route, also by saliva, blood and urine. [See also digestive system].

Immune System

Myalgic encephalomyelitis

Organic pathological CNS changes can be observed. The hallmark is muscle fatigue and exhaustion. Neuro-psychological effects include poor concentration and memory loss, depression, irritability. Lymphadenopathy. Cervical glands can be enlarged if upper respiratory infection is present. Musculoskeletal pain. Some 35 or so different symptoms are associated with ME. Some 25% of cases progress to a chronic form.

Treatment ME

Detoxification. Relaxation.

Medicine

Elutherococcus, Panax. Vitamin B1/2/6

Myasthenia gravis

Muscle fatigue associated with difficulty in maintaining muscle contraction. Shoulder muscles commonly affected. Eye, throat and respiratory muscles can be affected which give rise to respiratory difficulties. May be associated with disorders of the thymus gland.

Pancreas – diabetes which is insulin dependent

Primary biliary cirrhosis

Features an enlarged liver, spleen and pruritis. Xanthelasma of the hands/eyes.

Rheumatic disorders associated with allergy.
Ankylosing spondylitis

See musculoskeletal

Reiters disease

Associated with conjunctivitis and arthritis. It may occur after NSU or bacillary dysentery.

Rheumatoid arthritis

Associated with dry eyes & mouth, hepatic disturbance, raynauds, lymphadenopathy, neuropathy, pericarditis, pleurisy, renal amyloidosis.

Skin – rashes caused by allergies. [See dermatology].
Dermatitis herpetiformis

May be related to coeliac disease

Skin
Pemphigus vulgaris

Skin blistering [limbs and trunk], raw mucous membranes, malaise and fever.

Systemic lupus erythematosus - SLE
Affects the hair – hair loss, skin – erythema, scales, bones – arthritis, various eliminative organs and the nervous system. [See dermatology].

Scleroderma
A systemic sclerosis of connective tissue with fibrosis of tissue. Characterised by a tightening of the skin most noticeable on the fingers and face giving a mask like appearance. Most cases will produce oesophageal stricture. The heart and lungs can become affected.
Medicines
Capsicum, Centella, Cimicifuga, Colchicum, Glycyrrhiza, Oenothera, Peumus, Scolopendrum, Smilax, Symphytum, Zanthoxylum.

Stomach
Hydrochloric acid deficiency increases susceptibility and severity to bacterial and parasitic infections. Associated with hypoglycaemia.

Pernicious anaemia
Due to lack of intrinsic factor in the stomach from atrophy. It is associated with thyroid disease. Weight loss, anaemia and peripheral neuropathy. Jaundice, glossitis and angular stomatitis can be found.

Thyroid - Myxoedema. Goitre. Graves disease. Neonatal jaundice [can also occur from inadequate liver breakdown of RBC's causing jaundice]

Parathyroid – Hypoparathyroid.

25
Nervous system

Thurston says 'any continuous and persistent influence that alters cellular function will affect the functional capability of tissues and organs'.
Functional changes within the tissues including cerebral neurones will tend to change the psychological and emotional makeup of that temperament.

Nerve disorder medicines
Relaxant/antispasmodic medicines are more active when used with stimulants e.g. Capsicum, Zanthoxylum or Zingiber.
Too much relaxation may create a state of nerve exhaustion.

- **Nerve stimulant** - excites the nerves within physiological boundaries.
Cola, Hypericum, Ilex paraguensis.
- **Nerve sedatives/hypnotics** - decrease nerve activity and tension [anxiety], over excitement and irritation.
Anthusa officinalis, Chamomilla, Escholtzia californica, Gelsemium, Humulus, Lactuca, Lobelia, Melissa, Piscidia, Scutellaria, Tilia, Zizyphus, Valeriana, Viscum.
- **Nerve and cerebral tonics** - allay sensitivity, depression, exhaustion and neurasthenia.
Avena, Borago, Centella, Cola, Corydalis ambigua, Eleutherococcus, Ginkgo, Hypericum, Panax sp, Piper methysticum, Rosmarinus, Salvia, Scutellaria, Schisandra, Stachys, Turnera, Verbena, Viola odorata, Withania somnifera.
- **Nervine trophorestorative/Adaptogenic** - nourish the neurones.
Avena, Bacopa, Cola, Eleutherococcus, Panax, Passiflora, Polygonum multiflorum, Rosmarinus, Withania.
- **Nervine relaxant** – anodyne [analgesic] action with relaxation and antispasmodic effects.
Lobelia [affects all muscles], Artemesia vulgaris-neuralgia, Chamomilla, Escholtzia californica, Hypericum, Hyssopus, Lavandula, Papaver somniferum, Passiflora, Piscidia, Primula, Tilia, Valeriana, Viburnum opulus, Zizyphus, Dioscorea with lobelia is used in nervous tension.
Smooth muscle relaxants – Dioscorea, Lobelia, Melissa, Paeonia lactiflora, Viburnum prunifoleum.
- **Nerve antispasmodic** - spasmolytic
Artemesia absinthium - small doses, Atropa, Avena, Chamomilla, Chamaemelum nobile, Datura, Dioscorea, Gelsemium, Hyoscyamnus, Hyssopus, Lavandula, Leonurus, Lobelia, Nepeta, Passiflora, Piper methysticum, Pulsatilla, Ruta, Scutellaria, Viburnum opulus, Viscum.

- **Sympathetic stimulant**

Cinchona, Cola, Ilex, Salvia.

Nutritional therapy for nerve disease [See Ch on Naturopathy & Food regime].

Formulary of nerve prescriptions

Mist antispasmodic. Antispasmodic mixture
Viscum, Scutellaria and Valerian aa equal parts.
Tincturae antispasmodic Antispasmodic tincture
Scutellaria 7.5g Symplocarpus 7.5g Lobelia 15g Capsicum 7.5g Alcohol 550ml.
Sig 4ml et aqua.

Nervine relaxant formula
Gentiana, Humulus, Scutellaria, Valeriana and Viscum.

Nerve tonic
Stachys acts as a neutral remedy and can be used when unsure of the patients
causative disturbance. Further analysis upon a subsequent consultation will reveal
the causative conditions of the patients distress when a relaxant or tonic can be
used to advantage.
Stachys 30g to 500ml. Sig 30ml TDS or frequently.

Neuritis mixture
Humulus 15g Arctium 15g Scutellaria15g Menyanthes 15g Viscum 15g.
Simmer [covered] in one litre of water 15 minutes. Strain when cold.
Sig 30ml QDS

Liniment Camphor Co. [Compound Camphor liniment]
Ol Camphor   1ml
Ol Origanum   1ml
Ol Rosmarinus   1ml
Ol Sassafras   1ml
Tr Capsicum   1ml
Alcohol   100ml
External application for neuritis, ovaritis and pleurisy.

Tissue salts
Deficiencies of tissue salts create disturbances within the cells, aberrant function
ensues when the cell is no longer able to maintain its homeostatic balance.
Disordered conditions follow deficiency states and symptoms follow from the
altered physiological condition. Biochemic tissue salts are mineral salts and

Nervous system

support cellular function. For instance calcium is indicated for nerve transmission, magnesium is a nerve antispasmodic and potassium is a constituent of nerve fibre.

Coming off drugs

Synthetic drugs used for anxiety, depression or as sedatives are not to be tolerated they act as a chemical cosh. Chemical drugs suppress the vital reactions of the nerves and brain and benumb nerve action. Such drugs are never curative and often have serious side effects and may cause addiction. Addiction can be psychological, emotional or drug induced. Sometimes synthetic drugs are a prop for the patient. There are patients who just dont have it within themselves to get better and require long term support. Adverse drug reactions are common and lists of the reactions can be found in the Mims and British National Formulary. *Withdrawal symptoms* are often found when reducing drugs. A general rule of thumb is to reduce one drug at a time and always slowly. So take your time and reduce at the rate of one month for each year the patient has been on the drug, it may take longer. The major tranquillisers, only if it is possible, should always be carefully reduced e.g. lithium, chlorpromazine to reduce the possibility of unwanted withdrawal reactions. However it is often much better to give a herbal mixture to support the nervous system in the first place.

Difficulties arise when the patient wants to come off the drugs from:
1] the illness itself
2] family pressures
3] doctors/psychiatrists
There may be a lack of family support when the family expect the patient to take the drugs as sometimes it is an easier option than progressing through the sometimes difficult path towards recovery and health.

Predispositions towards nerve disease

Typology - body types
The body habitus typology will predispose the individual towards their neurosis or psychosis.
Manic/panic reactions are more likely in the asthenic and athletic.
Depression is more common in the pyknic.
Organ disturbances
Organ disturbances can affect and add to nervous system disorders. It is commonly known that functional problems within the eliminative organs will cause a build up of unreleased toxins. Toxins and free radicles cause damage to the organ and are carried by the blood to all areas.
Liver and gall bladder problems cause uneliminated biliary salts to remain in the blood their effect can cause depressive illness. Liver and gall bladder action can become sluggish from chronic anxiety. Anxiety causes contraction of smooth

261

muscle in the duodenum and bile ducts resulting in spasm of the gall bladder and reabsorption of bile salts.

Uric acid from renal inactivity irritates the blood, unbalances the blood pH and is detrimental to neurotransmitters. Anxiety and fearful sensations are created by an excess of uric acid within the blood. Renal and adrenal disorders occurring from trophic weakness can underlie many chronic anxiety and fear problems. Adrenal exhaustion causes weakness, tiredness and lack of energy. It is necessary to treat the organ area and the nervous system together in the prescription.

Computer effects.

Researchers in Japan have found that workers sitting over a computer screen for more than 5 hours a day have been found to be more susceptible to anxiety and depression [BBC radio 2, item. 31.12.2002].

The four pillars of mental health

1] Eliminate allergies –
    allergic reactions to food can affect anxiety and depression.
2] Regulate blood glucose - hypoglycaemia affects the mood.
3] Avoid pollution - pollutants create cellular toxins.
4] Optimal nutrition - adequate nutrients are essential for restorative nerve action
    [trophic response].

Treatment of nerve disorders implies the need to:

[1] Cleanse and detoxify the tissues.

[2] Support the vital organs in their work to restore and trophorestorate. Disorders of the eliminative organs allow a build up of impurities within the blood. Impurities then detrimentally affect nerve function. Liver disorders can affect depression. Renal [uric acid] and adrenal disorders can affect ones level of fear. Pancreatic disorders are known to affect mood and are a cause of obsessive behaviour.

[3] Equalise the circulation. Enhance the blood supply to all areas of the body. The brain is one of the first areas to become affected by ischaemia. Symptoms may not become apparent until there is sufficient ischaemia to disturb function. Iridology [diagnosis from the iris] shows cerebral sclerosis in all its stages.

[4] Balance the nervous system as healthy nerves are neither over tense or depleted in their functional activity. Trophorestoration means a balanced nerve supply subject to adequate nutrition and vasorelaxation of the blood supply that is relaxation supports neuronal vasomotor function and trophic response.

Examination procedures

Neurological examination begins with a careful history and physical examination. The patient should be encouraged to answer questions put to them. Answers provided by the patient will support the analysis of the patients state of mind, memory and level of concentration. Cognitive function can be examined by asking direct questions that lead to an analysis of mental function most patients can remember their address and telephone number. Does the patient know where they are? Can the patient explain their symptoms? These questions will further determine their level of cognitive function.

Examination: physical examination of the nervous system follows - gait, cranial nerves, motor system including muscle tone, involuntary movements, fasciculations, muscle strength, sensory testing and reflexes.

Rombergs test for coordination.
A test for co-ordination of the lower limbs.
Stand with the feet together and close the eyes. This procedure is made more sensitive by asking the patient to mark time.
Result: if the patient sways about or falls the test is said to be positive. Stand close to the patient when this diagnostic test is performed to prevent falls or injury.
Aetiology
1] Sense of position of limbs is defective.
2] Aural vertigo.
3] Cerebellar lesion.

Observation and examination of the patient for:
level of consciousness/pupil size/limb response.
Coma scale and response level to stimulus 5 is the best response, to 1, a diminished response.
Eyes open or closed [closed due to swelling]
Verbal response [either orientated or confused]
Motor response [obeys commands, localisation of pain]
Pupil scale. Size - diameter in mm. Reaction to light; right and left pupils - eyes open or closed.
Blood pressure and pulse rate. Temperature.
Limb movement arms and legs.
Consider whether there is normal power, mild weakness, severe weakness, spastic flexion, extension, no response. Record both sides and note any difference. [153]

Mental and emotional conditions
Symptoms usually fluctuate during illness and in accordance with the vital force. Continuous symptoms or those patients complaining of one problem after another with little ease in their symptoms inspite of treatment suggest a psychosomatic or neurosis effect.

Herbal Medicine - Keys

Mental and emotional disorders

Attitude

The difference between positive and negative mental attitude is how we interpret it. Samel [259] says that loss of nerve balance creates three mind poisons. These are Greed – Hate and Blindness [ignorance]. Wrong thinking makes you sick and in Tibetan medicine is seen as the cause of many illnesses. Further causes of illness are diet related. Climate, the amount of light or dark affect some patients.

Fear

Fear is a common accompaniment of living. When the fear goes out of control then we are said to be in a condition of fright, fearfulness, panic or terror. Sympatheticotonia is the term used to describe a condition of fear or panic which is one of negativity: a dry mouth, palpitations, stomach churning, trembly knees, sleep disturbances are typical symptoms. Overcoming fear is advantageous to the organism. Confronting our fears allows us to face the fear. Facing fear is seen as a positive way to handle a challenge. Fear will always be around. Everyone feels frightened in unfamiliar surroundings. Compromised individuals with an underlying fear occurs from a feeling of helplessness. The only way to be rid of the fear of doing something is to do something about it. Pushing out the barriers and taking small risks. Many people take risks everyday. So why is it that some can and others cannot? It's not the fear itself but our attitude to it. So what are you afraid of? Perhaps we are afraid we may not be able to handle the consequences - we may not be able to cope. Feeling secure with oneself is important too. Relaxation techniques such as Yoga or Tai chai are beneficial. Deep breathing is a must to adequately supply the body with oxygen. Deep breathing slows the mind and body, re-balances the vital force energy and produces relaxation. It may be useful to make a list of the fears that surround the patient. It is then possible to work through the fears that are amenable to treatment. Panic attacks are an extreme form of fear in which the patient is so terrified they can injure themselves or others. Deep and slow rhythmical breathing can control a panic attack.

Saying positive *affirmations* regularly is very useful as it focuses the mind on a positive aspect of life. Affirmations filter through to the subconscious mind where they are acted upon. The more constant repetition of the affirmations the more benefit it will bring. Affirmations are a useful aid to the medication. It gives the patient something to do other than worry as these types tend to do. Take a deep breath and release the resistance. No person has any control over us except for what we allow. Examples of affirmations include the following: I am willing to release the need for this condition. I feel safe. I release the past. I release all old hurts. I forgive myself. I am willing to release the need for fear. I am open to happiness.

Nervous system

Rage

Rage is the result of undealt with anger. A bit like trying to cap a volcano - we try to push painful, anger causing thoughts and events down inside us until there is no room for anything but an explosion. Lack of trust can eventually create rage. Whenever trust seems impossible life becomes a fortress for concealment and defence. It is true to say 'many people are trapped within their own minds because of addictions and unresolved pain. You have to untangle yourself from addictive patterns. Love and forgive yourself into freedom.

Take responsibility and take care of yourself.

Shock is an acute [sudden] disturbance of the nerve current within the body. Sometimes a scream or shout will release and neutralize the effects of shock.

Fear causes a paralysis of the vital functions and disturbs nerve balance. Hyperfunction of the nerve is the result, for example hairs stand on end, the gut tightens up etc. You are said to be in sympathetic dominance which is a sympatheticotonia of the autonomic nervous system. It is very depleting to the vital force to have long standing fears or chronic worry. Organs also become affected by becoming contracted and tense through nerve excitability. Cannon's classic phrase fight or flight is the mechanism that occurs in sympathetic dominance. Humans feel in their solar plexus and reactions come from here to affect the body. It depends where we have holding points for the discharge of nerve impulses and where the symptoms emerge in the tissues. A person will reflect their anxiety in certain forms of disease: migraine, asthma, peptic ulcers, irritable bowel, psoriasis etc. Depending upon their nerve holding points, will reflect upon the condition and symptoms experienced. Treatments for shock in the acute phase: Antispasmodic tincture, Bach flower remedy - Star of Bethlehem. Flower remedies can be used for acute and chronic conditions.

Memories from the past can indirectly affect todays thoughts and behaviour in an individual. Dr Robert Winston explains how to assess an individuals emotional state by asking them to list five happy memories and then to list five unhappy memories. Those cases easily able to remember happy memories are more happy than those easily remembering unhappy memories from the past. The tendency with the unhappy person is they tend to feel depressed in the present day. Creating happy memories for a baby occurs when a bond is formed between baby and mother. Considering around 50% of post pregnant women are unhappy or depressed treatment of hormonal levels together with Avena or other suitable tonics are required.

Problems signal that you are being called upon to change your life, it also follows that the greater the problem, the greater the change that calls you. You don't have to know how to change your life because you will be shown a way. You don't even have to know what the change will look like as that too, will all come to you in time. We don't have to feel impudent in our lives, in the face of illness. By changing our thoughts we can re-create our future. Our thoughts create our lives and our future. We all suffer from fear, guilt, self hatred etc in varying degrees. These are only thoughts and can be changed. Resentment, guilt and criticism are damaging thought patterns. Releasing any negative feelings will dissolve disease patterns. Releasing the feeling from the mind will clear the problem at its source. Say to yourself 'I release my negative feelings of: depression, anxiety, worry, guilt or fear of ? rage/pain. Together with love of yourself and your life - love yourself. Releasing the past and forgiving others is a useful place to start. No matter what they think - we have control over our lives and our thoughts. You control your thoughts, no - one else. Others can influence you but have no power over you. Self approval and self acceptance are the keys to positive change in yourself. Seeing yourself as basically good reduces the need for other peoples approval. There is so much good in the worst of us and so much bad in the best of us, that it will behold any one of us, to find any fault with another.

Partnership problems
- Criticism
- Contempt
- Defensiveness
- Withdrawal

These can lead to divorce or break-up of a relationship if not checked.
One answer is to trade complaints and listen to each other, try to make changes.

Listening
Attention and listening to the patient indicate a genuine interest in the problems brought to you. Listening is a skill and cannot be learnt quickly. However, a caring disposition together with good eye contact are the most important ways of communicating. Facial expression, posture and tone of voice are non verbal behaviour, they will signal the quality of your interest in the person talking to you. Explain that you will be taking notes during the meeting.

ANTS - automatic negative thoughts require cognitive therapy. That is replacing negative thoughts with positive affirmations. Often quite a feat but always worth it. It is surprising to find so many of us holding onto negative thought patterns. Negative thoughts are often put in place when we are young and continue into adult life. Of course changes can be made, it takes time and energy to make changes - will power too.

Nervous system

Disorders of the nervous system

Alzheimers disease
In 1906 a German neurologist Alois Alzheimer linked specific brain pathology to behavioural changes. A lack of neurotransmitters consequent upon atherosclerosis encourages alzheimers. Increasing age is a factor for the development of organic brain disease, around 50% of cases are over 85 years of age. Retrogenesis and poor memory occur, a sort of 'back to birth' effect with agnosis affecting all the senses. Cases are always worse from fatigue and at the end of the day. [See Parkinsons disease].
Treat as dementia.

Amnesia [Memory loss]
Is the amnesia short or long term? Has there ever been a head injury?
A poor memory has many causes from simple functional to organic pathological and the treatment will vary considerably depending upon the cause.
Aetiology includes anxiety, depression, diabetes/hypo/hyperglycaemia, alcoholism, drug intake, ageing process – dementia, atherosclerosis, CVA., thyroid disturbances, ME.
Medicine
Capsicum, Carduus, Centella, Cola, Crataegus, Eleutherococcus, Ephedra, Euphrasia, Ginkgo, Lavandula, Melissa, Mentha pulegrum, Panax, Rosmarinus, Scutellaria, Stachys, Verbena, Zanthoxylum, Zingiber. Phosphorus.

Anxiety – hypertonic nerves
Short term anxiety requires strong relief with a relaxing remedy. Whereas long term anxiety requires tonic nervines.
Relaxing nervine
Humulus, Hyssopus, Passiflora, Pulsatilla, Scutellaria, Tilia, Valeriana,
Viscum - nervine antispasmodic tonic with a sedative effect upon the solar plexus.
Tonic nervine
Cola, Rosmarinus, Scutellaria, Turnera, Verbena.

Anxiety and panic
Anxiety and panic can be controlled with the following prescriptions.

Flower remedies allay suffering, they can be added to the prescription - Aspen, Cherry plum, Mimulus, Rock rose ease fears. Star of Bethlehem is used for shock. Many of us are unaware and carry the damaging effects of shock. It is very helpful to neutralise any suspected shock as it allays tension. Tension can result from holding shock in the nerves.

Herbal Medicine - Keys

Sedative Px 1
Humulus 2ml Salix nigra 1ml
Valeriana 1ml Pulsatilla 0.5ml
Sig 5 ml PRN aq cal. Indicated for pain, sedation and spasm.

Sedative Px 2
Passiflora 1ml
Pulsatilla 0.5ml
Salix nigra 1ml
Stachys 1.5ml
Valeriana 1ml Sig 5ml TDS aq cal.

Bechets disease
Signs and symptoms: Iritis urgent action is required as it can cause blindness.
Aphthous ulceration. Oedematous vulva or penis.
Medicines
Arctium, Calendula, Colchicum, Commiphora, Echinacea, Hydrastis Urtica,
External
Dilute Apple cider vinegar, Sempervivum. Ung Allium. Collyr Hamamelis.
Hydrastis.

Breakdown [Nervous breakdown]
Nervous breakdown is where the nerve cells are overworking and using up all the
available nutrients more quickly than they are receiving it. A nervous breakdown
develops when the system blanks out certain brain cells at the expense of others
the remaining nerve cells may have their full quota of available nutrients supplied.
Medicines
Feed and nourish the nerve cells - Avena and Zanthoxylum are used singly or
together.
Avena is a nerve trophorestorative. Trophorestorative is a remedy which has the
power to enter directly into the nerve cells and to supply all the necessary
nourishment to sustain them. Exhaustion is the condition where millions of brain
cells are using up nourishment energy more quickly than they are receiving it and
a nervous breakdown develops.
Avena gives remarkable results in - nervous tremors, severe headaches that
accompany the wastage of phosphates in the urine during nervous exhaustion.
Nervous palpitation of the heart. Panic arising from ovarian or uterine disorders.
Avena gently inhibits the smoking habit.
Sexual impotence/sexual dysfunction is Avena's secondary selective action upon
the nerve structure of the genito urinary tract. Zanthoxylum enhances all the
functions of Avena. Zanthoxylum is an invaluable nerve tonic in its own right.

Nervous system

Zanthoxylum can produce a tingling through the whole body when taken as it acts upon the nerves.
Dose for nerve disorders: three parts of Avena to 1 part of Zanthoxylum.
Liquidum extractum Sig 20gtt in water QDS PC. Compound tinctures give the best results. Avena is considered a useful insurance for your nervous system.

Cerebral ischaemia
Occurs as a result of a shortage of blood to the cerebral cortex or labyrinth. Ischaemia can cause a sudden loss of consciousness
Aetiology
Atherosclerosis
Cervical osteoarthritis
Cerebro vascular accident
Hypotension and hypertension
Lack of exercise

Cerebral sclerosis
Sclerosis of arterial blood vessels can start at a very early age and is seen in the iris of the eye as an arcus that is a silver or white ring on the upper part of the iris. Sclerosis causes cerebral ischaemia.

Cerebro vascular accident - stroke
See cardio vascular system

Coma
Unconsciousness may be superficial or deep. Common aetiology includes head injury, drug or alcohol intoxication, diabetes, epilepsy, stroke, syncope.
Medicines
Capsicum and Commiphora are used as powerful vasostimulants.

Cranial nerves
Medicines
Cimicifuga and Scutellaria are used in the long term prescription for cranial nerve disorders.

Dementia
Decline in memory of recent events with cognitive dysfunction signals dementia. Cardiovascular disease is often implicated. Main causes are depression, CVA and Alzheimers. Stimulate vasomotor, liver and pancreatic function together with dietary adjustment. [See Parkinsons disease]
Treatments
Vitamin B1,6,12.Vitamin C, Folic acid. Antioxidants. Selenium.

Herbal Medicine - Keys

Depression -hypotonic nerves -Neurotransmitter imbalance

In the healthy brain neurotransmitters are constantly being released, reabsorbed and broken down. This leads to a healthy stimulation of the nerve cells and normal activity.

There are fewer neurotransmitters then normal in depression which leads to a reduced stimulation of nerve cells this results in feeling depressed.

Anti depressants [nervine tonics] work in one of two ways either:

a] by increasing the levels of neurotransmitters by **blocking their reabsorption**
or

b] increasing the levels of neurotransmitters by **blocking the action of enzymes** e.g. [MAOI inhibitors] which destroy the transmitters.

5 hydroxytryptophan [5HTP] is a precursor of serotonin. Serotonin is a neurotransmitter.

5 HTP is derived from Griffonia simplicifolia seeds and comes from West Africa.

Serotonin inhibitors block the reuptake of serotonin at receptor sites this increases its availability. It has been used for: depression, anxiety, hyperactivity, SAD syndrome, autism. Dose 50mg daily.

Other causes of depression – continuous anxiety that causes depletion of nerve force this leaves a depleted, exhausted and hypotonic, underfunctioning nervous system, thyroid disturbances [hypothyroid] can also cause depression. Thyroid hormone levels should be checked. Hormonal imbalances e.g. PMS, menopause, post natal.

Elevating mood medicines:

Arnica – 2-5gtt [188p143], Artemesia sp, Avena, Borago, Cinchona, Cola, Eleutherococcus, Escholtzia, Ginkgo, Hydrocotyle, Hypericum, Melissa, Panax sp., Passiflora, Piper methysticum, Rosmarinus, Salvia, Scutellaria, Stachys, Tanacetum, Turnera, Verbena.

Capsicum with Scutellaria in nervous exhaustion and depression. The effects of Capsicum are diffused with the addition of Scutellaria.

Epilepsy

Aetiology

Infections, genetic factors, heart disturbance [mitral], CVA, excess acidity, brain conditions causing increased EEG activity, epilepsy, menstrual disturbances, tumours, head injuries.

Medicines

Anticonvulsants/antispasmodics – Antispasmodic Tr, Capsicum, Convallaria, Crataegus, Humulus, Hyssopus, Lobelia, Passiflora, Scutellaria, Valeriana, Verbena, Viscum.

Nervous system

Grief
Medicines
Avena, Chamomilla, Leonurus, Melissa, Pulsatilla, Strychnos ignatii, Strychnos nux vomica, Valeriana. Flower remedy: Sweet Chestnut.

Guillain barre syndrome
A disease of the peripheral nervous system with sudden weakness, loss of sensation, tingling and numbness of the fingers and toes leading within a few days to weakness of the arms and legs. Sometimes severe pain leading to paralysis. Some cases lead to complete paralysis of the legs. In 25% of cases the chest is affected and a ventilator is required to enable the patient to breathe. The syndrome has been associated with previous vaccine use.
Medicines
Avena, Capsicum, Echinacea, Nepeta, Panax, Scutellaria, Viscum.

Hangover
Included here as it affects the nervous system. Alcohol poisons the neurones and dehydrates causing typical symptoms of thirst, irritability, depression.
Treatment
Rehydration. Vitamin B complex. Potassium – Bananas, Grapes. Honey.
Medicines
Avena, Capsicum, Cola as a stimulant, Erythraea/Filipendula as antacids, Panax, Scutellaria, Zingiber.

Hyperactivity
An overactive condition which can occur in children and adults. Colourings have been implicated and are a cause.
Treatment
Check the blood sugar levels. Provide adequate fluids and a regular balanced diet. Relaxation and overall trophorestoration provides improvement.
Medicines
Eleutherococcus, Humulus, Lobelia, Oenothera, Panax, Passiflora, Piscidia, Scutellaria, Valeriana. B vitamins. Manganese, Magnesium, Phosphorus, Zinc.

Hypochondriasis
Chronic worry, anxiety, unhappiness.

Nervine tonics
Avena, Scutellaria, Turnera. Relaxation may be required to assist the tonic process as relaxation is required for trophorestorative processes e.g. Valeriana.

Insomnia & sleep disturbances

There are four stages to the sleep pattern 1, 2, 3 REM and 4. Serotonin is found at level 4.

Chronic unrelenting stress is a major factor in sleep disturbances as is depression. Synthetic drugs numb nerve sensibility. Such numbing will produce sleep - it is not natural sleep that ensues.

Treatment

Avoid caffeine and nicotine.

Medicines

Chamaemelum nobile, Gelsemium, Humulus, Passiflora, Piscidia, Primula, Pulsatilla, Scutellaria, Tilia, Valeriana.

Panax helps to prevent adrenal suppression due to stress causing insomnia. Borago and Glycyrrhiza are useful adrenal tonics.

Tension and Insomnia prescription and to aid relaxation.

Chamomilla, Nepeta, Scutellaria, Valeriana, Verbena aa of each.

Sig 15ml TDS and 30ml on retiring.

Learning disorders

The diet was studied in children with learning disorders and the EFA's were found to be low. Trans fatty acids on red blood cells are high which also accounts for some learning disorders. Insufficient B vitamins are often implicated. Mercury toxicity and vaccines can be detrimental to brain function, memory and concentration.

Treatment

The diet is often lacking nutrients and will always need analysis.

Removal of all additives from the diet especially colourings. Reduction of sugar.

Medicine

Oil Oenothera starting with small doses of 500mg, gradually increasing the dose.

Masturbation [See Chapter 22].

Memory [See amnesia]

Meniers disease [See EENT].

Meningitis

An inflammation of the meninges of the brain lining and commonly associated with an infection which may be of either bacterial [rare] or viral origin. The organism that causes bacterial meningitis is common and lives in the nose and throat, it cannot live outside the body. Meningococcal forms live in the throat of 10% of people. Bacterial meningitis has an incubation period of between 2 and 10 days. Some meningitis cases progress to permanent deafness or brain damage.

Nervous system

There are around 3000 cases of meningitis each year.

There are three main forms of meningitis.
[1] haemophylus influenzae, [2] meningococcal and [3] pneumococcal.
Meningococcal - a number of strains commonly found are known as B and C strains. There are hundreds of strains of the B meningococcal bacteria. B strains cause 6 out of every 10 cases. The B strain can change to a C strain and vice versa. At risk groups are children under 5 and teenagers.
All signs and symptoms are indicative of an infective process in action.
Signs and symptoms in **babies** - feeding difficulties, fever, fretful, high pitched cry, drowsy. A stiff body or floppy lifeless body. Septicaemic rash with pale or blotchy skin – red or purple bruised appearance, eccymosis. When pressed firmly with a glass a septicaemic rash will not fade.
Adult symptoms include headache and neck stiffness, fever, vomiting, photophobia, drowsiness which can lead to unconsciousness or coma. Rash with purple spots [eccymosis]. The rash indicates septicaemia and can occur anywhere on the skin.
In all cases septicaemia can be a serious life threatening condition.
Treatment
Detox the system with an enema. Diaphoretics and Vasotonic alteratives.
Medicines
Aconite, Allium, Asclepias, Baptisia, Capsicum, Chamomilla, Cimicifuga, Cypripedium, Echinacea, Gelsemium, Lobelia, Nepeta, Passiflora, Thymus.

Migraine
Some 2% of migraine sufferers are intolerant to cheese, chocolate or red wine. More common is an intolerance towards wheat or oranges. Migraine has been associated with an increased risk of CVA [stroke]. Chronic headaches are a predictor of stroke [418].
Treatment
Avoidance of the offending article using an elimination diet may clear the migraine. There may be a flare up of the migraine while on the diet. Gastro intestinal bloating is often associated with migraine. Check the biliary function.
Anodyne medicines
Chrysanthemum, Cola, Gelsemium, Piscidia, Rosmarinus, Stachys, Valeriana.

Motor neurone disease
Hypotrophic degeneration of the central nervous system resulting in paresis and paralysis. Muscle wasting occurs in the limbs. Speech and swallowing eventually become difficult.

Herbal Medicine - Keys

Medicines for Motor neurone disease
Avena, Cimicifuga, Cola, Eleutherococcus, Ginkgo, Oenothera, Panax, Scutellaria, Turnera, Verbena.

Multiple sclerosis – disseminated sclerosis
Onset often at puberty. Aetiology includes myelin sheath damage from auto immune conditions and the poor conversion of fatty acids. It is suggested that a viral infection is a causative factor. Chronic viral infections lead to excess fatty acid and prostaglandins. Intestinal microvilli damage is suspected and has often been present for many years. Infection affects the phagocytes this produces sensitivity in the microvilli. Intestinal disorders with leaky gut syndrome are one effect. Gluten found in wheat, oats, barley and rye is a sticky substance and causes further damage to the intestine. Genetic factors and errors in fat metabolism are implicated. Thrombus formation in the capillaries cause obstruction to the blood supply.
Deficiency of fatty acids causes MS. MS affects the hands and legs causing parasthesiae. Eventually blindness with loss of central vision. The bladder and bowel are affected later on giving rise to repeated infections and eventually incontinence. Depression can occur.
A lack of essential fatty acids [EFA's] causes damage to the cell membranes. Dietary deficiency of EFA's - of the two main types Linolenic acid and Linoleic acid. Linoleic acid converts to gamma linoleic acid. Then into arachidonic acid.

Treatment
An astringent diet to help rebuild cellular structure. Prostaglandins E1 and E2 would be not be absorbed without insulin.
Dietary adjustment
Gluten free diet - avoidance of wheat, oats, barley and rye. Avoid sugar.
Avoid dairy produce and animal fats. Reduce blood cholesterol - Lecithin.
Avoid meat and eggs. Avoid soft drinks. Limited alcohol intake.
Flour can be made from - corn flour, cornmeal, potato flour, rice flour, soyabean flour, maize flour. Various mixtures are available on NHS prescriptions.
Fresh unprocessed food. Use green leafy vegetables. Protein from fish is beneficial. Spinach, turnips, peas, broccoli, cauliflower, rice, strawberries, asparagus, green beans, parsley, radishes, tomatoes, melon. Limited intake of salt.
Whole grains. Soya, millet, lentils, azuki beans, kidney beans, lima beans,

Medicines
CNS trophorestoratives - Do not use Avena as it contains gluten.
Cola, Cimicifuga, Humulus, Passiflora, Scutellaria, Verbena.
Circulation and blood condition - Baptisia, Echinacea, Eucalyptus, Zanthoxylum.
Hepatics - Berberis, Chelidonium, Leptandra. Condurango, Jateorrhiza,

Nervous system

Renal factors - Uva ursi.
Eyes - retrobulbar neuritis, Spigelia [pinkroot], Vaccinum.
Vitamins and minerals are essential - B6, B12, Zinc, EFA's.

Muscular dystrophy
Muscular weakness of the facial, shoulder girdle and pelvic muscles. Proximal muscle weakness produces foot drop. Ambulation is rarely lost. Individuals have chromosome damage.
Medicines for muscular dystrophy
Nervine trophorestoratives – Avena, Cola, Eleutherococcus, Ginkgo, Panax, Scutellaria, Turnera.

Myasthenia gravis – see musculoskeletal

Narcolepsy
Check for thyroid disorders, diabetes/hypoglycaemia, liver/gallbladder problems, alcohol, anxiety.

Neoplasms [See Malignancy/oncology]

Neuralgia [See Emergency herbal medicine]
Pain along the course of a nerve.

Neuritis
Inflamed nerves resulting from injury, degeneration or toxicity.

Pain relief [See Emergency herbal medicine]

Paranoia
Obsessive disorder of the personality. Associated with alcoholism and depression. See depression.

Parkinsons disease [See also dementia]
Apoptosis or death of cells is a normal process however the process breaks down due to [1] insufficient cerebral blood [2] eliminative dysfunction [3] neurotransmitter reduction [4] nutrition related disorders.
Risk factors include hypercholesterolaemia, diabetes and hypertension. Animal protein in the diet increases the risk of parkinsons disease by 1.3 times.
Treatments
Co enzyme Q10 and glutathione are important antioxidants. Vitamin C, E and beta carotine. Antioxidants regulate mitochondrial function. Vitamins B6 and B12 reduce the risk of vascular dementia.

Herbal Medicine - Keys

<u>Medicines</u> - Parkinsons
Atropa, Avena, Capsicum, Centella, Cimicifuga, Cola, Datura, Ginkgo, Hyoscyamnus, Hypericum, Panax, Passiflora, Paullinia, Stachys, Rosmarinus, Viburnum opulus, Viscum, Zanthoxylum, Zingiber. Care in the use of Atropa, Datura and Hyoscyamnus as they tend to cause the CNS to become somewhat depressed, this can aggravate any residual depression as is often found in these cases.

Psychosexual disorders [See Chapters 22 & 30]

Schizophrenia
Sometimes disorders of will, intellect and emotion are set off by a stressful experience invoking a chronic anxiety behaviour pattern. Hallucinations, fatigue, fears, depression and delusions can appear.
<u>Medicines</u>
Flower remedies for shock are indicated.
Avena, Centella, Cypripedium, Ginkgo, Oenothera, Panax, Piscidia, Pulsatilla, Rauwolfia serpentina, Rosmarinus, Scutellaria, Valeriana, Viburnum opulus.
B complex. Magnesium, Manganese, Zinc.

Shingles
Previous infection with varicella can provide some immunity. Neuritis from a dormant virus produces a very painful condition it may recur.
<u>Medicines</u>
Sedative prescription for the inflamed nerves.
Local application of Hypericum crem or oleum.

Shock [See Emergency herbal medicine]

Spongiform disease - brain disease from varient CJD
It has been found that animals suffering from BSE can infect humans. The human brain prion - this is a protein which as it's affected by a disease process changes the prion and affects further protein molecules. The animals with BSE have been found to have high levels of manganese together with low levels of copper and zinc. Pesticides make the animal more vulnerable to the disease process.

Stupor
Unresponsiveness but conscious patient briefly arousable by repeated stimulation.
Aetiology
Shock, grief, head injury, heart failure, drugs.

Nervous system

Suicidal thoughts
Aetiology
Depression.
Medicines
Capsicum, Cinchona, Ginkgo, Hypericum, Passiflora.
Bach flowers – Agrimony, Aspen, Cherry plum, Clematis, Mimulus, Rock rose.

Sydenhams chorea
Known as St Vitus dance. A CNS disease characterised by involuntary muscular movements that disappear with sleep. Lasts up to 12 months. Associated with rheumatic fever or streptococcus infection.
Medicines
Allium, Avena, Baptisia, Crataegus, Echinacea, Gelsemium, Humulus, Leonurus, Lobelia, Passiflora, Piscidia, Rosmarinus, Scutellaria, Stachys, Turnera, Tabebuia, Viscum.

Tabes dorsalis [Locomotor ataxia]
A Syphilitic condition of the nerve in advanced cases occurring some 25 years or so after the initial infection.

Flower healing
Flower remedies are available from retailers. However it is quite easy to make one's own flower remedies here is the recipe according to Dr Edward Bach promoter of Bach flower remedies.
The sun method of potentising.
One crystal glass bowl
A handful of flowers
Sunlight
750 mls of water
    Method
In the morning put the water into the bowl and place in the sun. Pick the flowers, avoid touching the flower head, and put them into the water stem side up. Repeat this until the whole surface is covered with flowers. They must all be in contact with the water. Leave the bowl in the sun for three hours then remove the blooms by using the stem of the flower so that the fingers do not touch the water. Half fill a bottle with the potentised water. Fill the remaining half with alcohol to act as a preservative.
Doses
Sig 4gtt QDS.
In acute cases four drops every half an hour.
More than one remedy being used Sig 1gtt aa in 20ml aqua. Sip throughout the day and replenish as required.

How to combine the remedies
Flower remedies may be given singly or combined together, up to six remedies can be combined. They are given as a dose directly onto the tongue. They can be applied to the skin in the form of a cream.

Flower remedies with herbal medicine
Add the flower remedy to the herbal prescription one drop of each remedy required. Noticeable improvement will occur within four weeks. On a follow up visit, the patient will often reveal other emotional disturbances; the remedy can then be adapted. The remedies work through the layers to bring to the surface and into consciousness deeper feelings from the past. Psychotherapy can then be used as you work together to bring about a healing reaction.

26
Dermatology
Including Hair & Nail Disorders

Skin is an organ of elimination
It should be remembered that the skin is an organ of elimination and toxins are often released through the skin when some other channel of elimination is obstructed in its function. The skin will increase its function to help the system to health. Capillary action is crucial for normal circulation. Dilating the capillaries will relieve internal congestion. Astringing the capillaries increases dermal blood.

Dermal absorption
Raising the temperature of the skin by **covering it with a dressing** allows a faster absorption of the medicament. Thus relief of itch, irritation, pain, hydration, and lubrication can all be improved by covering the area of skin having applied the medicament. Transdermal absorption is thus increased using this method.

Dermal medication [Including diaphoretics see Chapter 22]
Aloe vera gel – indicated for all damage to the skin e.g. burns
Arctium – cleansing vasotonic alterative. Capillary stimulant
Armoracea rusticana – vulnerary. Capillary stimulant
Carica papaya – vulnerary. Antimicrobial
Centaurium erythraea – vulnerary
Centella - allays inflammation in the skin where infection is present. Skin affections – wounds, infected ulcers.
Curcuma longa - antimicrobial
Echinacea - cleansing vasotonic alterative
Eupatorium perfoliatum - diaphoretic
Hydrastis – abrasions, abscess, furunculosis, lacerations
Iris – hepatic atony causing skin disease
Ledum latifoleum – astringent and vulnerary
Lobelia – all round relaxant for tense contracted or inflamed skin
Oenothera – corrects dry skin, omega acid deficiency, allergic skin, vulnerary.
Rumex acetosella - vasotonic alterative
Rumex crispus - cleansing vasotonic alterative
Sambucus – relaxing and cleansing vasotonic alterative
Sanicula europaea – astringent
Scrophularia - vasotonic alterative
Scutellaria – antipruritic
Simmondsia chinensis [Jojoba] –
        the wax oil is used in dermal disturbances - Acne, Dandruff,

Herbal Medicine - Keys

Dry scalp, Dry skin, Eczema, Psoriasis, Seborrhoea, Tinea, Warts, Wrinkles.
Smilax ornata – antipruritic and cleansing vasotonic alterative
Stellaria – antipruritic
Stillingia sylvatica - stimulating vasotonic alterative
Taraxacum – promotes alterative release via the liver
Trifolium - vasotonic alterative
Urtica – antipruritic and cleansing vasotonic alterative
Valeriana – antipruritic

Anaesthetic [local] – Aconitum napellus, Adonis vernalis, Gelsemium, Lobelia, Piper methysticum, Solanum dulcamera. Ice compress.
Antipruritic – Arctium, Echinacea, Hydrastis, Lobelia, Rumex, Sambucus, Scutellaria, Smilax ornata, Stellaria, Urtica, Valeriana.

Formulary for dermal prescriptions

Aerosol spray – see spray

Herbal Bath therapy
Hydrotherapy treatment using hot and alternating with cold stimulates the circulation.
Salt rubbed over the body will release toxins. Loofer to uninflamed skin encourages skin elimination and the discharge of toxins.

Balneum - Baths [See also Chapter 16]
Three types of bath are used
[a] Infusion/decoction, [b] aromatic floral waters [c] essential oil baths.

[a] Consists of making an infusion or decoction, allowing it to cool then adding to the bath water, then immerse the part to be treated.
Application - Typically 60g for a bath. Or put a handful of the herb into muslin and allow to soak.
[b] Aromatic floral waters are composed of volatile oils produced by distillation. Water distillation appears to produce a better product than the faster steam distillation process. Steam distillation using excessive heat damages the hydrosols or hydrolats which are the by products of steam distillation when essential oils are produced. Lower temperatures and lengthened distillation time always give a better product.
Application - Aromatic floral waters, adult bath up to 500ml. Child bath up to 100ml. Babies 20ml.
[c] Essential oil baths with 5-10 drops of preferable oil.

Dermatology, Including Hair & Nail Disorders

Medicated baths
Avena [baths are soothing in inflamed conditions e.g. eczema]
Achillea [baths in psoriasis]
Calendula – allays irritation.
Equisetum - connective tissue strengthener, weak feet - dropped arches, musculoskeletal disorders, neuralgia, dermatitis.
Quercus - astringent, hyperhidrosis, infected skin conditions/pustules.
Urtica - allays inflammation and itching.
Vulnerary medicines are suitable for baths.

Balneum with essential oils
Chamomilla, Cinnamomum [analgesic, stimulant, antimicrobial]. Cajuput [stimulant & antispasmodic].
Lavandula – relaxing.
Melissa-relaxing. Mentha piperita and Rose - relaxing and antispasmodic.
Melaleuca – antiseptic.
Rosmarinus - tonic.
Salvia - stimulating, antimicrobial. Szygium – stimulant and antiseptic.
Thymus - antiseptic, antifungal, antimicrobial.

Lotions
Lotions are [1] alcohol, [2] oil, [3] distilled, [4] aromatic waters.
Lotions can be alcohol based but tend to be fully absorbed so it is best to add some fixed oil to the lotion.
Oil & alcohol lotion. Essential oil 1ml. Fixed oil 20ml and alcohol to 50ml.
Sig Apply as required.

Crem & Unguentum [Creams and ointments]
Creams
Aqueous cream
Emulsifying wax 10g and water 50ml.
Heat to 60C add 10ml of a fixed oil. Mix and allow to cool a little before adding 5gtt essential oil.
Cream base
A simple cream base is available from typical herbal suppliers. Various LE's and Tr's can be added to the base cream as medicament. By far the easiest way to make a cream and far quicker than making from scratch.

Cold cream
Soothing, cleanser and as a night cream.
To make 300ml
Beeswax 60ml Ol almond 150ml Elderflower water 90ml Borax powder 2.5 ml.

Melt the beeswax and the oil. Heat the elderflower and pour over the borax. Remove both from heat. Pour the elderflower mix over the melted wax. Beat the mixture until smooth. Pour into jars and label.

Crem Calendula [Calendula cream]

Emulsifying wax	150g
Infused oil of Calendula	150ml
Glycerine	50ml
Infusion Calendula	550ml
Sodium benzoate	5ml

Melt the wax and then add the infused oil. Mix the glycerine, infusion and sodium benzoate together. Pour slowly into the oil mixture, while stirring continuously until the cream is cool.

The above cream can carry other medications e.g. Hypericum, Plantago, Symphytum.

Hair cream
Use coconut oil to soothe the scalp; dry scalp, eczema, psoriasis and cradle cap.

Skin softener lotion
Coconut oil 10ml, sweet almond oil 5ml with 5gtt essential oil.

Feet softening cream
Lanolin 30ml, sweet almond oil 10ml, glycerine 10ml.

Unguentum [Ointments]
Examples are here given of different methods of making ointments.

- Lard base. 250g of cut herb is added to 500g of lard and the mixture is simmered until the herb is crisp. Strain through muslin and pour into a jar. Keep stirring the mixture otherwise the ingredients tend to separate out.
- Paraffin molle base. Paraffin molle 15g and lanolin 5g Heat beeswax separately and add together. The herbal extract is added last and always slowly. Fill a jar and stir the mixture until cool. If too much beeswax is used the resulting ointment will be too hard.
- Mixed base

Herbal infusion	200ml	[Oenothera oleum can be used]
Beeswax	15g	
Emulsifying ointment	120g	
Ol Almond	120ml	Ol Wheatgerm 5ml
Borax	4g.	Ol Lavandula for aroma 5gtt

Dermatology, Including Hair & Nail Disorders

Obtain two containers. Melt the beeswax and add the emulsifying ointment. Mix the wheatgerm and almond oil - add these slowly to the beeswax. Keep mixtures warm. Add the borax to the warm infusion. Slowly combine the infusion with the beeswax and emulsifying ointment mixture. Stir slowly in one direction. Add the Ol Lavandula.

- Paraffin molle base. Melt the paraffin add the essential oils at the rate of 10 drops of each oil up to a maximum of 30 drops and pour into jars. Stir all the time while cooling.
- Oil base. An oil such as Almond, Sunflower, Olive or Rapeseed can be used. Mix and melt 240ml oil with 120g marc finely cut herb. Priest recommends 3 hours in an oven at 140 degrees C this is only a warm temperature. Strain and bottle.

Unguentum Gynocardia [Chaulmoogra ointment]
Ol. Gynocardia   1ml
Paraffin molle   60g
Melt the paraffin and stir in the oil. Pour into jars and stir until cool.
Used in scaly skin diseases, anal fissure and leprosy.

Unguentum Eucalyptus
Ol Eucalyptus   1ml
Paraffin molle   60g
Melt the paraffin and stir in the oil. Pour into jars and stir until cool.
Used as an antiseptic dressing.

Unguentum Peruvianum [Balsam of Peru ointment]
Balsum of Peru   12g
Paraffin molle   88g   Mix together.
Use against scabies and for varicose ulcers.

Dermal preparations
Fomentation [compress]
Fomentations are used hot upon an area for:
1] Visceral pain
2] to allay irritation or inflammation
3] ease painful joints and muscle groups
4] soothe skin damage and wound healer.
Medicines
Powder or mashed - Achillea, Althea, Calendula, Chamomilla, Chondrus, Fucus, Linum usit, Plantago, Sambucus, Stellaria, Symphytum, Trigonella, Ulmus.

Herbal Medicine - Keys

Method for making a compress
Make an infusion/decoction, strain the marc. Using a tea towel or flannel soak in the menstrum and apply hot to the treatment area.

Poultices
Althea & Ulmus – drawing poultice [abscesses], Bran – sciatica, Capsicum – stimulation, Humulus – pain, Linum – chest infections, burns/scalds. Lobelia – pain, Mango and Potato - wounds, Symphytum – fractures and ulcers, Ulmus – drawing and soothing to ulcers, Zingiber - stimulation. Usually muslin is used to contain the herb used for the poultice.

Pulv Ulmus fulva co. Pulverised Ulmus fulva compound.
Pwd Ulmus, Pwd Linum, Pwd Zingiber, Pwd Lobelia
Mix with a little water into a stiff paste. Apply to the site and cover with lint. Renew poultice every 2 hours.
A fine drawing and stimulating poultice for sepsis, furunculosis, wounds.

Spray [Aerosol spray]
Tincture Benzoin compound spray. Compound Benzoin tincture 15% with alcohol. Aerosol spray: for reducing skin sensitivity, irritation, infections and as a vulnerary – chilblains, dermal ulcers, eczema, fissure, gingivitis, herpes, nipple fissure, eczema, wounds [formula see Styrax benzoin].

Steaming
Steaming of the face, sinus disturbances, infection.
1] Infusion method
Two handfuls of fresh herb or 45g of dried herb into a bowl of boiling water lean over the bowl, cover your head with a large towel, then breathe in the vapours.
2] Essential oil method
Put one litre hot water and 3gtt essential oil into a bowl. Cover the head and bowl with a towel. Close the eyes and inhale.
Steaming is used to great advantage in sinusitis, catarrh and respiratory infections.

Herbal liquid soap
To make 750ml of soap
1 tablet of pure castille or glycerine soap – grated
600ml of rain water, 75ml of glycerine
4 gtt of essential oil, 15g of dried herba/fresh herba
Put the soap and water together, bring to the boil, stir in the glycerine, remove from heat. Stir in essential oil and herba.
When cool pour into bottles, cover and label.

Dermatology, Including Hair & Nail Disorders

Talcum powder
Add a few drops of essential oil to an unperfumed pure talc and shake.
Rice flour can be used instead of talc add 10% orris powder then the essential oil.

Tar preparations
Tar preparations are healing and disinfectant to the skin.
Using a concentration of up to 1% Oleum Cade [from Juniperus] or Oleum Pinus in a cream or ointment base. Zinc and Castor oil ung is suitable to carry the Oleum. Add an aromatic to cover the odour of the oil. Sig apply PRN.

Vinegar mist [Aromatic vinegar mixture]
Apple cider vinegar 100ml, essential oil O.5ml. Shake vigorously.
Used to cleanse the dermis of grease, infection, perspiration.

Nutritional therapy for skin disease
Bioflavonoids. Vitamin C, E
Selenium [toxicity garlic breath/rash]. Zinc.

Lesions associated with skin disease
Macule – reddening of the skin. [Erythema is another term used].
Papule – raised area of skin
Pustule – an area filled with pus.
Vesicle – fluid filled area. [Bula are large vesicles].
Wheal - a raised area of skin with a pale centre.

Dermatological considerations include the following:
1] Promote eliminative action
2] Cleanse and detoxify the blood - Vasotonic alterative
3] Cellular restoration - nutrients
4] Dermal treatment.

Skin conditions

Acne
Comedones and pustules located on the face, shoulders and back.
<u>Treatment</u> is to promote intestinal elimination, one way is to increase dietary fibre. Balance the hormones if required.
<u>Medicines</u>
Arctium, Berberis aquifoleum, Echinacea, Rumex, Taraxacum, Trifolium, Vitex, External - Oleum Tea tree, Vitamin E crem.

Acne rosacea
Butterfly symmetrical redness of the face, like a blush, enlarged red nose, and occasionally blepharitis, conjunctivitis. Aggravated by alcohol, allergy, menopause, hypochlorhydria.
Treatment
Avoid sun and heat directly on the face. Cold compress may help. Avoid niacin.

Acne vulgaris
Comedones and pustules are found on the face, chest, back and arms.
Treatment
Attention must be given to the bowel as inadequate elimination is always present in acne.
Medicine
Arctium, Iris, Smilax.
Vitamin A, C, Zinc.

Actinomycosis
Infected tissue that promotes elimination of toxins through the skin, these are seen as sinuses on the skin surface. Sinuses are found in the skin, gastro intestinal tract and lungs.
Medicines
Baptisia, Comiphora, Echinacea, Hydrastis, Rumex, Smilax. Vitamin C. Zinc.

Aids
Many skin manifestations can occur with aids: infections, seborrhoeic dermatitis, eczema, red scaly areas on the hairline, tinea, candida, pityriasis vers. acne, impetigo, shingles, ano rectal warts, human papilloma virus [HPV], herpes zoster, sarcoma.

Alopecia – see hair

Angio-oedema
Can occur as an anaphalactic reaction and could be fatal. Burning of the skin, absence of itching,
For treatment see urticaria

Burns [see emergency herbal medicine]

Candidiasis
Candida needs to be treated as a constitutional disorder. Maculopapular or nodular lesions.

Dermatology, Including Hair & Nail Disorders

Cellulitis see erysipelas

Colour changes
Purple striae is found in Cushings syndrome [adrenal trouble].

Brown [liver] spots on the skin
Treat the liver/gall bladder. Apply castor oil night and morning to the spots [macules and papules].

Dandruff [see hair]

Depurative prescription
Medicines
Arctium, Echinacea, Galium, Rumex, Scrophularia, Stillingia, Urtica, for eczema/erythema/papules/scaly skin/urticaria.

Dermatitis
Erythema with papules, vesicles, and bullae. Crusting may occur. In chronic cases scaling, fissuring and thickening occur. Lesions are sharply defined. Often aggravated by make up or drugs.
Treatment
Check the gastro intestinal, liver and biliary function.
Medicines
Allium, Arctium, Calendula, Echinacea, Galium, Iris, Plantago, Scrophularia, Sambucus, Scrophularia, Smilax, Stellaria, Taraxacum, Trifolium, Viola. Rhus toxicodendron Tr 1:10 Sig 0.12ml. External lotion 5% [BHP].

Eczema
Distribution - flexures of the arms, legs, ankles, buttocks.
Eczema patients show low levels of prostaglandins, raised histamine and reduced ability to clear infections.
Eczema of an allergic nature require dietary checks. Trigger foods are found commonly from dairy produce, wheat, corn, citrus fruits and sugar.
Breast feeding may help eczema. Some foods the mother eats could pass through the milk and aggravate baby or childhood eczema.
Treatment
EFA's may help if fed to the mother they will pass to the milk. Vitamin A 25,000 – 200,000iu
Medicines
Vaso tonic alteratives - Arctium, Berberis aquifolium, Hydrastis, Scrophularia, Stellaria, Stillingia Trifolium, Urtica, Viola tricolor.

Herbal Medicine - Keys

Erysipelas
Cellulitis characterizes this streptococcal condition. The face is most commonly involved with a presenting acute erythema. Pyrexia, pain, and drowsiness result from the infection.
<u>Medicines</u>
Achillea, Allium, Baptisia, Cnicus, Echinacea, Eupatorium perfoliatum, Galium, Phytolacca, Populus tremuloides, Sambucus, Smilax, Stillingia, Syrupus figs.
<u>External</u>
Aloe, Calendula, Symphytum, Ulmus.

Feet conditions
Perforating ulcers, varicose ulcers, corns.
<u>Medicines</u>
Calendula, Hypericum, Ruta, Rosmarinus, Tagetes, Thuja.
Tagetes is antiseptic, analgesic and anaesthetic when used as a compress to the ulcer/corn etc.

Foot odour
Rule out fungal infections. Detoxify the blood and treat the kidneys.

Fungal infections
Some fungal infections can occur with diabetes. General run down conditions of the immune system.
<u>Medicines</u>
Azadirachta, Echinacea, Phytolacca, Tabebuia, Thuja,
<u>External</u>
Allium, Aloe, Azadirachta, Calendula, Commiphora, Lavandula, Melaleuca, Thuja. Apple cider vinegar. Oleum Ricinus.

Purpura [See circulatory system].

Furunculosis
<u>Treatment</u>
Dietary changes - reduce sugar.
<u>Medicines</u>
Stimulation with strong vasotonic alteratives:
Commiphora, Echinacea, Phytolacca. Linum poultice.
A drawing powder can be used in bad pustules [see start of chapter].

Greasy skin see oily skin.

Dermatology, Including Hair & Nail Disorders

Hair disorders

Hair condition and quality are dependent upon the condition of the blood and any general health disturbances. Dandruff and falling hair are often caused by the elimination of systemic impurities through the scalp. Systemic disorders can affect hair health e.g. diabetes, nervous anxiety, depression, heart disease [mitral dysfunction], malnutrition, insufficient circulatory function to the head. Thyroid disease. Infection - Trichophyton. Skin conditions – eczema, psoriasis. Hormonal levels - post menopause, pregnancy. Vitamin A deficiency. Zinc deficiency.

Dandruff, Dry hair, Alopecia and scalp itch

When dandruff is found this is known as a vicarious elimination. Whereby impurities are being eliminated through the scalp skin. Treatment must include cleansing of the skin and detoxification through eliminatory channels.

Medicines

Arctium, Artemesia abrotanum, Artemesia absinthium, Capsicum, Chamaelirium luteum, Cimicifuga, Equisetum, Fucus, Iris, Leonurus, Medicago, Oenothera, Urtica, Rosmarinus, Rumex, Scutellaria, Stachys, Thuja, Viburnum prunifloeum, Vitex, Zanthoxylum. Vitamin A, E.

Px Hair loss. Alopecia - Tr Ceanothus 15ml, Tr Iris 8ml. Sig 5gtt TDS.

External treatment

Wash the hair less frequently as washing removes the natural oil from the hair and scalp. Do not use hair dryers. Do not use any rollers or anything that will pull at the roots of the hair. Rain water is good for the hair. Use a natural shampoo and conditioner. Only use natural hair colour e.g. Henna.

External rinses:

1] Arctium, Jojoba, Lavandula, Salvia, Thymus, Urtica – infusium rinse.
2] Rosmarinus adds a sheen to the hair.
3] Artemesia abrotanum [Southernwood] and Rosmarinus stimulate hair growth.
4] Chamomilla lightens the hair colour.
5] Quillaja saponaria bark shampoo.
6] Apple cider vinegar helps relieve scalp itching.
7] Vit A deficiency may also be a cause of hair loss or dandruff.

Lotions:

Achillea, Adiantum, Aloe, Althea, Arctium, Arnica, Bambousa arundinacea, Chamomilla, Equisetum, Foeniculum, Geranium, Lavandula, Melissa, Nepeta, Petroselinum, Picrasma, Pilocarpus jaborandi, Rosmarinus, Salvia, Sambucus, Saponaria, Simondsia [Jojoba], Symphytum, Urtica, Yucca, Laurus nobilis [Bay rum 127 p464].

Oleum Eucalyptus, Oleum Olea, Oleum Rosmarinus, Oleum Ricinus.

Herbal Medicine - Keys

Hair colouring
Chamomilla, Citrus limoneum, Lawsonia inermis [Henna available in 3 colours] – neutral, black or red, Quercus, Rosmarinus, Salvia.
Zinc deficiency causes and treats grey/silver hair.

Head lice [see pediculosis]

Herpes genital
Genital herpes is infectious when the lesions are open and active.
Medicines
Vaso tonic alteratives, Allium, Aloe, Baptisia, Commiphora, Echinacea, Hydrastis, Hypericum, Larrea, Piscidia, Rumex, Smilax. Cucumber juice, Lycine.

Herpes simplex
It is estimated that 80% of the population are carriers. Herpes is a viral condition of the mucous membranes. Painful vesicles that may become fissures are found. They affect the lips and nose and may spread over the face. Any area where the skin is broken can become infected. Once the infection is active it can be spread by touching the sore or by kissing. Tingling, burning or itching are the first signs and can last 24 hours. Redness and swelling results in a vesicle that is often painful. After a few days the area can break down to form an ulcer. They eventually dry up and crust over. It is advisable to treat constitutionally as Herpes occurs from lowered vitality.
Medicines
Baptisia, Chamomilla, Commiphora, Echinacea, Filipendula, Hydrastis, Hypericum, Melaleuca and Phytolacca. Vitamin C.
External use
Aloe, Cade oleum, Eucalyptus oleum and Hypericum, Szygium oleum.

Herpes zoster
Treatment [see also under nervous system].
Use remedies that will ease the pain.
Medicines
Baptisia, Calendula, Daucus, Echinacea, Humulus, Hypericum, Hydrastis, Lobelia, Melissa, Phytolacca, Piscidia, Stillingia, Urtica, Valeriana.
External use
Aloe, Fucus, Glycyrrhiza, Rininus oleum, Sempervivum juice [houseleek], Ulmus. Zinc.

Ichthiosis
Dry scaly skin which is prominent on the extensor surface of the extremities

Dermatology, Including Hair & Nail Disorders

Medicine - Ichthiosis
Arctium, Centella, Echinacea, Fucus, Galium, Lycopus, Oenothera, Phytolacca, Rumex, Sambucus, Stillingia, Trifolium.
Blackcurrant juice. Ol Oenothera. Ol Borago.

Impetigo
An infectious skin condition associated with a feeling of being run down.
Medicines
Vasotonic alterative – Allium, Althea, Arctium, Baptisia, Barosma, Calendula, Carbena, Commiphora, Echinacea, Galium, Iris, Larrea, Melaleuca, Phytolacca, Ricinus, Rumex, Saponaria, Smilax, Symphytum, Thymus, Trifolium.
Vitamins - B complex, C, E and minerals Zinc.

Inflammatory conditions of the skin
Medicines
Arctium, Sambucus, Urtica. Sempervivum juice applied locally.

Intertrigo
Damage and excoriation of the skin from excessive moisture and friction rubbing against two surfaces is found when clothes rub against the skin; under the breasts and scrotal areas.
Treatment
Keep the area dry and reduce friction. Talc with Lavander.
Calendula crem. Hamamelis dist. Melaleuca oleum spray. Ulmus powder.
Medicines
Sambucus.

Keloids
Treatment
Settle the immune system and allay nervous anxiety where this is found.
Medicines
Aloe, Juniperus sabina, Hypericum, Ricinus communis, Zanthoxylum, Zingiber.
Vitamin E locally and internally.

Leprosy [See tropical diseases]

Lichen planus [See also oral conditions].
Papules distributed in the mouth, sacrum, wrists or legs.
Medicines
Allium, Arctium, Berberis sp, Chionanthus, Echinacea, Ephedra, Fumaria, Iris, Smilax. Ricinus communis externally.

Herbal Medicine - Keys

Lupus erythematosus
An auto immune disease that affects the hair, skin, heart, spleen and kidneys.
Medicines
Aloe, Arctium, Baptisia, Calendula, Centella, Echinacea, Ginkgo, Iris, Phytolacca, Rumex, Smilax, Stillingia, Taraxacum.
External – Allium, Aloe, Calendula, Chelidonium, Ricinus communis.

Malignant conditions
1] Rodent ulcer
Carcinoma affects the naso labial folds. It often starts as an ulcer that is slow growing and weeps.
2] Squamous cell carcinoma
Featuring an ulcer with a scab at the centre. The sides of the ulcer are raised and have a rolled appearance to its edge. Face, neck and hands are areas affected.
3] Malignant melanoma
Pigmented naevi [mole] sometimes turn malignant. They are found in the face, neck and hands. Any mole that changes its character should raise suspicion – bleeding, colour change, increase in size, ulceration, an increase in pigmented patches. Metastases are rapid.

Milaria Heat rash
A rash resulting from sweat retention due to blocked sweat ducts primarily from perspiration and excessive heat. Secondary types occur from dermatitis. Blotchy redness, papules, vesicles or pustules may be seen. Symmetric distribution on the trunk, neck and friction sites.
Treatment
Increase fluids and keep cool with tepid sponging. Vitamin C. Sedatives, Antihistamines.
Medicines
Aloe, Arctium, Calendula, Chamomilla, Ephedra, Oenothera, Stellaria, Urtica.

Molluscum contagiosum
A viral disorder affecting the face, extremities or groin. Papules or nodules are 2 – 10 cm diameter and appear in small crops. Treat the blood.

Nevus
Benign common mole found within the dermis. Dome shaped, flat or elevated papules of a flesh, brown or black colour. Hairy moles never turn malignant. Any part of the skin may be affected.
Treatment
Externally apply – Allium, Chelidonium, Podophyllum, Ricinus communis, Taraxacum succus or Thuja.

Dermatology, Including Hair & Nail Disorders

Oily skin
Check the hormonal levels, liver function and diet.
<u>Medicines</u>
Allium, Berberis aquifoleum, Hydrastis, Iris, Oenothera, Stillingia, Vitex.
Essential fatty acids: Blackcurrant juice.

Onychosis - diseases of the nail
1] Blue nail
Fallots tetralogy is diagnosed when the nail is blue.
<u>Aetiology</u>
Associated with poor circulation or congenital heart disease.

2] Clubbed nail
Clubbing is when the nail curves over the finger end. It is caused by fluid build up from impaired circulation.
<u>Aetiology</u> It may signify chronic lung disease or congenital heart disease.

3] Lifting of the nail - oncholysis
The nail lifts off the nail bed.
<u>Aetiology</u>
Psoriasis, poor circulation and fungal infections.

4] Lines on the nail
Horizontal white lines appear as a ridge and occur when the nail stops growing because of an illness. [Beaufs lines].
Longitudinal lines from the ridge to the tip are seen in arthritis, age, lichen planus.

5] Malignant nail
Melanoma of the nail gives a brown yellow streak. A mole underneath the nail gives a similar appearance.

6] Pitting nail
Irregular dimples are a sign of psoriasis.

7] Splinter haemorrhage
Longitudinal red streaks.
<u>Aetiology</u>
Lung or heart infection [endocarditis or heart valve infection].

8] Spoon shaped nail
Thin at the end of the nail. Iron deficiency anaemia.

9] White patches
Large white patches on the nail bed could indicate hypoprotinaemia. Which impairs the development of the nail

10] White lines – leuconychia
Aetiology
Zinc deficiency or damage to the nail.

11] Yellow nail
Aetiology
Sinus disturbances, bronchitis, pulmonary oedema, hepatic disease.

Medicines to strengthen nails
Arctium, Avena, Centella, Chondrus, Commiphora, Equisetum, Galium, Medicago, Oenothera, Plantago, Rumex, Sanguinaria, Smilax, Stillingia, Taraxacum rad, Thuja.
Apple cider vinegar. Calcium. Magnesium. Silica. Zinc.

Papilloma [warts]
Treatment
Lotions
Allium, Chelidonium – fresh or Tr/LE, Echinacea, Juniperus sabina – small doses only, as a dressing to blisters in order to promote discharge, Podophylum, Oleum Ricinus communis apply BD., Ruta graveolens, Sempervivum tect [houseleek], Solanum dulcamera – face, Podophyllum, Staphysagria, Taraxacum juice, Thuja – venereal.

Wart lotion
Commiphora	1 part
Podophyllum	1
Ol Sassafras	1
Ol Ricinus communis	2

Applied upon a plaster and renewed BD.

Pediculosis Lice
An infestation by Pediculosis capitis.
The lice pass from one head to another by direct contact. Lice cannot jump, fly or hop. They prefer clean hair in which to lay eggs. The female louse lays around 8 eggs a night. Untreated the infestation can become severe. The eggs stick to the base of the hair. Head lice lay eggs in the hair and suck blood from the scalp. Itchyness is common.

Dermatology, Including Hair & Nail Disorders

Treatment - Lice
Wash the hair daily and rinse with a decoction of quassia chips [1:20] leave to dry. Combing through all the hairs with a fine comb to remove the nit eggs paying particular attention to behind the ears. Removal of the eggs is _essential_ to prevent the eggs hatching. Medication will only kill the nits in the hair. The eggs, if unremoved would ripen to produce more nits.

Medication - Pediculosis
Use a shampoo/lotion to kill the nits it can be made from one of the following:
* Azadirachta in a shampoo base.
* Essential oils:
  Chenopodium ambrosiodes, Mentha pulegium, Origanum compactum, Thymus broussonetti. Application kills lice in 15 minutes [389].
* Quassia of either species e.g. Quassia amora or Picrasma excelsa, Lippia multiflora [African verbena] kills body and head lice,
* Sassafras oleum @ max 2% into the lotion, if the oil is too strong it tends to burn.

Crab lice
In the sexually active appear in the groin hair.
Treatment
Treat both partners. Comb the hair to remove the eggs and nits and treat as above.

Pemphigus vulgaris
An autoimmune disease producing vesicles [blisters] on mucous membranes, trunk, limbs and genitals.

Petechia
Skin haemorrhage.
Medicines
Calendula, Fagophytum esculentum, Hamamelis, Ruta, Urtica.

Pityriasis
Fungal infection. Light brown plaques, up to 2cm diameter with fine scales. Collarate of loose scales along the border. Cheeks, upper arms, legs and trunk are commonly affected. May spontaneously disappear.

Pruritus
Allaying nervous irritability is often helpful. Hepatic disorders. Haemorrhoids. Check for icterus.
Treatment
Stimulate elimination. Cold compress.

Herbal Medicine - Keys

<u>Medicines</u> - pruritus
Humulus, Hypericum, Rumex, Stellaria, Scrophularia, Urtica.

Psoriasis
Distribution - elbows, knees and scalp, although it can occur anywhere. Silvery scales [which bleed upon removal] on red plaques, pitted nails. Always a very difficult condition to clear permanently.

<u>Treatment</u> - psoriasis
Vegetarian diet is best because animal protein irritates psoriasis.
Avoid citrus fruits, tomatoes, red meat, milk and coffee.
<u>Medicines</u>
Aloe, Arctium, Berberis aq., Echinacea, Galium, Glycerrhiza, Hydrastis, Iris, Larrea, Linum usit., Oenothera, Phytolacca, Rumex, Scrophularia, Smilax, Stellaria, Stillingia, Taraxacum, Thuja, Trifolium, Valeriana.
Zinc, chromium, EFA's.

Vasotonic alterative prescription for psoriasis.

LE Arctium	4 parts
LE Echinacea	6 parts
LE Galium	4 parts
LE Juglans	4 parts
LE Stillingia	2 parts
Decoctum Rumex 8 parts.	
Sig 5ml TDS.	

<u>External treatments</u>
Aloe. Oleum Oenothera, Oleum Ricinus, Oleum Vitamin E. Ulmus paste.

Unguentum Ol Cadini [Cade oil ointment is extracted from Juniperus].
Oil of Cade   2g [Oleum Juniperus can be used instead]
Paraffin molle 60g mix well together
Used for healing ulcers. Psoriasis. Scaly skin disorders.
Balneum
Achillea, Chamomilla or Sambucus baths - place Achillea into muslin and rub over the patches. An infusion can be added to the bath for dermal absorption.
Dead sea salt put into the bath
Oleum
Castor oil applied to the skin night and morning.
Crem
Cream made from: Berberis aquifolium, Calendula or Tagetes.

Dermatology, Including Hair & Nail Disorders

Talc
Dust the skin with Ulmus.

Scabies
Contagious and very itchy skin condition affecting the elbows, hands, feet, axilla, nipples.
Treatment
Ung 12.5% Balsamum peruvianum is parasitic and insecticide.

Treatment - Scabies
Lippia multiflora [African verbena] lotion of the oleum @ 20%. Sassafras 2% lotion. Tabebuia. Tanacetum vulgare balneum.

Seborrhoeic dermatitis
This is seen as cradle cap in infants. Dandruff in adults. Usually distributed on the head, eyebrows, nasal folds, buttock, axilla and groin folds. Red, greasy/glazed and scaling skin.
Treatment
Biotin and folic acid for infants. Adults require vitamin B complex, E, Zinc, EFA's.
Apply oil to soften the dryness.
Medicine
Arctium, Artemesia abrotanum, Iris, Phytolacca, Rosmarinus, Rumex, Smilax, Stellaria, Taraxacum, Urtica.

Swelling/bruises/sunburn [See emergency herbal medicine Chapter 36].

Tinea
Tinea is caused by a fungus [ringworm] of three varieties Epidermophyton, Trichophyton and Microsporon.
Ringworm has scaly red patches with a paler centre. The organism needs warmth and a moist environment in order to breed. Fungal spores are transmitted from person to person by infected skin fragments.
Tinea cruris
Affects the groin creases
Nail tinea
Produces thickened nails which are of a brownish colour.
Tinea - athletes foot
Fissures present in between the fourth and fifth phalanx are evidence of the active stage. The skin can become white and slough off. Pallor and itchiness are common. The whole foot may become affected in severe cases.

Cleanliness of the feet is essential to prevent re infection. Feet should be kept dry. Socks or stockings should be changed daily.

<u>Treatment</u> for all areas of tissue.

<u>External use antifungals</u> - After washing the area use a lotion, oil or cream preparation three times daily.

Allium, Aloe, Arum maculatum [cuckoopint], Azadirachta, Calendula, Commiphora, Eucalyptus, Grape seed extract, Juglans, Melaleuca, Plantago, Oleum ricinus, Saponaria, Sanguinaria.

Talc containing powdered Commiphora or Melaleuca is useful.

<u>Medicine</u> - antifungals

Constitutional remedies in resistant cases using vasotonic alteratives enable detoxification of the blood and tissues.

Baptisia, Calendula, Centaurium, Centella, Echinacea, Galium, Iris, Phytolacca, Rumex, Sempervivum juice, Stellaria, Stillingia, Tabebuia sp., Thuja, Trifolium.

Ulcers see wounds below

Urticaria

Itchy rash distributed anywhere on the body.

<u>Medicine</u>

Sambucus. Urtica - full dose.

Vitamin C.

Verruca

Linimentum Verrucae

Essential Ol Limonum	2.5ml
Ol Castor	2.5ml
Fresh plant Chelidonium	3ml
Fresh plant Allium	2g

Mix all together and apply BD. Applied upon a plaster it will have a prolonged effect otherwise it tends to be rubbed off.

Vitiligo

Loss of dermal pigment causing the skin to become white, it can affect all the skin surface.

<u>Medicines</u>

Juglans sem, Psoralea corylifolia and Piper nigrum - contains piperine it acts upon the protein kinase pathway, externally it stimulates melanin production.

Warts - see papilloma

Dermatology, Including Hair & Nail Disorders

Wounds/ulcers/cuts/abrasions/minor wounds
See emergency herbal medicine Chapter 36.

Xanthelasma
Yellow to white plaques on the skin surface by the inner canthus associated with cholesterolaemia.

Xeroderma see ichthyosis

27
Musculoskeletal System

Musculoskeletal medicines

Aegopodium podagaria - [Goutwort], used for gouty and aching joints.

Aesculus - for strained muscles, spinal lesions, and sacro iliac strain combined with Hypericum.

Agrimonia - general constitutional tonic with Fucus to aid digestion.

Angelica archangelica - when poor peripheral circulation is present.

Apium - a diuretic for the removal of uric acid.

Bryonia (white) - for muscular rheumatism. It seems to act most profoundly for cases that are worse on movement. For rheumatic pain. Small doses only should be used. Large doses are irritating and cathartic. Dose of 5 gtt.

Cimicifuga - stimulating the removal of uric acid

Dioscorea - allays inflammation

Drosera - acts upon the muscles, cartilage and fibrous tissues. Remove acid accumulations around bone injury

Dulcamara - bone, ligaments, cartilage and periosteum.

Filipendula - general antacid for the blood

Fucus – rheumatic disorders with thyroid disturbance [low], and obesity.

Gaultheria - allays inflammation

Guaiacum has an affinity with connective tissues.

Inula has an affinity for fibrous tissue. Combine with Drosera for better effect.

Juglans for strained ligaments and tendons. Combine with Hypericum.

Menyanthes - allays inflammation

Mullein - best in syrup form. Poultices for swollen joints. Tr for sciatica and rheumatism.

Phytolacca - stimulating for deep arthritic disturbances

Salix alba - allays pain and inflammation

Stachys palustris - [Wound wort] - relieves cramp, and pains in the joints.

Urtica - antacid, diuretic, rheumatic pain

Viburnum opulus - muscle antispasmodic

Viola odorata – activity on fibrous tissue and acts to remove growths on fibrous tissue. Fresh leaves or fresh plant Tr.

The following act upon the:

Muscles, Ligaments, Tendons and Periosteum:

Bryonia, Cimicifuga, Colchicum, Dulcamara, Hypericum, Juglans, Symphytum.

Musculoskeletal system

Formulary for external musculoskeletal treatments

Liniments

Herbal oils and tinctures that have penetrating, soothing and rubefacient qualities can be combined to advantage, always bearing in mind the desired end to be achieved by the application either as a medium for gentle application soft massage or deep soft tissue work. Oils are either stimulating relaxing or a combination depending upon the patient. Most oils are prescribed in a base of fixed oil. The base oil is of your own choice - Almond, Arachis, Linseed, Rape seed, Sambucus, Sunflower and Wheat germ oils are examples.

Essential oils

Are used to ease pain – Cajuput, Camphor, Chamomilla, Fucus, Hypericum, Lavandula, Mentha pip, Rosmarinus, Szygium, Symphytum.

Counter stimulants to improve circulation and allay inflammation –
Capsicum, Mustard, Ulmus.

The following liniment serves as a typical liniment. Just change the oil as required to suit the purpose.
Compound liniments can also be used.

Methyl Salicylate liniment

Methyl salicylate 5ml
Fixed oil to 100ml
Apply as required. [painful joints].

Liniment Szygium [stimulating]

Ol Cajuput
Ol Szygium
Ol Origanum
Ol Green Sambucus fol

Shake well before use. Used for stimulating and relaxing the skeletal muscle and easing pain.

Liniment relaxing

Ol Cedarwood
Ol Gaultheria
Ol Pinus sylvestris
Tr Lobelia
Tr Capsicum
Ol Almond

Mix and shake well. More intense application for stubborn complaints with pain.

Nettle liniment completely absorbable

Fresh dry nettles in small pieces. Place in a bottle cover with surgical spirit. Macerate for 7 days shaking each day. Strain and filter. An excellent liniment for backache. This liniment prescription could be used for many different plants. The addition of a little oil makes the liniment spread.

Diagnostic discriminators

Pain, stiffness and swelling are prime symptoms of rheumatic disease.

Pain may be related to trauma or an inflammatory response.

Ask about referred pain, onset, character, urethritis and duration of the pain.

Stiffness – distribution, duration, and circumstances.

Swelling – bony or peri articular.

Ankle pain is most likely from an inflammatory cause.

Bodily reactions in musculoskeletal disease

Mast cells anchored to the tissue walls e.g. blood vessels:

1] release histamine and bradychymin

2] release leucotrines which are inflammation producers and found in animal fats.

3] responsible for inflammatory prostaglandins - Prostaglandins series three occur more often in arthritis.

4] produce chemical mediators in inflammation

5] involved in chemotaxis - attract WBC's from a wider area into a local area. Chemotaxis is valuable in the healing process.

Inflammatory response

Inflammation discourages movement and creates pain to make you aware of trouble.

Inflammation is necessary to increase blood flow through tissues. Inflammation stimulates chemotaxis, along with WBC's. Protracted inflammation makes chemicals within the joint synovial membranes - lysosomal enzymes [which break down foreign debris], in the short term cleanse the synovial fluid and long term - attack bone and cartilage, then inflammation is perpetuated, which creates further damage.

The collagen matrix in the muscle and synovial membrane becomes damaged from

1] advancing age

2] with circulatory reduction

3] free radicle activity

4] excessive sunlight.

Free radicles are either super oxides or peroxides - they attack synovial membrane, anti oxidants fight off free radicles.

Musculoskeletal system

Free radicles are created from animal fats, beef, pork, poultry, hydrogenated fats, peroxides occur from rancid oil, fried foods in a rancid oil and hydrogenated vegetable fats.

Dietary changes encourage improvement in arthritis

Diet is very important for the arthritis sufferer. A reduction in animal meat is essential for improvement. So is avoidance of refined white sugar and flour products. Coffee, tea and excessive alcohol all provoke an acid state of the blood. Whole foods should be eaten together with fruit and salads. Increase prostaglandins - fish liver oils. PGE 3 from EFA's are obtained from fish. Reduce foods containing histamine. The pineapple enzyme Bromelain reduces inflammation and atherosclerosis.

Digestive enzymes help to breakdown proteins. In an arthritic process there is an incomplete breakdown of these proteins. Betaine hydrochloride increases the acidity of the stomach. Increased acidity of the stomach will improve the enzyme process. At a daily dose of 300-600 mg with meals. It is contraindicated where ulceration is suspected. [See also Chapter 18].

Movement and hydrotherapy.

Treatment for rheumatic conditions include hydrotherapy and mobility. Movement of joints is essential to avoid stiffness and swelling.

Exercise and relaxation using e.g.. Yoga, Eeman technique together with mobilisation techniques. Put the joints through a complete set of movements to encourage mobilisation. Hydrotherapy with cold wet compresses will support movement. The addition of herbal infusions to the compress will greatly support the healing process e.g. Seneco jacobaea.

Liniments to allay excess inflammatory activity - Oleum Cajuput, Camphora, Capsicum, Fucus, Lobelia, Juniperus.

Treatment

Chondroitin, Essential fatty acids, Glucosamine sulphate [a constituent of cartilage, tendon and ligament], Omega 3 fatty acids - fish oils, flaxseed, soya, walnuts.

General supportive Chondroitin, Essential fatty acids, Glucosamine sulphate [a constituent of cartilage, tendon and ligament], Omega 3 fatty acids - fish oils, flaxseed, soya, walnuts. **evidence is required for the successful treatment of any musculoskeletal condition.**

1] check the secernants for evidence of adequate elimination and detoxification particularly the kidneys, liver, gall bladder and intestine. The intestine can be affected by synthetic drugs – NSAI's, ageing, alcoholism, constipation and dysbiosis, intestinal infection and malabsorption, allergy to foodstuffs and trauma.

2] blood condition - impurities

3] joints never forgive injuries - osteoarthritis frequently follows damage to a joint area, albeit some years later
4] rheumatic and arthritic conditions are often caused by an excess of uric acid within the blood and joint area
5] internal prescriptions are supported by local applications of hydrotherapy and liniments.

Rheumatic conditions

Ankylosing spondylitis
A chronic and progressive inflammatory disease. Low back pain in the lumbar and sacroiliac areas are common. Pain in the mid back, neck, hips and shoulders.

Bursitis
Inflammation of a bursa. A bursa is a sac lined with synovial membrane and filled with synovial fluid. Bursa are interposed between bone and muscle or tendon and have a protective function.
Bursitis is commonly found in the shoulder, elbow, knee and hip. Pain is common as is a decreased range of motion in the joint.

Carpal tunnel syndrome
A trapped and compressed median nerve within the carpal tunnel. It can be aggravated by other conditions of the elbow, fractures in the wrist, fluid from pregnancy/ PMS, Acromegaly.
Signs and symptoms.
Numbness of the thumb, middle or ring finger. Pain on sharp flexion of the wrist. Thenar eminence atrophy [TEA also occurs with arthritis].
Treatment
Gelsemium, Humulus, Lobelia, Scutellaria, Viburnum opulus.

Corns [bunions]
Treatment
Avoid pressure on the painful area with felt pads.
External
Oleum Hypericum, Lobelia, Sambucus, Symphytum.

Costrochondritis
Pain in the chostrochondral junction of the 3rd 4th and 5th joints.

Cramp
Common in the lower limbs. A painful involuntary contraction of a muscle. Sometimes associated with excessive salt intake and fluid deficiency.

Musculoskeletal system

Dupuytrens contracture
Contraction of the palmar fascia. Associated with arthritis.
<u>Treatment</u>
Local application of Ol. Lobelia help to ease the contraction.

Epicondylitis
Known as tennis elbow. Strained and inflamed lateral forearm extensor muscles.
<u>Medicines</u>
Arnica, Apium, Cimicifuga, Guaiacum, Harpagophytum, Zanthoxylum.
External liniment of Hypericum, Lobelia, Urtica, Symphytum.

Facet joint syndrome
Articular facet joints guide vertebral motion. They can become inflamed due to trauma from a [whiplash] injury or incorrect twisting or lifting. Pain occurs from muscle spasm. Localised tenderness can be palpated. Swelling around the diseased joint.
<u>Treatment</u> internal and external: local for pain and damage to the muscle, tendon and bone applied twice daily.
Antispasmodic tincture. Gaultheria. Hypericum. Ruta. Symphytum.

Fibrositis
Tender spots or nodules on a muscle.

Fractures
Immobilize the fracture.
<u>Treatment</u> - external and internal.
Hypericum. Symphytum.

Frozen shoulder - capsulitis
Shoulder muscle spasm gives rise to restriction of movement. Often the arm is severly restricted in its movement. Pain is often severe and aggravated with elevation of the limb.
<u>Treatment</u>
Antispasmodics: Lobelia with Capsicum [20:1] Sig 10 drops two hourly.
Antispasmodic tincturae Sig 20gtt.
Massage with Oleum Cajuput, Oleum Camphor and/or Ol Lobelia.

Ganglion
Commonly found on the dorsa of the wrist. A ganglion is a fluid filled tumour, which is soft and often tender.
<u>Treatment</u>
Aspiration of the tumour gives relief, it may refill.

Herbal Medicine - Keys

Gout
Most commonly found in the feet. Acute gout - pain and inflammation can be severe.
Treatment
Avoid all red meat and alcohol. Apple cider vinegar drink/lotion. Increase fluids. Elevating the limb will ease the pain.
External
Hydrotherapy - Cold water foot baths. Epsom salt foot baths. Ol/Tr Arnica.
Medicine
Apium, Cimicifuga, Colchicum, Eupatorium purpureum, Filipendula, Guaiacum, Harpagophytum, Salix alba, Viburnum opulus, Zanthoxylum.

Hallux rigidus
Stiff or rigid great toe often due to osteo arthritis secondary to injury or damage.
Treatment
Apium, Cimicifuga, Guaiacum, Menyanthes, Symphytum.
External
Ol Chamomilla, Ol Hypericum, Ol Symphytum, Oleum Ricinus.

Hernia
Hernia are protrusions through the abdominal wall. Inguinal hernias are common in males. There are three main types - inguinal, femoral and umbilical.

Intervertebral disc lesions
Commonly called slipped disc by patients. The lesion is a herniation of the disc, a rupture of the annulus fibrosus. Sites affected are the 4th or 5th lumbar discs. Cervical discs 5/6/7 can also be affected. Sudden, severe pain aggravated by movement, if the patient is able to move at all. Nerve compression from the disc lesion may affect the muscle with characteristic effects of muscle weakness, spasm or atrophy. **Straight leg raising** is used as a test in sciatica. When the extended leg is raised pain restricts movement if the sciatic or spinal nerve roots are compressed.
Treatment
Rest and warm compress. [See emergency herbal treatment].

Low back pain/Lumbago/sacro iliac strain
Commonly occurs from **lumbosacral strain, trauma and degenerative** joint disease. Sciatica can result from lumbar joint degeneration. Pain, tenderness of the muscles and reduced movement occur. Muscle spasm is produced in a vital effort to protect and allow healing of the damage. [See emergency herbal treatment].

Musculoskeletal system

Marfans syndrome
Relaxed connective tissue resulting in joint prolapse and dislocation.
Medicines
Astringents.

Myasthenia gravis
An autoimmune disorder with muscle weakness. Cranial nerve involvement affecting the ocular muscles causes diplopia, ptosis and slurred speech. Weakness of the proximal limb muscles are involved in some 10% of patients. Other auto immune disease can be associated with myasthenia. Thymic hyperplasia is common, benign or malignant tumours may be found.
Medicine
Avena, Capsicum, Centella, Cimicifuga, Ephedra, Ginkgo, Panax, Scutellaria, Smilax. Vitamin E.

Myofibrositis
Scar tissue adhesions occur from: postural strain, trauma, inflammation or spasm. Pain, gritty muscles, painful local trigger points and diminished movement.

Osteoarthritis
Wear and tear arthritis. Articular degeneration gives rise to aching, stiffness, crepitus on movement and weakness.
Medicine
Externally - Symphytum liniment.

Osteomyelitis
Bone marrow infection. Unhealthy condition of the blood leading to osteomyelitis can occur from wounds, fractures and oropharyngeal conditions.
Medicine
Avena, Baptisia, Capsicum, Cimicifuga, Commiphora, Echinacea, Fucus, Galium, Harpagophytum, Plantago, Ruta, Thuja, Urtica, Zanthoxylum.

Osteoporosis
According to Webb in his article on 'the danger of evidence based advice' he spells out the oversimplification of using bone mineral density as a measure of estimating osteoporosis. It is a highly complex and dynamic physiological process that lends itself to naturopathic treatment. He considers proactive patient involvement in treatment is vital [388].
Reduction in bone strength associated with osteoporosis results from loss of collagen framework onto which calcium and other minerals are deposited [199]. Loss of collagen makes the bone appear like a 'crunchie chocolate bar'. Loss of collagen and calcium occur together. Peak bone mass attainment is reached at

307

around 25 years of age and muscle mass predicts strength of the bones. Some 1 in 3 women and 1 in 12 men may develop osteoporosis. Thyroid hormone increases osteoclast activity. Loss of 35-40% of bone mineral loss is necessary in order for osteoporosis to be detected by x rays.

Osteoporosis becomes a problem when the bone mass decreases which make bone more fragile and liable to fracture. Vertebral osteoporosis reduces the height of an individual. Vertebra can become crushed as a result. It only takes 5-8% increase in bone mineral density to reduce the risk of fracture.

Fracture sites [1] kyphosis in over 75's [2] thoraco lumbar junction [3] hips.

Some determining factors for osteoporosis:

Post menopausal, elderly, genetic factors, stress, endocrine causes – cushings, diabetes, thyrotoxicosis, infirm patients; on bed rest/disabled, lack of exercise, diuretics, renal disturbances.

Lack of sunlight, malabsorption, drugs, **antacids** reduce calcium, caffeine and alcohol increase calcium loss, alcohol, pregnancy, contraceptive pill. The contraceptive pill affects copper which it raises in the blood and has an indirect effect upon bone.

Nutrition – high protein – increases uric acid and uses calcium to buffer and eliminate it, high fat, sugar – refined and high sugar intake induces calcium loss, phosphate intake e.g. soft drinks affect bone metabolism. Refined grains lose 85% of magnesium and 60% of calcium. Salt increases urinary calcium loss. Phosphorus, sodium and calcium loss occur together

It could take 24 months in order for changes to be seen on a scan following treatment

Increase exercise like walking or swimming. Regular exercise lowers the incidence of osteoporosis.

Osteoporosis treatment to increase calcium absorption

HRT will stop bone density loss but will not replace bone that has been lost.

Check gastric acid levels as hypochlorhydria = poor calcium absorption.

A] Reduce fat intake, reduce protein. Use a vegetarian diet. Only small amounts of red meat may be consumed.

B] Check the Ca/Mg ratio. Magnesium and calcium balance should be 2:1. Consider daily dose of 600mg Calcium, 300mg Magnesium, Copper 1mg, Boron 2mg [Boron metabolises oestrogens], Folic acid 800mcg, Betaine Hydrochloride 20mg, B6 25mg, B12 20mg, Vitamin C 200mg, Vitamin K 300mcg.

Calcium gluconate and magnesium orotate are preferable. Milk once pasturised binds the calcium this makes it less absorbable by the body. Phytates found in bran also reduce the absorption of calcium in the body.

Musculoskeletal system

Vitamin D from sunlight and betaine hydrochloride increase calcium absorption. Excess Vitamin E can leach out calcium from the bone.

Hormonal Medicine

Chamaelirium luteum, Oenothera, Vitex, Cimicifuga and bone herbs: Symphytum, Ruta.

Medicine

Capsella, Cimicifuga, Equisetum, Filipendula, Fucus, Medicago, Symphytum, Trigonella, Urtica.

Pagets disease
Treat as osteoporosis

Polymyalgia rheumatica
Auto immune condition that may affect arteries too.
Medicines
Capsicum, Cimicifuga, Crataegus, Filipendula, Gaultheria, Salix alba, Zanthoxylum, Zingiber.

Pott's disease
Tubercular bone disease.
Medicines for tuberculosis are found in the respiratory chapter.

Reiters disease
Signs and symptoms – conjunctivitis, oral inflammation, psoriasis, arthritis of the sacro-iliac joints, knees and ankles. Urethritis if found is associated with sexually transmitted disease this induces Reiters disease.
Medicine
Arctium, Centella, Echinacea, Eupatorium purpureum, Filipendula, Gelsemium, Guaiacum, Juniperus, Menyanthes, Piper methysticum, Rumex, Smilax, Taraxacum, Uva ursi, Valeriana, Zea.

Tenosynovitis Repetitive strain injury
Inflamed tendon sheath.
Treatment
Liniment – Oleum Arnica, Camphor, Cajuput, Gaultheria, Lobelia.
Medicine - Tenosynovitis
Antispasmodic Tr., Arnica, Astragalus, Avena, Eleutherococcus, Gaultheria, Lobelia, Salix alba, Valeriana, Viburnum opulus.

Rheumatic pain see under gout for medicines.

28
Paediatrics

Prescribing for children
Infants and children require a lower dose of medicine compared to adults because children have lower body weights.
Dosage of the medicine would be calculated using the formula of age and weight ratios. Children have high metabolic rates as compared to adults and utilise the medicine more quickly. The liver in children is large in comparison to the rest of the body. Hence medicine breakdown is faster.

Babies in their first six months of life have poor elimination via the kidneys and liver. Nutriture would be best through breast milk that is easily digested. In order to give the medicine an oral syringe or dropper will provide an accurate fractional dose for infants.

Proportional doses according to age
The following are some of the methods available for calculating the dose for a child.

Formula for measuring a child's dose of medicine, for children under 12
Youngs rule

$$\frac{Age}{Age + 12}$$

Divide the child's age by the child's age + 12 to give the required proportion.

e.g. $\dfrac{age\ 4}{4 + 12}$ $\dfrac{4}{16}$ $\dfrac{1}{4}$

Quantity to be given is 25% of the adult dosage

Dillings formula – correlates dose with body weight

$$\frac{age}{20}$$

Paediatrics

Maximum dose range – using age and weight ratios

Age	approximate weight	% of adult dose
6 months	8 k	10%
1 year	10 k	20%
3 years	14 k	30%
5 years	18 k	40%
7 years	23 k	50%
12 years	37 k	75%

Carminative, antispasmodic and anodyne prescription:
Px Chamomilla, Foeniculum and Nepeta.

Colic, Diarrhoea, Insomnia, Restlessness, Teething pain.
<u>Medicines</u>
Anethum, Foeniculum, Melissa. Mentha piperita/Spicata, Nepeta, Passiflora, Plantago, Potentilla.

Paediatric conditions

Biggest killers of children
1] Infantile diarrhoea
2] Measles
3] Poverty

Colic can be caused by allergy to cows milk, nervous children, excess fibre in the diet.
<u>Medicines</u>
Nepeta, Calendula, Foeniculum [Fennel] or Anethum [Dill] water.

Cradle cap
A catarrhal condition with elimination of impurities through the scalp skin.
<u>Treatment</u>
- Oat scrub to scalp, put a handful of oats into muslin and clean the scalp. Bathe with shampoo containing
- Fixed oil applied to the scalp and wash off next morning.
- Urtica wash.

Diarrhoea
<u>Medicines</u>
Diarrhoea may be gently restrained with Hamamelis, Rubus.

Herbal Medicine - Keys

Feeding troubles - use the colic medicines.

Heat rash
Many babies are covered up too much.
Treatment
Use less clothing and give an infusion of Urtica or Mentha piperita to cool.

Night crying or night terrors
Is there a cause for the pain? Is baby wet, hungry, too hot or cold.
Medicine
Chamomilla, Nepeta, Passiflora.
Terrors at night the Bach remedy - Rock rose soothes fretfulness and fears.

Sticky eyes
Bath eyes with cotton wool, water and a pinch of salt [to make a saline solution].

Cord
The cord detaches in 5 - 7 days. It is usual for a small amount of infection to occur around the cord this encourages separation.
Treatment
Clean the area with Aloe or Calendula. Non stick dressing is applied to the cord.
Ricinus communis - Apply to the navel of a newborn infant if for any reason it shows difficulty in healing.

Urine suppression
Immerse the pelvis into warm water

Vomiting
May be postural.
Projectile vomiting - allergy, possible stomach pyloric spasm/stenosis.
Treatment
Sit the baby up.
Medicine
Atropa, Dioscorea.

Human brain development
A number of disorders can be helped says Dr Udo Erasmus in his book Fats that kill. He says 'a right fat diet is the requirement for health'. He mentions that children with learning difficulties, dyslexia, attention deficit disorders and hyperactivity 'could benefit from a right fat diet'. He further says 'if our foods are not right for our brains biological requirements, then our behaviour cannot be

right'. Hypoglycaemia can also affect the thought processes and ones actions. The brain cannot work effectively because it is not being fed correctly.

Essential fatty acids support neurone function and trophic state. Take EFA's before 8pm as they enhance energy, any later and sleep disturbances could result. Allergy to oils is rare because oils are protein free. EFA's can be used to treat fungal infections. EFA's are required for mineral transportation and metabolism they are also required for protein metabolism.

EFA's are found in Evening primrose and blackcurrants.

Dyslexia
Scans are not without risk. Ultrasound scanning before birth can lead to delayed speech development. In a 1982 research paper Liebeskind says that permanent hereditary defects can occur after just one scan. Foetal cells are altered by ultrasound scanning, the behaviour and motility of cells was found to be abnormal.

Haemolytic disease of the newborn Erythroblastosis foetalis
Impregnation of a woman with Rh -ve blood by a man with Rh +ve blood leads to haemolytic anaemia in the foetus. Transplacental mixing of blood during pregnancy and childbirth causes RBC's to be transferred to the mother with destruction of RBC's.
Treatment
For the baby's liver and blood where jaundice is present.
Medicine
Berberis sp, Calendula, Collinsonia, Gentiana, Hydrastis, Myrica, Silybum, Taraxacum.

Infancy
Gastro intestinal milk intolerance of infancy can cause haematochezia – bright red blood in the stool.

Low birth weight
There is good evidence that low birthweight is linked to a greater risk of infant mortality, ill health in childhood and an increased risk of adult degenerative disease. Low birthweight children need more hospital care, have higher rates of neurological problems, disability, poor attention span, lower academic achievement and more behavioural difficulties. They have more days off school because of illness and are greater users of the GP's services.

Low birthweight is closely linked to cardiovascular disease, hypertension, stroke, obesity and diabetes later in life.

The mothers nutritional status and diet during pregnancy are linked to birthweight [27, 28].

Herbal Medicine - Keys

Mortality
Infant mortality rate is 5.5 deaths per 1000 live births [2001 figures].

Pyrexia [Influenza]
<u>Medicines</u>
Eupatorium perfoliatum, Nepeta, Sambucus, Szygium.

Reys syndrome
Rare condition. Tends to follow an acute viral illness such as influenza or varicella. Aspergillus flavus, alfatoxin ingestion and salicylate ingestion may all cause Reys.
Signs – acute nausea & vomiting progressing to coma in severe cases. Affects the under 18 year age group. Encephalopathy and fatty liver infiltration occur, returning to normal within 16 weeks.
<u>Treatment</u>
Baptisia, Capsicum, Echinacea, Oenothera.

Rheumatic fever
Follows a streptococcal sore throat [tonsil infection] and affects the joints. Generalised erythematous rash. Check the renal activity.
<u>Treatment</u>
Bedrest. Fluids. Apple juice. Restrict food intake.
<u>Medicines</u>
Achillea, Agrimonia, Baptisia, Carduus, Chamomilla, Commiphora, Crataegus, Echinacea, Eupatorium perfoliatum, Filipendula, Harpagophytum, Menyanthes, Phytolacca, Sambucus, Salix alba, Tabebuia. Vitamin C.
<u>External</u>
Camphor, Gaultheria, Lobelia, Plantago, Seneco jacobaea, Stellaria, Symphytum.

Teething
<u>Medicine</u>
Chamomilla - Gel application or infusion.

Zinc is required for growth. During a growth spurt zinc needs to be increased. The usual dose is 15mg daily. Zinc citrate is well absorbed.

Specific paediatric disease conditions together with medicines for their treatments are covered in the appropriate sections chapter [17-31] of this work.

29
Tropical Diseases/Acute Infectious disease
Helminthic Infections/Parasitic Disease

As an historical note the following is quoted at length from Florence Nightingale, notes of 1858 [p128-133].
It is a vulgar error to suppose that epidemics are occasioned by the spread of disease, from person to person by infection or contagion for it is an ascertained fact that before any person is attacked epidemically the disease attacks individuals in a milder form one at a time at distant intervals for weeks or months before the epidemic appears. Before an epidemic of cholera these cases consist generally of diarrhoea of more or less intensity followed by a rapidly fatal case or two very much resembling cholera. .... without this preparatory stage the occurrence of an epidemic is impossible - the epidemic being the retributive stage of a succession of antecedent phenomena extending over months or years and all traceable to the culpable neglect of natural laws. It is simply worse than folly after the penalty has been incurred to cry out contagion and call for the establishment of sanitary cordons and quarantine, instead of relying on measures of hygiene. Epidemics are lessons to be profited by: they teach, not that current contagion's are inevitable but that unless natures laws be studied and obeyed, she will infallibly step in and vindicate them, sooner or later. Many of the following infectious diseases vindicate Nightingales words.

Infectious disease
Infectious diseases kill nearly 17 million people a year [130].
The most ruthless killer of all is poverty. Many people have no clean water or adequate sanitation along with poor housing and inadequate nutrition. Following armed conflict or economic collapse, conditions worsen for the populus. Drought with resulting crop failure often worsens the situation.

Signs and symptoms of infections
Constipation, diarrhoea, abdominal pain [colicky], flatulence and bloating, blood and mucus in stool, foul smelling stool
Nausea, vomiting.
Headache, fever, fatigue.
Skin rash, pruritis.

Rehydration mixture
Treatment
One pinch of salt, one teaspoonful of honey together with 200 ml of water. Mix together and drink.

Tropical disease conditions

Anthrax
An anaerobic infectious disease caused by a gram positive bacilli. Contracted through the soil, by touch, airborne or through contaminated meat. Red brown itchy papule or influenzal like symptoms. Lymphadenopathy. Pyrexia and respiratory distress [pneumonia] follow, leading to cyanosis, shock and coma.
Medicines
Baptisia, Capsicum, Commiphora, Echinacea, Tabebuia, Uncaria.

Blackwater fever
A complication of malaria. Characterised by fever, haemolysis, haemoglobinuria. Poor prognosis.
Medicines
Hepatics also Cinchona, Combretum micranthum, Echinacea, Mareya micrantha, Microglossa pyrifolia, Plumbago zeylandica.

Botulism
Contracted from animals through broken skin or mucous membranes. Incubates over 36 hours. It tends to be fatal if contracted.
Signs and symptoms - Diplopia, loss of accomodation, dry mouth and throat, dysphagia, vomiting, abdominal pain, diarrhoea with eventual respiratory arrest, cranial nerve palsies. May follow wound infection. Clostridium toxins block the release of acetylcholine.
Treatment
Isolate the patient.
Medicines
Baptisia, Capsicum, Commiphora, Echinacea.

Cholera
A new form of cholera has been found. Cholera spread is encouraged by inadequate and poorly maintained water and sanitation systems. In 1831 cholera was prevalent in overcrowded, dirty and unsanitary dwellings particularly among the poor. Carrier: water borne. Symptoms - Extreme diarrhoea with dehydration and electrolyte imbalance. Cardiac failure. Infective for up to 2 weeks until stool samples are clear.
Treatment
Rapid rehydration and antimicrobials – Allium, Cinnamomum, Eucalyptus, Iris, Psidium guajava - fol, rad, fructus [astringent].

Tropical Diseases/Acute Infectious disease, Helminths/Parasites

Dengue fever
Abrupt onset, acute febrile infectious disease lasting about a week - caused by a dengue virus transmitted by the Aedes mosquito.
Symptoms – headache, vomiting, muscle and joint pain or weakness, measles like rash, lymphadenopathy, pyrexia, depression and weakness.
Medicines
Achillea, Allium, Chionanthus, Echinacea, Eupatorium perfoliatum, Guaiacum, Sambucus, Thymus.

Diarrhoea
E coli is blamed for anything between 300,000 and 700,000 deaths a year among children under 5 and is the most common cause of diarrhoea in developing countries.
Medicines
Allium, Cinnamomum, Echinacea, Hamamelis.

Dracunculiasis [Guinea worm]
A small ulcer appears at the site of emergence of the adult female worm. This is usually on the lower limb. This is preceded by the appearance of a blister which ruptures and liberates swarms of eggs. It is possible to extract the worm but if care is not taken and the worm is broken cellulitis results.
Treatment
Removal of the worm if possible by threading it around a cotton wool bud or similar and gently extracting the worm.
Medicines
Boerhaavia diffusa - root softened and used as a poultice.
Cassia occidentalis - crushed leaves. Combretum micranthum - decoction.
Elaeophorbia drupifera. Hilleria latifolia - fol.
Jatropha curcas - leaves burned and a poultice applied.
Monodora myristica. Olax subscorpioidea - oral leaf decoction. Powdered rad to the dermal opening. Ricinus communis - boiled leaves put on the skin opening.
Spathodea campanulata

Dysentery - amoebic/bacillary
Amoebic type is infective for years if untreated. Bacillary is infective for up to 4 weeks until the stool is negative, even negative results can still produce symptoms. Both can cause colitis and intestinal abscess.
Treatment
Rapid rehydration and antimicrobials:
Medicines
Acacia catechu, Agrimonia, Allium sativa/ursinum, Artemesia annua, Baptisia, Cinnamomum, Cydonia oblongata [188 p364], Dioscorea, Echinacea, Eugenia,

317

Eucalyptus, Euphorbia sp., Geranium maculatum, Haematoxylon campechianum Sig 8ml [188], Hydrastis, Juglans regia, Monsonia ovata, Myrica, Picraena, Picrasma, Piper cubebs, Plantago sp., Polygonum, Rheum palmatum, Rubus, Sclerocarya birrea, Ulmus.

Ebola haemorrhagic fever
Highly contagious infection that causes the victims to bleed to death. Haemorrhage occurs from all orifices.

Filariasis
Roundworms. See helminthic.

Giardiasis
Sometimes associated with over growth of candida.
Medicines
Allium, Artemisia annua, Berberis species, Hydrastis, Origanum vulgare, Quassia, Trigonella. Grapefruit seed extract.

Hepatitis
Infective types A, B, C. [See under GIT].
Medicines
Allium, Berberis vulgaris, Mycobacterium smegmatis, Staphylococcus aureus, Uvaria chamae is an effective antimicrobial against Bacillus subtilis.

Lassa fever
A viral disease. The vector is a rodent and once infected humans carry the virus which incubates in 3-30 days. Mortality is up to 50%.
Symptoms include pyrexia, headache, muscular pain and leucocytosis.
Treatment
Rest. Fast on nourishing vegetable juices.
Medicines
Achillea, Allium, Centella, Glycyrrhiza, Guaiacum, Larrea, Trifolium.

Leishmaniasis [Kala azar]
Affects 10 million people and is found in Spain, Portugal, North Africa and Turkey.
Clinical signs develop two to twelve months after the initial bite of a protozoan parasite. Cutaneous signs - following a bite the macule ulcerates then heals. The parasite can erode the bones and skin. Mucous membrane ulcers of the nose and throat.

Tropical Diseases/Acute Infectious disease, Helminths/Parasites

Medicines - Leishmaniasis
Allium, Berberis species, Cassia acutifolia, Chasmanthera dependens, Commiphora, Echinacea, Hydrastis, Iris, Picrorrhiza kurroa, Picralima nitida.

Leptosporosis [Weils disease]
Rats urine contaminates water. Fairly rare ailment, 1988 produced 106 cases with 8 deaths. Rivers, canals and slow moving water are worse for contamination. Bacteria enter the body through cuts, grazes and open sores also through the mucous membranes of the eyes and nose.
Symptoms are flu like. If untreated can cause hepatitis and kidney failure.
Medicines
Antibacterial agents – Allium.

Leprosy [Hansens disease]
Insidous infection by Mycobacterium leprae.
Clinically divided into two types [1] lepromatous – nodular, symmetric dermal lesions, ulcers, pyrexia, neuritis and orchitis.
[2] tuberculoid – macular dermal lesions, asymmetric nerve involvement of sudden onset. Keratitis, iridocyclitis, epistaxis, nasal ulcers, anaemia, lymphadenopathy. Nerves swell and become anaesthetized.
Medicines
Acacia senegal, Afzelia africana, Albizia, Alchornea cordifolia - powdered root, Antiaris africana, Asphaltum, Cassia occidentalis, Centella [188 p214], Chlorophora, Corynanthe pachyceras, Echinacea, Erythrina mildbraedii, Ficus capensis, Hilleria latifolia, Hydrocarpus laurifolia [Gynocardia or Chaulmoogra oil rediscovered by botanist Joseph Rock in 1920. Seed oil is used externally also as an injection and emulsion [189 p72]. Hydrocotyle asiatica, Ledum, Lonchocarpus cyanesens, Melia, Momordica charantia – ampalaya [metabolic stimulant, fat burning dissolving body fat, diuretic, anticonstipation], Morinda lucida, Nauclea latifolia, Piliostigma thonningi, Plumbago zeylandica, Pycnanthus angolensis, Ricinis communis, Securidaca longepedunculata, Smilax, Spondias mombin, Synedrella nodiflora, Tabebuia, Tamarindus indica - rad. Terminalia glaucescens, Thymus, Treculia africana, Vitex doniana, Zanthoxylum sp.

Lyme disease
Infection by Borrelia burdorfer following a tick bite. Treatment see rickettsial.

Malaria
The parasite mutates, adapts and changes therefore it is immune to drugs. Malaria is the single largest disease in Africa and Asia. The Red Cross tells us 3000 children die from malaria daily and 500 million cases have been reported. It now is endemic in 100 countries.

319

Herbal Medicine - Keys

As a matter of interest more US soldiers died in Viet Nam from malaria than from any bullet.

Carrier: Female Anopheles mosquito bites its victims and lays eggs. Circular bodies are produced these burst out of the blood.

Symptoms: Recurrent fever, rigours, enlarged spleen. Cerebral malaria kills around 90% of cases.

Treatment

Avoid being bitten. Some remedies can be burnt to destroy the mosquito. Sleep under bed nets.

Spray the skin every three hours with Oleum Azadirachta [neem], Eucalyptus, Rosmarinus, Cymbopogon nardus [Citronella] and Citrus bergamia [Bergamot].

Medicines useful as use in a spray.

Achillea, Artemesia vulgaris, Basilicum, Chamomilla, Cedar, Cymbopogon nardus - effective for 1 hr. Eucalyptus, Hyssopus, Juniperus, Rose geranium, Sassafras and Santalum.

Herbal treatment - Antiprotozoals:

Acanthospermum hispidum, Alstonia boonei, Aristolochia bracteata, Artabtrys uncinatus, Artemisia annua, Azadirachta indica, Brucea javanica.

Carissa edulis, Chrysophyllum albidum, Cinchona officinalis, Citrus paradisi, Clausena anisata, Clutia abyssinica, Croton zambesicus, Cryptolepis sanguinolenta.

Dichroea febrfuga.

Eucalyptus globulus, Eupatorium odoratum [Osmia odorata].

Holarrhena floribunda [also as a steam bath]. Hoslundia opposita.

Khaya senegalensis, Kigelia africana tree [Bignoniaceae].

Mitragyna ciliata, Morinda lucida.

Nauclea latifolia, Newbouldia laevis, Nigella sativa

Ocimum sp. [oil to prevent mosquito bites, burning the leaves as a mosquito repellent]. Olea europaea leaves.

Picrorrhiza kurroa, Picralima nitida [sem, stem, bacc and fruit rind], Prunus mahaleb.

Psidium guajava, Quassia, Ricinis communis - seed oil destroys mosquitoes.

Sclerocarya birrea, Sesamum indicum.

Tabebuia sp., Tephrosia apollinea, Tamarindus indica, Tetrapleura tetraptera. Tinospora cordifolia.

Uvaria lucida and U. scheffleri - stem and root bark.

Warburgia ugandensis - also antifungal - candida and antiyeast - Saccharomyces cerevisiae, Sclerotina libertiana, Spadoptera littorialis and S. exepts.

Cinchona

Cinchona bark is a source of quinine and was discovered in 1834. It yields up to 16% quinoline alkaloids. Tannins and resin.

Tropical Diseases/Acute Infectious disease, Helminths/Parasites

Chewing on the bark of cinchona is an effective febrifuge for intermittent fever. Quinine is structurally similar to the quinoline antimalarials. Quinine has a more complex side chain containing carbons and one nitrogen atom in a two-ring structure. The amount of quinine varies in the bark [0.3-8%] and variable amounts of other antimalarial alkaloids such as cinchonine.
Dose
Short half life of 10 hours.
Sig 2g to start treatment then
1-2g every 6-8 hours for three doses each day and then daily for seven days. Overdosage [Cinchonism] of quinine causes tinnitus, headache, visual and aural dysfunction, vertigo, GIT and CVS effects.

Rickettsial diseases [Quassa fever, Typhus – spotted fever]
Characterised by opthalmia, rash, pyrexia, pneumonia, renal failure, encephalitis, coma. Infection is of bacterial origin transmitted to humans by ticks.
Treatment
Clear the bacteraemia together with the toxins.
Medicines
Allium, Aloe, Andrographis, Asclepias, Baptisia, Borago, Chamomilla [235], Capsicum, Chionanthus, Cinnamomum, Commiphora molmol, Commiphora erythraea [bisabolol myrrh] [272, 1994, 5 [5] p44]. Echinacea, Eucalyptus, Eupatorium perfoliatum, Hydrastis, Leptandra, Melilotus, Opopanax, Phytolacca, Potentilla. Vitamin C. Fasting.

Rift valley fever
Rift valley fever is caused by a virus. Symptoms are similar to Ebola. In 1998 an area in Kenya was flooded and people were falling ill with acute fever, headache and bleeding. Spontaneous abortions and deaths of domestic animals from haemorrhaging were reported. Mosquitoes harbour and transmit the virus to humans and animals.

River blindness [Onchocerciasis]
Carrier: black fly.
River blindness is a filarial disease [parasite] of humans caused by Onchocerca volvulus it lives in the lymph nodes. It migrates behind the eye and destroys the retina. Resulting in severe visual loss and eventual blindness.
Onchocercal chiroretinopathy has characteristic signs in the fundi. Loss of pigment that shows as grey/yellow mottling. Retinal pigment epithelium loss occurs in an arc around the macula. Atrophy and subretinal fibrosis follow. Changes are seen on the nasal aspect of the optic disc.
Symptoms: Itchy rash, nodules all over the body, blindness. Elephantiasis – occurs from blockage of the lymphatics from the worms.

Herbal Medicine - Keys

Schistosomiasis [Bilharzia]
Effects 200 million people. It is a human blood fluke. From the egg form development progresses into a microcidium then snail. It lives in water and penetrates the skin.
Few patients die however it does make patients ill.
The swimmers itch is a papular eruption caused by the penetration of the skin by cercariae of various schistosomia parasites. Skin nodules are seen after aborted attempts of schistosomiasis to infect the body.
Planting of Balanites aegyptiaca along the river banks of infested rivers helps to control infestation.
Medicines - Anti Biharzials
Balanites aegyptiaca is a tree found in Africa, the root and bark is lethal to freshwater snails and the intermediate stages of the schistosomes. The snails are hosts to Bilharzia. Chrysophyllum albidum, Citrullus colocynthis Sig 500mg, Citrus limoneum, Coriandrum sativum, Evodia rutaecarpa dried sem contain atanine this kills cercariae, the larval stage of the parasite, Morus nigra, Phytolacca, Ricinus communis, Tabebuia, Thymus, Vitis vinerifa and Zingiber.

Smallpox
Variola pox virus infection. Spread is by a coughing through droplet infection or dermal ulcer contact.
Medicines
Achillea, Allium, Berberis vulgaris, Echinacea, Hydrastis, Polygonum bistorta, Rubus, Salvia officinalis, Thuja. Vitamin C.

Snake bites [See emergency herbal chapter]

Tetanus [Lockjaw]
Acute infectious disease caused by Clostridium tetani bacteria. Wounds, drug abusers, surgery and neonates [cord infection] in developing countries are at risk. The toxin travels along the nerves to affect the jaw.
Medicines
Control toxins, muscle spasm and hypertonicity - Allium, Echinacea, Gelsemium, Lobelia, Scutellaria.

Toxocara
The worm infects dogs and cats. Transmission from animal faeces. There are around 40 cases a year and 3/4 cases are serious. Once in the human it moves about the body. Attacking the eyes, the parasite migrates across the retina and can cause blindness.
Medicines
Allium, Chamomilla, Picrasma, Stachys, Thymus.

Tropical Diseases/Acute Infectious disease, Helminths/Parasites

Toxoplasmosis
Febrile illness with rash. Lymphadenopathy. Hepatosplenomegaly. Myocarditis. Encephalomyelitis.
Medicines
Melilotus.

Trachoma
Trachoma an infection of the eye by Chlamydia trachomatis which can cause blindness. There is extreme light sensitivity.
Medicines
Allium, Berberis sp., Centella, Commiphora, Echinacea, Hydrastis, Phytolacca.

Trypanomiasis [Sleeping sickness]
Trypanosoma cruzi - the Tetse fly bites its host the toxins produced in the blood affect the brain and causes malaise, and sleeping sickness. It affects 35 million people worldwide.
Medicines
Baptisia, Berberis aquifoleum/vulgaris, Hydrastis, Garcinia kola, Kigelia africana [Bignoniaceae] fol, rad and wood contains dihydro - isocoumarins, flavonoids, iridoids and napthoquinones and is antibacterial, Mitragyna ciliata, Picralima nitida, Tabebuia sp. Selenium.

Tuberculosis
Tuberculosis is increasing worldwide and has a close association with HIV infection.
Medicines [inhibiting the growth of Mycobacterium tuberculosis]
Adhatoda vasica, Agave americana, Allium, Aloe, Berberis vulgaris, Buxus sempervirens, Centella, Cetraria islandica, Chondrus, Drosera, Echinacea, Embelia schimperi, Equisetum, Eriodictyon californicum, Eucalyptus globlus, Euphorbia pilulifera [191], Geum urbanum, Ginkgo, Glechoma hederacea, Glycyrrhiza glabra, Guaiacum, Hydrastis, Hydrocarpus laurifolia, Inula, Iris, Larrea tridentata, Lycopus, Myrica, Oplopanax horridus [Devil's Club] active against Mycobacterium tuberculosis and Mycobacterium avium, [278, 1997, 60], Plumeria sp [Frangipani] - 275, 1998, 57 p17-20. Sutherlandia frutescens, Symphytum, Tinospora cordifolia, Veratrum album/viride.

Typhoid
Watery diarrhoea results from the ingestion of infected food by Salmonella typhi. Intestinal haemorrhage can follow.
Medicines
Allium, Andrographis, Angelica archangelica, Apocynum, Aristolochia, Asclepias, Atropa, Baptisia, Bryonia, Capsella, Cinnamomum, Echinacea,

Herbal Medicine - Keys

Medicines for typhoid
Eucalyptus, Hydrastis, Menyanthes, Picrasma, Podophyllum, Potentilla, Sassafras, Strychnos nux vomica, Tephrosea, Veratrum sp.

Typhus see rickettsial

Helminthic infections - Worm infestations
Threadworms – Enterobius
Minute human parasites that live inside the bowel for a short time. Threadworms do not come from animals. They are harmless but as the eggs are deposited at the anus they tend to cause a lot of anal itching. Scratching causes the eggs to be trapped under the finger nails. The eggs are passed from the fingers to the mouth and swallowed.
Treatment
All the family must be treated for around six weeks to prevent re-infection. Cleanliness is of paramount importance. Scrubbing under the finger nails with a nail brush removes the eggs. Bedlinen must be changed frequently. Towels are for sole use only.
Medicines
On an empty stomach give night and morning - Artemesia species, Tanacetum mixed with syrup or honey.

Taenia - Tapeworm
Nematodes - Ascarides [Roundworm], Ancylostoma [Hookworm] and Filariasis.
Filariasis affects 50 million people worldwide.
Treatment
Fast. Enema. Oral anthelmintic.
Medicines
Allium, Carapa procera, Dryopteris [toxic], Embelia schimperi, Hoslundia opposita, Mallotus philippinensis, Melilotus, Morinda longiflora, Portulaca oleracea, Punica granatum – pomegranate, Spigelia.

Yellow fever
Viral infection caused by a mosquito bite.
Medicines
Capsicum, Chrysophyllum albidum, Eupatorium perfoliatum,
Trema guineensis [bacc].
Spray - Acorus calamus in combination with Curcuma longa or Pinus.

Yaws

An infectious disease caused by Treponema pertenue. Skin manifestations of the granulmatous type destroy the skin and bone.

<u>Medicines</u>

Carapa procera, Lonchocarpus cyanescens, Trichilia emetica,

Prescription: Guaiacum 1k, Sassfras bark 120g, Pimpinella 120g, sugar 500g. Boil in 4400 aqua until the volume reduces to 3300ml.

Sig 550ml daily with 1500 ml aqua daily. [131]

30
Obstetrics & Gynaecology

Anti nausea medicines
Ballota, Chamomilla, Cetraria, Chamaemelum, Cinnamomum, Dioscorea, Filipendula, Foeniculum, Lavandula, Mentha piperita, Rubus, Zingiber.

Medicines used in obstetrics and gynaecology
Alstonia boonei - expels retained placenta.
Archangelica archangelica - expels retained placenta.
Armoracia - expels retained placenta.
Artemesia species - oxytocic.
Asarum canadense - Parturition where there is pain and weak expulsive power.
Sig Tr 5gtt aqua 100ml Sig 5ml every 10 minutes for pain and weakness.
Capsicum - equalises the circulation, antihaemorrhagic.
Caulophyllum - relaxes tension of the sphincters, and lower circular fibres of the uterus. Vaginal and cervical rigidity.
Chamaelirium luteum - a uterine tonic and trophorestorative.
Cimicifuga - antispasmodic, anodyne. Partus preparator. Os rigidity.
Coriandrum – oxytocic - sem poultice to vagina – drawing action [228 p 111].
Dioscorea - smooth muscle antispasmodic, anodyne.
Dong quai - pelvic vasodilator
Erigeron canadense - uterine astringent, post partum haemorrhage.
Fraxinus - voluntary muscle stimulant. Uterine hypertrophy. Uterine tonic.
Gelsemium - antispasmodic, Os rigidity, anodyne.
Hamamelis - analgesia following episotomy.
Helleborus niger - eclampsia
Hydrastis - uterine tonic. Oxytocic.
Leonurus - parturient, anodyne.
Lobelia - antispasmodic, spasm of the Os cervix. Perineal or vaginal rigidity.
Mentha pulegrum - stimulates contractions. Oxytocic.
Mitchella - slow parturition, antispasmodic.
Piscidia - antispasmodic, anodyne. Parturient controls erratic or spasmodic pain.
Pilocarpus - rigid Os, puerpural eclampsia.
Rubus - contracts uterine smooth muscle and stimulates expulsive power.
Ruta - oxytocic.
Seneco aureus - as a general vaso relaxant to the uterus.
Szygium - stimulates uterus. Locally anodyne.
Tanacetum parthenium - anodyne, parturient,
Trillium - parturient and oxytocic.
Trigonella - oxytocic. Stimulates and tones the uterus.
Veratrum album/viride – eclampsia.

Obstetrics and Gynaecology

Antifungal

Albizia lebbeck, Alchemilla arvensis, Allium, Aloe gel, Angelica archangelica, Azadirachta, Baptisia, Berberis sp., Boscia senegalensis, Calendula, Cinnamomum zeylandicum, Citrus aurantium, Commiphora molmol, Curcuma longa, Echinacea, Hydrastis, Jateorrhiza, Juglans, Lavandula, Larrea tridentata, Myrica, Phytolacca, Szygium, Tabebuia, Tetrapleura tetraptera, Thuja, Thymus, Vitex, Warburgia ugandensis.
Ol Oenotherus Melaleuca – external. Ol Eucalyptus – external.

Antihaemorrhagic

Capsicum, Chamaelirium luteum, Cimicifuga, Composition essence, Erigeron canadense, Geranium maculatum, Myrica, Viscum, Zingiber.

Sphincter relaxants

Caulophyllum, Cypripedium, Cimicifuga, Pulsatilla, Valeriana, Viburnum opulus.

Medicines for hormonal imbalances

Alchemilla vulgaris, Humulus, Salvia, Geranium maculatum, Rubus.
Oestrogenic – Salvia, Smilax, Trifolium
Natural HRT - Vitex. Alchemilla vulgaris.
Prostaglandin balancer – Ol Oenothera.

Anti ovulatory, anti-implantation and antioestrogenic medicines

Antifertility activity has been shown in the following medicines from 60%-100% activity has been ascribed. Activity is related to percentage amounts.

Medicines

Abroma augusta rad 95% active, Acrostichum aureum herba 70%, Adhatoda vasica fol 66%, Albizzia lebbeck sem 60%, Aloe barbadensis fol 80%, Areca catechu nut 80%, Aristolochia indica rad 100%, Artabotrys adoratissima fol 67%, Artemesia scoparia herba 100%, Butea frondosa petals, sem 62-100%, Carica papaya unripe fruit 100%, Codonopsis ovata herba 80%, Cuminum cyminum sem 100%, Curcuma longa rhiz 70-100%, Daucus carota sem 40-100%, Embelia ribes bacc 100%, Ensete supebum sem 100%, Ferula yaeschkeana herba 100%, Hibiscus rosa-sinensis flos et herba 100%, Hyptis suaveolens 100%, Hyptis suaveolens fol, 100%, Juniperus communis sem 60%, Lepidium inermis herba 100%, Lygodium flexuosum herba 70-100%, Mentha arvensis Fol 100%, Ocimum sanctum fol 80%, Plumbago zeylandica rad et fruct 100%, Polygonum hydropiper rad to 80%, Pueraria tuberosa tub 100%, Punica granatum herba 75%, Randia dumetorum sem 100%, Rubus ellipticus herba 60-100%, Tabernaemontana heyneana rad 100%, Vitex negundo sem 100%, Sida cordifolia herba 85% [276].

Herbal Medicine - Keys

Uterine tonic prescription
Px   Avena
        Chamaelirium
        Dioscorea

Obstetrics
Foetal
Foetal abnormalities arise from:
- genetic predispositions
- faulty implantation of the ovum
- placental disease
- faulty hormonal balance
- dietary deficiency
- insufficient maternal blood supply
- foetal encumbrance [toxicity] from hepatic/renal/endocrine deficiency
- radiation damage e.g. ultrasound
- injury, falls.

Abortion spontaneous
A very distressing condition for both parents. Sometimes it is the bodies way of rejecting an unviable foetus. It occurs up to 20 weeks gestation. Bleeding or cramps should raise suspicion. Or the passing of the foetus may occur.
Intra uterine pollution is causing major changes in the whole of humanity. Oestrogen mimickers are the most dangerous substances to affect the tissues. Lowered sperm count and hypospadius are found in boys subject to intra uterine pollution from oestrogens.
Treatment
Rest the patient.
Antispasmodic tincture, Chamaelirium, Mitchella, Viburnum opulus, Viburnum prunifoleum.

Miscarriage
One quarter to one third of all pregnancies end in miscarriage. The symptoms are vaginal bleeding, sometimes uterine cramps. Examination reveals an open cervix, through which the uterus will clear the contents. Foetal death may be anticipated if high fever, eclampsia, or nephritis occur.
Make several checks on the patient e.g. thyroid.

Signs and symptoms of foetal death
1. Cessation of foetal movements
2. Sudden cessation of toxic symptoms in the first trimester.

Obstetrics and Gynaecology

3. The development of toxic symptoms in the later months.
4. Absence of foetal heart sounds.
5. The cessation of uterine growth. The uterus may become smaller and firmer. Cessation of breast growth. Loss of weight.

Medicine

Chamaelirium luteum [large doses] reinforced with Myrica [positive astringent tonic] or Viburnum prunifoleum for threatened miscarriage, corpus luteal insufficiency - bleeding or spotting.

An habitual loss within 9 weeks or so suggests a lack of hormonal effect from the corpus luteum – Vitex Sig 5ml BD in luteal insufficiency.

Ultrasound

Ultrasound exposure varies from one machine to another. Physiotherapists handling ultrasound equipment are more at risk of spontaneous abortion. Could it be that an abnormal set of sound waves disturbs the natural equilibrium within the uterus? The scan utilises around 3.5 to 5 megahertz as electromagnetic radiation to create sound waves while this is considered no more than a mobile telephone, it is to the sound waves produced that we must pay our attention.

The developers of ultrasound advised against its use in early pregnancy, under three months. This advice has been ignored.

Wide variations occur in detection rates using ultrasound for foetal abnormalities. Variations are due to the experience of the operator or old equipment.

It is also possible for a mistaken diagnosis to be made of abnormalities which dont exist. When abnormalities are diagnosed it takes an average of seven scans. Even so the diagnosis using scans was at best only 1 in 4.

Growth retarded babies were often wrongly diagnosed. Having an average of 4.7 scans, only 28 out of 72 severly retarded babies were detected before birth.

Caesarean section was performed more routinely often the result of medical intervention because of suspected foetal distress and was not related to rupture of membranes or premature labour.

The emotional impact upon a mother awaiting test results can affect her response to love her baby in case she may have to part with it. Minor foetal abnormalities can have serious implications for the family.

Ultrasound exposure can affect foetal germ cells, however it may not become apparent until some years after exposure. Currently more cases of ovarian cysts and carcinoma are seen. With behavioural changes, changes in reflexes, IQ and attention deficit disorders becoming more prevalent. Are these conditions related to ultrasound exposure?

Stark in 1984 found more evidence of dyslexia in ultrasound exposed children. Another study in Calgary in 1993 evidenced children with speech problems were twice as likely to have received ultrasound exposure. Present day ultrasound uses small levels of energy that would appear to be safe, there may be safety threshold

Herbal Medicine - Keys

levels possibly different for different tissues [Donald 1979]. Machines used today are more powerful and each scan appears to last longer. Foetal tissue grows at different rates during development.

When a woman is scanned her babies and her own ovaries and lifetime supply of eggs are also scanned.

Placenta praevia
A condition when the placenta is low in the uterus and may be obstructing the Os. The uterus stretches during pregnancy with consequent movement of the placenta. Placenta praevia may not occur as time moves towards delivery.

In vitro fertilisation IVF
Australian research argues that babies conceived by IVF methods are twice as likely to have birth defects e.g. cleft palate or heart problems [180].

Vitamins in pregnancy
Premature babies are often vitamin A deficient.
Vitamin A synthesizes corticosteroids and testerone, used for undescended testes
Vitamin B2 - Riboflavin deficiency causes hepatic disturbance, enzyme changes and toxin build up in the foetus.

Indications of pregnancy
Check the temperature orally in the morning a sustained rise may indicate pregnancy.
Blood testing of hormonal levels reflects pregnancy.
Amenorrhoea
Estimate the length of pregnancy as 280 days from the date of the last period.
Gums may bleed and become spongy.
Nausea often occurs with vomiting. This occurs from increase in plasma levels of oestrogen. After 3 months, nausea should stop. Check for toxaemia or a psychological cause if nausea persists. Heartburn and acidity may be troublesome. Small meals should be advised with nourishing drinks.
Nausea of pregnancy is due to a higher level of circulating oestrogens during the first three months.
Treatment
Ballota, Chamomilla, Cetraria, Chamaemelum, Cinnamon, Filipendula, Foeniculum, Rubus, Zingiber.
Frequent micturition in the initial stages.
Appetite increases for certain foods. Bodily requirement for specific elements results in a sort of craving for that food which provides the necessary element.
Intestinal constipation may occur from progesterone increase. Later in pregnancy it is due to the foetal position.

Obstetrics and Gynaecology

Tiredness can occur from anaemia and a higher metabolic rate.

<u>Anaemia treatment</u> - green leafy vegetables and vitamin A.

Dyspnoea often occurs when the foetus presses upon the diaphragm. Anaemia can cause dyspnoea

Breasts enlarge in preparation for breast feeding. Tenderness may occur. Veins are seen on the skin this is due to an increased blood supply. The nipples enlarge and the areola darken. From 29 weeks colostrum may leek from the breasts. Leakage is natural and is produced before the milk.

Breast pain

<u>Treatment</u>

Calendula, Chamomilla, Oenothera, Symphytum. Cabbage poultice.

Softening of the cervix and vagina from the 8th week plus.

Change in the form of the uterus to a pear shape. Increase in size and shape of the uterine walls. The pregnant uterus is soft and spongy. The uterus positions itself into anteflexion onto the bladder.

Skin can become greasy due to hormonal changes. A dark line on the skin is sometimes seen down the linea alba. It occurs from separation of the linea alba.

Backache is common due to stretched ligaments.

<u>Treatment</u>

Massage, Cimicifuga, Piscidia, Viburnum opulus.

Contractions may be sporadic and isolated during pregnancy. Real labour provides more regular contractions.

Vaginal discharge – some is normal also check for infection and perform a urinary test.

Development of the uterus during pregnancy

12 weeks - above the symphysis pubis, along with foetal heart monitoring.

16 weeks - half way between symphysis and umbilicus.

20 weeks - 2 cm below the umbilicus

24 weeks - at the level of the umbilicus

28 weeks - 3 cm above the umbilicus

32 weeks - half way between the umbilicus and the xiphisternum

36 weeks - at the level of the xiphisternum

40 weeks - foetus drops into the pelvis at around 14 days before term.

Stress can restrict the growth of the foetus in the uterus.

Second trimester

Quickening from the 16th week. Intermittent uterine contractions from the 10th week onwards. These may be present irrespective of the life or death of the foetus. Softening of the pelvic tissues can give rise to joint and pelvic ache.

Active foetal movements from the 12th week plus.

Ability to palpate the foetal body from 20 weeks onwards.

Herbal Medicine - Keys

Auscultation of foetal heart sounds from 12 weeks.

Third trimester

Uterine contractions become more noticeable and foetal movements are easily felt. Long and powerful contractions completely dilate the cervix. Cerebral symptoms can occur such as nausea, vomiting or shaking. Mental symptoms include irritability and/or anger.

In normal circumstances the foetal position by the end of this trimester is as during labour. Perform regular foetal heart monitoring.

Thyroid

Hypothyroid conditions of the foetus could create changes in the cerebral cortex and lead to defective myelination.

Uterus and Rubus

Rubus tea is often indicated for the last trimester of pregnancy. However Rubus will increase the tonicity and trophicity of the plain muscle fibres of the uterus and is consequently contra indicated in athletic [sthenic] conditions. The use of Rubus could increase the pain of childbirth or contribute to the dangers of precipitate labour in the athletic.

Lightening occurs when the foetus drops into the pelvis.
Lightening is absent in
- Contracted pelvis
- Large foetus
- Twin pregnancy
- Occipito posterior foetal position [OP, Baby faces the mothers back].
- Placenta praevia

Foetal position

Encourage foetal positioning by leaning forward and sit upright or lie on the left side with a cushion between the knees. Malposition of the foetus as in breach or posterior then crawling for 20 minutes a day encourages the foetus to turn. Sit and face the back of a chair and lean forward is also helpful.

Pre eclampsia

Insufficient placental blood flow with consequent hypertension, fluid retention, and albuminuria [nephritis]. Left untreated its very dangerous for mother and foetus.

Treatment
Sitz bath. Rest with the legs elevated.

Obstetrics and Gynaecology

<u>Medicines</u> – pre eclampsia
Cimicifuga, Helleborus niger, Leonurus, Veratrum album/viride, Zanthoxylum.
Diuretics – Agrimonia, Apium, Hydrangea, Parietaria, Uva ursi, Zea.

Pregnancy
Delivery stages of labour
1st stage
Oxytocin makes the uterus contract. Oxytocin is released as the vagina distends and the perineum stretches. The vagina and external genitals swell. Monitor the foetal heart.
The first stage is complete once the cervix is fully dilated. The cervix will gradually dilate to around 10 cm. Timing varies with each individual mother. Labour can be accompanied by worry and fear. Foetal distress can be minimised by movement and upright positioning. The mother is often aware that something is wrong long before anyone else is - encourage her to say how she feels. Meconium is the babies first bowel movement and varies in colour, seen when the waters break. Meconium before 40 weeks requires investigation. After 40 weeks there is unlikely to be a difficulty in an otherwise normal pregnancy.

2nd stage
The discharge of the liquor amine [breaking of the waters] indicates the start of labour it may occur at any stage. Foetal bradycardia may occur and is acceptable in the late second stage of labour for up to three hours.
The contractions become expulsive in character. Breathing should be slow and light. Pain becomes almost continuous. Braxton hicks contractions [usually painless and occur from 16 weeks] occur for up to a few hours at a time and indicate that labour has begun. These contractions indicate the uterus is contracting and become more powerful as labour unfolds. Contractions become more intense and regular. It is important the woman follows her body's needs and adopts the position that she feels is most comfortable. She may wish to adopt the kneeling or standing positions.

Pain killers
Birth pool eases pain along with massage and hot compresses together with correct positioning. Transient numbness may occur in the extremities.
After a while there is what is known as the 'rest and be thankful stage' it is a rest period for the body before the final stage. The second stage may last several hours. After five hours in the second stage it is unlikely the delivery is going to be spontaneous. It will be necessary to stimulate the uterus after two hours in the second stage. Empty the bladder as required.
Foetal rotation, into the OA [occipito anterior] position, occurs as it passes through the pelvis. As the foetus moves along the pelvic floor muscles have to dilate and the contractions are strong and mild. Atony of the pelvic floor muscles

reduces the efficiency of the uterine contractions. As does an epiosotomy. Cord prolapse is unlikely if quickening has occurred. Check the foetal heartbeat for signs of distress. No distress indicates adequate oxygen to the foetus.
Bearing down pains are of shorter duration and further apart. During crowning the fontanel's are watched - anterior four sutures and posterior three sutures. Pain may be felt as a ring of fire around the vagina.
The position of the mother affects the birth process. Mothers position for birthing should be encouraging gravity - so standing, squatting on a stool, kneeling, on hands and knees are all suitable positions. These positions encourage a shorter and pain-freer time. They also increase pelvic diameter by up to 2cm. Debility and tiredness lie the mother on her left side. This is suitable for delivery too. Mothers fear can be helped with Rescue remedy.

Delivery
Crowning is the showing of the foetal head at the vulva. Wait and observe the position of the foetal head. Guard the perineum with one hand and prevent the head from too rapid a descent. Restitution and external rotation of the head now occurs. Hold and lift the foetal head with the other hand. Hold the head, the baby will rotate to one side then lift the baby out by its shoulders. Where the cord is found around the babies neck it may be possible to slacken it and allow the shoulders to pass through. If the cord is very tight it will be necessary to clamp and cut the cord before delivery. Bathing in Calendula infusion is soothing and emollient to the skin of baby and mother.
Second and multiparous labours are usually faster then the first.

3rd stage - expulsion of the placenta. The placenta carries blood to the baby after the birth, it may be advantageous to the baby to keep the cord unclamped especially if the baby is premature or appears anoxic. African Bantu women do not cut the cord until after the birth of the placenta. In Britain it is usual to clamp the cord in two places at 4cm from the baby. However the cord should not be clamped until one minute after birth as the babies iron stores will be depleted. When the cord is clamped and cut too soon it interferes with placental separation and encourages blood clots to form and increases the risk of infection.
The third stage lasts from 5-15 minutes up to a maximum of 90 minutes [Cronk & Flint 1989]. Hasty expulsion of the placenta or traction on the cord could give rise to uterine inversion. It is suggested that before applying traction to the cord is to wait until the cord has lengthened and fresh blood has been seen - this will indicate the placenta has separated from the uterine wall. Excessive traction can cause pain, tear the placenta or cause involution. There is no urgency and quiet peaceful surrounds will enable the mother to deliver her placenta naturally. Natural oxytocin enables the uterus to contract and is produced in a quiet atmosphere, encouraging the baby to suck is also beneficial [62, 84].

Obstetrics and Gynaecology

Treatment during labour

Pre natal care

Caulophyllum during the last month of pregnancy [188], as required to allay rigidity of the Os. Sig 1ml every half hour or PRN.

Hypertension

Treat the cause.

Malpresentation

Baby is not in the correct position for descent. Manual movement of the foetus is possible.

Medicine

Pulsatilla.

Uterus

Hypertonic labour

Caulophyllum as required to allay rigidity of the Os.

Sig 1ml every half hour or PRN.

Medicine

Cimicifuga, Lobelia, Piscidia, Tanacetum parthenium, Viburnum prunifoleum in uterine contractions and uterine irritability.

Hypotonic labour

Weakness or pain – LE Pulsatilla. Sig 1ml every 15-30mins [188].

Medicine

Composition essence, Hydrastis, Rubus, Viscum.

Parturition slow with backache

Medicine

Cimicifuga, Commiphora, Hypericum, Turnera.

Labour pain/Emotional stress

Medicine

Cimicifuga, Lobelia, Piscidia, Ruta, Scutellaria, Viburnum prunifoleum, Viburnum opulus.

After pains

Colicky and gripy pain can affect the uterus following childbirth. Restlessness.

Medicine

Chamaelirium, Mitchella, Piscidia, Viscum.

External application of a compress to the lower abdomen and feet supports relief from pain. Compress - Artemesia, Szygium, Lavandula, Chamomilla.

Post partum - immediate

Two conditions that may arise [1] retained placenta

[2] post partum haemorrhage-more than 1000ml.

The retained placenta must be expelled and post partum haemorrhage stopped.

Herbal Medicine - Keys

Retained placenta
Alstonia boonei, Angelica archangelica, Composition essence.
If the medicines fail to expel the placenta then it must be removed manually and will require an anaesthetic.
Check the haemoglobin levels rather than estimating the level of blood loss which are frequently inaccurate.

Antihaemorrhagic medicines
Chamaelirium luteum, Cimicifuga, Composition essence, Erigeron canadense, Geranium maculatum, Myrica, Viscum, Zingiber.

Post natal care
Involution of the uterus following delivery

Day   1 - 11 cm height above the pubis
           2 - 11
           3 - 11
           4 - 10
           5 - 9
           6 - 8
           7 - 7.5

Uterine involution and recovery depends upon careful management.
Normal involution following childbirth is dependent upon the restoration of full local function and tone. Where this is never recovered, then passive hyperaemia develops. Fibroid induration is due to a gradual increase in the connective tissue around the blood vessels and is one of the most important effects of passive hyperaemia.
Use tonic astringent medicines: Aletris, Chamaelirium, Hydrastis, Mitchella.

Breast feeding and Lactation disorders
Ergometrine used to contract the uterus post partum can be antigalactogogue. Breastfeeding for more than four months provides long term protection against haemophyllus influenzae infections, otitis media and diarrhoea [196].
Dairy produce often produces signs of allergy and intolerance to the protein in the milk. Cows milk also has too much fat. Breast fed babies may also show signs of dairy intolerance if their mother drinks cows milk. Breast feeding is considered the best way to start feeding a baby. Immunity is stimulated from the mothers milk, this is particularly important because babies have very poor immune resistance in the early months. Colostrum is the first breast secretion which contains lactobacillus bifidus bacteria. The bacteria colonises the baby's intestine. Colostrum aids digestion and helps to support the manufacture of the vitamins, minerals and enzymes within the intestine. Breast fed babies have increased levels of Bifidobacterium bifidus which helps in the formation of vitamins B 1, 6 & 12.

Obstetrics and Gynaecology

Milk is produced within 2/4 days. Excessive congestion can be controlled with small frequent doses of Tr Pulsatilla or Nat sulph 3x.

Sore or fissured nipples
Apply: Althea ung, Calendula crem, Plantago herba, Stellaria. Vitamin C.

Insufficient breast milk
Stimulus to breast feeding occurs from the sucking action upon the breast. Prolactin from the pituitary is thus stimulated this produces milk.
Treatment
Galactogogue [to increase breast milk].
Anethum, Atriplex nummularia, Atriplex vessicaria, Borago, Carum, Centaurium, Cnicus, Foeniculum, Galega, Humulus, Medicago, Ocimum basilicum/sanctum, Pilocarpus, Pimpinella sp., Ruta, Trigonella, Tribulus terrestria, Urtica, Verbena, Vitex.
Apricots, barley water to drink, carrots, green leafy vegetables, watercress, peas, pecans and soya beans.
Antigalactagogue - milk depressor – Digitalis, Petroselinum, Rosmarinus, Salvia.
Prolactin depressor – Rosmarinus. Salvia.

Mastitis
Swelling and tenderness of the breast and sometimes a discharge occur with [early] pregnancy. Mastitis may sometimes accompany tumour growth.
Treatment
Aloe, Baptisia, Calendula, Chamomilla, Echinacea, Iris, Oenothera, Phytolacca, Symphytum, Thymus, Trifolium, Vitex.
External treatment
Alternating hot/cold compresses of Ulmus fulva/Seneco jacobea. Calendula crem.
External poultice
Althea, Hamamelis, Linum usit., Plantago, Ricinus communis, Symphytum, Stellaria or Ulmus powder.

Unguentum Uvedalia - ointment of bearsfoot root
LE Polymnia uvedalia   5ml
Paraffin molle   60g
Melt and mix together.
Apply in mastitis. Enlarged glands. Spinal soreness.
Caution - Discontinue use once the inflammatory process has cleared - it's continued use will stop milk production.

Basic principles in the aetiology of pelvic disorders
Physiomedicalism considers that wrong living habits lead to functional imbalance. Functional imbalance is at the root of all pathological conditions. Diagnosis

depends upon tracing the aetiology of the pathological condition as pathological physiology eventually becomes organic pathology.

Review the following aspects to determine the course of treatment.
1. Biochemical - relating to deficiency of cellular elements e.g. trace elements, vitamins and minerals or toxicity. Tissue salts calcium or potassium.
2. Physiological - balance of the circulatory and nervous supply.
3. Hormonal - adjust the hormone levels
4. Structural - pelvic and lumbar spine
5. Psychological - psychosomatic problems.

Biochemical
Disturbances of menstruation and discharges reflect the blood condition. The mucous membrane of the genital tract may act as a discharge shute for the excretion of catarrhal and toxic materials from the blood. Vaginal discharge is known as leucorrhoea. It is important to exclude malignant change when leucorrhoea is found. Many vaginal leucorrhoeas are due to infection by Candida or Trichomonas.
Electrolyte disturbance involving sodium chloride may give rise to a serous discharge. Lack of potassium chloride gives a viscous discharge. Both disturbances are the direct result blood changes.
Vaginal discharge may be from a toxic focus and the aim of treatment is to the cause of that toxicity. It is not considered good therapy to allow the vagina to eliminate waste. However if the discharge is secondary to an inflammatory condition e.g. endometriosis the discharge may be encouraged. It is important not to suppress the elimination of local toxic material which is secondary to an original suppression e.g. from the use of antibiotics, anti fungals etc.
Uterine haemorrhage can occur from anaemia and electrolyte disturbances. Also muscular laxity, ligamentous fixation of the uterus or fibroid changes.

Physiological
Pelvic drainage is dependent upon venous return. There are no valves in the vena cavae, muscular action and breathing support the return of blood. Tight clothes and shallow breathing inhibit the aspirating action of the thorax in its action upon the venous return. The pelvis is a location for dependent oedema: in males the scrotum and females the labia, can become congested.

Pelvic nerve supply is dual from the sympathetic and parasympathetic divisions. They have opposing actions.
Sympathetic supply is from L 2,3,4. They activate the sphincters and lower circular fibres of the uterus. Sympathetic effects are **vasoconstriction**.

Obstetrics and Gynaecology

Parasympathetic supply is from S 2,3,4. They are motor to the longitudinal expulsive fibres of the uterus and inhibitory to the circular fibres e.g. uterine colic in the presence of local sympatheticotonia. Parasympathetic effects are **vasodilation**.

Long term uterine trophic changes depend upon ANS balance as it affects the local blood supply to the uterus. Long continued stress during puberty may adversely effect uterine development and the uterine circulation. Developmental anomalies can occur; usually anteflexion.
In health the uterus is in a normal anteverted position.

Hormonal

Levels of the hormone oestrogen and progesterone fluctuate throughout the fertility cycle. Oestrogen at ovulation time and progesterone during the pre menstrual phase of the fertility cycle. A reduction in the levels of either hormone will create in the simple case inability to ovulate. Oestrogen reduction affects the whole body. Progesterone reduction encourages pre menstrual syndrome.

Structural

Structural disturbances can affect the dorso-lumbar spine and pelvis, it can lead to uterine and ovarian pathology. Any structural condition affecting the apex of the lumbar curve may affect the uterus. Lumbar sacral strain, lordosis and sacro iliac lesions encourage pelvic disorders. High heeled shoes also cause pelvic tilt.
Visceroptosis is common and is affected by restriction from corsets and tight clothing. Breathing becomes inhibited and eventually results in the loss of connective tissue tone.
The asthenic type produces asthenic intra - abdominal visceroptosis.
Pyknic types with a gross accumulation of fat produce ptosis and lumbar lordosis.
Pelvic floor muscular integrity, especially of the levator ani muscles are responsible for supporting the uterus.
Uterine ligaments give little uterine support [6].

Psychological

Fears and stress activate the sympathetic nerve that increases the activity of the sphincters including the lower circular fibres of the uterus - resulting in functional dysmenorrhoea [spasm].

Clinical approach - aetiology

1. Check the composition of the blood e.g. anaemia.
2. Pelvic drainage/mechanics - observation of the pelvis and lumbar spine.
3. Sphincter tone can indicate the ANS effects as a gauge of the para/sympathetic balance.

Herbal Medicine - Keys

4. Visceroptosis [also respiratory mechanics]. The uterus is in health found in an anteverted position [that is slightly tipped forward].
5. Pelvic floor integrity

Gynaecological conditions

Gynaecological conditions causing backache
Aetiology
Pregnancy,
Renal disturbance, Cystitis,
Endometriosis, Uterine malposition, Pelvic tumours.

Breast underdevelopment
Treat as [1] Hormone deficiency [2] Nerve deficiency [3] Diet.
Anethum, Avena, Borago, Carbenia, Foeniculum, Galega, Glycyrrhiza, Panax, Smilax, Oenothera, Serenoa, Pueraria mirifica [kudzu vine], Trigonella, Vitex.

Gynaecomastia – breast enlargement.
Associated with liver disturbances and the inability to clear toxins. Testicular tumours and drugs including Cannabis use.
Medicines
Centella, Rosmarinus, Serenoa, Smilax, Taraxacum, Trifolium, Vitex, plus liver medication.

Cervical dysplasia/cervicitis/erosion/cervical polyp
A cervix that bleeds upon palpation or after intercourse should be suspected of malignant change. The typical cervical smear is diagnostic of changes to the cervix.
Treatment
Local douche of Aloe, Althea, Calendula, Chamomilla, Oleum Melaleuca, Propolis, Salvia, Tabebuia, Thymus or Ulmus. Live yoghurt injection.
Douche
Lie down and administer 30ml of medicament via the douche. Retain for up to 10 minutes. Dose usually BD or PRN.
Tampon
Soak tampon and insert immediately. Or use a pessary.
Use the above medicaments for the pessary and tampon. [See also vaginitis].
Diet
Short fruit or vegetable fast. Fresh juices of carrot, cucumber. Zinc.

Obstetrics and Gynaecology

Endometriosis
Endometrial tissue can grow in the abdomen and pelvic cavity. It is subject to the hormonal changes of the fertility cycle. Endometriosis can create chronic pain.
<u>Treatment</u>
Rebalancing of the hormones. Blood vasotonics to clear residual impurities.
<u>Medicine</u> – Arctium, Astragalus, Boswellia, Chamaelirium luteum, Crataegus, Curcumin. Sig 3/500mg and Bromelain enzyme both allay inflammation in the uterus. Echinacea, Frankincense Sig 400mg, Hydrastis, Pulsatilla, Taraxacum, Verbena, Viburnum prunifoleum, Zingiber.

Inflammatory disease of the vagina, uterus, fallopian tubes and ovaries.
Enlarged mass may be palpated within the pelvis. Vaginal discharge. Severe pain is noted upon moving the cervix when inflammation is present.
Vaginitis, endometritis, salpingitis, oophoritis are all treated constitutionally.
<u>Medicine</u>
Achillea, Alchemilla vulgaris, Allium, Althea, Baptisia, Chamaelirium, Commiphora, Echinacea, Gelsemium, Humulus, Hydrastis, Krameria, Pulsatilla, Rubus, Turnera, Viburnum opulus, Vitex, Zea.

Fibrocystic breast disease
Cysts are often palpable in breast tissue. Hormonal levels affect the breast creating an aggravation at ovulation.
Aetiology includes factors like the material of the bra. Wearing a bra which is badly designed and often ill fitting can obstruct the venous drainage from the breast. Breasts drain into the axillary lymph nodes. Some women with a fuller breast wear bras that are too small. Compression of the breast tissue and nipples lead to a build up of toxins. Women living in non bra wearing areas are less prone to breast lumps than those wearing bras.
<u>Medicine</u>
Calendula, Iris, Phytolacca, Scrophularia.

Hormonal disturbances
Oestrogenic excess is associated with breast tumours. Thyrotrophic hormone - oxytocin plays a part in insufficiency of progesterone. Oxytocin inhibits oestrogen and progesterone. The neuro hormonal axis via the ANS is affected by thyroid and gonadotrophic hormones.
Breast massage and nipple stimulation activate neuro hormonal reflexes - oxytocin has a particular role in preventing breast cancer. Inverted nipples predispose to the development of carcinoma of the breast. By using a niplette [it produces a sucking action] inverted nipples can be made more responsive.
<u>Treatment</u>
Oestrogen precursors - Soya, Trifolium, Smilax, Dioscorea.

Herbal Medicine - Keys

Hormonal disturbance medicine
Progestogenic – Vitex.
Hepatic deobstruents. Blood vasotonics – Arctium, Phytolacca
External
Hamamelis compress.
Naturopathic treatment
Avoidance of caffeine.
Liver foods support detoxing and include – beetroot, carrots, lemons, watercress.
Oils from Linum, Oenothera, Blackcurrant are hormonally and neuro supportive.

Fibroids

Fibroids within the uterus are common. Sub mucus fibroids give rise to irregular bleeding. The uterus appears to be acting as a sort of waste collection point for toxins. A fibroid may in fact occur following an abortion. Treatment is dependent upon the type of fibroid. Only the sub mucous varieties will have to be eliminated via the vagina. The other types - interstitial, and subserous must be reabsorbed into the blood.

Fibroid treatment
For fibroids general systemic detoxification is required.
Capsella, Trillium – fibroids with uterine haemorrhage.
Conium maculatum in small doses
Fraxinus americanus – uterine fibroids
Chimaphilla umbellata, Phytolacca, Scrophularia – mammary.
Juniperus sabina small doses only of this powerful emmenagogue
Famous prescription is Iris/Rubus/Chelone/Smilax for sub mucous type fibroids

Haemorrhage vaginal - pre puberty

Vaginal trauma/foreign body, Precocious bleeding.
Leukaemia, Purpura.

Haemorrhage - vaginal

Hormonal, HRT., Menopause.
Uterus as a cause of haemorrhage
Abortion, Ectopic pregnancy.
Endometrial – clotting problems, pelvic inflammatory disease – endometriosis.
Neoplasms
Cervix as a cause of haemorrhage
Carcinoma. Erosion. Polyp
Vagina as a cause of haemorrhage
Carcinoma. Foreign body. Trauma. Vaginitis.
Fresh bleeding, a boggy uterus and an open cervix are seen in an incomplete abortion.

Obstetrics and Gynaecology

Menstrual disturbances

Amenorrhoea

The first question to ask - is the patient pregnant?
Secondly have there been periods in the past. Stress, shock and anorexia may be found. Ovarian failure, hypothalamic and pituitary disorders could account for amenorrhoea.
Is the patient menopausal? Have they been taking HRT? Absence of periods increases the chances of uterine carcinoma.

Medicine

Aletris, Glycyrrhiza induces ovulation, Chamaelirium luteum.

Dysmenorrhoea

Aetiology

- Physiological causes - ANS imbalance
- Endocrine imbalance - which may arise from endocrine or psychological imbalance.
- Psychological disturbance affecting the ANS.
- Structural disturbance - lumbar sacral problems that may only be apparent during menstruation because this is the time of physiological activity. Palpate the spine to reveal the local segmental sensitivity.
- Local structural pathology - fibroids, prolapse, uterine displacements, ligamentous contraction. IUD's. Stress. Uterine pain referred to the back is diffused - it cannot be localised and deep pressure does not increase it.

With uterine pain - two types exist:
1. Congestive premenstrual pain which is up to 10 days before the onset of menses and is hypogastric, dull and constant.
   Aetiology of congestive pain - prolapse, retroversion, fibroids, cysts, salpingitis, infections all produce localised oedema and congestion.
2. Colic spasmodic pain results from some obstruction to the flow. Any accumulation of blood in the uterine cavity will clot. Large clots will be accompanied by severe pain and possible shock [fainting, clammy skin etc]. Aetiology of spasmodic pain include uterine malposition, adhesions, contractures of the supporting ligaments, small Os cervix.

Excessive sympatheticotonia causes undue contraction of the circular retaining sphincter fibres at the cervix, this results in colic. The vagina and anal sphincters may also be affected.

Treatment

Relax the sphincters - Caulophyllum, Cimicifuga, Pulsatilla, Valeriana, Viburnum opulus.
The exact choice depends upon the patient

343

Herbal Medicine - Keys

[a] ANS imbalance secondary to anxiety suggests Pulsatilla reinforced by Scutellaria

[b] Sympatheticotonia second to asthenia suggests Caulophyllum with Viburnum and Zingiber

[c] Excessive tension associated with hypersthenia requires lobelia

[d] Increased fibrous tissue within the uterus - fibroids/endometriosis require the long term use of Cimicifuga.

Magnesium can be used as an antispasmodic.

Essential fatty acids - PG2's. Up to 3000mg Ol Oenothera daily.

Animal products create arachadonic acid so reduce meat. It is better to eat a vegetable, fruit and a grain diet to rebalance. Eat fish, salmon, cod, mackerel or fish oils as these make PG2 & PG3.

Other causes of pain include:
Polyps uterine/vaginal - Sanguinaria
Pregnancy – including ectopic gestation
Salpingitis
Ovarian tumours - haemorrhage, rupture, torsion

Elixir Viburnum prunifolium
Used as a uterine sedative in dysmenorrhoea and ovaritis.
Px   LE Viburnum prun.   20ml
        Tr Pulsatilla   20ml
Sig 35gtt hourly.

Infertility
Make checks upon the patient after 12 months of regular intercourse.
Check the male for a sperm count first. Females must have the hormone levels checked. Ensure the fallopian tubes are clear of infection, obstruction or stricture.
Ingested fluoride in toothpaste and water can damage the ability of sperm to swim properly. Fluoride is accumulative.
Treatment
In uncomplicated cases use – Chamaelirium luteum, Aletris, Panax, Vitex.
Vitamin E.

Obstetrics and Gynaecology

The Fertility cycle

Cycle in Ovary

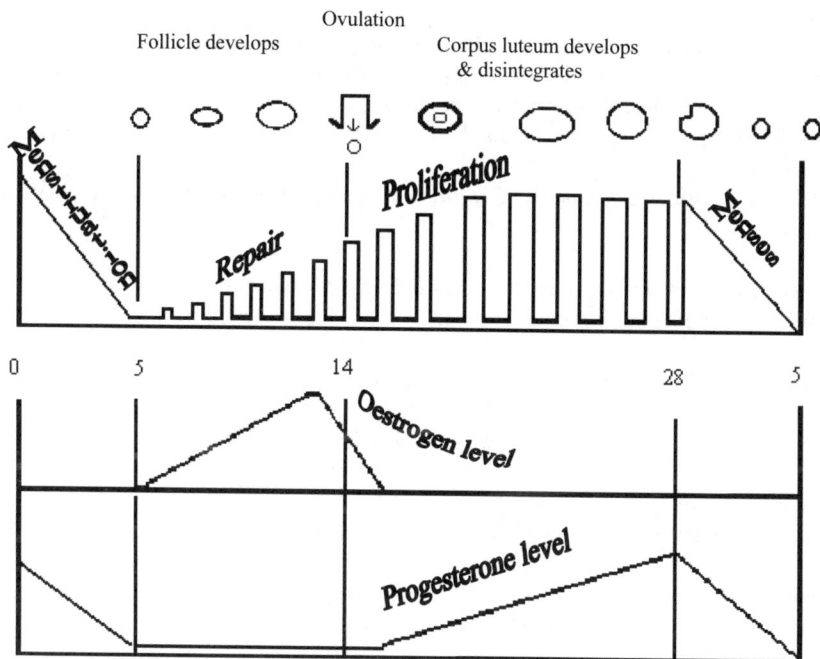

The numbers refer to the days of the cycle.
The first column across the page indicates oestrogen from the follicle.
Second column across the page the level of progesterone from the corpus luteum.
Day 14 is ovulation day with fertilisation and implantation.

Menorrhagia
Menstrual bleeding which is prolonged, excessive or irregular.
Many causes are attributed to this condition and treatment is directed to the cause.
Hormonal reduction at the menopause, fibroids. Chart the bleeding, pain and flow in the diagnosis.
Treatment
Haemorrhage – Achillea, Alchemilla vulgaris, Capsella, Cimicifuga, Composition essence, Geranium maculatum, Myrica, Rubus idaeus, Trillium, Vitex.
Prescription
To raise the tone of the musculature of the uterus, sustain the uterine circulation and promote a healthy menstrual cycle. LE Artemesia vulgaris Sig 5ml TDS.

Herbal Medicine - Keys

Uterine haemorrhage prescription [After Dr. Sarah Webb. USA].
Trillium 30g. Geranium maculatum 30g. Composition essence 30g. Myrica 30g.
Capsicum 4g. Sig 3g.

Metrorrhagia
Uterine bleeding that occurs outside of the normal menstrual period.
Aetiology includes carcinoma, endometriosis, fibroids, hormonal disturbances,
IUD's, polyps, polycystic ovaries – more hair growth due to increased androgens,
raised LH. Specific treatment must be followed and depends upon the cause.
Treatment
Alchemilla vulgaris, Capsella, Geranium maculatum, Hydrastis, Trillium, Vinca,
Vitex.

Prescription advice for patients with pelvic disturbances
There are seven areas for consideration:

1] Hepatic/gall bladder cholagogue, choleretic.
Where hormonal disturbances are affected by biliary conditions.
Berberis species, Carbena, Chionanthus, Silybum, Taraxacum rad.

2] Uterine tonic
Uterine tonics as indicated for atonic, underfunctioning uterine endo and
myometrium.
Angelica sinensis - CI heavy bleeding, pregnancy, Chamaelirium luteum,
Cimicifuga, Mitchella, Trillium.

3] Medicines for hormonal imbalance.
Hormonal regulation natural HRT – Vitex. Given as 5ml daily for 10 days pre
menstrually.
Flushes – Salvia, Trifolium, Vitex - small doses stimulate the pituitary.
Prostaglandin balancer – Alchemilla vulgaris, Ol Oenothera.

4] Tonics. These nervines settle over anxious states.
Hypericum, Turnera, Leonurus, Salvia.

5] ANS balancer – Dioscorea

6] Adrenal support – Borago, Glycyrrhiza

7] Increase unsaturated fatty acids – Oenothera, pumpkin seeds, linseed,
sunflower seeds, sesame seeds, artichoke – hepatic and diuretic.

Obstetrics and Gynaecology

Ovaries
PMS is often associated with fatty acid deficiency. Fatty acids are required to make three kinds of prostaglandins. Prostaglandins lower blood pressure and cholesterol levels, help wound healing and repair skin damage. Prostaglandins depend for their manufacture upon gamma linoleic acid [GLA]. GLA is found in Oleum Oenothera, Oleum Borago and blackcurrants. These prostaglandin medicines help as a replacement to a hypotrophic ovarian condition.
<u>Ovary treatment</u>
Chamaelirium luteum - stimulating to the ovaries
Dioscorea - for pain in the abdomen arising from ovarian disorders
Mentha pulegium - for painful or obstructed menses, large doses in amenorrhoea, small doses in ovarian hypotrophy. Ovarian tonic, oestrogenic.
Vitex – progestogenic.
Zanthoxylum - stimulating to the vasomotor function and encourages tissue nutrition and catabolic waste removal.

Oestrogen
Menopause affects oestrogen, the most potent is oestradiol and is synthesized from cholesterol in the ovaries. Plant oestrogens bind to oestrogen receptor sites in target cells. When production of cellular oestrogen is low, dietary oestrogens, vitamins and minerals will support oestrogenic availability. Low circulating levels of oestrogen leave more receptor sites free in bodily tissues. Plant oestrogens bind with the receptor sites, exerting a mild oestrogenic activity.
Phyto oestrogens
Phytoestrogens are plant oestrogens [lignans] and are selective to certain tissues in the body. Plant oestrogens [Po's] are hydrolysed in the gut before they can be utilised. Lignans found in fibre rich food stimulate the production of SHBG in the liver and therefore reduce the levels of free oestrogen. Po's are selective receptor oestrogen modulators. They are anti progesterone compounds. Breast, heart, bone and uterus each have different receptors. After the menopause the ovaries continue to produce small amounts of testosterone which is converted to oestrodiol. The amounts produced are less than before the menopause.
<u>Sources of Phytoestrogens</u>
Are found in flaxseed, legumes such as soy, chickpeas, clover, lentils, whole grains, fruit, vegetables and beans.

Ovarian cancer - a palpable ovary is always pathological.
Becoming a more common condition. Tumours are relatively silent and changes in the fertility cycle may herald ovarian degeneration. Palpation of an enlarged ovary in a post menopausal patient could suggest a tumour. A smear test could prove the diagnosis.
[Treatment see chapter on malignancy].

Herbal Medicine - Keys

Ovarian cysts [polycystic ovarian syndrome - PCOS].
Cysts can be single or multiple, benign or malignant.
Common signs and symptoms are infertility in 75%, excess body hair in 60%, amenorrhoea in 30%, metrorrhagia in 30%.
The tendency is to produce too much androgen. Androgens cause erratic ovulation or amenorrhoea.
Aetiology includes excess

- Adrenal androgens. Androgens can be aggravated by stress when they are converted to oestrogens. LH would then increase ovarian androgen production.
- Ruth Trickey argues that dysfunctional uterine bleeding - irregular periods occur in about 90% of cases.
- ACTH can also lead to increased androgen production producing excess body hair in around 60% and Virilisation in 20% of cases.
- Liver and gall bladder disturbances, pancreatic insufficiency are also implicated. Hyperinsulinism leads to excess androgen levels.
- Hypothalamus disorder could create elevated LH and reduced FSH. Elevated LH causes the increase of androgen production in the ovaries. Reduced levels of FSH in the ovary are less able to convert the androgens back to oestrogens.
- Excess testosterone itself the result of enzyme dysregulation also elevates LH.
- Obesity is found in some 40% of cases. Excess adipose tissue provides for further conversion of androgens to oestrogens.
- Associated conditions - adrenal hyperplasia/tumours, cushings disease, hyperprolactinaemia, insulin disturbance.

Treatment is required for the constitution
[a] blood condition - Arctium, Echinacea, Iris.
[b] adrenals – Glycyrrhiza glabra
[c] nerves – Elutherococcus, Humulus [reduces LH levels], Panax.
[d] ovaries/hormonal levels - Cimicifuga, Paeonia lactiflora
    [acts upon the ovary and reduces androgens], Serenoa, Smilax.
[e] weight/blood sugar - dietary adjustment. Cynara scolymus and Galega
    officinalis - glucose tolerance. Trigonella foenum-graecum,
[f] Diet & exercise
    Avoid sugar and salt. Increase fibre. Eat small frequent meals.
    Exercise. Reduce stress.

Pain - acute lower abdominal
Appendicitis
Endometriosis

Obstetrics and Gynaecology

Fibrotic degeneration

Ectopic pregnancy/ovarian cyst – diffuse lower abdominal pain, shoulder tip pain [particularly left], Vaginal examination reveals tenderness on cervix movement. Salpingitis – unilateral abdominal pain, right sided rectal tenderness. Left sided tenderness is an indicator of fallopian tube or ovary disease. Tenderness on movement of the cervix is a more useful sign in ectopic pregnancy and salpingitis.

Pain - chronic lower abdominal
Adhesions
Endometriosis
Infections
Menstruation - see under acute pain.
Ovarian tumours
Salpingitis - chronic
Uterine fibroids – haemorrhage, rupture,
Uterine malpositions/prolapse

Pre menstrual syndrome
It is a mistake to view all cases of PMS improving with Vitex. Look at the lifestyle. Some 15% of cases have eating disorders. There may be body dysmorphia.
Four types of PMS exist to date and patients may have one or more of the types in an admixture of symptoms.
PMT A – tension of the nerves, irritability
PMT C – cravings often for sugar/chocolate
PMT D – depression, crying, confusion
PMT H – weight gain
Various symptoms can accompany PMS – migraine, panic attacks, acne, disorientation etc.
Some sufferers have homicidal or suicidal tendencies. In such cases look for raised sodium and reduced Mg and Mn.
Congestive conditions give pain as the uterus engorges with blood. The pain is dull, constant and hypogastric. It occurs no more than ten days before blood loss.
Treatment
Congestive conditions require stimulation to the uterus body with uterine tonics. Myrica, Pulsatilla, Vitex. Nervine remedies.
Reduce caffeine containing substances – chocolate, tea, coffee, alcohol.

Prolapse
Usually a surgical outcome is required here. However for the very elderly or unwell patient conservative treatment with herbal medicine may provide relief.

349

Herbal Medicine - Keys

Medicine - prolapse
Muscular and mucous membrane remedies help support tone –
Acacia, Alchemilla vulgaris, Capsicum, Equisetum, Geranium maculatum,
Myrica, Nymphaea, Polygonum bistorta, Tsuga canadensis.
Medicines containing silica, calcium, iron are helpful e.g. Anethum, Capsella,
Equisetum, Helianthus and Zea.
Galium verum - Ladies bedstraw - for retroversion and prolapse of the uterus, it
acts upon the broad ligament and combines well with Hamamelis and Aletris
Douche
Juglans sp., Nymphaea, Quercus, Rubus, Rumex, Trillium.
Pelvic floor muscle exercises.

Toxic shock syndrome
Tampons are a cause for a severe infection with Staphylococcus aureus [SA].
Death has resulted from toxic absorption into the blood from the vagina. Toxins
can be absorbed into the blood stream from a vaginal infection. Found mainly in
the 13-21 age group. Older females carry immunity against Staphylococcus
aureus. Some 9% of asymptomatic women are carriers of SA. Only 1% of these
cases produce symptoms as a result of toxins from the infection. Nearly 35% of
all women are persistent carriers of SA.
Treatment
Avoid tampons use towels instead. Inspect the vagina. Douche with Melaleuca,
Thymus [217 – 219].

Uterine carcinoma
Uterine bleeding after the menopause should raise suspicion of a malignant focus.
A mass may be detectable upon examination. [See chapter 31 Malignancy]

Vaginismus
Spasm of the vaginal muscles restricting intercourse. Associated with the fear of
sex, or the fear of pain.
Medicine
Antispasmodic Tr., Chamomilla, Caulophyllum, Lobelia, Pulsatilla, Valeriana,
Viburnum opulus/prunifloeum. Bach flower remedy – Mimulus, Rock rose.

Vaginitis and vulvovaginitis
Check for a sexually transmitted infection.
Medicines
Calendula, Chenopodium vulvaria [Arrach], Cimicifuga, Copaifera langsdorffii,
[Copaiba], Pulsatilla, Rubus, Rosmarinus, Santalum album, Thuja occidentalis,
Trillium, Vitex.

Obstetrics and Gynaecology

<u>Treatment</u> vaginitis
The following lotion can be used for thrush or vaginitis with infection. Where one preparation is unsuitable change the medicament.
<u>Lotion per vagina</u>
Low alcohol Tr Hydrastis/Calendula/Baptisia or Thuja 10ml, FE Althea 10ml. Ol Origanum/Ol Thymus/Ol Melaleuca 1gtt.
Sig 20gtt diluted in aqua 50ml. Test with a small amount first.
Apply on a tampon or use the gel/lotion/douche application.
<u>Other medicaments suitable for application.</u>
Aloe, Calendula, Chamomilla, Hydrastis, Lavandula, Melaleuca, Oenothera, Ulmus.

Candida – [see also digestive conditions]
It is possible to become infected by thrush during sex. Known as a yeast infection. Often produces intense itching of the genital or anal area and a white cheesy discharge, which smells yeasty. Swelling of the vulva, itching may be intense. Dysuria. A Low neutrophil count encourages candida proliferation [414].
<u>Treatment</u>
Alchemilla arvensis, Allium, Aloe gel, Calendula, Echinacea, Hydrastis, Lavandula, Myrica, Phytolacca, Syzygium, Tabebuia, Thuja, Thymus, Vitex, Ol Oenotherus. Vitamin A or beta carotene. Vitamin C in large doses up to 3g daily. Magnesium, selenium, zinc.
<u>External</u>
Wear cotton underclothes. Allow plenty of air to the area when this is possible.
Bathing use a saline wash - add salt to the bath water.
Cider vinegar added to the bath water, or as a douche is effective.
Yoghurt live as a douche. Avoid sugar.
Oleum to be diluted and used as douche - Ol Szygium, Eucalyptus, Melaleuca, Ocimum sanctum, Olea europaea, Origanum vulgare.

Sexually transmitted diseases
Chlamydia
A bacterial infection causes urinary burning and cervicitis. Untreated it can cause pelvic inflammatory disease. Symptoms – discharge from the vagina, penis or anus. Inflammation around the genitals. Frequency, dysuria or burning on micturition. Some cases may be asymptomatic.

Gardnerella [haemophilus vaginalis]
Abnormal vaginal odour.

Genital herpes
<u>Medicine</u> Sutherlandia frutescens

Herbal Medicine - Keys

Gonorrhoea
Dysuria may be the first symptom. Purulent discharge. Infection can spread to the bladder and vagina. Sore throat. Joints, abdomen - pain [pelvic inflammatory disease] and eyes. Anal discharge. Around 10% of gonorrhoea cases are symptomless.
<u>Medicine</u> - gonorrhoea
Acacia, Althea, Barosma, Cimicifuga, Echinacea, Equisetum, Gelsemium, Guaiacum, Hydrangea, Piper guineense, Piper methys., Smilax, Thuja, Uva ursi.
<u>External</u>
Melaleuca.
Injection to the bladder – Hydrastis 10gtt and Piper methysticum in Dist. Hamamelis to 100ml.

Hepatitis B
The virus is present in the blood and body fluids of an infected patient. It can be spread by sexual contact, blood, saliva and urine. The infection can cause liver damage. Symptoms - flu like, cough, sore throat, severe tiredness, loss of appetite and joint pain. Jaundice which can last up to 8 weeks. Weight loss may occur with jaundice.
<u>Treatment</u>
Rest and fluid.
Artemisia species, Commiphora, Glycyrrhiza uralensis, Leptandra, Lobelia, Silybum.

Herpes see under skin
Vesicles are found on the penis, vaginal labia and cervix. There may be itching in the genital area. Pyrexia, headache and backache, burning sensation during micturition. Vesicles appear 4-5 days after infection and clear within 1-2 weeks.

Pubic lice
Small lice can live in the pubic hair and are spread by close bodily contact. Severe itching in the genital area. Small nits on the pubic hair or the louse may be seen. [See dermatology].

Syphilis
Historically syphilis was found in the USA and Europe. Excavated wooden coffins found at York dated around 1300-1420 BC - this was some 70 years before Columbus set sail for the USA. It was previously thought syphilis was imported from the USA to Europe and that the American Indians were the cause of the infection. It has been proved untrue by analysis of the coffins found at York. Skeletons found within these coffins had been infected by syphilis as were the babies born from parents with syphilis. The teeth of infants showed a

Obstetrics and Gynaecology

transverse fissure of the incisor teeth some incisor teeth were completely damaged.

Syphilis is a transmittable disease and is common. Skin to skin contact is all that is required for infection to take place. The indigenous population of American Indians were all infected as children. Immunisation was provided, against the venereal form later on in life. The Spirochaete mutates towards a venereal form. As with all infections they must mutate to survive.

Various stages follow an infection by this Spirochaete organism. Initially there is a chancre [ulcer] on the penis, vagina, cervix, sometimes in the mouth or anus. Ulcers appear up to 12 weeks after contact and last up to 3 weeks. Fever, headache and sore throat can last up to 6 weeks. Rash on the hands and body, fever and arthralgia follow. In the later stages [10 years on] neurosyphillis destroys the posterior tracts of the spinal cord and brain – damage to nerve pathways produce pinpoint pupils.

Treatment

Arctium, Baptisia, Berberis vulgaris, Betula alba/pendula, Capsicum, Commiphora, Desmodium, Echinacea, Guaiacum, Iris, Juglans, Phytolacca, Piper guineense, Rhamnus purshiana, Smilax, Stillingia, Thuja, Trifolium.

Urethritis see kidney and urinary system.

Vaginal trichomonas

Yellow, frothy, purulent, smelly vaginal discharge, vulval itching, colpitis macularis [strawberry cervix], vaginal and vulvar erythema. Symptoms can appear up to three weeks after the infection. Men have few or no symptoms so they may be carriers without even knowing. Trichomonas can only survive in heat and with an acid medium.

Treatment

Allium, Chenopodium olidum [goosefoot or arrach], Hydrastis, Melaleuca, Piper methysticum, Santalum album, Thuja, Raphanus [black radish], Vitex.

Douche – Allium, Melaleuca, Propolis.

Venereal warts [condylomata]

Genital warts are sexually transmitted. The warts are cauliflower shaped and often have an irregular border appearing anywhere on the genitals or anus. It could take a year following infection before the warts appear.

Podophyllum is painted upon the warts. Protect the skin around the warts as it tends to excoriate

31
Malignancy & Oncology

Cancer is not a symptom that is treated, nor a specific disease but the reactions and functions of the entire body that have to be transformed and restored.

Max Gerson, MD. A Cancer Therapy. 1990

William Russell [1852-1940]. A pathologist at Edinburgh university identified microbes in cancer slides from tumours. Variable in shape and size, these were intracellular and extracellular. The Russell bodies [large cell wall deficient bacteria] are immunoglobulins [proteins]. Microbes mutate according to natural phenomenon. Microbes are affected by antibiotics, this also causes mutation.

Wilheim Reich [120] He discovered the T-bacilli in cancerous conditions. Later on he would also find these T-bacilli in the blood and excreta of healthy people. Reich concluded

'the disposition to cancer is therefore determined by the biological resistance of the blood and the tissues to putrefaction.'

Ernst explains: Herbal medicine use against carcinoma is high with some 34% of Australians and 75% of Americans using it [227]. Cancer patients generally report satisfaction with herbal medicine treatment.

Aetiological factors that influence the predisposition to cancer
1] Genetic mutation – unstable genes.
2] Infection.
3] Lymph stasis.
4] Toxic conditions – free radicles, radiation damage, pesticides.
5] Faulty nutrition – dietary factors.
6] Psychological impacts – emotional trauma.
7] Synthetic drugs, oestrogen hormones.
8] Cell adhesion molecules – are proteins on the surface of the cell which receive
   signals from the nucleus. CAM can create free radicles.
9] Tobacco, alcohol.
10] Ultraviolet and ionising radiation.
11] Occupational exposures.

Malignancy & Oncology

Aetiology of Cancer

Cancer is caused by a pleomorphic micro-organism. Pleomorphic means it is able to change its size and become a virus, bacteria or fungus and such an infection is always present in every case of a cancer. Aids is another form of cancer. A bacterium can change its form and be filterable, known then as a filterable form. In 1969 the **New York Academy of Sciences** published its report: 'Micro organisms of various sorts have been observed and isolated from animal and human tumours, including viruses, bacteria and fungi. There is however, one specific type of highly pleomorphic micro-organism that has been observed and isolated consistently by us from human and animal malignancies of every obtainable variety for the past 20 years...The organism has remained an unclassified mystery, due in part to its remarkable pleomorphism and its stimulation of other micro-organisms. Its various phases may resemble viruses, micrococci, diptheroids, bacilli and fungi.

Gruner argues: 'Viruses in the strict sense are mostly discredited where cancer is in question. The virus form is one phase in the life history of many if not all bacteria. The bacterial forms do not produce cancer but the virus form does. The existence of virus forms of typhoid bacillus, colon bacillus, tubercle bacillus cannot seriously be disputed'. Mr **Royal Rife** explains this phenomena in his works. The bacteria are often unobserved due to the infective organism being killed before observation under the microscope. Once killed the pleomorphic changes could not be observed. Rife proved in 1931 that a virus could cause cancer [be associated with] and that it was possible to cultivate it artificially. He stated that the cancer microbe had four forms [one form identical to mushrooms]. Rife confirmed the work of Bechamp [see Chapter 6]. Rife maintained that pig meat and mushrooms cause cancer and were a medium in which cancer liked to grow. Mr O Cameron Gruner of Canada in 1942 saw the fungus of cancer [114]. Rife explains that pathogenic organisms carry different vibratory rates and his frequency treatment machine was able to treat the patient using light rays of varying vibratory rates to knock out the pathogenic organisms and cure the disease. A scientist named Rous found the first cancer causing virus in 1911 but wasn't awarded the Nobel prize until 1966 when he was 85 years of age. Virginia Livingston Wheeler confirmed the cancer micro-organisms ability to change from a bacteria to a virus depending upon what it has been fed. Such pleomorphic changes are the cause of cancer and aids. Cantwell asserts, 'the idea of a cancer microbe is still taboo. There is little doubt that aids is a pre cancerous disease. One possible reason for the emergence of the new epidemic of aids is the widespread use of antibiotic therapy' [115/9].

Up to 60% of gastric cancers are attributable to Helicobacter pylori and infections run in families [229].

Herbal Medicine - Keys

Principal factors

The principal factors concerned in cancer are: faulty nutrition, inadequate elimination of waste products, lymph stasis/reduced immune responses. Suppression of vicarious eliminations e.g. catarrh, diarrhoea, skin rashes. Suppression of acute diseases. Environmental chemicals including those added to food and water. Toxic effects of vaccines, smoking and alcohol. Sodium chloride [common salt] is an active provoker of cancer [122].

Lowered auto immunity can be produced by toxic states within the body. Lymph stasis, spleen congestion, blood impurities and extracellular fluids create lymphangitis in the smaller lymphatic vessels that affect the epithelial cells. Chronic inflammation within these lymphatics leads to fibrosis and congestion of the tissue. Insufficient exercise combined with over nutrition [excess protein, sugar, CHO] encourage lymph congestion. Constipation provides the focus for the absorption of toxins into the blood.

Lindlair states 'whenever morbid secretions accumulate inevitably will be found the seat of chronic disease.' 'Where inflammation, fever or acute manifestations of disease are suppressed consequences result from the accumulation and storage of metabolites'. 'If every time the vital force attempts to establish a normal homeostatic balance, by the development of some form of acute disease [during which process these stored toxins might be removed], the condition is effectively suppressed, then it is not to be wondered that after a period of time a suitable environment is formed for the development of a malignant condition'.

Suppression of discharges

Suppressing the natural secretions of the skin, axilla or feet forces the secretion into the tissues to be carried around by the circulation. In this way much harm can be done and while the local suppression may be entirely successful, the constitutional manifestations are inimical to health.

Suppression of other secretions and discharges such as nasal catarrh, purulent discharges from the ears [otitis], or vagina [leucorrhoea], bladder [cystitis], intestine [diarrhoea] or skin [acne], often lead to more serious disease either immediately or at some later date. Attempts at elimination through some other channel will often be made. When the vital force is ineffective at removing the toxins those very same toxins are tolerated in some other area, often far removed from the seat of the original action - cysts arise in this way. Lipoma of the skin is another example.

Many disease states found today result from the suppression of an acute disease by arresting elimination of toxins. Cancer grows from this medium of suppressed reaction – blood impurity – cellular congestion – immune depletion – poisoned cellular environment – cancer. These stages of disease provocation are often to be found. 35% of all cancers are diet related with high fat, alcohol, smoking, alfatoxins on food, toxic products from food e.g. nitrosamines and rancid fats. Treatment is aimed at the re establishment of the initial discharge to effect a cure. Surgery sometimes has its place in the treatment of cancer as when the cancer is causing obstruction to function or elimination in the rectum, stomach, bladder, kidney or bronchus.

Genetic considerations
Genetic mutations can cause cancer to develop. Suppressor genes inactivate the cancer cells. Mutations in the suppressor genes, allow changes to occur and set up the cancer condition. The tumour suppressing gene known as gene p53 is found to be mutated in 70% of colon cancers. Individuals inherit gene deficiencies, this makes the gene defective and encourages the predisposition to develop cancer. Gene p53 is a repair gene and damage to the gene allows altered DNA to move about in the blood.

Research undertaken by Dr Kamilla Czene of the Karolinska Institute, Stockholm examined a database of 10 million people including 700,000 contracted cancer cases. They looked at environmental factors, diet, habits and links between family members.

The report was published in the International Journal of Cancer in April 2002. They found that environmental causes were the most important factors. [201]

Percentage of cancers caused by environmental [e] and genetic [g] factors:

Thyroid	[e] 47%	[g] 53%
Breast	[e] 75%	[g] 25%
Lung	[e] 92%	[g] 8%
Stomach	[e] 99%	[g] 1%
Colon	[e] 87%	[g] 13%
Rectum	[e] 88%	[g] 12%
Testes	[e] 75%	[g] 25%
Bladder	[e] 93%	[g] 7%
Kidney	[e] 93%	[g] 7%]
Melanoma	[e] 79%	[g] 20%
Leukaemia	[e] 99%	[g] 1%
Non Hodgkin lymphoma	[e] 90%	[g] 10%
Cervix	[e] 75%	[g] 25%
Endocrine	[e] 72%	[g] 28%
[Adrenal, parathyroid and pituitary].		
Nervous system	[e] 87%	[g] 13%

Herbal Medicine - Keys

The above figures are from the Swedish family cancer database. The researchers conclude that environmental and hereditary factors cause cancer. Environmental factors include diet and lifestyle. Reliable modelling of the aetiology of cancer is found when the researches linked familial relationships. Shared environmental factors are found with lung and stomach cancers.

Treatment programme

Gerson uses coffee enemas four to six times a day initially to detoxify and help relieve pain and spasm. The enemas are gradually reduced. Castor oil is given by mouth, and a castor oil enema every other day. Gerson says that frequent enemas as prescribed above, completely eliminate the need for sedation. Coffee enemas are used to stimulate the liver. During exacerbations, detoxification of the blood is required. Hepatic stimulation with a cholagogue, Peumus, Berberis, Chelidonium [all stimulant] would be required. Mentha piperita helps relieve nausea from metabolites, take freely.

A positive approach to the treatment of malignant conditions involves the use of a whole food diet. Potassium is required for cellular function and elimination of fluids and toxins. Potassium washes from the cellular environment sodium and with it, fluids containing **cellular** waste. Metabolites from the cell in cancer, poison the nearby cells so potassium must be increased to force water from the cell and tissues. The cancer patient has a tendency to increased blood clotting - this requires consideration.

Protein must be decreased as it holds water within the cell. Preferable to use almonds, rice, sunflower and pumpkin seeds as a source of protein. All the food factors within the diet require to be looked at.

Metabolites and infective processes

Reducing the level of metabolites and infection within the blood will support cancer cases.

Medicine

Baptisia, Echinacea, Origanum, Phytolacca, Usnea barbata.

World cancer research fund stated in 1997 after a review of 4000 recent scientific papers, concluded in its advice to patients, for minimally processed food and to ingest a plant based diet rich in fruits, vegetables, wholegrains and pulses. There is a reduced risk of developing cancer in vegetarians. Evidence needs to be convincing or probable when looking for nutritional aetiology of cancer.

Noticeably a low level of folic acid increases women's cervical abnormality x 5 times [197].

Meat consumption carries health risks due to contamination. Reading in the European Journal of cancer explains that there is a role for fruit in combating cancer. A 20% reduction in breast cancer is found with vitamin C, and beta carotine.

The mortality of non vegetarian and vegetarian cases [198].
Lung cancer 33%, preventable by increasing fruit and vegetables.
Colorectal cancer up to 75%, preventable by increasing fruit, vegetables and increasing exercise.
Prostate cancer up to 20%, preventable by reducing meat and fat.
Breast cancer up to 55%, preventable by increasing vegetables, reducing calories and alcohol.

Conservative treatment is preferred to the cut, burn and poison treatments the hospitals use. It will be seen by the figures [210] that some 260,000 people get cancer each year and 151,000 will die of the disease in spite of the orthodox treatments. Cancer research UK figures compiled by the UK Association of Cancer Registries for 1999 give breast cancer as 40,900 new cases a 15% rise over five years. Bowel cancer shows a similar pattern 35,600 an increase of 7%. Testicular cancer has increased to 2000 a rise of 24%.

Herbal medicine and Naturopathic regimes
Regular blood and urine tests will be carried out for the patient.
Full blood count, ESR
Serum electrolytes
Urinalysis

Diet and nutritional support
An optimum body mass index ranges from 18.5 – 25.
Avoid alcohol, salt, tobacco, limit fatty foods, avoid charred meat.
Unprocessed fresh fruit and vegetables - 800g [five portions] of pulses, grains, veg, salads, fruit daily.
Vitamin B6 combined with Inositol hexaphosphate [IP6] also known as phytic acid is a component of fibre found in legumes [peas and beans] and wholegrains. IP6 is antioxidant and antineoplastic it is found in most mammalian cells. IP6 reduces free radicle damage [200].
Daily exercise – movement for one hour a day.
Banana research
Kashivade of South Carolina university evaluated Oligomeric tannins against cancer, the major compounds from bananas, against cancer cells, that included malignant melanomas, carcinoma of the bronchus, ileocoecal adenocarcinoma, epidermal carcinoma, and medulloblastoma. Bananas were found to be effective in cancer treatment. Useful in hypertension.

Herbal Medicine - Keys

Juices for health
Gerson recommends fresh juice that should be organic.
Orange juice, Apple juice and carrot juice, Grape juice, Grapefruit juice
Green leaf juice, Tomato juice
Daily portions of each juice is 250 ml. One portion taken 12 times daily.

Avoidance of environmental toxins. Aluminium utensils. Avoid all animal products – dairy produce, meat and eggs. Forbidden - salt

Injections of liver extract, niacin, acidol pepsin, pancreatin, linseed oil. Selenium, vitamin A, C @ 3g daily and E. Co enzyme Q10. Lipoic acid. Glutathione.

As the patient improves the following are added:
Fibre, antioxidants, whole grains, fruit.
Anthracins from beetroot is used for radiation cancer.
Artichokes. Bananas.
Bioflavonoids are found in the pith of oranges etc., buckwheat spaghetti and tea.
Chlorophyll from green plants; spinach, cabbage, nettle, brassica.
Lactobacillus acidophyllus has a powerful stimulating effect upon the immune system and is helpful in the regime to combat cancer.
Anticancer foods include the cruciferous - broccoli, raw cabbage, sprouts.

Tumour medication [including benign tumours]
Remedies are carried to the site by the inclusion of a specific organ/area remedy. Medication is indicated to:

1] Neutralise and eliminate the cancer.
2] Support immune responses.
3] Support the intestinal elimination of waste
4] Give full hepatic support – bile salts are cytotoxic.
5] Detoxify the tissues and blood
6] Restore metabolic functions

At the cellular level antimitotics act by:
[1] Making cancer cells differentiate and have a more normal form and function,
[2] Prevent cancer cells from entering the cell cycle,
[3] Induce cell death through apoptosis or necrosis [170].

Malignancy & Oncology

Oncology treatments used to support the body and help resist malignancy are known as: Antimitotics

Antimitotics
Antimitotics inhibit cell division and are useful in treating cancer conditions.

Agrimonia - general tonic.
Allium [also Ransom] detergent, anti viral. Allium cepa – neuroma.
Aloe - leukaemia.
Anemarrhena asphodeloides – gastric carcinoma growth inhibition and apoptosis.
Armoracia - dissolves internal tumours.
Artemesia annua – Artemisinin – breast cancer.
Andrographis paniculata – andrographolides are immune stimulating. Cytotoxic.
    Leukaemia. Stomach, breast and prostate carcinoma. Non Hodgkins
    lymphoma. Lymphocytic leukaemia. Melanoma.
Arctium – benzaldehyde; anti tumour activity. Contains-B factor [Burdock
    factor]. Arctigenin inhibits leukaemia.
Aristolochia – aristolochic acid stimulates NK cell activity [226].
Artemisia abrotanum – angioma.
Artemisia annua - leukaemia
Astragalus - increases interferon levels and T cells. Immunemodulator.
Attractylodes macrocephala – atractylin, atractylon and butenolide B.
    Oesophageal cancer.
Bellis – tumours occurring from a traumatic cause.
Berberis - stimulates mucous membranes.
Boswellia – [Boswellic acid] nasal tumours, liver & intestinal carcinoma,
    leukaemia, brain tumours.
Bupleurum chinense – induces apoptosis and inhibits angiogenesis. Breast, liver
    and colon cancers.
Calendula – neuroma. Mucous membranes.
Camptotheca acuminata – camptothecin anteoplastic to leukaemia and solid
    tumours.
Camellia sinensis – epigallocatechin-3-gallate [192 p254]
Cardius marianus - hepatic.
Catharanthus rosea [Vinca] – vincristine and vintblastine are cytotoxic. General
    vasotonic alterative. Leukaemia.
Ceanothus americanus - T cell activator. Splenic tonic. Lymphadenopathy.
    Ovarian cysts [194p50]. Decongests the lymphatics, spleen and liver.
Centella asiatica - slows the growth of tumours.
Chelidonium - hepatic, cholagogue, slows mitosis.
Chimaphila – lymph cleanser and deobstruent. Vasotonic alterative.
    Breast cancer.

Herbal Medicine - Keys

Colchicum autumnale - leukaemia.

Combretum micranthum – solid tumours.

Conium maculatum - stony hard indurations - small doses.

Cordyceps sinensis – enhances immune activity. General tonic – anaemia, debility and an hepatitis C treatment. Lung tonic – anti asthmatic, coughs. Renal tonic – impotence/sexual dysfunction [around 1g daily]. Tiredness.

Coriolus versicolor - [known as Trametes versicolor] stimulates NK cells [261].

Coriolus versicolor is a mushroom, is non toxic an well tolerated. Two Proteoglycans: [1] PSK – Polysachharide K and [2] PSP – Polysachharide-peptide appear to be responsible for the effects. Used in carcinoma of the oesophagus, stomach, lung, ovary and cervix. Lowers telomerase activity and encourages cell mediated TH1 immune response. Average dose is 4.5g daily [395].

Corydalis formosa – vasotonic and analgesic.

Crocus sativus - cell oxygenator.

Curcuma longa - Curcuminoids are found in the yellow pigment and are antioxidant. Anti neoplastic. Has been used against cervical cancer. Dermal carcinoma.

Cydonia japonica [Quince] [192 p454].

Daphne mezerium – bone tumours/chondromata, dendrobium.

Drosera – antiviral.

Echinacea - immune stimulant.

Eleutherococcus – immune stimulant with an overall enhancing of tissue resistance.

Eucalyptus - respiratory conditions.

Eupatorium cannabinum – Immunostimulant and antineoplastic. Cytotoxic [189 p142].

Fucus - general supporter and mineral enhancer. Breast carcinoma.

Galium - nodular lesions in the mucous membranes or skin. Bladder carcinoma.

Ganoderma lucidem - Polysaccharides – Lentinan, Triterpenes [antitumour].

Geranium robertianum – [Herb robert -Venus] carcinoma of the cervix [246 p212]

Ginkgo – antioxidant activity.

Harpagophytum – skin carcinoma [192]. Hepatoma. Sarcoma. Inhibits platelet aggregation

Glycyrrhiza – flavones, mucous membrane cleanser and demulcent.

Grifolia – Maitake D fraction. Antitumour.

Hydrastis - tumour of any mucus membranes and of the stomach and breast.

Hypericum – hypericin, anti tumour - colon. Leukaemia.

Lavandula - cancer of the breast, colon, ovary, pancreas and prostate [150].

Ligustrium - stimulates natural interferons.

Lentinus edodes – antineoplastic.

Loquat leaves - general activity.

Malignancy & Oncology

Iris versicolor - for blood disorders [autotoxaemia] affecting the skin.

Larrea tridentata - general vasotonic alterative.

Lentinus edodes - Shitake mushroom [261], antineoplastic.

Marsdenia – supperative ulcerations, stomach cancer.

Melilotus officinalis - melanoma. Prostatic carcinoma. Renal cell carcinoma.

Muntingia calabura found in Thailand and Philippines. Action - colds, liver disease, headaches, antispasmodic, tranquilliser. Cytotoxic - cancer cell lines with cultured P-388 cells. 12 new flavanoids isolated with cytotoxic activity. Flavans are more active than the flavones. [278, 1991, 54 [1] p196].

Nerium oleander [Oleander] - antineoplastic, antiparasitic [192 p391].

Panax ginseng – direct action increasing resistance against malignant cells.

Perilla frutescens - stimulates interferon and inhibits tumour necrosis factor 281, 1999, Vol. 15, No. 3.

Petasites officinalis – antineoplastic anodyne.

Pfaffia paniculata - Pfaffic acid and the associated Pfaffosides inhibit the growth of tumours and melanomas

Podophyllum - liver and gall bladder deobstruent.

Polyporous umbellatus – [Zhu ling] mushroom.

Phytolacca – [adenoma, lipoma], hard/painful tumours, leukaemia, lymphoma, osteosarcoma, breast dysplasia, carcinoma of the breast and uterus.

Porea cocos – [mushroom] polysaccharide - pachymanese. Immunostimulant.

Pinellia ternata - cervical, mammary, gastric, lymphoma.

Prunella vulgaris - astringent.

Rabdosia rubescens - terpenes. Oesophageal tumours. Breast tumours.

Rheum palmatum - cholagogue

Ricinus communis - supports elimination from the intestine and aids hepatic function by allowing the latter to rest.

Rosmarinus officinalis - breast tumours. Antioxidant.

Rumex acetosela - oral pre cancerous lesions [contains carotene], melanoma.

Ruta – chondromata, used orally and as a compress.

Sambucus – skin carcinoma.

Scrophularia – adenoma.

Schizandra - protects against toxins, antioxidant, antitoxic, hepato protective.

Scutellaria baicalensis – flavonoids inhibit reverse transcriptase and inhibit the HIV virus. Increases serum immunoglobulins. Cervical carcinoma. Sarcoma. Bronchial carcinoma.

Sempervivum - poultice for breast tumours [228 p345].

Seneco jacobaea – Fetrow mentions use in cancerous ulcers [192].

Seneco vulgaris - detergent, cleansing to mucous membrane surfaces.

Serenoa - prostate.

Silybum - carcinoma of the skin, ovary and breast.

Herbal Medicine - Keys

Solanum - breast tumours. Beta-Solamarine is a tumour inhibitor [236].

Spirulina - carotenoids. Phycocyanin. GLA. Inhibits cancer colony formation.

Staphysagria - papilloma. Vasotonic alterative.

Stephania tetandra - destroys lymphatic and myeloid cells.

Sutherlandia frutescens – antineoplastic.

Symphytum - bone tumours/chondromata. Breast carcinoma – fol poultice.

Tabebuia - Lapachol is antineoplastic and suppresses tumour formation. Vasotonic alterative. Solid tumours.

Tanacetum parthenium – nasopharyngeal, fibrosarcoma, lymphoma, cervical.

Taraxacum - hepatic, breast carcinoma.

Teucrium scordonia – cleansing vasotonic alterative.

Thuja - stimulates T lymphocyes, increses interleukin production. Lung, breast, colon, rectal and uterine cancers. Papilloma/polyps/epitheoliomata/lipoma.

Tinospora cordifolia – antineoplastic [265, 2001, 13].

Tremella fuciformis [Bai Mu Er] mushroom.

Trifolium - coumarins, general vasotonic alterative which has emphasis upon the liver/intestine and throat.

Ulmus - absorbs and eliminates toxins.

Uncaria - cancer preventing properties. Immunostimulant.

Viola odorata - throat/larynx/lymphatics/intestinal tumours.

Viscum - viscumin and viscotoxins are cytotoxic. Polypeptides are cytotoxic. Increases T cells. General vasotonic alterative.

Vitis vinifera [grapeseed] – proanthocyanidins [192 p252]

Withania somnifera - increases WBC's. Immunemodulator. Antineoplastic.

Zanthoxylum americana - adenoma/lymphomata.

Vitamin C and Selenium are necessary in all neoplastic conditions.

Prescriptions that have stood the test of time

Essiac – an old American Indian remedy -
Arctium 720g, Rumex acetosella 480g, Rheum officinalis 30g, Ulmus 120g.
Sig 30g et aqua PRN. [269 1991 Vol.XII,No.III].

General blood prescription
Viola odorata herba, Trifolium and Phytolacca.

Hoxey formula

Arctium	9%	Rhamnus cathartica	17%
Baptisia	4%	Stillingia	9%
Berberis aquifoleum	9%	Trifolium	17%
Glycyrrhiza	17%	Zanthoxylum	9%
Phytolacca	9%		

Malignancy & Oncology

Hoxey is an vasotonic alterative and depurative medicine. Activity via the lymphatic and glandular mucous membranes. Breaks down catabolic waste.

Cancer syrup – [Dr Eli Jones. USA]

Dicentra cucullaria	Rumex
Guaiacum	Scrophularia
Juniperus	Solanum dulcamera
Phytolacca	Zanthoxylum
Podophyllum	

Carcinoma sites – treatment

Listed in system order – eent, pineal, pituitary, blood, respiratory, gastro intestinal, genito urinary, adrenal, dermal and bone, breast, pelvic organs, lymph, nerve.

Oral carcinoma
Medicine
Allium, Aloe, Althea, Commiphora, Curcuma longa, Epilobium, Hydrastis, Larrea, Marsdenia [188p89], Phytolacca, Rumex, Salvia, Sempervivum, Stellaria, Symphytum, Thuja, Trifolium, Ulmus, Verbascum, Viola, Viscum.

Pineal/pituitary medicine
Centella, Dioscorea, Hydrastis, Phytolacca, Sassafras, Trifolium, Verbena, Viscum.

Respiratory
Laryngeal carcinoma
Medicine
Allium, Althea, Centella, Echinacea, Glycyrrhiza, Hydrastis, Iris, Phytolacca, Plantago, Salvia, Trifolium, Ulmus, Verbascum, Viola odorata.

Bronchial carcinoma
Tr Sanguinaria [contraindicated in haemorrhage]
LE Inula
LE Piscidia
LE Lycopus
LE Glycyrrhiza
Other medicine
Cetraria islandica, Chondrus crispus, Echinacea, Glycyrrhiza, Inula, Lycopus [188p92], Marrubium, Rumex, Taxus, Thymus, Trifolium, Ulmus, Verbascum, Viola.

Gastro intestinal
Stomach carcinoma
LE Viola odorata
LE Trifolium
LE Phytolacca
Succus Taraxacum
Medicine
Acorus, Hydrastis, Lavandula, Marsdenia, Plantago, Ulmus, Verbascum.

Intestinal carcinoma
Medicine
Hypericum, Lavandula, Trifolium, Ulmus, Viola odorata.

Ano rectal carcinoma
Medicine
Capsicum, Dioscorea, Echinacea, Galium, Glycyrrhiza, Hydrastis, Myrica, Phytolacca, Scrophularia, Stellaria, Ulmus, Viola odorata, Viscum, Zingiber.

Liver carcinoma prescription
Tr Hydrastis
LE Euonymous
LE Viola odorata
Qs Succus Taraxacum

Liver carcinoma
Medicine
Agrimonia, Bupleurum chinense, Chelidonium, Galium, Hypericum, Myrica, Silybum, Taraxacum, Viola, Vinca.

Pancreas carcinoma
Medicine
Chelidonium, Chionanthus, Glycyrrhiza, Mentha piperita, Myrica, Smilax, Taraxacum, Ulmus.

Spleen carcinoma
Medicine
Bellis, Ceanothus, Chionanthus, Myrica, Polygonum multiflorum, Scolopendrum.

Prostate and Testicular carcinoma [prostate and ovarian medicines are interchangable]

Malignancy & Oncology

Medicine for prostate and testicle
Agropyron, Althea, Capsella, Echinacea, Equisetum, Hydrangea, Hydrastis, Myrica, Phytolacca, Plantago, Piper methysticum, Serenoa, Solidago, Symphytum, Thuja, Trifolium, Trigonella, Ulmus, Uncaria tomentosa, Vinca, Viola, Viscum, Zea.

Adrenal tumour
Barosma, Glycyrrhiza, Panax, Smilax, Viscum.

Dermal and bone
Dermal – epithilioma - tumours, breast tumours
Arctium, Centella, Chelidonium, Curcuma longa, Echinacea, Larrea, Linaria vulgaris, Petroselinum, Phytolacca, Plantago, Rumex acetosella/crispus, Stillingia, Symphytum, Thuja, Trifolium, Ulmus, Viola odorata.

Dermal carcinoma px
Commiphora gum resin 1, Styrax benzoin gum 1, Sanguisorba officinalis hb 1, Iris rad 2
aqua 800 ml.
Apply liberally to an inflamed surface Its cleansing properties are carried to all parts of the system [59].
External poultice:
Chelidonium, Oleum Ricinus, Podophyllum, Sanguinaria, Sempervivum.

Bone myeloma/sarcoma
Medicine
Capsicum, Echinacea, Galium, Phytolacca, Plantago, Rumex, Ruta, Stephania tetranda, Symphytum. Tabebuia, Vinca, Viscum, Zanthoxylum.

Pelvic carcinoma
Ovary and uterine medicines
Allium, Calendula, Chamaelirium, Echinacea, Geranium robertianum, Hydrastis, Lavandula, Nymphaea, Phytolacca, Plantago, Serenoa, Thuja, Trifolium, Viola, Vinca, Viscum.

Breast carcinoma
A lump will often be the first symptom complained of. Skin changes – orange peel effect. Discolouration and changes to the shape of the breast with nipple retraction. Lymphadenopathy. Nipple bleeding. Eventual metastasis to the axillary lymph nodes.

Herbal Medicine - Keys

<u>Medicine</u> - breast
Althea, Arctium, Bupleurum chinense, Centella, Commiphora, Curcuma longa. Echinacea, Galium, Iris, Larrea, Phytolacca, Rosmarinus, Rumex, Scrophularia, Serenoa, Solanum, Stillingia, Symphytum, Taraxacum, Taxus, Thuja, Trifolium, Viola odorata, Vinca, Viscum, Zanthoxylum.
<u>Poultice</u>
Althea, Carrot – grated, Podophyllum, Phytolacca [176], Plantago, Sanguinaria, Seneco jacobaea, Sempervivum, Symphytum fol/rad, Ulmus, Urtica.

Leukaemia
<u>Medicine</u>
Allium, Camptotheca acuminata, Centella, Echinacea, Iris, Larrea, Phytolacca, Plantago, Rumex, Tabebuia, Thuja, Trifolium, Vinca rosea, Viscum, Zanthoxylum. Beetroot juice.

Lymphoma
Lymphatic carcinoma
<u>Medicine</u>
Andrographis paniculata, Echinacea, Galium, Hydrastis, Phytolacca, Pinellia ternata, Stephania tetranda, Tanacetum parthenium, Vinca rosea, Vitex, Zanthoxylum,

Hodgkins disease
<u>Medicine</u>
Centella, Echinacea, Glycyrrhiza, Hydrastis, Iris, Phytolacca, Smilax, Thuja, Trifolium, Vinca Rosea, Viscum.

Neuroblastoma
<u>Medicine</u>
Allium cepa, Calendula, Cimicifuga, Passiflora, Tabebuia, Vinca rosea.

32
Nutritional regime

What this Chapter is about.
Various kinds of diet are explained in this chapter. Through exclusion diets to normal eating. During a disease process the diet needs to be simple or there may need to be a fast, where food is eaten, it must be light and easily assimilated. Fruits, salads and vegetables together with juices are best for nourishment. Acute disease requires little food or only water as thirst dictates. Too much or the wrong kind of food will delay healing, it will not be properly assimilated. Eating will interfere with the elimination of tissue waste. It forces the digestive organs to work on digestion instead of elimination. While still eating, the vital force is diverted from its work of combating disease to digest food thus delaying recovery.

There are two types of diet:
catabolic
anabolic

Catabolic diet - breaking down waste matter, clearing toxins etc. Catabolic reactions occur with fasting.
Anabolic diet - a building up regime. Anabolic diets strengthen tissue and provide increased muscle stamina. They are used if there is a low vitality or a need to improve ones vigour and muscle bulk.
The anabolic and catabolic diets are interchangeable and variable.

Fluids – the quantity of fluid intake is regulated by the patient. Drink when you are thirsty is the safest rule. Eat dry, without fluids, favours better digestion. A *minimum* of 1000 ml fluid is required each day for an adult.
Fasting - the digestive processes need to be engaged in the processes of elimination not digestive assimilation during disease processes. Because fasting takes a lot of vital energy from the tissues it is preferable to build up the tissue strength before commencing the fast.
Acute disease and inflammatory processes call for a selected fast or restricted food intake.
In acute disease the body discharges large amounts of toxic waste. The vital energies are concentrating on the cleansing and healing processes. Kuhne claimed that disease consists of an accumulation of waste and morbid matter in the body, the fastest way to clear the tissues is to fast. In many cases of weakness, lowered vitality and low resistance the tendency towards encumbrance of the tissues increases. There is a greater need to cleanse and detoxify the tissues of waste matter. During a fast the body has a greater need to eliminate toxins. Toxins that

are not eliminated would be a cause of autointoxication - where toxins produced from cellular processes are reabsorbed into the tissues. In order to keep the elimination active the secernants are stimulated to remove the toxins. Secernants are the bowel, skin, liver and kidneys.

Extra elimination often creates new symptoms. It is quite natural for the tissues concerned to produce eliminative symptoms. Gastro intestinal symptoms may include a coated tongue, nausea, sometimes vomiting and increased intestinal elimination. Nerve symptoms often accompany the elimination of toxins such as fear, depression, irritability and irritation, these are common effects.

Emotional temperaments and sensitive/negative people often require support with fasting as they have nerve sensitivity. Lindlahr suggested great care with treatment of the asthenic types. More robust athletic types can fast more easily, they have less nervous fragility.

Sometimes it takes around six weeks of treatment before the healing crisis occurs. Following the fast use non citrus fruits, vegetables, allergen free diet, millet, cous cous, bulgar wheat, sesame, brown rice. Avoid sugar as it depletes.

Mono diet/juice fast
A single or multiple variation of juices may be used depending upon the disorder being treated. A mono diet uses single items of a specific fruit or vegetable. Grape diet is an example, whereby the potassium encourages the elimination of fluid from the cell and extracellular spaces.

Food used as drinks
Regular small drinks of juice throughout the day advantages the patient.
Pulp and extract the juice using a liquidiser. In the case of vegetables they are used raw.
Apple - natural stimulant, blood purifier, constipation, sluggish liver, skin eruption, anaemia.
Banana - contains barium, boron, cobalt, iron, manganese, magnesium, nickel, selenium, silicon, strontium, zinc. Highly efficacious in gastro intestinal disorders of an inflammatory nature.
Beetroot – used in the treatment of carcinoma. Increases haemoglobin. Liver, gall bladder stimulant, renal stimulant. Best combined with carrot juice.
Cabbage – Cleanser of mucous membranes of the GIT as it helps to destroy pathogens and is anti neoplastic. Soothes peptic ulcers. Gum infections. Diarrhoea and diverticulitis – use ¼ cabbage with 2 tomatoes. Best mixed with other juices e.g. carrot.
Carrot - provides beta carotine, vitamins B, C, D, E, G. It helps to promote the appetite and aids digestion. Raw carrot juice is a natural solvent for ulcerous conditions. Digestive aid – and helps to clear infections of the tonsils, appendix, colon. Skin cleanser. Solvent for cancerous growths.

Nutritional regime

Apple and carrot - an aid in jaundice, gastric catarrh, arthritis, neuritis, cystitis, skin eruptions, constipation sluggish liver.

Carrot and coconut - provides calcium, magnesium and iron, helps heal ulcers of the gastro intestinal tract.

Carrot, dandelion and lettuce - for poor appetite, nerve tonic, mildly diuretic. For kidney, bladder and liver disorders. Blood cleanser. High in magnesium

Celery and lemon - eases flatulence if used before a meal. Serves as a tonic for nerve relaxation.

Carrot, celery, spinach and parsley - rich in potassium, this combination of foods virtually covers the entire range of organic minerals and salts.

Carrot, beetroot and cucumber - heals gall bladder and liver disorders.

Carrot, beetroot and coconut - cleanser of the kidneys and gall bladder. Contains alkaline elements. Potassium, sodium, calcium, magnesium and iron.

Carrot, celery, endive and parsley - iron, sodium and calcium. Asthma, skin disease, gall stones, gall bladder irritation, diseases of the urinary tract, stomach ulcers, otitis media.

Carrot, apple and beet top - rich source of iron. Anaemia, constipation, arthritis, obesity, low vitality.

Carrot, celery and turnip leaves - rich in minerals. Anaemia, acidosis, impure blood, tumours, hypertension, poor appetite, torpid liver.

Celery – contains potassium, calcium and phosphorus and is used in diabetes, varicose veins, calculi, ulcers. Celery and carrot for ulcers.

Cherry and strawberry juice – neutralise uric acid.

Cucumber – stimulates hair growth. Hypotensive agent. Anti uric acid effect through diuresis. Removes excess sodium. Combines with carrot and beetroot. Detoxifier to the liver and kidneys.

Grapefruit - improves liver function.

Lettuce – high in chlorophyll and iron. Soothes the stomach. Diuretic.

Lemon juice – High in calcium @ 86mg per 100g.

Pyorrhoea, and recession of the gums use 1 part juice to three parts spring water after meals and before retiring. Anticatarrhal. Stimulates the liver. Cleansing to the alimentary tract. Sluggish renal function. Stimulates bowel action. For sore throat and tonsillitis gargle with lemon juice. Skin blemishes and discolouration, abscesses, erysipelas, ringworm - apply lemon juice. Cleanses the blood. Poultice of lemon pulp is good to reduce swellings. Dysentery. Diarrhoea. Obesity. Depression. Virus infections.

Parsley – supports the adrenals, thyroid, kidneys, eyes, CNS and ANS. Combines best with carrot and celery.

Spinach – Mucous membrane cleanser. Speeds up digestion and peristalsis. Due to oxalic acid content dilute with other juices.

Watercress – intestinal cleanser. Contains sulphur. [181. p82-103]

Herbal Medicine - Keys

Stimulant, astringent and relaxant foods

In the treatment of disease, make your patient's food subservient to your medication says Cook.

Fruit such as **citrus fruits are antacid** when taken into the body they never produce acid. However a drink of lemon juice may appear to create acid due to it's strong alkaline effect and indicates the need to reduce acid levels within the blood.

Food may be stimulating: apple cider vinegar, beetroot, capsicums, parsley, sour apples and watercress.

Astringent foods are arrowroot, crab apples, cranberries, flour, milk, rhubarb.

Relaxing foods are asparagus, bananas, pears, peaches, sweet apples, turnips.

Although wholesome food given regularly is a necessity to maintain health. At times it is a requirement for health to omit food and rely on the vital force to heal, using other techniques as: fasting and special food diets e.g. Mono diets.

Foods leaving acid and alkaline residues

Protein foods - acid/nitrogen residue.

Fat/starch in excess - cholesterol residue.

Fruit leaves an alkaline residue.

Vegetables leave an alkaline residue.

Pulses and grains are alkaline.

Protein foods leave an acid residue which under normal circumstances is eliminated by the kidneys. Excess protein intake will create acidity of the blood and lead to a delicate homeostasis. Excess acids cause rheumatic conditions.

When carbohydrates [starch] are consumed as energy foods. Those unused calories will be stored as fat. Fat substances can deposit as cholesterol in the blood vessels and this will eventually lead to sclerotic changes [conditions of obstruction].

Pulses and grains are high in fibre and an excellent source of protein.

Fruit and vegetables, together with salads are alkaline and to be encouraged. Fruit intake is known to reduce mortality among men [205].

Dietetic advice to a patient for a whole food diet - an example

Try to eat five portions daily made up of fruit/salad/vegetables/pulses.

Breakfast

Fruit – prunes, stewed apple or grapefruit with

Soya yoghurt or

Muesli with pumpkin seed or

Organic cereal

Lunch

Jacket potato with butter and/or

Nutritional regime

Salad – lettuce, chives, cucumber, radish, tomato, celery, sweet corn, olive, watercress, beetroot, peppers, sauerkraut, red or white cabbage.
Fresh fruit – single type
Dinner
Soup.
Main course:
Chicken, lamb, beef, fish, omelette, pasta dish, nut roast, or bean dish,
Steamed vegetables – aubergine, cabbage, carrot, cauliflower, onion, peas, sprouts, spinach, swede, turnip. Potato as desired.
Sweets:
Fruit, macaroni, semolina or brown rice pudding.
Organic soya yoghurt.
Jelly - natural crystals [made from seaweed].

Snacks in between a meal e.g. for hypoglycaemia - nuts, pumpkin seeds, sesame seed bars, fruit and nut bars, raisins, fruit, yoghurt, oat milk, rice milk.
Ideally all the above should be organic.
Potatoes are best eaten with vegetables and salads.
Drinks
Eat dry is the rule. So the digestive juices are not diluted.
Condiments
Salt is to be used sparingly, biosalt is the most balanced. Do not cook with salt as it lengthens cooking time, it makes beans harder in the finished product. Pepper – in small amounts only. Herbs like rosemary, basil, dill, chives, garlic, horseradish are all suitable for flavouring. Put onto the meal late in cooking otherwise the goodness may be lost. Apple cider vinegar is the only type of vinegar to be used. Malt vinegar is acid forming.

Research items
Vegetables protect against genetic damage. Tomato, carrot and spinach produced a significant decrease in DNA damage as measured in white blood cells. [21]
Broccoli and brassica vegetables appear to halt breast cancer cells. These contain sulphur and inactivate oestrogen in the liver. [25]
Research has shown that an estimated 90% of women and 12% of men in the UK do not receive adequate iron nutriture. MAFF 1994
Banana contains acitan which contains fatty acids; palmitic, oleic, pentadecanoic, myristic and stearic acids, phenolic compounds and tannins. Bananas are a useful treatment in gastro intestinal disorders: enteritis, colitis, diverticulitis, IBS.

Soya beans
The consumption of soya foods can lead to a reduction in the incidence of coronary heart disease, carcinoma of the breast, prostate and colon, osteoporosis.

Herbal Medicine - Keys

This is due to the presence of isoflavones which have health protective effects [185].
Isoflavones influence oestrogen receptor binding and have antioxidant effects. Isoflavones are metabolised in the GIT prior to absorption. Isoflavones possess weak oestrogenic activity. LDL and serum total cholesterol is reduced. There are three main isoflavones present in soya as genistein, daidzein and glycitein. Genistein inhibits thrombin formation and platelet activation [58].

Cabbage – raw juice or raw green cabbage, raw sauerkraut produce health effects which is *lost in cooked cabbage.*
Cabbage contains antioxidants, Vitamins A and C. 75% of the Vitamin C was still present after two months in cold storage. It contains iodine but depletes another substance which may lead to goitre if concentrated juice is taken for too long a time [use for two weeks only at a time]. Sauerkraut does not adversely affect the thyroid and contains:
Indoles which neutralise metabolic toxins
Histidine and sulphur inhibit the growth of cancerous cells
Protect against radioactive damage
Amino acid – glutamine is an anti ulcer remedy, and a powerful antacid.
Vitamin U, the anti pepsin factor protects the gastric membrane.
Anti infectious, resistance to typhus, upper respiratory infections, candida.
Protecting against carcinoma of the stomach, intestine and rectum.
Wound healer [228 p345], varicose veins, gangrene.
Reduces LDL cholesterol
Cabbage produces hydrogen sulphide which is a by product of the cleansing process when eliminated by the intestine.
Local action of cabbage
Apply every other day to inflamed joints and alternate with clay poultices. Both remove uric acid impurities from the area.
One part to three parts water for a wash in fungal infections and vaginal candida.
Poultice of cabbage helps to prevent sepsis, eliminate pus formation, reduce swelling, tonsillitis, gangrene, piles, colitis, sprains.
RDA is 480ml for peptic ulcer treatment over two weeks [62].

Cabbage poultice for all inflammatory conditions of the GIT [Crohn's disease, ulcerations, colitis]. Alternate with potato poultices.

Pineapple
Bromelain derived from pineapple is a proteolytic enzyme and inhibits pro inflammatory prostaglandins. Allforms of arthritis are benefitted by its use.

Nutritional regime

Obesity
Pear shaped obesity in patients have fewer complications as compared to apple shaped people; those with an increased waist to hip ratio. Apple shaped patients suffer from altered hormonal levels e.g. increased cortisol, from chronic stress that promotes fat absorption and a Cushing appearance [moon face].

Weight assessment
For body mass index ones weight must be considered as a guide to treatment using diet and lifestyle habits. The body mass index is an accurate assessment of weight.

BMI normal range is up to 25 and the greater the index as it rises above this figure the more obese the patient.

The formula given by Budd is as follows:
Height divided by weight x weight divided by 3.35 = BMI

33
Pharmacy

What this Chapter is about.
Pharmacy governs:
Preparations and prescribing methods.
Dosage of remedies for infants and the elderly.
Detoxification and deamination of remedies.
Formulary of external and oral compound prescriptions. [See also Chapter 17-30].

Herbal classification
The old classification of herbs into diuretic, diaphoretic, hepatic etc is unspecific as far as the herb is only related to the organ or area of influence. Using physiomedicalism the herb action is refined and we are able to select a relaxing or stimulating diaphoretic, pulmonary stimulant or tonic, astringent or tonic stomachic, tonic or relaxant/antispasmodic nervine, hepatic tonic or relaxant, renal relaxant or tonic etc. The prescription reflects accurate clinical correlation with the physiological state and is balanced by correct physiological medicine.

Preparations and abbreviations with meanings

Capsules	Capsulae	Caps.
Creams	Cremores	Crem.
Decoction	Decoctum	decoc.
Draught	Haustus	Haust.
Dusting powders	Conspersi	Conspers.
Ear drops	Auristilae	Aurist.
Elixirs	Elexiria	Elix.
Emulsions	Emulsiones	Emuls.
Enemas	Enemata	Enem.
Eye drops	Guttae pro oculus	Gutt.
Eye lotions/eye drops	Collyria	Collyr.
Eye ointment	Oculenta	Oculent.
Extract	Extractum	Ext
Gargle	Gargarismata	Garg.
Glycerine	Glycerina	Glyc.
Infusion	Infusium	inf
Injection	Injectiones	Inj.
Irrigations	Irrigationes	Irrig.
Liniment	Liniments	Lin.
Linctus	Linct.	Linctuses
Lozenge	Trochisci	Troch.

Pharmacy

Lotions	Lotiones	Lot.
Mixtures	Mistura	Mist.
Mouth washes	Collutoria	Collut.
Nasal drops	Naristillae	Narist.
Ointment	Unguentum	Ung.
Oil	Oleum	Ol.
Paints	Pigmenta	Pig.
Pastes	Pastae	Past.
Pessaries	Pessi	Pess.
Pills	Pilulae	Pil
Plaster	Emplastrum	Emp.
Poultice	Cataplasma	Cataplasm.
Powders	Pulveres	Pulv.
Solutions	Liquores	Liq.
Solution tablets	Solvellae	Solv.
Spirit	Spiritus	Sp.
Spray	Nebulae	Neb.
Suppositories	Suppositoria	Supp.
Syrup	Syripus	syr.
Tablets	Tabellae	Tab.
Tincture	Tinctura	Tinct.

Take the prescription	Sig/Mitte	Dispense
Mixture	Mistura	mist
Dose	Dosis	dos.
At once		Stat
Every hour	omni hora	o.h.
Twice daily		BD
Thrice daily		TDS
Four times daily	quarter in die	QDS
As required	Pro re nata	PRN
Morning	Mane	M.
Nocte	nocte	Noct
Water	Aqua	aq.
With water	cum aqua	cum aq.
Fill up with warm water		Aqua cal
Fill up with cold water		Aqua frig
Without water	sine aqua	s.aq.
Diluted	dilutum	dil.
After meals		PC
Before meals		AC
With meals	cum cibos/ciburn	c.c.

Herbal Medicine - Keys

Between meals	intercibos	I.c.
Drops		Gtt/gtt
Before	ante	a
Of each	ana	a.a
Affected parts	partibus affectis	p.a.
By mouth		per os

Botany shorthand

Baccae	Bacc.	Berries
Bulbus	Bulb	Bulb
Cortex	Cort.	Bark
Flos/Flores	Flos/Flor	Flower/s
Folium	Fol.	Leaf
Fructus	Fruct.	Fruit
Gemmae	Gem	Buds
Lignum	Lign.	Wood
Radix	Rad.	Root
Rhizoma	Rhiz.	Rhizome
Semen	Sem.	Seed
Stipites	Stip.	Stem
Stigma	Stig.	Stigma
Turiones	Tur	Young growths

Prescribing for the patient

Prescriptions assembled by herbalists require for the medicines to be written and kept on a suitable record card. The dose and medication must be clearly stated on all prescriptions. The above system is in operation amongst medical herbalists this provides for the statutory cover in prescription writing.

Bartrum explains that a prescription should only contain four medicines in combination [p123].

Delivery of medication

- Herbal tea [infusium, decoctum] provides a quick and satisfactory delivery of the medication.
- Sublingual delivery is faster as the medicine by passes the liver without undergoing changes by liver enzymes. Medication comes into contact with oral blood vessels more quickly than at any other site.
- Dermal or intravenous injection gives prompt relief.
- Dermal patches. Impregnate lint with remedy to be used and apply to the area, cover with adhesive plaster. Anti smoking patches are an example of this.

Pharmacy

Dosage and mode of application for the medication

Finding the correct dose.

The adult dose of a remedy is given in each condition. The dose range is dependent upon the patient and the condition being treated. The quantity administered is shown as one single dose. Prescriptions are usually dispensed in weekly amounts for ease. A single dose multiplied accordingly to give the amount for the required number of weeks [for one week x 21 doses].

Consider starting with a small single dose and adjust as required.

Prescribing for the elderly

As a person becomes older so their is a diminished functional efficiency of bodily organs. Elimination is affected, detoxification and excretion is less efficient.

Bodily changes in the elderly patient

a] diminished functional efficiency of bodily organs
b] loss of lean body mass
c] delayed enzyme induction [reactionary]
d] cell membrane alteration [hypotrophicity]
e] altered salt and water content of tissues [hydration level]

Proportional dosage according to age – elderly patients.
Appropriate for many elderly patients is to use the lowest dose, say around 50% to start with.

age	maximum %
60-70	80%
70-80	75%

Small dosage of the remedy will excite less vital activity within the tissues demonstrated and explained using the principle of potentisation.

Give small doses of medicines often so that a concentration is achieved within the tissue.

Alcohol in medicines

Alcohol is formed from the starch of grain [barley, maize] potatoes or fruit which undergoes alcoholic fermentation. Alcohol is ethyl alcohol or ethanol both terms are synonymous. During fermentation, starch in grain and potatoes is converted into glucose and then yeast forms to produce ethyl alcohol. Fruit is fermented by yeast into alcohol.

Alcohol is broken down in the liver by the enzyme - alcohol dehydrogenase. Acetaldehyde forms from the breakdown of alcohol. Intoxication from alcohol causes euphoria and eventual depression.

Herbal Medicine - Keys

Deamination of alcohol
Breakdown of alcohol in the blood for:
- men is 15mg per 100ml per hour
- women it is 10mg per 100 ml per hour.

Preservation
Alcohol is used as a preservative in medicines. It has anti microbial action. 25% alcohol will preserve a liquid preparation. Where the alcohol content is lower mould will grow.

Absorption
Alcohol extracts those constituents otherwise only very partially extracted in water e.g. essential oils, resins and gums. Alcohol supports absorption from the stomach and intestine of the medication.

Alcohol in the medicine
Tr 5% alcohol content gives 0.0015g of alcohol in 0.4ml of medication.
Tr 25% alcohol content gives 1.5g of alcohol in 7ml of medication.
Tr 45% alcohol content gives 7g of alcohol within 20ml of medication.
Tr 70% alcohol content gives 25g of alcohol in 45ml of medication [182].

Prescriptions
Always ensure the bottle is clearly labelled with the instructions for use, the name of the patient and the dispensing date.

Oral compounds
Tincturae Antispasmodic [Antispasmodic tincture]
Lobelia 15g Scutellaria 7.5g Symplocarpus 7.5g Capsicum 7.5g
Alcohol 96% ethanol 400ml, aqua 150.
Macerate for 10 days. Shake menstrum each day. Extract and filter.
Dose 1-2 ml TDS aqua frig.
For severe spasmodic states use the tincture hourly. It can be used externally.

Compound tinctura Lavandulae [Tincture Lavender compound]
Ol Lavandula 5ml
Ol Rosmarinus 0.5ml
Cinnamon bruised 10g
Red sanders root in fine powder 20g
Alcohol 60% aqua to 1000ml and macerate for 10 days.
Sig 2-4ml. For conditions of flatulence, intestinal spasm, colic, pain.

Pharmacy

Composition essence - Myrica cerifera
Myrica cerifera [Bayberry bark] is the main ingredient of composition essence. Equal proportions of stimulating and astringent qualities are combined within the root bark.
Physiological effects
It has a tonic effect upon the system. Myrica does not dry up the secretions but promotes glandular activity and tones and stimulates the system. It restores the mucous secretions. Circulation through the arteries and capillaries is improved. Relaxed conditions and feebleness of the circulation are improved.
Combined with diaphoretics it is used for colds. Hypothermia could benefit from its use. A strong infusion is nauseating. Large doses contract the stomach resulting in emesis. Myrica is more tonic in cold than hot preparations.

Composition essence [two formulas exist]

Myrica	240g
Zingiber [African is stronger]	120g
Zanthoxylum berries	60g
Asarum canadense	90g
Capsicum	

[2]

Myrica	240g
Pinus canadensis	120g
Zingiber	120g
Szygium	30g
Capsicum	30g

Use the same method for both formulas. Mix the powders or finely ground herb with a 1:5 mixture of water and alcohol 45%.
Second prescription is used in diphtheria – leaving out Asarum and substituting with Pinus canadensis, Szygium are added and Capsicum is increased.
Indications – with emetics, in colds, colic, diarrhoea, menorrhagia, delayed parturition.
Contraindicated in typhoid fever.
Cook says 'Thomson eventually stopped using Pinus canadensis as he found it too drying to the mucus membranes'. [111]

Herbal Medicine - Keys

Decoction
Compound decoctum Smilax Compound decoction of Smilax

Smilax	12ml
Sassafras	2ml
Guaiacum	2ml
Glycyrrhiza	2ml
Daphne mezerion	0.5ml
Aqua to	100ml

Sig 5ml TDS
A glandular and Vasotonic alterative [detoxing and depurative] prescription.

Elixir
Using an LE or tincture - dilute with vegetable glycerine at the rate of 0.5 – 1ml per 4ml respectively. Dose 5/10 ml TDS. This creates an elixir which can be produced in seconds. While it is not considered good practice to use this method often. Correct elixir making enhances the herb.

Elixir simplex [Simple elixir]
    Px   Tincturae Auranti 10ml
             Syrupus   90ml
    Mix the tincture with the syrup and shake.
    Used as a flavouring mixture.

Elixir aromaticum. [Aromatic elixir]
Oleum orange 2ml. Oleum Lemon 0.5ml. Oleum Coriander 0.25ml. Oleum Anise 0.06ml. Alcohol 250ml. Syrupus 375ml. Aqua to 1000ml.
Dissolve the oils into the alcohol then slowly add the syrup.
Shake before use Sig 8ml.

Elixir Paullinia [Elixir of Guarana]
Tr Paullinia 800ml. Oleum Cinnamomum 0.5ml. Syrupus 100ml. Alcohol to 1000ml. Sig 8ml.

Elixir Valeriana. [Elixir of Valerian]
Tincturae Valeriana 150ml. LE Glycyrrhiza 50ml. Aromatic Elixir to 1000ml. Mix and filter. Sig 8ml.

Essence
Essence of Sassafras
First make a strong essence of Sassafras. Ol Sassafras 1ml, EA 135ml, Aqua 135ml, mix first the EA and oil, then add the water.
Use 5ml of essence to 500 ml of mixture/syrup for the flavouring of medicines.

Pharmacy

Concentrated Mentha piperita [Peppermint water]
Ol Mentha piperita 20ml, Alcohol 90%   600ml, Purified water to   1000ml
Dissolve the oil into the alcohol, add water in small quantities to produce 100ml.
Shake vigorously after each addition. Sig 0.25 - 0.5ml.

Infusions

In acute conditions the hot infusion is best. Always cover the container to prevent
loss of volatile oils. Hot infusions work quicker than tablets or tinctures.
Planta Medica quotes that a bark decoction of Salix purpurea shows that the
extraction strength of water for salicin derivates and flavonoids is high. Water
extracted about 50% of total flavonoid glycosides of Ginkgo.
Decomposing of secondary metabolites could be stopped in Hypericum by hot
extraction at 50 degrees C. A secondary effect of heating was a higher yield of
hypericin, without any changes in the TLC-fingerprint of flavonoids compared
with the herbal drug. 263, 1991 57 (8) Suppl. 2 A26

Infusium Mentha piperita. [Peppermint infusion]
Peppermint herb 3g. Aqua 150ml. Cover and leave for ten minutes.
Strain and drink.

Linctus [See Chapter 18]

Mixtures

Preparations of herbs in a base ready for dispensing.
Mistura Concentrated Composita Gentian infusion
                                          [Concentrated Compound of Gentian]
    Gentian infusion 1ml.
    Auranti/Citrus 4ml. Aqua to 10ml.
    Sig 10ml. To stimulate the gastric secretions and appetite.

Mistura Composita Rheum palmatum [Compound Tincture Rhubarb]
Compound Tincture Rhubarb 1ml
Tincture Zingiber forte 0.5ml Aqua to 10ml
Sig 10ml. Prepare fresh.

Pastilles

Glycero gelatine 50% medicament 50%. Melt over a water bath and stir. Run
into moulds.
Sig Suck one pastille every two hours. Indications – oropharyngeal conditions.

Solid/Soft and dry extracts
A solid, soft or dry extract represents the plant constituents with a minimum amount of inert material. Method: make a tincture and evaporate until a soft dry extract is produced. In general such extracts are given in a 0.06g dose.

Syrupus – medicinal syrups. [See also Chapter 18]
Syrup makes all internal medications relaxing. This is suitable for irritable and inflamed conditions. Respiratory and gastro intestinal conditions are often best served with a medicinal syrup. Syrup is contraindicated in diabetes.
To make a syrup take 10g of herb, 250ml aqua, 250g sugar.
Bring to the boil and simmer for around 5 minutes. Strain when cold and bottle.
Sig 30ml

Syrup Allium [Garlic syrup]
Garlic juice 20ml. Sucrose 80ml. Cider vinegar 20ml. Aqua 20ml. Mix together.
Sig 8ml

Succus Allium [Garlic juice]
Crushed garlic 80g. Aqua 80ml. Express and mix with Alcohol 20ml. Filter.
Sig 4ml

Throat nebulae [Throat spray]
Althea   20ml
Commiphora   5ml
Echinacea   10ml
Piper methysticum 15ml
Salvia   20ml
Mix the above and dispense 70ml. Put into a spray bottle.
Sig spray the throat PRN.
Use: for inflammatory throat disorders where an antiseptic and anaesthetic action is required.

Tincture Tincturae
Many firms supply tinctures as a 1:2, 1:3, 1:4. Prescribing with this array of different strengths is confusing when the practitioner wants to obtain some degree of standardisation within their practice. Using fewer numbers of different strength preparations makes prescribing much easier. There are exceptions to this hypothesis. Some medicines are too strong as a 1:5. The materia medica explains which remedies fall into this category.
It is known that 1ml of a Liquid extract 1:1 equals 5ml Tincture 1:5 and equals 1000mg or 1g in [dry] weight. While 1ml LE equals 5ml Tr and this is for water, it is a useful base line when thinking about standardisation. Standardisation in

Pharmacy

this work means standardised for the whole of the part of the remedy as outlined in the materia medica on the parts of the plant to use as medicine.

Tinctures are preparations containing the active ingredients of the plant to be used as medicine. Prepared with an alcoholic menstrum as low as possible, this is usually 25% of an ethyl alcohol [Ethanol] at 96%. DRF or doubly rectified fermentation alcohol is used for extraction processes. It will dilute oils. Vodka could be used but tends to cost more as the duty has to be paid. Good quality tinctures are made cold so as not to damage the plant constituents.

Method to prepare a Tincture using 25% alcohol.
Remedy to be used 200g dry fine cut material, Alcohol 250ml Aqua 750ml. Shake the mixture for ten days to distribute the contents. Extract using a centrifuge or press and filter then bottle and label. The marc [mixture remaining after extraction] is recycled. An example of a centrifuge is a spin dryer. Upon extraction it is usual to lose up to 20% of the extract especially with the aerial parts as they tend to keep hold of more of the menstrum. Starting with one litre expect around 750ml as the finished product. Keep a record of the use of alcohol amount and concentration with date and remedy used.

Fresh plant tinctures
Start with a 1:5 extraction using twice the fresh herb to one litre menstruum. The alcohol content needs to be increased to 45% because the water in the herb will require the extra alcohol. Failure to take this into account will create a water saturate mixture and leave less alcohol in the final mixture – mould will grow if there is not a minimum 25% alcohol in the final product.

Prescription example

Make up medicine 100ml for a patient with anxiety.
Px
Scutellaria 40, Dioscorea 10, Passiflora 40, Elettaria to 100 ml
Sig 5mls TDS aq cal pc. Mitte 100ml.
[This equates to 5ml thrice daily in warm/hot water after food].
Dispense in an amber glass bottle with a label to give clear instructions.

Liquidum extractum [Liquid extract/Fluid extract]
Liquid extracts are made using a similar process as in tincture making.

Method to prepare a liquid extract using 25% alcohol.
Exactly the same as for the tincture. The only difference is the amount used.
Remedy to be used 1000g [1k]. Alcohol 250ml. Aqua 750ml. Mix together.

Herbal Medicine - Keys

There are two methods of extraction of the marc. One method is the same as the tincture. The second is by percolation. A percolator is funnel shaped with a tap at the lower end. Large enough to hold 1 kilo of material and the menstrum. After macerating the marc is transferred into the percolator together with all the menstrum. The tap is opened and allowed to drip through slowly; 120 drops per minute. Once the menstrum has passed through pour more menstrum over the marc until 1000ml have passed. Always add extra menstrum slowly and at the same concentration as that started with. Filter, bottle and label. The advantage of using the percolator means that 1000ml is extracted – there is no waste. The exhausted marc can be used with glycerine or syrup to further extract and make a syrup.

External prescriptions

Individual external prescriptions are found under the chapter for which you are seeking e.g. eye lotions & ointments chapter 17. Inhalations chapter 18. Chapter 21 for enemas and emulsions. Chapter 26 dermal preparations.

Dressings

Green surgical dressing for wounds
Poultice the area with the appropriate remedy or cover wound with sterile gauze, medicament and a dressing. [See chapter emergency herbal medicine].
Sterile dressing – when a sterile dressing is unobtainable a freshly laundered sheet is considered sterile and will be suitable for cutting up to required sized dressings.

Emplastrum [plasters]

Preparation method 1.
The following can be used to incorporate medication for dermal absorption.
Plaster base

Beeswax	50g
Castor oil/Sunflower oil	25ml
Anhydrous lanolin	25g
Soft paraffin	100g

Melt and mix together. Add the LE or powdered remedy and mix together. Use an open wove cotton bandage which can be put into the warmed and fluid base and slowly withdraw. The bandage will soak up the base with medicament. Allow to cool on a flat surface and roll up ready for use. Strips can be cut to the required size for use.
Method 2
Powdered or crushed fol, herba or rad. Moisten dry material. Place inside muslin and apply.

Pharmacy

Medications for emplastrum
Calendula, Althea, Symphytum. [See emergency section for more remedies].

Fixed oils
Fixed oils used in herbal practice are of vegetable origin and consist of triglycerides of glycerol.
Fixed oils carry medicaments and are often used as liniments, dermatological agents as an emollient or vulnerary.
Oleum [oils]
Almond, Arachis [peanut], Coconut, Cottonseed, Linum, Olive, Rape, Ricinus, Safflower, Sesame, Soya, Sunflower.

Inhalations. [See Chapter 18].
Liniment. [See Chapter 27].

Pessaries
Use an 2 gram pessary mould. Melt powdered cocoa butter/gelatine on a water bath. Add the medicament and stir. Lubricate the moulds with almond oil and pour in the mix. Leave to cool.
Sig Advise - insert one pessary three or four times daily.

Poultice
Applied to the skin or joint to encourage local dermal or rubefacient activity.
Method
Put powdered, cut or crushed herb into muslin. Dried herb must be mixed with water or oil. Broken skin must have a sterile dressing.
Suitable medicaments for poulticing are:
Althea, Arnica, Calendula, Chamomilla, Humulus, Hypericum, Linum usit., Stellaria, Symphytum, Ulmus.

Powder [Pulv]
Powder can be used in capsules or teas. The delivery to contact medicine time is short due to the fibrous material having been crushed. Powders do not keep as well as tinctures. Once the cell walls have been crushed the important volatile constituents are lost fairly quickly.

Spray [Aerosol spray]
Compound Tincturae Benzoin Tincture Benzoin compound spray. 15% with alcohol @ 25%.

Aerosol spray: for reducing skin sensitivity, irritation, infections and as a vulnerary – chilblains, dermal ulcers, eczema, fissure, gingivitis, herpes, nipple fissure, eczema, wounds [formula see Styrax benzoin].

Suppositories
Preparation
Example one using Glycero gelatine. Glycero gelatine combines easier mixing with a liquid extract. First make a glycero gelatine base using powdered gelatine, glycerine and water one part of each. Lubricate the moulds with almond oil. Then mix three parts [60%] of base with two parts [40%] of the medicament. Run into moulds and allow to set. Keep cool.

Example two using Theobroma oil. Melt Theobroma Oil and mix in medicament.

Example three using chocolate. Obtain sugar free cooking chocolate [Theobroma]. Break up the pieces and warm until soft. Mix with the medicament and run into moulds. Add the medicament: powder add 40% volume to the mix, essential oil [add 1gtt to each mould] or liquid extract 40% allow to cool. Chocolate can be used as a faster method – just melt.
The mould used is 1 gram size [15grains].

Local medicaments for use in suppositories
Belladonna extract, Conium extract, Hamamelis extract, Lobelia extract, and Solanum dulcamara.

Soothing haemorrhoidal preparations
Anodyne for painful conditions – anal fissure, cystitis, vomiting, colic, diverticulitis, colitis, proctitis, haemorrhoids, anxiety.

Suppositorium Hamamelis [Hamamelis Suppository]
LE Hamamelis 0.33ml
Glycero gelatine base
Mix and pour into a mould.

34
Pharmacology

Bioavailability Oral drug delivery.
Variation in the serum level of the drug [herbal medicine] apart from patient individuality, disease severity and level of vital force, the difference in remedy action/response is due to variation in the metabolic handling.

How much drug reaches the target site is dependent upon two factors:

solubility and absorption

Drug metabolism of the [herbal medicine] before absorption depends upon:

[1] surface of the intestine/gut motility
[2] inside of the intestinal cell walls/enzymes
   Medicines are more effective in some patients and not in others with the same condition – one factor determining the clinical response to medicine is the ability of the patient's digestive system to degrade the product to liberate bioactive low molecular compounds from repeating polymers
   263, 1991 57 [4] 299-304.
[3] liver function – high metabolic rate – loss of drug by liver enzyme mechanisms.
[4] alcohol/food intake
[5] pH and remedy form - molecular size and solubility

Variation in the serum level occurs with the following
Distribution
Binding to serum – some of the remedy will bind to blood protein, the unbound free particles would then become active in the body. The half life of the remedy is determined by the rate of metabolism and excretion of that remedy.

Metabolism
Remedy group
                    - hydroxyl
                    - carboxyl - conjugated to from glucuronide [an etheral sulphate]
or a glycine/acetyl derivative.

Remedies lacking the above group will be:
oxidised, dealkylated, deaminated, hydroxylated with subsequent conjugation.

Pharmacology

Excretion

When disease of the **liver** exists medicines will be broken down more slowly and can lead to more plasma bound drug affecting the tissue.
Renal excretion, if impaired would allow a build up of remedy particles within the blood. Actual **renal** disease can lead to protein loss in the blood, the loss of protein increases the proportion of active remedy within the body.

Mechanisms of drug absorption are:

molecular and
cellular

Diffuse across lipid membrane of intestine – diffusion
Carrier mediated – active or passive [passive is the most important].
Paracellular – filtration through pores
Endocytosis – particles are engulfed by cells of the bowel wall.

A molecule passes between cells not affected by cell enzymes. It may pass neatly across the intestinal barrier. Bioavailability of the drug compound is assisted by increasing the process by getting the cell to accept the compounds.
Endocytosis has a minor quantity role. Drugs entering the endosome system are macromolecules. The lysozyme system destroys the drug. Lysozyme enzyme is further activated in intestinal hurry. Hepatic enzymes act upon some drugs and alter their chemical structure and assist remedy particles to enter the tissue fluid as a simpler substance. Some remedies are not converted but remain unaltered. Hepatic enzymes induce or inhibit the remedies action.
Serum estimation of drug level tell us little about the amount crossing over the membrane. Blood entering the liver in the portal circulation carry remedy particles to be acted upon by liver enzymes. Some of the drug will enter the liver cells.
Alcohol slows down the emptying of the stomach contents into the intestine. Alcohol is absorbed in the stomach.
After food or drink absorption of the drug will be delayed because the remedy becomes diluted. Few remedies are absorbed by the stomach. Most remedies will be absorbed from the small intestine. Some remedies are not absorbed but act by reflex action via a nerve plexus or mucous membrane connections.
pH - in solution remedies are weak acids or weak bases.

Insitu perfusion technique
Cellular level – common technique, cell culture system. Cells are grown in a chamber and the transport of molecules across the cell layer can be measured.

Pharmacology

Advantages of a cell culture system: human cells used for screening
measured resistance
runs for several hours [12]
Disadvantages: no mucus
very slow rates of growth

Monitoring a sugar – marker molecule, transports across the wall and it crosses in a linear fashion with concentration apparent permeability.
Polymers enhance absorption to increase the absorption of the drug.

Some drugs have absorption windows in the gut and some drugs enter only through certain windows. If there is poor absorption then make substances hang around longer. Small intestinal transit time is 2/3 hours. So an increase in the transit time could make substances stick to the intestinal wall. Absorption is enhanced.
Lectin is a plant protein. Lectin binds to the surface of intestinal rings. Uptake by sacs of the intestine to tissue was increased as a compound, compared to a control by endocytosis.

Remedy form
Tablets have to be dissolved in the stomach and intestinal fluid. Large tablets dissolve more quickly than smaller ones. The hardness of the tablet affects its solubility. Fluid medication would absorb faster than tablets. Infusions and decoctions produce readily available mixtures of sufficient strength to give reliable results in the tissues. Even a high gum resin within the plant will be sufficiently soluble in boiling water to give the desired effect. It is possible to extract enough gum resin for tissue medication.

What are medicines ?
Healing effects of any medicine is dependent upon three factors.
1] The solubility and absorption of the medicine.
2] Active constituents within the plant.
3] Uptake, utilisation and beneficial effect to produce a healing action within the tissues.

The active constituents are standardised in the preparation of some herbal extracts. While this will give a certain effect it is questionable whether the standardised remedy is appropriate for the condition being treated. Standardised remedies are based upon only known constituents. Once a single constituent is used as a base for medication it is the writers view that a medication is changed by this approach. It is the whole plant which creates the tissue change towards health. A single constituent is wholly certain in it's action and becomes orthodox in this approach with subsequent side effects. The whole herb is preferable in treatment. Whether as a solid extract, simple, Tr or Le - all the required elements of the drugs action from the plant are balanced and give a better action for the patient.

Pharmacokinetics
Plasma concentrations of medicine determine its activity. Two models describe the pharmacokinetic data - these are compartment and non compartment types. Plasma is viewed as one large compartment within the body. The compartment has input and output channels for the medicine.
The volume of medicine has variable levels within the plasma. Tissue concentration and distribution provides an estimate of the amount of remedy within the tissues. Plasma – 4 litres. Interstitial fluid – 13 litres. Intracellular fluid – 28 litres. It follows that the amount of medicine required to activate a target tissue will need clearance through the gastro intestinal tract and liver. Volume distribution is dependent upon the volume of fluid within the tissue analysed.
Non compartmental models as shown within the whole body, show the elimination rate of the medicine under observation. The estimated oral clearance is 30 litres per hour for many of the medicines described in this work. Dose administered is every 4-8 hours. Multiple dosing of medicine must take into account the plasma concentration. Plasma level is determined by dose, dose interval and oral clearance.

To determine the required dose of medicine - known as the Emax model.
Using 15 micrograms [15uM] as a test dose of medicine. We arrive at the following result whereby an average of 1.3g per dose is required every 8 hours. However for practical purposes a four hourly routine is adopted. Phenolic compounds are eliminated between 4-9 hours. When longer dosing intervals are used it is necessary to increase the dose.

Using *Hypericum* as an example for molecular absorption. The dose level of 300mg, 900mg and 1800mg represent examples used as test doses. It was found that hypericin and pseudohypericin plasma concentration was active within 30 minutes of ingestion and continued for six hours. Both compounds exhibited interesting results. Pseudohypericin is found in higher levels than hypericin. However pseudohypericin plasma levels were lower than those of hypericin. Tissue levels are higher in the GIT within one and half hours falling after 6 hours.

Concentrations of compounds - hypericin and pseudohypericin, in the tissues.
The times given represent a level of action in various tissues.
GIT - active within 1 and maximum activity up to 5 hours. Maximum level at 4½ hours.

Pharmacology

Liver - maximum action at 6 hours after ingestion.
Kidney - maximum action at 6 hours after ingestion.
Muscle - maximum level at 6 hours.
Blood - maximum level at 6 hours.
Brain - maximum level at 6 hours.
The half life of a 300mg dose was 10 hours, while that for 1800mg was 21 hours.

Whole fresh plant extracts
Analysis of fresh plant extracts made within two hours of harvesting gives interesting results.
Of the herbs tested, all produced, in the fresh plant extracted and then analysed by spectroscopy, increased levels of active constituents.
Fresh *Echinacea* alkylamide content was 79.9 and in the dried 30.
Fresh *Crataegus* procyanidins content was 330 and in the dried 270. The stability of procyanidins remained constant in the fresh berries over 2 years storage. Whereas in the frozen and dried berries kept for 2 years there was a marked reduction in the procyanidins.
Fresh *Symphytum* rad allantoin content was 1.1 and in the dried 0.34. Pyrrolizidine alkaloids were also found in greater quantities in the fresh plant, these could be removed from the final product.
Fresh *Valeriana* essential oil content 1050 and in the dried 630. Valerianic acid derivatives fresh plant 230 and dried 170.
Fresh *Achillea* millefoleum essential oil content was 0.436 and dried 0.349.
Fresh Hypericum gave interesting results - flavonoid glycosides 1.94 and dried 2.47. Flavonoid aglycones fresh 0.814 and dried 0.870. Dianthrones fresh 0.140 and dried 0.150.
Fresh *Chamomilla* recutita essential oil content 98 and dried 86. Matricine fresh plant 97 and dried 29. Bisabolol fresh plant 100 and dried 97. Apigenin-7-glycoside 105 and dried 100.

Standardisation of the extracts depends upon controlled organic growth techniques. Batch pooling will help to minimise the variables of growth changes within the plant. In this paper one years batch pooling of extracts was carried out [134].

When a remedy is standardised upon a certain constituent there is a danger the other constituents would become out of balance within the preparation. The part of the plant being used is more appropriately extracted into the menstrum and macerated for ten days. Pressed or centrifuged to give a first class product standardised as nature intended. An example of a centrifuge is a small spin drier. The herbs and menstrum are put into a pillow case and the unit switched on. The extract is collected and filtered. Much easier than using a press and it is often faster than pressing. Mixing batches could provide improved efficacy.

Randomised, double blind, placebo-controlled trials 'Only 5 randomised, double blind, placebo-controlled trials have been found. Three trials found a positive effect of the herb compared with placebo, whereas the other two did not. One explanation for the negative findings is that these trials used extracts standardised for the concentration of parthenolides, thought to be Tanacetum [Feverfew's] active constituents. This could suggest that other compounds found in whole leaf preparations may be important - a potential blow to those who are promoting standardisation as the way forward in herbal medicine' [Lancet 1999].

Healing agents
Only those medicines which are herbal are covered in this work. No inference is given to synthetic drugs. If it is at all possible to heal the patient then herbal medicines are to be used. When improvement is not forthcoming after a reasonable time, [some improvement in the condition should be possible within four - six weeks in a chronic condition and within minutes or hours in an acute state, it may be necessary to consider using tissue salts 6x strength or Celloids. Celloids are produced by Blackmores. Tissue salts/Celloids are essential to correct cellular deficiencies.

Long term healing effects
Medicines act to restore the functional balance, promote elimination of toxins and rebuild the tissue [trophorestoration].
Functional balance utilises tonics and trophorestoratives. Elimination is always central to physiomedicalism. The elimination of toxins is paramount in the healing process. Where treatment is continued for some time, over three months, tissue cleansing and improvement in organ status will occur. So the longer the patient takes the medication the better are the chances of recovery. Even if the condition cannot be totally allayed at least the patient will be stronger and more able to cope with the condition that they have.

Detoxification
Hepatic and renal disturbances affect the way remedies are broken down and eliminated. Impaired function could lead to the cumulative effects of substances in the blood.

Pharmacokinetic interactions
Certain medicines contain constituents which act upon Cytochrome p450 [CYP]. CYP is a drug metabolising enzyme and is found in human liver microsomes. It is

Pharmacology

most fortunate that medicines like Allium sativum, Hypericum, Mentha piperita and Silybum have CYP ability to detoxify and rid the tissues of toxic substances.

Brain and nervous system

a] In the elderly patient brain atrophy occurs, which increase with age.
b] Significantly less neurotransmitters and fewer receptors are able to take up the medication.
c] Start with smaller doses of medication.
d] Memory deteriorates with age, one vital question is to find out if all the medication has been taken.
e] High blood concentrations of a medicine with a prolonged half life can occur with elderly patients.

Toxic effects

A yellow reporting card is now used by the profession for adverse reactions to medicines.

More potent medicines require for a level of caution to be observed in prescribing and observation of the patient. While the patient is advised to report any adverse reactions. When adverse reactions are reported at consultation the dose level is adjusted according to the condition, or the remedy is changed to one more suitable.

Finding the correct dose

Dosages are given in the pharmacopoeia for the specific medication being used. When one medicine is used it may be given to full dosage, or reduced if required, a useful rule is to start with the minimum possible dose to avoid cellular abreaction and build up the dose as improvement occurs. When more than one remedy is used in a compound prescription the dosage is adjusted accordingly. Carrier remedies are utilised by the vital force to take the other healing medicines in the prescription to their location. Agrimonia acts upon the stomach, intestine, kidneys and liver. The effect is bound to the organ area by combination with direct acting medicines e.g. Agrimonia with Berberis - liver/gall bladder, with Barosma – renal system, with Gentiana – stomach, Juglans – intestine. Other remedies can be given depending upon the preference and the effect.

Prescribing and dispensing contra indications

It is preferable to prescribe the medication together with a food regime as the quality and amount of food will enhance the medication. Much is spoken about of the incompatibility of drugs and herbal medicines. Whenever possible avoid the concurrent use of synthetic drugs. Where it is not possible care must be taken to make sure the herbal prescription and synthetic drugs are compatible.

Herbal Medicine - Keys

Plant properties
Priest comments 'the purpose of the physiomedical fluid extract is to represent the plant properties in their normal proportions, not to produce a preparation selective of the supposedly active constituents'.

Incompatibles
Avoid dispensing:
Alkaloids with tannins as precipitation is produced.
Digitalis with tannins.
Mixing a liquid extract with water causes precipitation.
Oils with water.

Precipitation
Prescription precipitation is commonly found and will not disadvantage the medication in any way. Except where alkaloidal or high resinous medications are prescribed which can precipitate, when it is necessary to suspend the resinous particles in an even suspension – an emulsion Powdered Compound Gum Tragacanth is used in the process.

Tragacanth Co. Compound Tragacanth powder
Powdered Tragacanth 50g
Powdered Acacia   50g
Powdered starch   50g
Powdered sucrose   150g
Mix together and use as required. Store in airtight containers.

Method
Mix the herbal medicines together. Using a pestle and mortar triturate a small amount of the medication with the compound Tragacanth powder. This makes a creamy mixture, then add the rest of the medication and continue to triturate. All the ingredients of the medication will be evenly suspended in the mixture.
Advise shake the bottle before use.
Medicines requiring suspension are Commiphora, Guaiacum, Myroxylum balsamum [Tolu], Podophyllum, Stryax benzoin.

Sterilisation method
Boiling
Boiling is not considered a safe practice to remove pathogenic organisms.
Soap
For washing of hands.
Alcohol
Suitable to clean and disinfect instruments e.g. isopropyl alcohol, surgical spirit.

Pharmacology

<u>Chemical</u>
Spores have been shown to grow in Savlon antiseptic.
<u>Herbal</u>
Essential oils that have been diluted e.g. Thymus, Szygium can be used to sterilise.
<u>Autoclave</u>
Preferred method to sterilise.
Autoclaving in a pressure cooker for 15 minutes will destroy micro-organisms.

Autoclave Method for medication, dressings, instruments etc.

- Put the nebulae, collyr, ung, crem, medication, into Pyrex glass or plastic containers and label.
- Put cotton wool, bandages, dressings into sealed waterproof paper bags and label.

Method
Add water, bring to pressure, turn down the heat and allow to gently simmer for 15 minutes. Result is a sterile product, free from pathogenic micro-organisms.

Professional autoclaves are available for purchase within clinics.

35
PRACTITIONERS PHARMACOPOEIA

Important note
The dosages given are standardised to the preparation being used.
Thus: **Infusions [Infusium] are 1:20**
         Decoction [Decoctum] are 1:20
         Tinctures [Tincturae] are 1:5
         Liquid extracts [Liquidum extractum] are 1:1
                                        [also called fluid extracts].

When dosage is mentioned this is a - <u>**maximum single dose at any one time**</u>.
Usual dosage for chronic conditions is three [TDS] or four times [QDS] daily
with dosing every 15 minutes in acute cases. Thurston was aware that alcohol
was toxic and it was considered beneficial to remove it from the final medication.
The most potent medication is considered to be the hot aqueous infusion or
decoction. Mills and Bone explain - glycosides in an *aqueous* preparation convert
to aglycones in the large bowel thus becoming more bio available. When alcohol
is used as menstrum use as lower level as possible - alcohol is hepatotoxic.
Modern science again confirms physiomedical viewpoints.

This Pharmacopoeia contains 420 medicines. Remedy constituents are not
conclusive as only information currently known has been added. The aim of the
pharmacopoeia is to give the physiomedical orientations of the particular remedy.
While researching this work one herbalist exclaimed with vigour to the writer
'how did the old physiomedicalists know that a medicine would work in a
particular way?' This was a thought provoking question how could they know
when at that time chemistry was in its infancy stage – the answer lies in the fact
that the clinicians of those days took elaborate case histories and similar to the
homeopathic drug pictures, built up a repertory of symptoms for that herbal
medicine. Modern analytical methods in chemistry and pharmacy continues to
prove the activity of plants used as medicines through the action of its
constituents. Take Foetida for instance as stated by Cook; used as a diffusive
relaxant, we now know this to mean an antispasmodic whereby the essential
volatile oil is antispasmodic.
Where inflammation is mentioned the word anti inflammatory is not used as it
suggests that inflammation is a disease producer this is not so, therefore the term
'allays inflammation' is used instead. The scientific term for blood cleansing
medicines is <u>vasotonic alterative</u> previously known as <u>alterative</u>. Several
medicines listed are potent and often indicated for acute medical emergencies, it is
required that further training on the use and application to prescribing habit is
necessary for full appreciation of the medicine together with its full effects.

Practitioners Pharmacopoeia

Medicines subject to restrictions are to be prescribed with care. All prescribed medicines are to be diluted and taken with water.

The Pharmacopoeia analysis of each medicine is as follows:
- Remedy name in Latin.
- Constituents.
- Primary pharmacological action is considered under this heading.
- Therapeutic classes - other actions enhancing the whole plant.
- Medicinal indications - are the conditions presenting. Medical Astrology.
- Tissue conditions - explains how the remedy works at a tissue level.
- Cautions - contra indications of the remedy.
- External use - preparations for the body cavities, musculoskeletal and skin.
- Preparations where combination of remedies is useful. Compounds and mixtures are included in this section.
  Also see Chapters 17-30 & 33 for preparations.
- Dosage - **given as a maximum** <u>single dose.</u>

The Pharmacopoeia contains medicines used in practice and accepts the facts of biological remedy activity. Activity and actions can be checked from pharmacological sources. Bibliography contains the herbal books used in this work as References – namely Felter, Cook, Ellingwood, Priest, Potters, Bartram, Grieve, BP, BHP, Pharmaceutical Codex and The Extra Pharmacopoeia - Martindale 27th edition. If further scientific proof is required by the reader refer to the end of the pharmacopoeia. Several medicines may be unfamiliar to the reader and occasionally these are unobtainable. It is hoped that unfamiliar medicine monographs are used for further research.

Mills and Bone have taken some orthodox principles and use these as relevant for a modern herbalist e.g. 'essential hypertension where there is no known cause'. Such a statement clearly shows the need for an holistic approach to the cause of hypertension unfortunately lost in the Mills and Bone book. Look at the aetiology of hypertension and treat accordingly because there is always a cause for any sustained rise in blood pressure. Physiomedically speaking Priest explains the requirement to clear obstructions within the eliminative organs as capillary obstruction causes congestion within the organ and its inability to eliminate impurities. The organ disturbance and resulting impurities are the <u>cause</u> of the hypertension. Quotes from Weiss are also interesting whereby he says that full doses are required for digitalisation of the patient. Gill says the major reason for Digitalis overdosage is that the dose is too high and therefore causes toxicity. All the literature tells the prescriber to give a loading dose of Digoxin which is often too high and immediately puts the patient into a toxic condition repeating the dose encourages further toxicity. Weiss is seen by some as an authority on herbal medicine but it must be realised he is an orthodox doctor prescribing herbs. There are major differences between holistic physiomedical herbalism and orthodox herbalism. You will read of conditions in this work that are no longer treated by medical herbalists. In the past all conditions were treated successfully by medical herbalists as there was no other form of treatment available. Successive governments have continued to strip the profession of its lawful and God given right to treat all disease conditions and to use all herbal medicines with discretion. The government agencies cite toxic effects of herbal medicines, while doctors are allowed to prescribe freely any poison they wish. There are several toxic medicines listed in the pharmacopoeia, it is considered by medical herbalists that such medicines be used in treatment as the benefits far outweigh the risks associated with prescribing of the medication.

Dosage of an individual medicine will be found in
[1] Practitioners Pharmacopoeia and
[2] the quick reference guide to dosage [Chapter 39].

Practitioners Pharmacopoeia

To navigate the Pharmacopoeia an example follows to make it easier for you to quickly read the monograph.

> Name of medicine

Acorus calamus [Sweet flag]

> Main constituents of the medicine

Constituents
Volatile oil - asarone. Amines. Terpenes –
eugenol, Humulene, Tannin 1.5%.
Bitters. Resin. 2.5%. Mucilage.

> Primary activity

Primary pharmacological action
Carminative, aromatic and stomachic tonic.

> Classes of activity of the medicine

Therapeutic classes
Antimicrobial. Sialagogue.
Aperitif. Carminative. Breath freshener.
Diuretic. Diaphoretic. Antiperiodic.
CNS sedative – gentle. Antispasmodic to smooth
muscle. Antineoplastic. Tobacco habit.

> Indications for use - from head to foot, through the systems

Medicinal indications
Halitosis. Anorexia. Debility. Flatulence.
Dyspepsia. Gastritis. Gastric ulcers. Gastric
atony. Gastric carcinoma. Nausea. Intestinal colic.

How the medicine works within the tissues - at a cellular level

Tissue conditions
Used in atony [loss of tone] or spasmodic conditions of the stomach. Stimulates saliva and gastric secretions. It tones the gastric mucous membrane and muscle layer. Prevents griping. Helps to antidote the effects of smoking due to its bitter taste.

External use With advice upon how to use the preparation

External use
Application to burns, scalds, ulcers.

Useful mixtures with other medicines

Preparations
Althea, Acorus and Gentian form a strong tonic prescription.
Stomach ulcerations use with Cetraria.
Intestinal antiseptic combine with Zingiber.

Dosage of medicine, with the part used. Dried/powder/infusion. decoction/tincture/liquid extract/liniment etc.

Dosage and mode of application
Dried rad Sig 3g
Decoctum 30ml
Tincturae Sig 4ml
Liquidum extractum Sig 3ml

Practitioners Pharmacopoeia

Citations of available research listing key clinical studies of the medicine. The writer conducted an exhaustive review of literature from around the world including rare research studies.

References.
BPC 1934. 43 p13. 142 p44. 246 p548.

Practitioners Pharmacopoeia

Abies alba [Silver fir]

Constituents
Resin. Volatile oil.

Primary pharmacological action: Rubefacient.

Therapeutic classes
Antiseptic. Anticatarrhal. Expectorant. Circulatory stimulant.
Diuretic.
Medicinal indications
Antiseptic in gum disorders. Catarrh. Chest infections.
Haemorrhoids.
Genito urinary disorders. Rheumatic affections. Impetigo.
External use
Respiratory disorders applied as a liniment.
Rheumatic disorders - liniment.
Impetigo – apply an oil.
Dosage and mode of application
Inhalation of volatile oil.
Linimentum Abies resin.
References. 127 p635.

Abrus precatoreus [Jequirity bean seed]

Constituents
The seed contains Abrin which is a toxic glycoprotein it is inactivated by heat - boiling at 100 C for 30 minutes. Flavonoids - abracatorin. Indole alkaloids. Phytosterols.
Medicinal indications
Ophthalmic. Fungicide. Anti microbial - Staphylococcus aureus, Shigella dis. Vermifuge.
Antineoplastic. Oxytocic
Therapeutic classes
Eye inflammation. Conjunctivitis granuloma. Trachoma.
Coughs, hoarseness, bronchial constriction.
Constipation. Colic.
Adrenal stimulant.
Epithilioma of the face, vulva, vagina and skin.
Abortifacient. Both the excitatory and inhibitory substances are uterotonic. Seed infusion hastens labour. Crushed seeds are used as a vaginal pessary to induce abortion. [124/5].
Entire plant decoction - venereal disease and snake bites. Effects upon smooth muscle. Inhibitory substance in low concentrations relaxes smooth muscle and stimulates uterine muscle. Excitatory effect of the glycoside [a pyridinium moiety] in high concentrations.
Tissue Conditions
The seed has been used for skin cancer. The seed oil is a uterine contractant. Poisoning has occurred with ingestion of the unripe or chewed seeds. No neuronally resident substance mediated the inhibitory action on the uterus.
Cautions
Restrictions apply. Dosage is determined by the relief of symptoms.
Dosage and mode of application
Collyr 1:12
Contraceptive –
a single dose 200mg of the powdered seeds give up to 13 months protection.
References. 127 p492. 189 p159.

Acacia catechu [Black catechu]

Constituents
Tannin - Catechin. Catechu tannic acid and acecatechin. Indole alkaloids.
Flavonoids.

Primary pharmacological action: Astringent.

Medicinal indications
Hypotensive.
Dermatological agent. Vulnerary. Anti fertility activity.
Therapeutic classes
Chronic catarrh. Pharyngitis. Epistaxis – as a snuff.
Relaxed spongy, sore gums. Aphthous ulcers. Tonsillitis. Dysentery. Diarrhoea.
Vaginal discharge/leucorrhoea. Menorrhagia. Nipple fissures. Gonorrhoea.
Cutaneous eruptions. Furunculosis. Ulcers.
Tissue conditions
Astringent without stimulation. Soothing demulcent for all irritated conditions of
the mucous membranes of the stomach, intestines, renal and respiratory systems.
Acacia is applicable in excessive and passive relaxations of the mucous
membranes e.g. catarrhs, spongy gums, aphthous ulcers, tonsillitis, pharyngitis.
Hepatitis. Acacia is used as a suspending agent.
External use
Powder for external application to ulcers, furunculosis, cutaneous eruptions.
Gonorrhoea - use a urethral injection.
Haemorrhoids - use the enema.
Dosage and mode of application
Powdered cort Sig 5g
Tincturae Sig 5ml
Acacia mucilage
Pwd Acacia with water 1:16 is used as an internal drink to allay inflammation.
Acacia syrup. Acacia 10g, sucrose 80g, aqua to 100ml
References
43 p53. 176 p192 p62/64. 262 p67.

Acacia senegal [Acacia gum]

Constituents
Gum Arabic is a glycosidal acid. Mucilage. The powder gum is used as a
suspending agent for medicines.

Primary pharmacological action:
Emulsifier to suspend medicines and for tablet preparation.

Therapeutic classes
Demulcent. Allays inflammation. Anti infective.
Anticholesterolaemic.
Medicinal indications
Colds. Coughs.
Oral plaque. Periodontal infection. Dysentery and diarrhoea.
Renal failure. Gonorrhoea.
Burns. Sore nipples. Leprosy.
Tissue conditions
Used as a demulcent for irritable and inflammatory conditions of any mucous
membrane.
Lowers serum urea nitrogen concentration.
Preparations
Recommended as a nutrient in malaria.
Inflammation with Althea or Glycyrrhiza.
External use
Dental plaque – chew gum.
Nodular leprosy and local inflammation.
Dosage and mode of application
Linctus
6% Acacia Syrup 74ml Aqua Auranti 20ml
Cough linctus Sig 15ml
Syrup Acacia
Gum Acacia 25% Syrup 75%
Employed as demulcent in linctus for mucous membrane inflammation-Sig 15ml
Cholesterolaemia Sig up to 50g daily
References
189 p1. 192 p261-262.

Achillea millefoleum [Yarrow]

Constituents
Volatile oil up to 1.4% containing azulene [allay inflammation]. A and beta
pinines. Sesquiterpine lactones [guaianolides], achilleine. Sesquiterpene lactones
[antibacterial, cytotoxic] are converted to chamazuline. Flavonoids - spasmolytic,
diuretic and hypotensive. Achilleine is haemostatic [given IV]. Thujone.
Alkaloids - betonicine, stachydrine, trigonelline. Sterols. Tannin up to 4%,
condensed. Amino acids. Vitamin C.

Primary pharmacological action:
Stimulating diaphoretic and tonic.

Therapeutic classes
Allays inflammation. Vasotonic alterative. Astringent. Antiscorbutic.
Antibacterial - Bacillus subtillus, Escherichia coli, Mycobacterium smegmatis,
Shigella flaxneri, Staphylococcus aureus.
Haemostatic - venous or contusion haemorrhage. Hypotensive. Peripheral
vasodilator.
Carminative. Aromatic bitter. Choleretic. Cholagogue.
Diuretic. Urinary antiseptic. Diaphoretic. Antipyretic.
Emmenagogue.
Antispasmodic. Vulnerary. Dermatological agent.
Medicinal indications [Venus]
Epistaxis. Hypertension. Thrombosis - vascular, cerebral, coronary.
Varicose veins.
Colds. Night sweats. Influenza. Pyrexia.
Anorexia. Dyspepsia. Diarrhoea. Dysentery. IBS. Haemorrhoids.
Amenorrhoea. Dysmenorrhoea. Menorrhagia. Vaginal discharge.
Intermittent fever. Pyrexia. Chicken pox. Measles.
Dermal inflammation. Wounds. Ulcers.
Tissue conditions
Mild, stimulating tonic. Used in treating the first stage of acute disease in hot
infusion it is a stimulating diaphoretic when the skin is cold and the pulse is weak.
Taken cold it tones the mucous membranes and stimulates the appetite. Relaxes
the gastro intestinal tract and relieves spasm and flatus.
Cautions
Contains thujone - not recommended in pregnancy.
Preparations
Pyrexia combine with Mentha piperita.
Haemorrhoids with Ranunculus and Verbascum.

External use
Many authorities suggest the fresh leaf poultice for dermal disorders.
Bruises and wounds – fomentation and/or poultice.
Psoriasis. Inflammation/Pain/Pyrexia – Balneum
Dosage and mode of application
Give the infusion in acute conditions.
Dried herba/flos. Sig 4g
Infusium Sig 2g
Tincturae Sig 10ml
Liquidum extractum Sig 4ml
Succus Sig 5ml
Balneum Sig 100g in muslin. Sitz [hip baths] are effective in supporting the removal of pelvic congestion – see the naturopathy chapter 16.
References
43 p145. 176 p355. 188 p459. 230 p105. 233 p227. 251 p163. 394 p419.

Acorus calamus [Sweet flag]

Constituents
Bitter volatile oil - up to 3%, acorin, asarone. Terpenes – eugenol, humulene.
Amines. Tannin up to 1.5%. Resin 2.5%. Mucilage.

Primary pharmacological action:
Carminative, aromatic and stomachic tonic

Therapeutic classes
Antimicrobial. Sialagogue. Aperitif. Carminative. Breath freshener.
Diuretic. Diaphoretic. Antiperiodic.
CNS sedative –gentle. Antispasmodic to smooth muscle. Antineoplastic.
Medicinal indications
Halitosis. Anorexia. Debility. Flatulence. Dyspepsia. Gastritis. Gastric ulcers.
Gastric atony. Gastric carcinoma. Nausea. Intestinal colic.   Tobacco habit.
Tissue conditions
Used in atony [loss of tone] or spasmodic conditions of the GIT. Stimulates saliva
and gastric secretions. It tones the gastric mucous membrane and muscle layer.
Prevents griping. Helps to antidote the effects of smoking due to its bitter taste.
External use
Application to burns, scalds, ulcers.
Preparations
Althea, Acorus and Gentian form a strong tonic prescription.
Stomach ulcerations use with Cetraria.
Intestinal antiseptic combine with Zingiber.
Dosage and mode of application
Dried rad Sig 3g
Decoctum 30ml
Tincturae Sig 4ml
Liquidum extractum Sig 3ml
References
BPC 1934. 43 p13. 111 p221. 142 p44. 189 p56. 246 p548.

Aconitum napellus [Aconite, Monkshood]

Constituents
Aconitine and di Terpenoid alkaloids.

Primary pharmacological action: Anodyne

Therapeutic classes
Ophthalmic. Allays inflammation. Pulmonary tonic.
Capillary astringent. Febrifuge.
Diuretic. Sedative. Anaesthetic – local.
Medicinal indications [Saturn]
Conjunctivitis and other inflammatory conditions of the eye.
Acute bronchitis. Pharyngitis. Laryngitis. Laryngismus stridulus. Acute
inflammation in pleurisy, pneumonia [1st stage]. Asthenic febrile and
inflammatory diseases.
Diminishes the force and rate of the pulse. Angina.
Reflex vomiting. Vomiting of pregnancy. Inflammation of the stomach, liver,
intestine, peritoneum and appendix. Cholera. Dysentery.
Nephritis.
Metritis. Mastitis. Amenorrhoea from cold of chill.
Meningitis. Spinal irritation. Neuralgia. Neuritis. Sciatica. Acute inflammatory
arthritis. Joint pain. Injury – bruising.
Tissue conditions
A circulatory and temperature controlling remedy. Stimulates the vagus with
subsequent vagal depression. Depresses the vasomotor centre. Professor Scudder
selects the remedy for dilated and atonic capillaries with enfeeblement or loss of
tone of the capillary circulation and pulse deficiencies it stimulates the circulatory
system to normal activity. Small frequent pulse with pyrexia is a direct indication
for its use. Inflamed mucous and serous membranes. Acute and irritable
conditions with pyrexia. Lowers the temperature and re establishes the secretions.
Helps prevent pneumonia resulting from complicated measles.
Cautions
Restrictions apply. Dosage is determined by the relief of symptoms.
Poisonous. Overdosage causes tingling of the tongue and mouth. Nausea and
vomiting. Intestinal spasm. Dyspnoea. Weak and irregular pulse. Cold and
clammy skin. Giddiness. Avoid in inadequate pyrexia.
Treatment give an emetic. Capsicum.

Pharmacopoeia

Preparations
Aphthous ulcers with Phytolacca.
Meningitis with Gelsemium. Cerebral congestion with Atropa.
Pleurisy with Asclepias.
Neuralgia and neuritis with Piper methysticum.
External use
Local anaesthetic in Pruritus. All painful rheumatic conditions, neuralgia, sciatica, joint injury causing pain.
Dosage and mode of application
Tincturae rad/fol. 5gtt aqua 120ml Sig 5ml
Tincturae 1:10 Sig 0.3ml [BPC 1949]
Linamentum Aconitum. Tincturae 2% qs Dist. Hamamelis to 100ml.
Ung 3%
References
43 p12. 126 p148. 176 p79. 188 p5. 189 p3. 224 p1716. 246 p114.

Adhatoda vasica [Malabar nut tree]

Constituents
Alkaloids up to 1% including Vasicine which is bitter. Essential oil.

Primary pharmacological action: Bronchodilator

Therapeutic classes
Vasotonic alterative. Expectorant. Antiallergic.
Diuretic.
Antispasmodic. Oxytocic - mild. Parturient. Uterine astringent tonic.
Medicinal indications
Asthma. Bronchitis. Bronchiectasis. Emphysema. Tuberculosis.
Gingivitis. Dyspepsia.
Post partum haemorrhage. Supports uterine sub-involution.   Intermittent fever.
Tissue conditions
Stimulating to the respiratory mucous membranes to soften thick sputum.
Cautions
Avoid in the early stages of pregnancy.
External use
Hair loss use an infusion as a lotion.
Periodontal disease - use the diluted LE.
Oxytocic effect may be increased by using a douche.
Preparations
Piper longum enhances effect.
Allergies with Euphrasia, Scutellaria baicalensis.
COPD – Euphorbia, Grindelia, Inula, Polygala or Verbascum.
Dosage and mode of application
Dried herba Sig 10g
Tincturae Sig 4ml
Liquidum extractum Sig 3ml
References
48 p91. 127 p506. 189 p182.

Adiantum pedatum [Maidenhair fern]

Constituents
Flavonoid glycosides. Rutin. Tannin. Mucilage. Terpenes.

Primary pharmacological action:
Demulcent with stimulating action to the mucous membranes.

Therapeutic classes
Anti tussive. Expectorant. Pectoral. Refrigerant [dect].
Galactagogue. Antipyretic.
Medicinal indications
Respiratory conditions - catarrh, laryngitis, influenza, bronchitis.
Detoxes alcohol. Pyrexia. Dandruff.
Tissue conditions
Leyel states it should be used fresh.
External use
Scalp tonic to improve hair growth and remove dandruff - lotion.
Dosage and mode of application
Dried herba Sig 2g
Infusium 10ml
Liquidum extractum Sig 2ml
References
43 p14. 111 p223. 148 p164. 188 p281. 246 p563.

Adonis vernalis [False hellebore, Golden pheasant's eye]

Constituents
Cardiac glycosides - Anodised, 16-hydroxy-strophanthidin [vasoconstrictor].

Primary pharmacological action: Cardiac tonic and diuretic.

Therapeutic classes
Antiepileptic.
Medicinal indications [Saturn]
Cardiac dyspnoea. Cardiac insufficiency, valvular incompetence - mitral stenosis
and oedema. Arrhythmia. Extrasystoles. Tachycardia. Endocarditis. Oedema.
Venous stasis from arterial insufficiency. Following myocardial damage. Raises
blood pressure. Nephritis.
Sedates ANS function. Epilepsy.
Tissue conditions
Adonis is cardio selective, it stimulates the vagus nerve, increasing arterial tension
[arterial contraction]. Motor stimulant. It slows the heart rate and is used for
arrhythmia. Heart strain from over exertion. Heart tonic for weak heart action -
feeble or irregular pulse with hypotension or venous congestion. Asthenics with
myocardial weakness.
External use
Local anaesthetic in chronic glaucoma, iritis and iridocyclitis use a 1% solution.
Cautions
Restrictions apply. Dosage is determined by the relief of symptoms.
Dosage and mode of application
Dried herba Sig 1g [Ref 390]
Infusium herba 1:40 Sig 15ml
Tincturae 1:5 Sig 0.9ml
Liquidium extractum Sig O.12ml
References
126 p156. 176 p233. 189 p141. 224. 288, Vol 4 No 3. April 1978.

Aesculus hippocastanum [Horse chestnut]

Constituents
Coumarins. Flavonoid glycosides - rutin [astringent]. Triterpene glycosides up to 6% as aescin [analgesic, antiviral]. Aescin binds to plasma protein where it protects against nephrotoxicity. Aescin, an astringent, inhibits elastase and hyaluonidase – these are both involved in enzyme protoglycan degradation. Condensed tannins. Allantoin. Sterols. Quinone.

Primary pharmacological action: Astringent and Absorbent.

Therapeutic classes
Allays inflammation. Antiexudative. Antioxidant. Immunemodulator.
Venous tonic in venous insufficiency of vascular disorders. Portal vein tonic.
Decreases capillary permeability.
Diuretic. Antioedematous. Prostatic tonic. Uterine tonic. Antirheumatic.
Vulnerary.
CNS stimulant. Febrifuge. Obstetric use as a venous tonic.

Medicinal indications
CVI. Phlebitis. Varicose veins. Spider veins. Venous congestion.
Deep vein thrombosis. Thrombophlebitis. Lower limb oedema. Heavy legs.
Respiratory disease.
Diarrhoea. Haemorrhoids – [including haemorrhoidal bleeds]. Proctitis [Rectal neuralgia]. Malaria.
Prostatic enlargement. Lymphoedema. Cramp.
Pain. Fatigue. Backache/strain. Rheumatism. Neuralgia.
Prolapsed disc. Ligamentous sprains and Strains.
Pruritus. Haematoma. Traumatic oedema. Intermittent fever. Breast soreness.

Tissue conditions
Half the remedy is excreted in 20 hours. Reduces vascular fragility and moderates inflammation leading to the absorption of excess extracellular oedema. Oedema from gingival haemorrhage, cranial fracture or trauma, meningitis, effusion around fractures. Dull aching pain from congested tissues with venous fullness. Increases leucocytes. Increases serum protoglycan hydrolase in patients with venous insufficiency. Indicated in venous insufficiency - portal congestion. Specific astringent to the rectal, pelvic and portal veins. Reduces painful haemorrhoids by astringent action.
The fruits have been used to treat rheumatism and neuralgia. Spinal injuries, strained muscles, sacroiliac strain. Uterine congestion, menorrhagia and cervical enlargement. Tones the skin, relieves cellulite and astringes veins when used dermally. Bells palsy where local inflammation and oedema compress the nerve.

Cautions

Avoid in pregnancy and breastfeeding.

External use

More effective than compression bandaging.

Reduces tenderness to pressure of haematomas.

Leg ulcers, contusions, haematoma, penetrating wounds, injuries with oedema, injuries to the ligaments or tendons:

Use as a cleansing and astringent wash then Gel.

Rheumatism and neuralgia.

Prolapsed disc – gel of concentrate LE direct upon the area.

Sunburn – ung.

Breast soreness – lotion.

Preparations

Combines with Hypericum in muscular strain and sprain.

Dosage and mode of application

Powdered sem. stripped of bark. Sig 2g

Dect. sem. Sig 15ml

Dry extract Sig 200mg

Tincturae sem Sig 10ml

Liquidum extractum sem Sig 2ml

Liquidum extractum cort Sig 4ml

References

111 p224. 126 p156. 176 p390. 179 p450. 192 p 277. 239 p128. 246 p227. 263, 1993, 59, no 5, p394. 270 6, 1996, p483. 271 no65, 1998. 394 p201.

Agaricus blazei [Sun mushroom]

Therapeutic classes
Bactericidal. Hypoglycaemic.
Anticholesterolaemic. Hypotensive. Antisclerotic.
Anti tumour. Immunostimulant.

Medicinal indications
Hypertension. Sclerotic arterial problems.
Diabetes.

External use
Used in burns and [acute radiation burns] ulcers and wounds.

Dosage and mode of application
Decoction Sig 30g
Succus Sig 25ml

Agrimonia eupatoria [Agrimony]

Constituents
Tannins up to 21%. Flavonols. Triterpenoids. Vitamin B2, C, K. Volatile oil.
Bitters.

Primary pharmacological action:
Mild astringent and gastro intestinal tonic.

Therapeutic classes
General tonic. A gentle tonic for all areas of the body. Antihaemorrhagic.
Anticatarrhal. Hepatic tonic. Antidiarrhoeal.
Diuretic. Renal tonic. Diaphoretic. Vulnerary. Antineoplastic.
Medicinal indications [Jupiter]
Pharyngitis. Laryngitis. Influenza. Bronchitis. Asthma. Tuberculosis.
Stomatitis. Aphthous ulcers. Stimulates the appetite. Hepatic atrophy and
cirrhosis. Jaundice. Diarrhoea. Dysentery. Visceral obstructions. Relaxed
intestines. Colitis.
Cystitis. Enuresis. Incontinence. Cystic or renal inflammation. Gout.
Skin eruptions - macules, papules, pustules. Malaria.
Tissue conditions
Agrimony aids remedies when an astringent action is required. It has a gentle
persistent action in catarrh as it astringes back excessive mucus.
For conditions of relaxation of the stomach and intestines with flatulence and
diarrhoea. A general tonic influence and supportive in urinary incontinence and
chronic inflammatory conditions of the bladder and kidneys accompanying deep
sediment with deep soreness and tenderness over the kidneys.
Sharp cutting deep seated pain in the lumbar region.
External use
Infusion used warm will soften hard ear wax.
Tonsillitis with Salvia.
Tonic mixture with Gentiana, Centarium, Jateorrhiza.
A wound herb used as a fomentation - ulcers.
Preparations
Agrimonia is expended to the stomach with other tonics. Intestinal mucous
membrane with hepatics in cases of diarrhoea and dysentery. Kidneys with renal
tonics/diuretics. Hepatic disorders with Centaurium and Berberis vulgaris.
Gargle for aphthous ulcers, inflamed mouth and throat.
Pyrexia in hot infusion.
With uterine remedies it relieves vaginal discharge/leucorrhoea.

Pharmacopoeia

External use
Externally for Tinea [ringworm] and ulcers.
Wounds, bruises and sprains.
Dosage and mode of application
Slow and persistent - the action is strengthened with other remedies.
Infusium herba Sig 4g
Tincturae Sig 4ml
Liquidum extractum Sig 3ml
References
6 p76. 43 p16. 111 p225. 176 p429. 246 p175. 251 p5. 289, 1993.

Agropyron repens [Couch grass]

Constituents
Contains around 10% mucilage - triticine is diuretic. Glucose and laevulose. Mannitol. Inositol. Gums and acids. An antibiotic essence formed from agropyrene present as a polysaccharide. Glucoside [glucovanillin]. Flavonoids - Tricin. Volatile oils - Agropyrene.

Primary pharmacological action: Demulcent diuretic.

Therapeutic classes
Vasotonic alterative. Stimulant. Haemostatic.
Aperient. Emollient.
Antirheumatic. Antineoplastic. Vulnerary.
Medicinal indications [Jupiter]
Jaundice.
Cystitis. Urethritis. Prostatitis. Prostatic hypertrophy. Renal calculi. Lithuria. Pyelitis. Gonorrhoea. Gout. Rheumatism.
Tissue conditions
A soothing, demulcent diuretic indicated whenever the urine causes irritation of the urinary system as in cases of cystitis, urethritis, prostatitis [both acute and chronic with enlargement, strangury and haematuria] and gonorrhoea. Renal calculi, lithuria with aching back, dysuria and tenesmus. Agropyron will remove uric acid, phosphates and gravel. Agropyron assists in the reduction of pyrexia.
Preparations
Combined with other genito urinary medicines activity is enhanced.
Cystitis/Prostatic enlargement with Barosma, Hydrangea.
Dosage and mode of application
Dried rhizome Sig 8g
Tincturae Sig 15ml
Liquidum extractum Sig 4ml
References. 43 p17. 188 p131. 189 p93. 246 p541.

Ajuga reptans [Bugle]

Constituents
Iridoid glycosides. Tannins.

Primary pharmacological action:
An aromatic and astringent tonic.

Therapeutic classes
Astringent. Antihaemorrhagic.
Cardioactive.
Bitter. Cholagogue. Laxative – mind.
Dermatological agent. Vulnerary.
Analgesic. Sedative.
Medicinal indications [Venus]
Slows and strengthens the pulse and equalises the circulation.
Allays coughs. Indicated for pulmonary haemorrhage [in TB].
Mild sedative action upon the stomach and nerves. Acts upon the gall bladder.
Bruising. Dermal ulcers.
Alcohol habit.
External use
Ulcers, wounds including stab wounds, haematomas and hernias - combine with
Sanicula [self heal], and Scabiosa [Devils bit Scabious].
Dosage and mode of application
Infusium herba Sig 30ml
Liquidum extractum Sig 4ml
References
189 p47. 228 p106. 246 p364. 262 p81.

Albizia lebbeck [Siris/Shirisha]

Constituents
Polyphenols. Saponins. Triterpenoids. Cardiac glycosides. Tannin.

Primary pharmacological action: Anti allergic.

Therapeutic classes
Antifungal. Antimicrobial. Bronchodilator.
Anticholesterolaemic.
Anthelmintic.
Medicinal indications
Gum inflammation. Allergic rhinitis. Asthma. Bronchitis. Hayfever.
Skin conditions - eczema, leprosy, pruritis.
Tissue conditions
Reduces the effects of allergens upon the mucosa thereby lessening the allergic
response. It has a better effect upon those with bronchoconstriction associated
with acute lung disease.
Inotropic effect upon the heart.
Intestinal smooth muscle relaxant.
External use
As an application in weeping eczema.
Dosage and mode of application
Powdered cort Sig 2g
Liquidum extractum Sig 3ml
References
48 p94. 271 No 71,1999.

Alchemilla vulgaris/mollis [Ladies mantle]

Constituents
Flavonoids. Tannin up to 6%.

Primary pharmacological action: Haemostatic.

Therapeutic classes
Astringent. Depurative. Tonic.
Emmenagogue. Uterine tonic. Febrifuge. Vulnerary.
Medicinal indications [Venus]
Circulatory tonic. Aids blood clotting in wounds.
Indicated for relaxed intestines with diarrhoea or enteritis. Specific in acute and epidemic diarrhoea.
Menorrhagia. Metrorrhagia. Progesterone effects. Fibroids. Pruritis vulvae.
Vaginal discharge/leucorrhoea. Tones the breasts.
Tissue conditions
Women's tonic enhancing conception.
External use
Haemostatic after tooth extraction – oral rinse.
Wounds – lotion.
Breast toner – lotion made from the infusium.
Vaginal discharge/leucorrhoea and pruritis vulvae – Douche.
Dosage and mode of application
Dried herba Sig 2g
Tincturae Sig 15ml
Liquidum extractum Sig 4ml
References
43 p19. 189 p166. 192 p 322. 251 p100.

Aletris farinosa [True unicorn root]

Constituents
Saponins. Volatile oil. Resin.

Primary pharmacological action: Stimulating uterine tonic.

Therapeutic classes
Stomachic. Bitter tonic. Flatulence. Colic.
CNS trophorestorative. Tonic.
Medicinal indications
Antinausea. Anorexia. Nervous dyspepsia.
Impotence/sexual dysfunction. Sterility. Prevents miscarriage. Promotes an easier confinement. Prevents subinvolution. Amenorrhoea. Dysmenorrhoea. Irregular menstruation.
Tissue conditions
Soothing to the stomach and relieves nausea, it stimulates the appetite. For atony of the uterus. Preventer of miscarriage, it can be given during any stage of pregnancy.
Preparations
Miscarriage with Viburnum species.
Dosage and mode of application
Dried rhizome Sig 0.6g
Liquidum extractum Sig 1ml
Elixir LE Aletris 0.25ml LE Glycyrrhiza 1ml Syrupus 3.75ml
Sig 5ml
References
43 p19. 126 p175. 176 p479. 188 p13/14. 189 p272.

Allium sativa [Garlic]

Constituents

Sulphur [around 1% dry weight] containing the amino acid – Alliin. Crushed bulb causes an enzyme reaction to create allinase. Allinase converts allinin to allicin [around 1.15%] or diallyl disulphide S oxide, imparting the typical garlic odour. Odourless preparations of Allium are less effective. The oleum stimulates the vagus to slow and strengthen the heart rate. Prostaglandins. Allicin acts upon neutrophils, platelets, vasomotor tone and lysosomal enzymes.

Primary pharmacological action: Anti infective.

Therapeutic classes

Stimulant. Antiseptic. Antimicrobial. Allays inflammation.
Antibacterial – Aeromonas, Bacillus genera, Brucella abortus, Citrobacter, Cryptococcus, Escherichia coli, Hafnia, Klebsiella, Mycobacteria [30 species], Mycobacteria tuberculosis [17 species], Proteus, Providencia, Pseudomonas aeruginosa, Salmonella typhi, Shigella, Staphylococcus, Streptococcus faecalis and Vibrio cholerae.
Antifungal - Aspergillius parasiticus, Candida and Tinea.
Antiprotozoeal – Plasmodium sp.
Antiviral – Coxsackie, Cryptococcal meningitis, Parainfluenza, Herpes Simplex. Hypotensive. Anticholesterolaemic. Anticoagulant. Antilipids. Reduces platelet aggregation. Vasodilator. Enhances leucocytosis. Antioxidant.
Catarrh. Colds. Rhinitis. Expectorant. Antihistamine.
Anthelmintic.
Diaphoretic.
Antispasmodic. Antineoplastic. Imunostimulant. Rubefacient. Vulnerary.

Medicinal indications [Mars]

Arteriosclerosis. Thrombosis. Hypertension. Hyperlipidaemia. Gangrene. Improves the coronary circulation. Reduces post MI infarction rate.
Colds. Asthma. Pharyngitis. Bronchitis. Pneumonia. TB. Pertussus. Influenza. Respiratory infections.
Toxic halitosis. Stomach carcinoma. Hypoglycaemic. Dysentery. Cholera. Typhoid. Acute and chronic infections of the intestines - enterocolitis. Fermentative and putrefactive dyspepsia. Cestodes and nematodes. Constipation. Stomach, liver and colon carcinoma. Sarcoma. Bladder tumour.
Heavy metal poisoning. Wards off evil spirits. Cryptococcal meningitis.

Tissue conditions

Half life in water of four days. Allium is a stimulating diffusive to the mucous membranes. It diffuses rapidly throughout the body. Allium increases microvascular diameter showing significant arteriole dilation of arterioles and venules in the conjunctiva. It dilates and increases capillary flow in nails. It raises the resistance of the body. Antiseptic expectorant in respiratory disease. Intestinal toxicity and auto intoxication, ulcers both internally and externally. Anti-infective action is very well documented. Smooth muscle relaxant in hypertension through potassium-channel opening and membrane hyperpolerisation. Where Allium is dried before being crushed it retains more Allicin activity.

External use

Local treatment for ear infections and otitis media. Lie patient on unaffected side, instil 2gtt oleum into the ear meatus and plug with cotton wool.

Wounds – Succus diluted with sterile water as an application to wounds.

Dermal ulcers/wounds – essential oleum [with] oleum Lavandula.

Laryngeal tuberculosis – poultice.

Dosage and mode of application

Dried/fresh bulb Sig 1.5g

Tincturae Sig 10ml

Liquidum extractum Sig 4ml

Succus Allium Sig 8ml [See Chapter 33 for syrup formula].

Ol. Allium Sig 0.12ml

References

BPC 1949. 43 p20. 176 p260. 192 p222/224. 206. 207. 208. 230 p41. 251 p80. 264, M22 Sep 91 [2nd International. Sym. on Garlic - Berlin 1991]. 273, 1996, [4]. 394 p144.

Alnus glutinosa [Alder]

Constituents
Bacc – Lignans, Tannin, Phenolic glycosides. Fol – Flavonoid glycosides, Resin.

Primary pharmacological action: Vasotonic alterative.

Therapeutic classes
Allays inflammation – buds. Astringent. Tonic. Antibacterial. Antiviral - Herpes.
Anti haemorrhagic - passive haemorrhage.
Emetic. Anti diarrhoeal.
Dermatological agent. Vulnerary. Lymphatic. Febrifuge.
Medicinal indications [Venus]
Blood and tissue cleanser. Rhinitis. The cones are astringent in haematuria and haemorrhage.
Sore throat. Debility of the stomach with indigestion or diarrhoea. Enteritis.
Secondary syphilis. Enlarged glands.
Skin conditions with pustular eruptions - acne, eczema. Furunculosis. Impetigo.
Scalp scurf. Mastitis.
Tissue conditions
Stimulates the mucous membranes. Stimulates gastric secretions. Indicated specifically for chronic, scaly or pustular skin disease.
External use
Aphthous ulcers, rhinitis, pharyngitis - spray Dist aqua Alnus.
Mastitis, bruises - poultice with folium.
Leucorrhoea – douche.
Gangrene - poultice with fol.
Inflamed dermis – lotion.
Dosage and mode of application
Infusium fol/bacc. Sig 30ml
Liquidum extractum Sig 4ml
References
111 p233. 127 p17. 147. 176 p274. 189 p6. 246.

Aloe vera [Aloes]

Constituents

The aloe leaf yields aloe resin and aloe gel. Resin is found in the fol tip and base and contains the anthraquinones. Gel is mucilaginous and found mainly in the centre of the leaf. Once the leaf is split into two halves the gel is peeled off. **Anthraquinones from the resin** is mainly barbaloin. Barbaloin up to 40% is an anthrone-c-glycoside. Anthraquinones are bitter and add a yellow or orange colour. **Acemannan** is antiviral, immunostimulant and enhances T lymphocytes. Increasing T lymphocytes enhances cytokines that destroy malignant cells. **Sterols** allay inflammation. Cholesterol, B Sitosterol, Campesterol, Lupeol. Lupeol is antiseptic and analgesic. Skin and mucous membranes are influenced by aloe. Aloe vera inhibits thromboxanes and prostaglandins. Thromboxanes are vasoconstrictors. Thromboxanes and prostaglandins affect platelet aggregation, leukocyte infiltration and vasoconstriction.
Vitamins: B1, B2, B6, choline, B12, C, Folic acid, E.
Minerals: beta carotene, calcium, chromium, copper, iron, magnesium, manganese, potassium, sodium, zinc.

Primary pharmacological action:
Resin/latex - Laxative. Gel – Demulcent.

Therapeutic classes

Ophthalmic. Allays inflammation. Demulcent.
Antibacterial – Citrobacter species, Corynebacterium, Enterobacter cloacae, Escherichia coli, Klebsiella pneumoniae, mycobacterium, Streptococcus agalactiae/faecalis/pyogenes, Staphylococcus aureus, Propionibacterium acnes, Pseudomonas aeruginosa and Serratia.
Antifungal – Candida albicans, Tinea pedis, Trichomonas and Trichophyton.
Anti viral - Herpes simplex, Herpes zoster, HIV/Aids.
Increases phagocytosis. Stimulant. Antihaemorrhagic. Vasodilator.
Stomachic. Choleretic. Purgative. Anthelmintic.
Analgesic. Anaesthetic. Emmenagogue. Antiarthritic. Antineoplastic. Immunostimulant.
Dermatological agent. Antipruritic. Radiation damage. Vulnerary. Antipyretic.

Medicinal indications

Full doses stimulate the circulation. Varicose veins. Asthma.
Aphthous ulcers. Peptic ulcers. Gum as - tonic cathartic, in dyspepsia and haemorrhoids. Colitis. Diabetes. Constipation. Hepatic carcinoma.
Headaches. Breast carcinoma.
Radiation burns. Cuts. Ulcers. Wounds. Insect bites.

Pharmacopoeia

Tissue conditions
The resin is effective for gastro intestinal conditions. It acts upon the lower bowel, improving muscular tone, stimulating peristalsis, increasing blood to the intestine. A visceral stomach tonic. Aloe is vasodilatory increasing blood flow to the skin encouraging healing. Skin conditions with inflammation, dermatitis, poison ivy dermatitis, urticaria. Dermal ulcers in diabetics.

Cautions
Resin/latex only - contraindicated in pregnancy, lactation and irritable conditions of the colon e.g. irritable bowel, colitis, haemorrhoids.

External use
Bites, pruritis, burns, ulcers, pruritis vulvae, psoriasis – Gel.

Dosage and mode of application
Powder Sig 200mg. Laxative dose of powder Sig 5g.
Tincturae fol. 1:10 Sig 2ml
Liquidum extractum resin Sig 1ml
    Succus gel Sig 10-15ml
    Laxative - Tincturae 1:10 with LE Glycyrrhiza Sig 0.5-2ml
    Laxative & tonic - Tinctura aloes 1:30 with Gentiana, Rhei and Zingiber
    Sig 4-8ml

References
192 p24. 230 p3. 233 p19. 246 p506. 262 p42. 263, 1991 57 [1] 38-40. 290, Vol. 6, No. ?, 1994, p40. 272, 1995, 7 [4] 70. 291, Vol 13, No. 1. 292 1999, 49 [447] p823-8.

Aloysia citriodora [Lemon verbena]

Constituents
Flavonoids [flavones]. Volatile oils. Mucilage. Tannin.

Primary pharmacological action: Antispasmodic.

Therapeutic classes
Antiseptic. Aromatic. Stomachic. Sedative. Antipyretic.
Medicinal indications
Colds. Asthma.
Indigestion. Flatulence. Diarrhoea. Fever.
Tissue conditions
A pleasant refreshing light herbal tea with a pleasant scent.
Dosage and mode of application
Infusium herba Sig 30ml
References
189 p173. 246 p357.

Alpinia officinarum [Galangal]

Constituents
Volatile oil. Acetoxychavicol acetate – antifungal. Resin

Primary pharmacological action: Tonic.

Therapeutic classes
Disinfectant. Antifungal – candida.
Aromatic. Carminative.
Antirheumatic.
CNS trophorestorative.
Deodorant.
Medicinal indications
Diphtheria. Bronchitis.
Dyspepsia. Flatulence. Nausea.
Motion sickness.
Tissue conditions
Alpinia a stimulating, aromatic, carminative with tonic action. It acts upon the stomach and intestines to prevent fermentation. Atony of the stomach or intestine is improved by the tonic action. Recommended as a remedy for motion sickness.
Preparations
With Dioscorea for flatulent colic.
Dosage and mode of application
Dried rhizome/rad Sig 2g
Infusium/decoctum Sig 15ml
Tincturae Sig 4ml
References
192 p219. 263, 62, 1996, 308.

Alstonia constricta/scholaris [Alstonia]

Constituents
Indole alkaloids –
Echitamine which lowers carotid pressure and increases renal output.

Primary pharmacological action:
Antimalarial - stem bark and leaves.

Therapeutic classes
Astringent. Vasotonic alterative. Tonic.
Hypotensive.
Diarrhoea. Dysentery. Anthelmintic.
Emmenagogue. Galactagogue.
Antipyretic. Antiperiodic.
Analgesic.
Dermatological agent.
Medicinal indications
Hypertension.
Atonic dyspepsia. Diarrhoea. Dysentery.
Debility. Febrifuge for relapsing fevers – malaria.
Bark decoction helps to expel the placenta.
Tissue conditions
Stimulates the secretions. Indicated for gastro intestinal conditions consequent
upon malaria with weakness, dirty tongue and sallow complexion.
External use
Leaves and latex for rheumatic pain.
Preparations
Most Alstonia species have antimalarial action.
Dosage and mode of application
Infusium powdered bacc 1:20 Sig 30ml
Tincturae 1:8 Sig 4ml
Liquidum extractum Sig 8ml
References
BPC 1934. 127 p258. 176 p175. 189 p9. 262 p64. 390 p323.

Althea officinalis/rosea
[Marshmallow/Hollyhock – Malva sylvestris has identical activity].

Constituents
Mucilage around 11% contains galacturonorhamnans, xylose and glucose.
Flavonoid glycosides - quercetin. Tannin 2%. Phenolic acids. Pectin – up to 11%.

Primary pharmacological action:
Demulcent action for all mucous membranes.

Therapeutic classes
Antiseptic. Allays inflammation. Antimicrobial against Proteus vulgaris,
Pseudomonas aeruginosa, Staphylococcus aureus. Stimulates phagocytosis.
Haemostatic.
Expectorant. Antitussive.
Oropharyngeal agent.
Diuretic. Antilithic.
Anodyne.
Dermatological agent. Emollient. Vulnerary.
Medicinal indications [Venus]
Catarrh. Oropharyngeal inflammation. Laryngitis. Pharyngitis.
Laryngopharyngeal irritability. Bronchitis. Pneumonia.
Sore mouth and gums. Inflamed gastro intestinal tract. Peptic ulcers. Dysentery.
Diarrhoea. Typhoid. Enteritis. Ulcerative colitis.
Cystitis. Urethritis. Urinary calculi. Nephritis. Gonorrhoea oral and local
treatment.
Eczema. Dermatitis. Furunculosis. Dermal pigmentation disturbances.
Tissue conditions
The herb is slightly more antiseptic than the root. A soothing demulcent which
affects all the mucous membranes. For inflamed or irritable conditions of the
respiratory, digestive and urinary tracts. Indicated for mucous surfaces which are
raw, sore or damaged by infective or inflammatory processes. Mucilaginous
compounds in small dose restrain peristaltic action of the gut, antidiarrhoeal
action as in enteritis. In large quantities they are laxative. Mucilage is a colloidal
compound and is effective in stopping coughs caused by irritation of the mucosa.
Althea inhibits melanocyte cell development in the skin according to a Japanese
study].
External use
Pharyngeal and oral inflammation - gargle or mouthwash.
Sore nipples, mastitis, abscesses, boils, ulcers, wounds, burns and scalds – apply
as a decoction fomentation. Added to the bath water it will soothe skin irritations.

A

Fomentation for bruises, sprains, aching in the muscles and tendons.
Mastitis – use as a poultice with Phytolacca, Chamomilla, Ulmus.
Abscesses and ulcers – use a poultice,
Burns and scalds – althea with Ol Linseed. Renew every 2/3 hours.
Inflamed/gangrenous wounds with Ulmus as a poultice. Use both as powdered roots and renew before it dries.

Preparations
Althea will be carried by other remedies to the preferred location.
Lung diseases use with pectorals/expectorants.
Pertussus with lobelia and antispasmodics.
Lung mixture – Althea rad 8 parts, Glycyrrhiza 3, Tussilago 4, Verbascum 2.
Gastritis with Filipendula and Symphytum.
Urinary disease with Zea or Agropyron.
Mucilage extraction is best prepared from a decoction of the root. However a tincture will extract the mucilage.

Dosage and mode of application
Dried rad/fol Sig 5g
Dried extract Sig 1g
Decoctum rad Sig 60ml
Tincturae Althea fol/rad Sig 25ml
Liquidum extractum fol/rad Sig 5ml
Syrupus Althaea Althea syrup
Syrupus 550ml Althea 30g Lobelia 15g
Sig 10ml. Indications - bronchial antispasmodic.
Ung extractum 10%

References
43 p22/23. 111 p236. 192 p351 & 344. 230 p77. 246 p243. 251 p108. 394 p246. 412.

435

Amenopsis californica [Yerba mansa]

Constituents
Essential oil.

Primary pharmacological action: Astringent

Therapeutic classes
Anticatarrhal. Anti-infective.
Carminative. Antiemetic. Antiulcerogenic. Amoebicidal. AntiGuardia.
Vulnerary.
Medicinal indications
Nasal catarrh. Sinusitis. Pharyngitis. Laryngitis. Bronchitis.
Ulcerations of the gastro intestinal tract. Dyspepsia. Stomach and duodenal infections. Giardia infection. Enteritis.
Cystitis. Urethritis. Vaginitis. Gonorrhoea.
Rheumatic disturbances. Uric acid disturbances.
Skin conditions - rashes, wounds.
Tissue conditions
Similar effects to Hydrastis.
External use
Apply to all internal surfaces to remove infections and ulcerations.
Tinea - powdered rad.
Preparations
Gonorrhoea with Piper cubebs.
Dosage and mode of application
Decoctum rhiz Sig 4g
Tincturae Sig 3ml
References
126 p188.

Ammi visnaga [Kella]

Constituents
Furanochromes up to 4% of which; Khellin [smooth muscle relaxant] up to 1.2%
Visnagin [vasodilator and hypotensive] up to 0.3%, Khellol up to 1%. Flavonoids.
Pyranocoumarin up to 0.5%.
Essential oil up to 0.03% primarily of camphor, carvone, linalool and alpha-
terpineol. Fixed oil up to 18%.

Primary pharmacological action: Antispasmodic.

Therapeutic classes
Antiasthmatic. Bronchodilator.
Coronary vasodilator. Hypotensive. Biliary spasm.
Antilithic. Diuretic. Sphincter relaxant.
Medicinal indications
Angina. Post Myocardial infarction. Arteriosclerosis.
Laryngismus stridulus. Asthma. Bronchitis.
Gall stone colic.
Renal colic. Urinary calculi.
Vitiligo. Psoriasis.
Tissue conditions
Khellin is a vascular smooth muscle relaxant. Supports the prevention of asthma
attacks. Spasmolytic to the coronary and cerebral circulation. Coronary artery
vasodilator with a slowing and strengthening activity to the myocardium.
Encourages recovery from MI. An anti allergic drug was developed from Amni
visnaga.
Preparations
Calculi with Agropyron.
Dosage and mode of application
Powdered sem/herba. Sig 30ml
Tincturae sem. Sig 5ml
Liquidum extractum Sig 0.5ml
References
224. 142 p179/221/338. 392.

Anamirta cocculus [Cocculus indicus]

Constituents
Picrotoxin consists of proportions of picrotoxinin and picrotin. Picrotoxinin is a highly oxygenated sesquiterpine. Fats.

Primary pharmacological action: Parasiticide.

Therapeutic classes
CNS stimulant. Antidote. Diaphoretic.
Medicinal indications
Checks night sweats in Tuberculosis.
Antidote in barbiturate and morphine poisoning. Destroys lice.
Migraine. Dysmenorrhoea.
Tissue conditions
Powerful stimulant to the CNS. Affects the medulla, increasing arterial blood pressure and stimulates respiration and slows the pulse. Increases secretions. Martindale [p1167] states 'Its effects are of brief duration and 20 minutes after injection only traces remain in the blood'.
Cautions
Restrictions apply. Dosage is determined by the relief of symptoms.
Overdosage can cause convulsions, coma, respiratory depression and death.
Avoid on open wounds. Antidote - stimulants and an emetic.
External use
Lice and scabies – crem or lotion.
Dosage and mode of application
Liquidum extractum Sig 0.06ml
Lotion @1%
Crem @ 1%
References
189 p81. 390 p1167.

Andrographis paniculata

Similar to Swertia chirata [Chiretta] see reference 43 p200, 189 p75, 246 p326.

Constituents
Bitter di Terpenoid lactones – Andrographolides are immune-enhancers.
Flavonoids.

Primary pharmacological action: Immunostimulant.

Therapeutic classes
Bitter tonic. Vasotonic alterative. Antibacterial. Antiviral - Herpes simplex and zoster. Antimicrobial. Allays inflammation. Antiplatelet.
Stomachic. Cholagogue. Choleretic. Hepatoprotective. Laxative. Anthelmintic.
Adrenocortical supportive. Antifertility. Antipyretic.
Anodyne. Antineoplastic. Antivenomous.

Medicinal indications
Inflammatory conditions. Limits myocardial ischaemia. Acute infections.
Respiratory infections. Colds. Sore throats. Influenza. Tonsillitis. TB.
Anorexia. Dyspepsia. Flatulence. Infective hepatitis. Diabetes. Ulcers. Gastro enteritis. Bacillary dysentery. Diarrhoea. Typhoid. Worms.
Acute pylonephritis. Pyrexia.
Malaria. Leptospirosis. Snakebite. Abscess. Stomach, breast and prostate carcinoma. Non Hodgkins lymphoma. Lymphocytic leukaemia. Melanoma.

Tissue conditions
Inhibits platelet aggregation. Inhibits histamine release. The leaf juice promotes the appetite. Lowers PSA counts. Active against E. coli. Anthelmintic against Ascaris.
Immunostimulant effects control infective processes.

Cautions
Contraindicated in pregnancy.

Dosage and mode of application
Dried herba Sig 2g
Liquidum extractum Sig 3ml

References
48 p96/98. 191. 209. 210. 239 p170. 265 1998, 10 [2]. 270, 1996/7, 3 [4] p315.
270 1997 4, [2], p101. 271, April 2001. 390 p323.

Anethum graveolens [Dill]

Constituents
Volatile oil in the seed up to 68% Carvone, up to 83% dihydro Carvone.
Anethum herba contains no carvone. Limonene.

Primary pharmacological action:
An aromatic and carminative which is stimulant,
diffusive and stomachic.

Therapeutic classes
Antiflatulent. Anti nausea. Galactagogue. Sedative.
Medicinal indications [Mercury]
Anorexia. Halitosis. Hiccups. Flatulence. Nausea. Stomach pain. Colic. Full
dosage for infant colic pains.
Headache. Insomnia. Muscle spasm. Nail strengthener.
Preparations
Combines with tonics and cathartics to prevent griping. Removes flatulence to
relieve hiccoughs and colic. Increases nursing mothers milk
External use
Headache apply to temples.
Dosage and mode of application
Dried sem Sig 4g
Aqua Anetha distillata. Distilled Dill water. Dill 1:10 Sig 4ml.
Oleum Anethi Sig 0.2ml
References
43 p24. 111 p246. 192 p186. 224. 228 p343. 246 p292. 293, 7, 1995, p11-20.

Angelica archangelica [Angelica].

[A. sinensis/polymorpha has similar activity].

Constituents

Furanocoumarins. Psoralen. Volatile oil up to 1.9% of which up to 90% are monoterpene hydrocarbons – beta phellandrene. Flavonoids. Resin up to 6%. Sitosterol. Volatile oil loss is around 0.10% per year.

Primary pharmacological action: Stimulating expectorant.

Therapeutic classes

Antifungal. Antibacterial – Mycobacterium avium Rad oleum. Antiseptic. Disinfectant.
Tonic. Circulatory diffusive tonic.
Expectorant. Bronchial tonic.
Aromatic bitter. Carminative. Gastric stimulant - Hypochlorhydria. Cholagogue. Diaphoretic. Diuretic.
Antispasmodic.
Emmenagogue. Oxytocic. Uterine tonic. Prostate tonic.

Medicinal indications [Sun]

Anaemia. Peripheral vascular disease. Intermittent claudication. Buergers disease – obstructed blood vessels. Raynauds disease.
Respiratory catarrh. Bronchitis. Colds. Asthma. Spasmodic coughs. Pleurisy. Anorexia nervosa. Heartburn. Nervous dyspepsia.
General debility. Rheumatism and arthritis. Backache.
Amenorrhoea. Expels retained placenta. Menopause. Osteoporosis. Acute febrile diseases. Infectious fevers [plague]. Typhoid fever. Malaria.
Useful in alcoholism. Headache. Eczema.

Tissue conditions

A circulatory diffusive tonic. In warm infusion angelica is a stimulating and relaxing diffusive. Appetite stimulant. Seeds are stronger and more diaphoretic. Smooth muscle relaxant. The disinfectant properties were deemed protection against the contagion of infectious diseases.

Cautions

Inflamed conditions of the GIT. Pregnancy. Skin sensitisation to light – furanocoumarins.

External use

Pleurisy and bronchitis use a leaf compress to allay inflammation.
Rheumatism – liniment.
Ulcers and wounds where there is a need for stimulation use a decoction wash.

Pharmacopoeia

Preparations
Pulmonary disturbances with Tussilago.
Indigestion with Filipendula.
Compound tincturae Angelica, Carminative guttae.
Carminative drops to ease griping pain in infants/adults.
Angelica rad 12g Dioscorea 3g Leonurus 3g Pimpinella 3g Anethum 3g
Renal with Galium, Uva ursi, Daucus.
Stomach tea – Angelica, Carum, Gentiana.
Angelica root can be candied and used as a **confection**.
Method 1
Remove roots. Beat an egg white until foamy then dip the stalks into the egg white then in sugar. Lay upon greaseproof paper on a cooling rack. Cover with greaseproof paper in a warm oven until dry.
Method 2
Cut into pieces 10cm long. Simmer in a closed vessel until soft and strip off the outer skin. Simmer again until tender. Add syrup then turn onto greaseproof paper, sprinkle with sugar and allow to dry.
Dosage and mode of application
Dried herba Sig 5g or infuse.
Dried rad/rhiz. Sig 2g or as a decoction.
Tincturae herba. Sig 5ml
Tincturae rad. Sig 2ml
Liquidum extractum Angelica herba. Sig 5ml
Liquidum extractum Angelica rad. Sig 3ml
References
BPC 1934. 43 p25. 111 p246. 251 p7. 246 p299. 251 p111. 262 p46.

Angelica sinensis [Dong quai]

Constituents
Volatile oil up to 0.7% – ligustilide. Sterols. Coumarin as ostheol up to 0.2% –
angelol, angelicone. Organic acid as ferulic acid.

Primary pharmacological action: Astringent.

Therapeutic classes
Allays inflammation. Vasotonic alterative. Antiviral – herpes zoster.
Circulatory arterial stimulant. Antiplatelet. Antiarrhythmic. Antisclerotic.
Hepatoprotective.
Diuretic.
Analgesic. Uterine antispasmodic with tonic activity. Hormone regulator.
Antineoplastic. Immunostimulant. Vulnerary.
Medicinal indications
Blurred vision. Toothache. Angina. Antiarrhythmic. Atrial fibrillation.
Palpitations. Buergers disease – obstructed blood vessels. Atherosclerosis.
Raynauds disease. Thrombocytopenia. Hypertension. Cramp. Catarrh. Asthma.
Ulcers. Hepatitis. Cirrhosis. Constipation.
Amenorrhoea. Dysmenorrhoea. Menorrhagia. PMS. Menopause – flushes.
Infertility. Toxic shock syndrome.
Abscess. Infections. Bruising. Malaria.
Insomnia. Nervous exhaustion. Headache. Herpes zoster.
Tissue conditions
Relaxes and dilates coronary blood vessels - angina.
Inhibits IGE antibodies in allergic conditions. Immunological function -
stimulates phagocytes and lymphocytes.
Amphoteric activity upon the uterus as it contracts the smooth muscle of the
uterus relieving spasm or dilation.
Cautions
Pregnancy and menorrhagia.
Preparations
Dysmenorrhoea with Paeonia.
Dosage and mode of application
Powder Sig 1g
Tincturae Sig 5ml
Liquidum extractum Sig 2ml
References
48 p4/5. 192 p188. 265, 1993, Vol. 5 [4] 87-91. 219.

Aphanes [Alchemilla] arvensis [Parsley piert]

Constituents
Tannin.

Primary pharmacological action: Demulcent diuretic.

Therapeutic classes
Allays inflammation. Hepatic. Antilithic.
Medicinal indications
Hepatic congestion. Obstructive jaundice. Ascites.
Bladder inflammation. Urinary calculi. Dysuria. Strangury. Renal oedema.
Tissue conditions
Soothes tissue where damage to the mucous membrane occurs from calculi or
infections. Removes obstructions in the liver and will relieve jaundice and
oedema from hepatic disorders.
Preparations
Combined with stimulating remedies – Barosma, Daucus or Parietaria. Demulcent
action is enhanced with Althea, Symphytum or Ulmus.
Dosage and mode of application
Dried herba 4g
Infusium 4g
Tincturae Sig 10ml
Liquidum extractum Sig 4ml
References
40. 43 p28. 246 p184. 251 p122.

Apium graveolens [Celery]

Constituents
Up to 3% volatile oil which is around 60% d-limonine - bactericidal and sedative. Phthalides - diuretic, spasmolytic and antineoplastic. Volatile oil, apiol - antispasmodic, uterotonic and diuretic. Limonine and phthalides stimulate glutathione s transferase and is antineoplastic. Furanocoumarin [bergaptine]. Flavonic glycoside - apigenin. Alpha linoleic acid – allays inflammation, antineoplastic and is immunostimulant. Coumarin. Flavonoids. Phenols. Resin. Fatty acids. Calcium.

Primary pharmacological action:
Diuretic and urinary antiseptic.

Therapeutic classes
Ophthalmic. Allays inflammation. Bactericidal.
Antioxidant. Hypotensive.
Aromatic. Carminative. Digestive tonic. Hepatoprotective. Splenic.
Urinary antiseptic. Antirheumatic.
Galactagogue. Emmenagogue. Aphrodisiac.
Antispasmodic. Analgesic. Sedative.
Antineoplastic. Antipyretic.

Medicinal indications [Mercury]
Eye disorders. Toothache. Hypertension.
Colds. Influenza. Asthma. Bronchitis.
Anorexia. Halitosis. Flatulence. Heartburn. Hiccups. Hepatic disorders. Jaundice. Vomiting.
Inflammation or infections of the urinary tract. Oedema. Calculi. Urinary retention.
Arthritis. Rheumatoid arthritis. Gout. Sciatica. Muscle spasm. Urticaria. Amenorrhoea.
Depression. Headache. Insomnia. Neuralgia. Panic. Restlessness.

Tissue conditions
Ulcerated throat. Strengthens the eyesight.
The volatile oil acts to produce a local vasodilatation and local reflex irritation to the prostate gland. Apium is a uric acid solvent diuretic and is most useful in rheumatic conditions - arthritis, neuralgia, sciatica. Antiseptic and allays inflammatory action of the urinary tract.
It promotes the appetite and clears wind. Apium is useful as a tonic nervine in debility. It promotes restful sleep, where the brain is debilitated from overwork or

excitement and it has a sustaining influence over the CNS. Apium vegetable is less stimulating than seeds.

Cautions
Pregnancy.

Preparations
Throat ulcerations - mix with honey and gargle.
Rheumatic disorders – combine with Taraxacum, Menyanthes or Guaiacum.
Nervous debility – combine with a tonic hepatic.
Eczema combine with Rumex and Smilax.

External use
Tumours, inflammation, bruises - leaf infusium for a poultice.
Bruised leaves have been applied to the feet in panic attacks.

Dosage and mode of application
Action is potentiated by Taraxacum.
Dried fruct/sem Sig 3g
Decoctum Sig 2g
Tincturae Sig 5ml
Liquidum extractum Sig 2ml
Apium vinegar - 1:20 with cider vinegar. Macerate for 10 days. Filter.
Sig 15ml.

References
43 p28. 111 p252. 192. 233 p56. 246 p294. 262 p91.

Apocynum cannabinum
& rosaemilfoleum [different plants with similar actions].

Constituents
Cardiac glycosides – Strophanthin, Cynarin [390]. Tannin. Resin.

Primary pharmacological action: Renal vasotonic.

Therapeutic classes
Stimulant. Detergent. Depurative.
Cardiac tonic.
Expectorant.
Emetic - large dose. Hydragogue cathartic.
Diuretic. Diaphoretic. Emmenagogue. Antipyretic. Antivenomous.
Medicinal indications
Pneumonia.
Arteriosclerosis. Dyspnoea. Cardiac atony. Angina. Valvular weakness. Cardiac
oedema.
Cholagogue. Choleretic. Jaundice.
Nephritis - congestive phase. Syphilis.
Rheumatism - acute. Neuralgia of the lumbar spine. Sciatica. Arthritis.
Meningitis. Pyrexia. Intermittent and remittent fever - typhoid, malaria
Dysmenorrhoea from congestion.
Tissue conditions
Given in atonic conditions of the circulatory system with oedema. Stimulates and
relaxes the stomach, intestines, liver, gall bladder and kidneys. It has a slow
persistent action. Weakness, atony with exudation of blood. Serous cavity
oedema. Slows the pulse and has a marked effect upon the vasomotor system.
Increases the strength and force of the heart beat. It lessens arterial tension.
Similar to Digitalis in activity.
Cautions
Restrictions apply. Dosage is determined by the relief of symptoms.
Similar in action to Digitalis. Bradycardia. Irritable conditions of the stomach and
intestines e.g. gastritis, ulcers. Irritant emeto-cathartic in excessive doses.
Preparations
Griping with Pimpinella or Zingiber.
Dosage and mode of application
Dried rad and rhizome Sig 0.3g
Tincturae Sig 0.5ml
Liquidum extractum Sig 0.25ml
References. 111 p253. 126 p193. 176p227. 188 p82. 189 p58. 235 p205. 390p623

Aralia racemosa [Spikenard]

Constituents
Glycosides. Essential oil.

Primary pharmacological action: Vasotonic alterative.

Therapeutic classes
Aromatic. Stimulant. Tonic expectorant. Diaphoretic.
Antirheumatic. Nervine tonic.
Medicinal indications [Venus]
Dry or irritable coughs in chronic bronchitis with excessive sputum. Tuberculosis.
Pertussus.
Rheumatic conditions. Cutaneous affections. Physical/mental exhaustion.
Tissue conditions
Tones and allays irritability of the respiratory mucous membranes and skin.
Nervine with tonic effects similar to Panax ginseng [188].
Cautions
Avoid in sensitive or depleted conditions.
Dosage and mode of application
Liquidum extractum rad/rhiz Sig 4ml
References
111 p259. 126 p201/2. 176 p185. 188 p399. 189 p256.

Arctium lappa [Burdock]

Constituents
Bitter glycosidal principle – arctiin a CNS stimulant. Lignan - Arctigenin inhibits leukaemia cells. Polysaccharide up to 50% Inulin. Polyacetylines are antimicrobial to staphylococcus and other gram + ve organisms. Acids. Volatile oils. Terpenoids. Mucilage. Tannin.

Primary pharmacological action: Vasotonic alterative.

Therapeutic classes
Antiseptic. Demulcent. Depurative.
Antibacterial to gram + ve organisms and gram - ve organisms, Bacillus subtilis, Escherichia coli, Mycobacterium smegmatis, Staphylococci. Salmonella typhimurium, Shigella flaxneri, Shigella sonnei and Staphylococcus.
Antifungal – Trichophyton.
Circulatory stimulant.
Bitter stomachic. Hepatic stimulant. Choleretic.
Diuretic. Antirheumatic. Diaphoretic.
Lymphatic stimulant. Antineoplastic. Immunemodulator.
Dermatological agent.
CNS stimulant. Analgesic. Antivenomous.

Medicinal indications [Venus]
Hordeolum. Catarrh. Feeble cutaneous circulation. Bronchitis.
Aphthous ulcers. Anorexia. Hypoglycaemic. Haemorrhoids.
Cystitis. Gout. Osteo and rheumatoid arthritis. Rheumatism. Sciatica.
Vaginal tissue laxity. Syphilis.
Dermatitis. Dermal ulcers. Eczema. Hair loss. Psoriasis. Erysipelas. Scurvy.
Plague. Furunculosis. Leprosy. Leukaemia. Ringworm.

Tissue conditions
The crushed seed has a better action on the skin, suderiferous and sebaceous glands. Arctium induces differentiation in cancer cells. Arctium is an eliminator of metabolic waste, it has a strong Vasotonic alterative action upon the blood stream drawing impurities from the extracellular spaces into the blood.
Bitter tonic action acts as an CNS stimulant The mucous membranes throughout are soothed. The glandular secretions of the stomach are normalised. It influences the respiratory passages when irritated from any blood disorder whereby it relieves irritable coughs. Cystitis with irritable conditions of the bladder or kidneys. The diuretic action promotes the elimination of waste impurities and urates, cleansing the mucous membranes, skin and serous membranes. A reduction in urates benefits rheumatic and gouty constitutions. It relieves

Pharmacopoeia

congestion of the lymphatics. Chronic glandular enlargements are reduced.
Chronic skin disease – acne, eczema, dermatitis and psoriasis.
Internal and external use for boils and inflamed skin conditions. Leaf infusion imparts tone to the stomach so aiding indigestion. Seed infusion is diuretic.
Supports the regulation of blood sugar levels.

Cautions
Arctium is very stimulating and should be used with caution. Small doses are best. Large doses promote rapid elimination of toxins.

External use
Dandruff – dect. wash.
Swelling and inflamed or infected skin e.g. boils, bruises, wounds - fol poultice is resolvent.
Panic attacks - bruised leaves can be applied to the soles of the feet.
Ulcers and scaly skin disorders - the root mucilage is soothing as a wash.
Fused joints – apply a poultice of the root.

Preparations
Hepatic action use with Taraxacum.
Oedema with Agropyron, Juniperus or Eupatorium purpureum.
Reproductive system use with Mitchella
Skin conditions with Rumex/Smilax/Trifolium or as an ointment or poultice.
Tonic effect with Hydrastis.
Venereal disease combine with more stimulating agents e.g. Guaiacum/Smilax.

Dosage and mode of application
Dried fol/ sem/radix Sig 4g
Decoction Sig 15ml
Solid extract Sig 1g
Tincturae Sig 6ml
Liquidium extractum Sig 4ml

References
BPC 1934. 43 p127. 111 p261. 176 p378. 230 p11. 236 p23. 246 p482. 251 p27.

Arctostaphylos uva ursi [Bearberry]

Constituents
Hydroquinone glycosides up to 18% - arbutin, methylarbutin. Tannin. The antimicrobial/antiseptic/disinfectant effect of uva ursi occurs by the hydrolysis of arbutin to hydroxyquinone in the renal tubules. Uva ursi stimulates the renal tubules. Hydroquinone [antibacterial to gram + ve organisms] can be detected by allowing the urine to stand, as oxidation takes place the urine takes on a dark to deep green or brownish colour. Triterpines up to 0.8% - Iridoids. Allantoin. Flavonoids. Polyphenolic tannins up to 20%, ellagic tannin, gallotannin. Phenolic acids. Triterpenes.

Primary pharmacological action:
Tonic, antiseptic and astringent diuretic.

Therapeutic classes
Antimicrobial - Bacillus subtilis, Enterobacter aerogenes, Enterococcus faecalis, Escherichia coli, Klebsiella, Mycobacterium smegmatis, Mycoplasma hominis, Proteus vulgaris, Pseudomonas aeruginosa, Salmonella typhi, Shigella sonnei, Shigella flaxneri, Staphylococcus aureus, Streptococcus genera, Ureaplasma urealyticum.
Antifungal - Candida albicans.
Antiseptic. Allays inflammation. Antihaemorrhagic [Haemostatic].
Soothing mucilaginous urinary tonic.
Mollusicidal.
Uterine tonic. Oxytocic. Antineoplastic.

Medicinal indications
Mollusicidal activity against Biomphalaria glabrata.
Bladder and kidney tonic. Disinfects the urinary tract.
Chronic inflammation/infection of the Genito Urinary Tract.
Cystitis. Dysuria. Enuresis. Incontinence. Gonorrhoea. Haematuria. Lithuria. Nephritis. Pyelitis. Bladder ulceration. Prostatitis. Urethritis. Acidic urine.
Rheumatic tendencies with backache. Lumbago.
Gynaecological conditions - menorrhagia, uterine prolapse, cervical erosion, vaginal laxity. Atonic vaginal discharge/leucorrhoea.

Tissue conditions
Maximum antibacterial effects occur after 3/4 hours. Astringent, antiseptic and tonic diuretic with soothing action to the genital and urinary mucous membranes. The bacteriostatic action occurs within three hours after ingestion. Uva ursi is primarily indicated for the urinary and genital structures where there is a relaxed condition allowing an excessive mucus discharge or haemorrhage which it

Pharmacopoeia

corrects by astringent and tonic effects. Tonic effect is better obtained from cold preparations. Prescribed for raised uric acid acidic urine with infection. Infection often accompanies excess urinary acidity. Soothing influence is useful in acute and painful inflammatory conditions of the urinary tract – acute catarrhal cystitis, urethritis, endometritis. It cleanses suppurative and offensive vaginal discharge/leucorrhoea. Cervical ulceration internal and external. Direct influence upon the pelvic mucous membrane - bladder, uterus and vaginal walls, exercising both astringent and tonic effects.

In chronic urethral irritation, aching through the bladder, prostate congestion and bladder ulceration, involuntary seminal emissions and incontinence of urine. Astringent in haemorrhage of the stomach, bowel or kidneys – being careful to redistribute blood to the surface e.g. diffusives.

Cautions

Pregnancy. Lactation.

External use

Cervical erosion - apply to cervix on a tampon or pessary.

Haemorrhoids – wash with a decoction or diluted Tr.

Preparations

Hydrangea, Eupatorium purp or Zea in urinary disorders.

Aletris, Calendula in gynaecological trouble.

Parturient combine with Zanthoxylum or Zingiber.

Cystitis with Agropyron, Althea, Populus tremuloides.

Dosage and mode of application

Dried fol Sig 4g

Dry extract Sig 210mg

Infusium Uva ursi conc. Sig 4ml

Tincturae Sig 2ml

Liquidum extractum Sig 4ml. [1ml = 70mg arbutin].

References

43 p29. 111 p263. 176p429. 192 p47. 224. 246 p310. 394 p389.

Areca catechu [Betel nuts]

Constituents
Alkaloid including arecoline [0.5%]. Arecoline is an anthelmintic. Tannins.

Primary pharmacological action: Anthelmintic.

Medicinal indications
Antiseptic. Astringent. Stimulant.
Aromatic. Sialagogue. Carminative. Antiparasitic. Antimalarial.
Therapeutic classes
Chewed sem are a tonic. Cardiac stimulant – sem.
Sore throats.
Nematodes. Cestodes. Constipation. Dysentery.
Para sympathomimetic.
Tissue conditions
Chewing the nut clears halitosis. Strengthens the gums. As a vermifuge mix with honey or syrup.
Cautions
Restrictions apply. Dosage is determined by the relief of symptoms.
A case is given of volunteers consuming 12 betel nuts experiencing bradycardia hypotension and increased perspiration as a result [390].
Dosage and mode of application
Powder sem [nuts] Sig 4g [390]
Decoctum 1:20
Liquidum extractum sem/fruct/rind Sig 4ml
Enema decoction Sig 1:20
References
262 p50. 390 p139.

Aristolochia serpentaria [Virginia snakeroot]

Constituents
Aristolochic acid – antibacterial. Volatile oil. Bitters.

Primary pharmacological action: Stimulating diaphoretic.

Therapeutic classes
Allays inflammation. Antiviral. Bactericidal. Immunostimulant.
Circulatory diffusive. Cardiac stimulant. Expectorant.
Sialagogue. Bitter stomachic. Hepatic – mild. Digestive tonic.
Diuretic.
Antispasmodic. Nervine tonic. Anodyne. Antipyretic.
Vulnerary.
Emmenagogue. Aphrodisiac. Antineoplastic [226]. Pesticide. Antivenomous.
Medicinal indications [Venus]
Enhances leucocytosis.
Dental fistula. Tonsillitis. Diphtheria. Dyspepsia. Nausea. Vomiting. Abdominal
pain. Typhoid. Anal fistulas.
Eruptive fevers - Scarlet fever, Typhoid fever. Smallpox. Measles.
Fistulas. Gout. Arthritis.
Amenorrhoea. Dysmenorrhoea. Parturient - pain relief. Contraceptive.
Fainting. Surgical shock. Depression. Panic.
Tissue conditions
Aristolochic acid stimulates NK cell activity.
Increases perspiration. Lessens pain. Allays excitability. Induces sleep. Indicated
for eruptive, febrile, typhoid fevers. Atonic conditions of the skin and viscera.
Stimulating and relaxing to the capillary circulation. Full doses increase arterial
and capillary circulation. Restores the secretions in inflammatory conditions.
Stimulates and tones the functional activity of the stomach, uterus, prostate,
kidneys and skin. Dental and anal fistulas. Genito urinary disorders from cold or
chills. Urinary phosphates, lumbar pain with a sense of weight in the loins. Renal
atony. Infected lochia post partum. May be used as an adjunct to quinine.
Cautions
Restrictions apply. Dosage is determined by the relief of symptoms.
Large doses are emeto cathartic. Diarrhoea.
External use
Tonsillitis - gargle.
Wounds, furunculosis, leg ulcers, osteomyelitis.

Dosage and mode of application
Powdered rad, rhiz. Sig 100mg
Concentrated infusium 2:5 Sig 4ml
Tincturae Sig 4ml. [Ref 390 p328]
Liquidum extractum Sig 2ml
References
111 p265. 126 p629. 176 p367. 188 p444. 224 p256. 226.

Armoracia rusticana [Horseradish]

Constituents
Volatile oil glucosinates are glycosides of mustard oil which yield allyl isothiocyanate [inhibit bacteria] which is responsible for the pungent taste and odour of the root. Bitter resin. Coumarins. Phenols [phenolic acids]. Vitamins A, B & C.

Primary pharmacological action:
Stimulant to the capillary circulation and the digestive organs.

Therapeutic classes
Antiseptic. Stimulant. Allays inflammation. Antibacterial – Gram +ve organisms, Salmonella. Circulatory stimulant.
Anticatarrhal. Respiratory infections. Expectorant.
Periodontal disease. Condiment. Sialogogue. Anorexia. Emetic. Stomachic. Cholagogue. Hepatic and splenic stimulant. Pancreatic stimulant. Aperient – mild.
Diuretic. Antilithic. Urinary antiseptic. Diaphoretic. Antirheumatic.
Dermatological agent. Rubefacient. Vulnerary. Antineoplastic.
Oxytocic. Thyroactive.
Medicinal indications [Mars]
Chilblains. Frostbite.
Enlarged tonsils. Catarrh [ears, lungs, stomach and intestine]. Sinus disturbances. Hoarseness. Asthma. Bronchitis. Influenza. Pertussus.
Tooth decay. Dental caries. Anorexia. Atonic dyspepsia. Atonic constipation. Nematodes.
Oedema. Urinary infections. Cystitis. Calculi. Gout. Arthritis. Rheumatism. Pyrexia.
Neuralgia. Palsy. Paralysis. Thyroid disturbances [hyperthyroid].
Scurvy. Retained placenta. Vaginal discharge/leucorrhoea. Tumours.
Tissue conditions
Arterial and capillary circulation is improved through greater firmness of the pulse. Armoracia breaks up catarrh and reduces sepsis by it's antiseptic action. Clears clogged viscid mucus where it clogs eliminative capability.
The dried root is a strong stimulant to the pancreas, liver and gall bladder, a fair portion of it's influence is expended to the stomach and the glandular secretions. Stimulates the kidneys. Tones the stomach tone. Aids digestion of oily fish
A general feeling of warmth is felt upon the skin surface when applied dermally. Armoracia is more useful in chronic and sluggish conditions. It can be used as an alternative to Capsicum when required.

Cautions

Best in chronic conditions when used locally. Avoid the fresh root as it causes blistering.

Avoid in acute conditions, arterial excitement, in sensitive patients. Pregnancy.

External use

Poultice or acetic acid solution is highly beneficial applied direct in cases of – bronchial trouble, chilblains, gout, joint aches and pains, laryngitis, neuritis, neuralgia, pneumonia, slow healing dermal ulcers or wounds, swelling of the liver and spleen.

Localised effects are produced by stimulating the nerve plexus to effect the local vasomotor function to the organ area by reflex action.

The fresh root and leaves blister the skin – do not leave on for too long.

Preparations

Atonic stomach or bowel with Gentiana, Taraxacum and Syrupus Citrus/Auranti.

Oedema with Brassica nigra or alba or Juniperus.

Take before meals for best effect. It is usual to give small doses.

Dosage and mode of application

Fresh rad Sig 6g

Powder Sig 250mg

Decoctum 1:20 Sig 120 ml BD

Tincture Sig 10ml

Liquidum extractum Sig 2ml

Oleum @ 2% strength.

Poultice - Grated fresh rad 15g and wrap in muslin then apply.

Acetum Armoracea Armoracea vinegar

Armoracea 30g Cider vinegar 550ml Macerate 7 days. Sig 5-10ml.

Spiritus Armoraciae compositus Compound spirit of Armoracia

Armoracea 45g, Auranti 45g, Myristica 10g Tincture as 1:5 Sig 4ml [administered as a carminative].

Tincturae Armoraciae compositus Compound tincture of Armoracia

Armoracia 30g Brassica 30g Juniperus 30g Myrica 30g Auranti 30g Cider 1500ml alcohol 500ml Macerate 7 days press and filter. Sig 30ml

References

111 p369. 142 p207. 188 p234. 189 p148. 192 p279. 246 p142. 294, 2000, 13 [1-4], p271-6. 394 p205.

Arnica montana [Arnica]

Constituents
Flavonoids up to 0.6% as isoquerciluteolintrin - reduce cytotoxicity. Sesquiterpine lactones helenanoidtype - allay inflammation. Volatile oil - thymol. Phenols. Coumarins – scopoletin, umbelliferone. Mucilage. Resin. Tannin.

Primary pharmacological action: Circulatory stimulant.

Therapeutic classes
Antiseptic. Antibacterial - gram positive and gram negative organisms - E. coli, Proteus vulgaris, Pseudomonas aeruginosa and Staphylococcus aureus. Antifungal - Candida, Epidermophyton sp, Microsporum gypseum and Trichophyton sp. Immunostimulant.
Antiphlogistic. Tonic. Inotropic. Respiratory stimulant.
Antineoplastic. Uterine.
Anti pyretic. Rubefacient. Vulnerary.

Medicinal indications [Sun]
Oropharyngeal inflammation.
Hectic fever in tuberculosis.
Cardiac debility. Chilblains. Apnoea. Respiratory depression.
Typhoid. Weak sphincters.
Spinal enervation. Paralysis. Rheumatic muscle and joint pain.
Acne. Furunculosis. Hair loss. Scalp itch. Insect bites.
Wound healer.
Bruising. Dislocations. Lacerations. Sprains. Oedema in fracture.

Tissue conditions
Deficient nervous response. Sluggish vascular power. Spinal and vagal enervation. Torpid or depleted nerve function. Sphincters weak or paralysed. Feeble respiration with dyspnoea.
Arnica induces increased perspiration. Establishes secretions. In small diluted dosage it is tonic to the heart and nervous system. Will remove ecchymosis from injury or haemorrhage e.g. CVA. Cardiac debility from over excitable nervous conditions. Enhances immune responses.

Cautions
Restrictions apply. Dosage is determined by the relief of symptoms.
Nervous excitability - discontinue. Gastric irritation, dizzyness, palpitation, collapse. Dermatitis. Dermal ulcers.

External use
20% gel applied TDS.
Muscular soreness, weakness and bruising.

Chronic venous insufficiency with heavy leg syndrome. Gel improves tone and reduces oedema.

Mastitis - dilute 1:20 and use as a compress.

Stimulates hair growth – dilute Tr.

Preparations

Local use to skin, muscles and ligaments. Dilute tincturae flos. with six parts aqua. Then apply as a fomentation or as a dressing for contusions, wounds and lacerations.

Dosage and mode of application

Advisable to start with a very small dose and observe the patient.

Potency of 3x or 6x.

Oropharyngeal treatment – 10% strength.

Dried rad Sig 2g

Tincturae 1:10 Sig 0.25ml [5gtt]. Safer dosage is 5ml aqua ad 100 Sig 5ml TDS

Liquidum extractum flos Mix LE 30gtt with Aqua 120ml. Sig 5ml TDS

Oleum 1:5 Dilute with five times the volume.

Ung. up to 25% Tr.

Oleum @ 15%.

References

BPC 1949. 43 p30. 126 p205. 142 p169. 176 p147. 476.246 p476. 262 p52. 271 No 15. 394 p7.

Artemisia abrotanum [Southernwood]

Constituents
Volatile oil.

Primary pharmacological action: Anthelmintic. Antiseptic.

Therapeutic classes
Ophthalmic. Stimulant. Tonic. Deobstruent. Detergent. Venous tonic. Expectorant
Aromatic. Carminative. Bitter. Stomachic. Cholagogue. Antiparasitic.
Diuretic. Diaphoretic. Antirheumatic.
Emmenagogue. Anodyne. Antispasmodic. Antivenomous. Vulnerary.
Medicinal indications [Mercury]
Raynauds disease. Peripheral vascular disease. Gangrene. Asthma.
Anorexia. Flatulent dyspepsia. Ascaris. Strongyloides. Tanea.
Cramp and spasm of the muscles and ligaments. Sprains. Sciatica. Rheumatism.
Nervine tonic. Amenorrhoea.
Dandruff. Hair growth. Itchy skin. Lice. Adder snake bite.
Tissue conditions
A warm infusion is a stimulating diaphoretic and tonic in febrile conditions.
Supports an increase in weight.
Cautions
Pregnancy.
External use
Eye soreness – poultice.
Anorexia with Chamaemelum.
Sprains, swellings, gangrene and wounds - fomentations for pain.
Sciatica fomentation with Artemesia vulgaris, A. absinthium and cider vinegar.
Skin itch and eczema - used as a final rinse it will remove dandruff if used
regularly.
Adder snake bites oral and ung.
Scalp and skin lice and parasites - Lotion or oleum. Stimulates hair growth.
Hung in a wardrobe it's pleasant smell will drive away moths.
Insect repellent – rub on dermis.
Preparations
Bronchial disturbances with Tussilago.
With Artemisia vulgaris, Mentha pul. or Chamaelirium lut. in delayed menses.
Dosage and mode of application
Dried herba Sig 4g
Liquidium extractum Sig 4ml
References. 43 p31. 188 p398. 192 p518. 228 p349. 246 p471.

Artemisia absinthum [Wormwood]

Constituents
Essential oil - antibacterial - alpha and beta thujone, alpha-pinene, terpinen-4-ol, linalool, nerol1,8-cineole. Bitter glycoside absinthe.

Primary pharmacological action: Stimulating and tonic bitter.

Therapeutic classes
Antiseptic. Allays inflammation. Antifungal – Trichophyton.
Aromatic bitter. Stomachic. Cholagogue. Hepatic. Anti emetic. Anthelmintic.
Diuretic. Lithuria.
Emmenagogue. Anodyne. Nervine. Immune enhancer. Febrifuge. Insecticide.

Medicinal indications [Mars]
Catarrh. Dimness of sight. Discharging ears.
Halitosis. Atonic dyspepsia. Anorexia. Gastritis. Flatulence. Nausea. Vomiting.
Jaundice. Diarrhoea. Ascaris. Nematodes. Trematodes. Faciola hepatica – sheep liver fluke. Gout pain.
Epilepsy. Depression. Nervous exhaustion and fatigue. Neuralgia. Drug withdrawal
Pyrexia. Hair loss. Varicose ulcers.

Tissue conditions
The intense bitterness acts upon the stomach, gall bladder and intestines.
Stimulates the CNS. Aids the assimilation of food, promotes the appetite and digestion removing flatulence, and halitosis. It stimulates the production of hydrochloric acid. Stomach debility with atony and sluggish digestion. Nausea and retching, acidity and bloated ness. Nervous stomach and pain from flatulence. For atonic vaginal discharge/leucorrhoea.
Stimulates the central nervous system and heart. In nervous and physical exhaustion with fatigue. Eases the alcohol hangover. Small dosage for spinal irritability.

Cautions
Always use a small dose – this is a very stimulating remedy. The oleum is a nerve depressant.
Pregnancy. Lactation.

External use
Fleas and lice use an infusion as a wash.
Septic sore throat – apply a hot fomentation or use with honey.
Hair loss use a scalp rinse.
Popular for the treatment of roundworms if taken on an empty stomach night and morning combined with syrup. An enema should be taken on day one and three.

Pharmacopoeia

Varicose veins and ulcers – decoction as a wash.
Spinal nerve irritability – use the oil.
Sprains and bruises, rheumatic affections, painful swellings – use the oil or a fomentation.
Keeps away moths if hung where there are clothes.
Preparations
Cathartic with Juglans.
Vermifuge with Juglans, Ruta or Tanacetum.
Dosage and mode of application
Dried herba Sig 2g
Infusium Sig 30ml
Tinctura Sig 1ml
Liquidum extractum Sig 2ml
References
43 p32. 111 p269. 142 p 79. 188 p188. 246 p470. 251 p160. 293, 7, 1995, p271.

Artemisia annua [Sweet wormwood]

Constituents
Sesquiterpine lactone - Artemisinin which is antimalarial and antineoplastic. It bonds with parasite proteins. Flavonoids. Essential oil.

Primary pharmacological action: Antimalarial.

Therapeutic classes
Anti infective: Clonorchis sinensis [Liver fluke], Enterobacter, Escherichia coli, Klebsiella, Leishmania major, Pneumocystis carinii, Proteus, Serratia marcescens, Shigella dysenteriae, Staphylococcus aureus, Streptococcus faecalis.
Anti schistosomal – Schistosoma japonicum, Schistosoma mansoni, Anti nematode - Clonorchis sinensis, and mansoni. Antiamoebicidal - Naegleria fauleria.
Febrifuge. Antineoplastic.

Medicinal indications
Enhances phagocytes. Breast carcinoma.
Systemic lupus erythematosus. Malaria.

Tissue conditions
Malaria - effective in removing cerebral malaria with cure rates up to 90%, pyrexia and coma associated with malaria infection. Antimalarial prescription can be given by IV injection and suppository.

Cautions
Pregnancy.

Dosage and mode of application
Dried herba Sig 3g
Liquidum extractum Sig 5ml
Larger doses to effect in malaria up to 13ml TDS

References
190p14. 295, 7051 [313] p240. 296, 1996, 347 [9016]. 297, 24.6.1995. 392 p3.

Artemesia tridentata [Big sagebrush]

Constituents
Essential oil up to 6%; Camphor 1'8 cineole, alpha pinene, alpha terpineol, artemiseole, borneol, camphene, pinene, thujone. Camphor and Thujone are CNS stimulants. Monoterpenes. Sesquiterpine lactones – artevasin, deacetoxymatricarin, dehydroleucodin, ridentin. Phenols – coumarin, flavonoids.

Primary action: Antimicrobial agent.

Therapeutic class
Ophthalmic. Antiseptic.
Antimicrobial – gram positive to 11 Bacillus species. Corynebacterium diphtheria, Pneumococcus, Sarcina lutea, Staphylococcus aureus, Streptococcus faecalis.
Gram negative – Aeromonas hydrophilla, Alcaligenes faecalis, E. coli, Neisseria gonorrhoea, Neisseria sicca, Proteus vulgaris/mirabilia, Pseudomonas aeruginosa/fluorescens, Salmonella enteritidis/gallinarum/typhosa, Serratia marcescens. Mycobacterium phlei/tuberculosis.
Antifungal – Alternaria solani, Aspergillus fumigatus/niger, Candida albicans/krusei/tropicalis, Cryptococcus neoformans/rhoboenhani, Helminthosporum sativum, Mucor mucedo, Nigrospora panici, Penicillium digitatum, Rhizopus nigricans, Saccharomyces cerevisiae, Streptomyces venezuelae, Trichophyton.
Antiprotozoal – Plasmodium gallinaceum.
Stimulant. Vasotonic alterative.
Bitter tonic. Carminative. Laxative. Parasiticide.
Diaphoretic. Febrifuge.
Emmenagogue.
Analgesic. Thyroactive. Antidote. Dermatological agent.

Medicinal indications
Conjunctivitis. Toothache. Colds. Laryngismus stridulus. Diphtheria. Influenza. Pneumonia. Tuberculosis.
Dyspepsia. Nausea. Vomiting. Diarrhoea. Gastro enteritis. Colic. Intestinal flatus. Constipation. Worms.
Arthritis. Rheumatic pain. Lumbago. Sprains. Ulcers.
Amenorrhoea. Dysmenorrhoea. Postpartum haemorrhage.
Abscesses. Contusions. Wounds. Pyrexia. Malarial fever. Erysipelas. Snakebite. Red ant bites.
Goitre. Poisoning – barbiturates, opates, mushrooms.

Cautions
Avoid in early pregnancy.

External use

Conjunctivitis - Collyr

Respiratory infections – poultice.

Ulcers – poultice of powder or decoction wash.

Sagebrush smudgestick - burn the herb as an aerosol for the sick room.

Dosage and mode of application

Liquidum extractum fol/flos Sig 4ml.

References

310, Vol 2, N03, 1991/92.

Artemisia vulgaris [Mugwort]

Constituents
Bitter glycosides. Treterpenoids. Sesquiterpine lactones. Volatile oil containing cineole. Resin. Flavonoids. Tannin.

Primary pharmacological action:
Stimulant and tonic emmenagogue.

Therapeutic classes
Antibacerial. Antifungal.
Aperitif. Stomachic. Cholagogue. Choleretic. Purgative. Anthelmintic.
Diaphoretic. Diuretic.
Emmenagogue. Hormone enhancer.
Sedative – mild. Antipyretic.
Dermatological agent. Antineoplastic.
Moxibustion. Opium antidote.

Medicinal indications [Venus]
Deficient circulation. Asthma.
Anorexia. Nervous dyspepsia. Vomiting. Diarrhoea. Intestinal cramp.
Nematodes - Roundworms, Threadworms.
Gout. Rheumatism.
Anxiety. Depression – mild. Headache. Insomnia. Epilepsy.
Amenorrhoea. Dysmenorrhoea. Retained placenta. Eases partum pain.
Menopause.
Inflamed skin. Abscesses. Bruises. Tumours. Whitlows.

Tissue conditions
Acute intestinal pain is relieved with an infusion and fomentation. In epilepsy with a feeble constitution. Improves uterine muscular tone by sustaining the uterine circulation.
Crushed leaves create a pungent aroma for use as an air freshener.
Mugwort is the prime ingredient rubbed and formed into a small cone it is used as moxa [moxibustion]. A quick burning herb and will produce a deeply penetrating heat. Moxa is burnt to induce a small blister upon the skin and thereby create vasodilation and rubefacient action, this draws blood to the surface and decongests the internal congested area. Used over any painful area to stimulate the circulation in pain and old injuries.

External use
Inflammatory swellings – apply a hot fomentation and renew when cool. Follow with a poultice of Ulmus or Stellaria.
Bruises, wounds, whitlows, abscesses, pustules – apply a hot fomentation.

Infusion added to the bath helps rheumatism and gout.

It has been used in dream pillows to encourage prophetic dreams.

Cautions

Prescribe small doses. Pregnancy.

Preparations

Menstrual irregularity with Mentha pulegrum or Artemisia abrotanum.

Worms – with Tanacetum and an enema on day one and three.

Dosage and mode of application

Dried herba. Sig 2g

Infusium herba Sig 15ml

Liquidum extractum Sig 2ml

References

43 p34. 192 p 368. 236 p93. 246 p469.

Asarum canadense [Wild ginger]

Constituents
Alkaloids. Volatile oil up to 4.5% – methyleugenol. Resin. Mucilage. Bitter-asarin

Primary pharmacological action: General vasodilator.

Therapeutic classes
Ophthalmic. Stimulant. Antiseptic.
Antibacterial - streptococci, staphylococci and pneumococcus.
Cardiac.
Expectorant.
Carminative. Antiflatulent.
Diaphoretic. Diuretic.
Antispasmodic.
Emmenagogue. Parturient. Uterine tonic.
Medicinal indications
Angina. Palpitations. Oedema.
Nasal catarrh. Conjunctivitis. Chronic chest. Asthma. Pertussus.
Flatulent colic. Relieves spasm of the intestine. Colic. Cholera.
Amenorrhoea - from chill. Dysmenorrhoea. PMS. Post partum depression.
Tissue conditions
Stimulates the mucosal lining of the GIT and uterus. Smooth muscle relaxant.
Fever and inflammatory affections with dry skin.
Parturition with pain and weakness of expulsive power. Menstrual disorders: pre
menstrual backache, dysmenorrhoea with cutting pain in the lower abdomen,
groin and thighs, from uterine atony. Taken hot it is a strong diaphoretic.
Cautions
Avoid in acute inflammatory conditions. Early pregnancy.
Dosage and mode of application
Restrictions apply. Dosage is determined by the relief of symptoms. Taken hot it
is a strong diaphoretic.
Infusium rad/rhiz. Sig 30ml
Parturition Tr 5gtt aqua 100ml Sig 5ml every 10 minutes for pain & weakness.
References
111 p273. 126 p221. 176 p274. 189 p128. 192 p565.

Asclepias tuberosa [Pleurisy root]

Constituents
Cardiac glycosides known as cardenolides. Resin. Flavonols - kaempferol, quercetin. Flavonic glycosides - rutin. Sterols. Triterpenes. Volatile oil.

Primary pharmacological action:
Relaxing diaphoretic. Vasorelaxant.

Therapeutic classes
Allays inflammation. Antiviral. Antimicrobial. Expectorant.
Carminative. Cathartic – mild [large dose] Emetic [large dose].
Diaphoretic – relaxing. Diuretic.
Antispasmodic. Nervine.
Medicinal indications
Spasmodic coughs. Bronchitis. Influenza. Laryngismus stridulus. Pleurisy.
Pneumonia.
Flatulent and bilious colic. Peritonitis. Typhoid fever. Inflammation of the serous tissues.
Amenorrhoea. Eruptive diseases - measles, chicken pox. Intercostal rheumatism.
Tissue conditions.
Asclepias produces a mild and persistent relaxing diaphoretic action. It's diffusive action upon the capillary circulation produces a full flow of blood to the skin dissipating the heat of inflammatory fever.
Asclepias has a specific action to the lungs – it will reabsorb serous exudate [pleural effusion] from the pleura, and allay inflammation. Given for pleuritic pain in the lung with a hard and painful cough.
The heart and arteries are released from undue tension by the promotion of excessive heat through the capillaries and skin glands.
Asclepias is indicated for a hot, dry skin with rigid pulse, It soothes the nervous system.
Asclepias has a slow, persistent and mild action.
Eruptive diseases give as a hot decoction.
Acute dysentery with fever.
Cautions
Depressed [atonic] or chronic conditions, excessive perspiration, cold skin surface, weak or small feeble pulse, suppuration, putrescence, congestion. Diphtheria.

Pharmacopoeia

Preparations
Pleurisy, bronchitis, peritonitis – give with Lobelia and Zingiber. Sig every 30 minutes.
For more stimulation with Grindelia, Lobelia and Capsicum.
Influenza – action is increased with Zingiber due to a more permanent diffusive action upon the capillaries.
Influenza mistura Asclepias, Solidago, Zingiber, Capsicum.
Diaphoretic – where more stimulation is required; Asclepias, Zingiber, Capsicum.
Amenorrhoea, dysmenorrhoea – Caulophyllum, Capsicum and Zingiber.
Equalise the circulation and induce diaphoresis in pleurisy use Angelica arch., Sassafras and Zingiber.
Intercostal rheumatism – with Ballota or Cimicifuga.
Eruptive diseases – Asclepias, Zingiber and Capsicum.
Dosage and mode of application
Dried rad Sig 4g
Infusium Sig 4g
Tincturae Sig 2.5ml
Liquidum extractum Sig 2ml
References
43 p35. 111 p277. 126 p222. 176 p250. 189 p219. 246 p333.

Asparagus racemosus [Shatavari, Wild asparagus]

Constituents
Glycosides – shatavarin, Saponins. Sitosterol. Mucilage. It has a sweet taste.

Primary pharmacological action: Nutritive Tonic. Adaptogen.

Therapeutic classes
Ophthalmic. Allays inflammation. Astringent. Demulcent. Nutritive. Refrigerant.
Cardiotonic. Antihaemorrhagic.
Expectorant.
Antacid. Antidiarrhoeal.
Aphrodisiac. Spermatogenic. Reproductive tonic to male and female [uterine tonic] .
Galactagogue. Antioxytocic.
Febrifuge. Immunostimulant.
Antispasmodic.
Anabolic.
Medicinal indications
Ophthalmic disease.
Leucopenia, neutropenia, leucocytosis, improves macrophage function.
Dry cough. Haemoptysis.
Sore throat. Gastritis. Heartburn. Hyperchlorhydria. Peptic ulcers. Crohns disease. Dysentery. Biliousness. Inhibits Entamoeba histolytica also E. Coli.
Cystitis. Dysuria.
Dysmenorrhoea. Menorrhagia. Fertility and menopausal difficulties – vaginal dryness, flushes and irritability. Increases milk flow. Memory loss.
Low sperm count with irregular forms.
Epilepsy.
Tissue conditions
Soothes and allays inflammatory conditions gastro intestinal mucous membranes.
Utilised as a prostate and uterine tonic rebalancing hormonal irregularity.
Anabolic activity supports tissue nutrition and increases muscle mass.
Preparations
Gynaecology – Curcuma and Zingiber.
Uterine tonic/infertility – Ashwaganda.
Dosage and mode of application
Tincturae Sig 8ml
Liquidum extractum Sig 4ml

Asperula odorata [Sweet woodruff] see Galium odoratum.

Aspidosperma quebracho blanco
[Quebracho]

Constituents
Indole alkaloids – aspidospermine and yohimbine, up to 1.4% are alpha adrenergic blockers. Sterols. Tannin.

Primary pharmacological action: Bronchial antispasmodic.

Therapeutic classes
Antimicrobial. Tonic. Cardioactive. Peripheral vasodilator.
Antiasmatic.
Bitter.
Diuretic. Febrifuge.
Antispasmodic.

Medicinal indications
Angina. Arrhythmia. Cardiac and respiratory stimulant. Cyanosis. Hypertension.
Emphysema. Chronic bronchitis. Asthma. Tuberculosis.
Malaria. Pyrexia.
Impotence/sexual dysfunction.

Tissue conditions
Stimulates the respiratory centre. Increases respiratory depth and rate. Relieves dyspnoea from cardiac and respiratory conditions - asthma, bronchitis and emphysema.

Cautions
Restrictions apply. Dosage is determined by the relief of symptoms.
Emetic in large dosage.

External use
Skin infections – use the latex.

Dosage and mode of application
Dried bacc/rad/fol. Sig 50mg
Tincturae Sig 4ml
Liquidum extractum Sig 2ml [Ref 390 p328]

References
BPC 1934. 126 p228. 176 p248. 188 p363. 224. 390

Asphaltum

Constituents
Benzopyrones and fulvic acid. Bitters.

Primary pharmacological action: Tonic

Therapeutic classes
Hepatic
Medicinal indications
Jaundice. Antidiabetic. TB.
Dysmenorrhoea/menorrhagia.
Arrests ageing process

Astragalus membranaceus
[Membraneous/Mongolian milk vetch]

Constituents
Triterpenoid saponins - astragalosides potentiate NK activity. Flavonoids. Sterols.
Essential oil. Polysaccharides are immune enhancers and potentiate NK activity,
lymphocyte and monocyte activity. Amino acids.

Primary pharmacological action: Immunostimulant.

Therapeutic classes
Stimulant. Anti viral – HIV., Parainfluenza, Coxsackie B2 and viral myocarditis.
Antibacterial. Antioxidant. Tonic.
Cardiotonic. Hypotensive. Increases leucocytosis. Vasodilator. Pulmonary tonic.
Hepatoprotective. Intestinal muscle tonic. Hypoglycaemic. Splenic tonic.
Nephritic. Diuretic. Antipyretic.
Antineoplastic. Immunostimulant. Adaptogenic. Dermatological agent.

Medicinal indications
Palpitations. Ischaemic heart disease. Hypotensive.
Chronic infections. Upper respiratory infections. Influenza.
Anorexia. Peptic ulcers. Diarrhoea. Rectocoele. Organ prolapse.
Cervical erosion.Uterine prolapse. Post partum haemorrhage.
Debility. Fatigue. ME. Senility. Malaria. Spontaneous perspiration.

Tissue conditions
It helps to restore immune function as an immunostimulant – it increases
interferon. Reduces blood viscosity. Inotropic action on the myocardium.
Improves the sodium pump activity to reduce intracellular sodium. Enhances the
white blood cell count. Enhances NK cell activity. Improves the tone of the
intestine. Balances the amount of perspiration on the skin - an adaptogenic skin
remedy. Promotes stamina. Allays the effects of chemotherapy and radiotherapy.

Preparations
Vitality tonic with Codonopsis pilusula.

Cautions
Dry mouth. Acute infections.

Dosage and mode of application
Dried rad Sig 2g
Liquidum extractum rad. Sig 3ml
Interferon effect Sig up to 8g daily
Oncology patients - Sig up to 20g daily

References
48 p13. 188 p235. 194. 239 p170. 271, 1999, No 67. 398.

Atropa belladonna [Deadly nightshade]

Constituents
Tropane alkaloids [around 0.3% - hyoscyamine] & hyoscine are anti cholinergic.
Scopolamine. Flavonoids. Coumarins.

Primary pharmacological action:
Smooth muscle antispasmodic

Therapeutic classes
Ophthalmic.
Antiasmatic. Anticholinergic. Antihydrotic. Inhibits glandular secretions.
Medicinal indications [Saturn]
Dilates the pupil. Dries secretions. Mydriatic. Acute inflammatory conditions.
Palpitations.
Asthma. Pertussus. Phlebitis. Scarlet fever.
Biliary colic. Intestinal colic. Strangulated hernia.
Enuresis. Renal colic. Nephritis. Urinary irritation. Lumbago.
Hyperhidrosis. Pyrexia.
Prolactin depressor.
Eruptive skin disorders, Measles.
Meningitis. Neuralgia. Parkinsons disease. Chorea. Epilepsy.
Tissue conditions
Paralyses muscles of accommodation, increases intra ocular pressure.
Impairment of the cerebral capillary circulation with congestion [dizzyness, drowsiness, coma].
An excitant to the cerebrum promoting active hyperaemia – a full active cerebral circulation. Depresses the CNS indicated in cerebral and spinal congestive states.
Atropa dilates the cerebral capillaries, stimulates the heart by 20-40 BPM and contracts the splanchnic capillaries. A powerful influence is obtained with passive hyperaemia [congestion] in any area. In full dosage the face becomes flushed and the skin bright red with dry mouth, and difficulty swallowing.
Paralyses the parasympathetic nerves.
Atropa will relieve pulmonary hyperaemia, clear cyanosis and promote full deep breathing.
It will allay palpitations.
Atropa quickly stimulates the capillary circulation in engorged [congested] organs, preventing the local effects of acute inflammation in diphtheria, tonsillitis, croup, bronchitis, pneumonia and peritonitis.
Atropa is indicated with the onset of inflammatory conditions. Reduces salivary and bronchial secretions. Reduces perspiration.

Pharmacopoeia

Used as an antispasmodic in pertussus, asthma, gall bladder, renal, or intestinal colic – given in drop dosage every two hours. It will relieve the griping of purgatives.

In fevers with cold skin – eruptive, scarlet and malarial, continued and typhoid, Atropa has an essential place in some stage of the fever. It will help protect from the infection of scarlet fever.

Meningitis – sub acute cases with a 2-3 degree rise in temperature, dilated pupils, eyes dull, head drawn back, eyes partly open, when the patient is asleep – Atropa is directly indicated to equalise the circulation.

Improves the speech, tremor, rigidity and gait of parkinsons disease.

Milk secretion will cease with Atropa, internally and locally. Dysmenorrhoea with cool skin and extremities given in drop dosage for the pain.

Cautions

Restrictions apply. Dosage is determined by the relief of symptoms.

Always give in small dosage.

Avoid with alkaline medicines.

Contraindications - Glaucoma, paralytic ileus, prostatic hypertrophy, tachycardia.

Discontinue if the following symptoms occur as result of overdose: restless excitation, headache, diluted pupils, intolerance to light, visual disturbances, hot dry skin, dry mouth, bradycardia, stertorous respiration, confusion, hallucinations delirium or coma.

Antidote with tannin.

Preparations

Neuralgia with Camphor.

External use

Dilates the pupil and paralyses the ciliary muscle. Used in anterior chamber inflammation.

Acute inflammation, it acts as a sedative and anodyne.

Will relax a rigid Os - apply to the Os.

Spasmodic urethral stricture – injection.

Inflammation [phlebitis] – plaster over the area affected.

Spinal tenderness, lumbago, neuralgia of the spinal and sacral nerves, rheumatism, sprained and painful joints - liniment or plaster.

Furunculosis.

Suppository for haemorrhoids.

Dosage and mode of application

Dried herba Sig 50mg

Dry extract – an alcoholic percolate evaporated and powdered. Sig 60mg

Dried rad Sig 30mg

Tincturae Atropa radix. 1:10 Sig 0.5ml

Liquidum extractum Atropae rad. Sig 0.2ml

Ung Atropa 2%

Oculentum Atropa 1%
Guttae pro oculus Atropa 1g Aqua sterile to 100ml. Sig 5gtt.
Mist Atropa paediatric [prepare fresh]
Tr Atropa rad 0.15ml, Tr Auranti 0.01ml, Glycerol 0.5ml, Syrup 1ml, Aq
add 100ml. Sig up to one year 5ml. 1-5 years 10ml.
5ml contains 45 micrograms of alkaloids.
Linimentum Atropinae – Atropa 1ml, Ol Olive 15ml, Ol Ricinus 15ml Ol
Lavandula 1ml Alcohol to 100. Apply with gentle friction.
References
BP 1980. 43 p36. 126 p239. 176 p178. 233 p31. 246 p395. 390 p282.

Avena sativa [Oats]

Constituents
Silicon dioxide up to 2%. Triterpenoid saponins. Carbohydrate. Protein.
Calcium. Iron. Magnesium. Vitamin B, E.

Primary pharmacological action:
Nervine tonic. CNS trophorestorative.

Therapeutic classes
Nutritive heart tonic. Anticholesterolaemic.
Hypoglycaemic.
Dermatological agent.
Immune stimulant. Alcohol and nicotine addiction.
Nerve antispasmodic. Sedative. Sexual tonic.
Medicinal indications [Mercury]
Palpitations.
Spasmodic and nervous disorders e.g. chorea. Nervous debility of convalescence.
Nervous exhaustion and tremors. Muscular feebleness. Nervous tachycardia and
excitement.
Gout. Spermatorrhoea. Impotence/sexual dysfunction. PMS.
Dermal irritation/inflammation . Pruritus. Seborrhoea.
Chorea. Excitability. Epilepsy. Enhances athletic performance. Insomnia.
Obsessive behaviour. Panic.
Paralysis. Schizophrenia. Shingles. Alcoholism.
Tissue conditions
Strengthens the nerve force by improving nutrition to the neurones. Exhaustion is
the key note to this remedy. Avena is selective to the genito urinary and cerebral
nerves. Allays nervous excitement, tachycardia and insomnia. Weakness of the
mind, debility and a tendency to excess indulgence – obsessive behaviour. As a
tonic in spermatorrhoea. Relieves spasmodic conditions of the bladder and
ureter. PMS with headache, exhaustion, panic or nausea. Blood and hair tonic.
Supports the withdrawal from tobacco. Children fed with porridge for breakfast
tend to be more alert and study levels improve.
Cautions
Avoid concurrent use with Passiflora.
External use
Balneum - put two handfuls sem or 100g herba into muslin then run hot bath
water allowing the milky solution to cover the skin - treatment for eczema, spots
and freckles.

Preparations
With Zanthoxylum or Capsicum it will assist its stimulating properties.
Cardiac weakness with Selenicerus.
Chorea with Scutellaria, Cimicifuga or Gelsemium.
Impotency/spermatorrhoea with Turnera and Serenoa.
Prostate trouble with Pulsatilla, Fucus, Serenoa, Salix nigra or Apium.
Dysmenorrhoea with Aletris or Mitchella.
Poultice made with oil of Bay leaves helps the itch, fistulas and Leprosy.
Dosage and mode of application
Tincturae herba or sem Sig 10ml
Liquidum extractum Sig 4ml
References
43 p37. 126 p235. 142 p287. 176 p204. 188 p315. 192 p390. 246 p543. 394 p281

Azadirachta indica [Neem]

Constituents
Quercetin. Triterpenes – [limonoids] meliacins, nimbin, azadirachtin. Tannin.
Chlorophyll.

Primary pharmacological action: Astringent & Bitter Tonic.

Therapeutic classes
Antiseptic. Allays inflammation. Vasotonic alterative. Antibacterial. Antiviral.
Antifungal – Candida, Epidermophyton, Geotrichum, Microsporum,
Trichophyton and Trichosporon.
Antimalarial - decoction inhibits Plasmodium berghei, Plasmodium falciparum.
Oral agent. Stomachic. Antidiabetic. Anthelmintic.
Antiperiodic. Antipyretic. Antimalarial. Parasiticidal. Antivenomous.
Analgesic.
Medicinal indications
Angina. Hypertension.
Bronchitis. Dyspnoea.
Dental caries. Gingivitis. Jaundice. Intestinal parasites. Diarrhoea. Haemorrhoids
Alopecia. Infected burns or skin. Eczema. Itchy skin. Psoriasis. Pediculosis.
Scabies.
Bruises and sprains. Snakebite. Sepsis.
Lymphadenopathy. Pyrexia.
Tissue conditions
Rebalances the intestinal microflora.
Preparations
Scabies with Curcuma.
External use
Dental antiseptic, antifungal - toothpaste.
Chronic eczema, tinea, furunculosis, dermal ulcers, pediculosis, psoriasis,
scabies – use ung, oleum 5% or soap.
Dosage and mode of application
Infusium fol/fruct/sem/bacc/rad. 1:20 Sig 30ml
Tincturae bacc, fol. Sig 4ml
References
272, 1993, 5 [3] p40. 284, January 2000, p36-8. 390 p323.
Martindale advises references for constituents from Bhandari P & Mukerji B
East Pharmst. 1959, 2 [No 16], 7 and 2 [No 19], 9. 392.

Backhousia myrtifolia [Myrtle]

Constituents
Essential oil. Tannin.

Primary pharmacological action:
Nervine relaxant to the Gastro intestinal tract.

Therapeutic classes
Astringent.
Carminative.
Topical anaesthetic.
Medicinal indications
Dyspepsia. Colic. Diarrhoea. IBS.
Nervous tension.
Tissue conditions
Used in bowel disorders with nervous irritability.
Dosage and mode of application
Tincturae Sig 4ml

Bacopa monniera [Herpastis monnieri]

Constituents
Saponins. Bramhine – cardiac tonic.

Primary pharmacological action: Cerebral and nervine tonic.

Therapeutic classes
Cardiotonic. Vasoconstrictor.
Anxiolytic. Sedative. Tranquilliser. Analgesic. Anticonvulsant.
Medicinal indications
Constipation.
Diuretic.
Anxiety. Stress. Nervous exhaustion/breakdown. Poor memory. Lack of
concentration. Aids memory and learning. Epilepsy.
Tissue conditions
Effects include improved memory and mental well being. Nervous disorders
with convulsions or unconsciousness. Nerve disorders due to depletion of
neurones e.g. alzheimers, CVA, concussion, injury, disorders of behaviour and
insanity.
External use
Chest conditions – poultice.
Rheumatism – ung.
Preparations
With Rosmarinus, Stachys, Withania or Panax.
Dosage and mode of application
Dried herba 2g
Liquidum extractum Sig 4ml
References
48 p101. 191 p29. 298, 1999, Vol. 5, No 2, p21-27.

Ballota nigra [Black horehound]

Constituents
Flavonoids. Diterpenes. Volatile oil.

Primary pharmacological action:
Gentle tonic to the circulatory, digestive, nervous and reproductive systems.

Therapeutic classes
Expectorant. Bactericidal - pneumococcus Mild astringent.
Cardiac neuromuscular relaxant.
Antiemetic. Anti dyspeptic. Vermifuge.
Antirheumatic. Diaphoretic.
Antispasmodic. Sedative.
Parturient. Uterine tonic.
Medicinal indications [Mercury]
Tachycardia. Tuberculosis. Coughs. Bronchial complaints. Pneumonia.
Vomiting of central origin. Nausea. Nervous dyspepsia. Nematodes. Ascaris.
Rheumatism.
Panic attacks. Migraine. Motion sickness.
Amenorrhoea. Dysmenorrhoea. Metrorrhagia. Parturient - labour pain.
Tissue conditions
Cardiac neuromuscular relaxant.
Resolves excess mucus secretions and acts as an vasotonic alterative and tonic upon the mucous membranes, cleansing and healing diseased membranes. It will allay irritable coughs. It corrects acidity. Relieves centrally induced vomiting. As a nervine in asthenia/nervous debility.
Preparations
Pulmonary complaints with Althea, Hyssopus and Lobelia.
Hypertension with Crataegus, Leonurus.
Nervous dyspepsia with Chamaemelum nobile.
Metrorrhagia – with Bidens and Zingiber,
Parturition with Leonurus.
False labour pain -with Leonurus.
Dosage and mode of application
Dried herba Sig 4g
Tincturae Sig 2ml
Liquidum Extractum Sig 3ml
References
43 p38. 189 p146. 246 p373.

Baptisia tinctoria [Indigo]

Constituents
Glycoside Baptisin. Alkaloid - Baptitoxin. Cytisine. Purgative glycoside Baptin. Isoflavonoids.

Primary pharmacological action:
Stimulating antiseptic and vasotonic alterative.

Therapeutic classes
Stimulant. Tonic. Allays inflammation. Antimicrobial – Bacillus coli, Coxsackie infection. Discutient.
Cardioactive [mild]. Circulatory tonic. Antihaemorrhagic.
Choleretic. Hepatic. Purgative.
Anodyne.
Antivenomous.
Antineoplastic. Antipyretic.

Medicinal indications
Ear, nose and throat infections. Otitis media. Suppressed secretions. Scarlet fever. Septicaemia. Circulatory deficiency. Gangrene. Infectious mononucleosis.
Catarrh. Diphtheria. Pharyngitis. Laryngitis. Influenza.
Aphthous ulcers. Gingivitis. Stomatitis. Tonsillitis. Stomach carcinoma. Peptic ulcers. Emetic.Diabetes. Amoebic dysentery. Hepatic disorders. Ulcerative colitis. Haemorrhoids. Typhoid.
Syphilis. Cervical ulceration. Ovarian cancer. Sore nipples. Mastitis.
Lymphadenitis. Sepsis. Smallpox. Scorpion bites. Furunculosis. Meningitis. Pyrexia.

Tissue conditions
Specific in toxic and septic conditions. Increases secretions. Stimulating to the intestinal glands, increasing glandular secretion. Choleretic and purgative in large doses. Suitable for asthenic conditions [with fever]. Combats protracted fevers.
Indicated in suppressed secretions with sepsis ulcerative colitis, intestinal toxaemia, suppuration with offensive breath and diarrhoea all indicate it's use.
Ulcerations of the mouth, throat, nipples, intestine, cervix and skin.

External use
Tonsillitis and mouth ulcers - gargle and oral.
Abscesses use a hot fomentation.
Skin ulcers, gangrene use with Ulmus.
Cervical erosion, vaginal discharge - saturate a tampon or paint the area.
Vulval pruritis - use the ointment.
Chancres - apply a dry powder.

Preparations
[Throat] conditions with Capsicum, Echinacea and Commiphora.
Stomatitis - Filipendula, Ipecacuana.
Gargle with Capsicum.
Aphthous ulcers with Cephalis.
Wounds, lymphadenitis - with Arctium, Commiphora, Capsicum, Viola odorata.
Furunculosis - Phytolacca.
Rheumatiod arthritis with Filipendula.

Dosage and mode of application
Small doses are stimulant and large doses are emetic.
Powder rad Sig 1g
Decoctum Sig 1g
Tincturae 5ml
Liquidum extractum Sig 1.3ml
Ung 1 Part LE to 8 parts base.

References
43 p38. 111 p288. 126 p237. 176 p367. 188 p132/454. 192 p286/567. 194p54.
279 Vol 46, 1996

Barosma betulina [Buchu]

Constituents
Flavonoids including rutin. Volatile oils. Mucilage. Resin. Essential oil up to 2%.

Primary pharmacological action:
Genito urinary tonic stimulant.

Therapeutic classes
Stimulating, tonic and antiseptic diuretic. Urinary tract disinfectant. Antilithic.
Aromatic. Diaphoretic.

Medicinal indications
Urinary infections. Dysuria. Cystitis. Urethritis. Renal infections. Pyelitis.
Enlarged prostate. Prostatitis. Gonorrhoea. Gravel. Suppression of urine. Muco
purulent discharges. Acidic urine with frequency of micturition.

Tissue conditions
For atonic conditions of the genito urinary tract [GUT]. Mucous membranes of
the bladder, stomach and uterus are influenced by its tonic action as are the
pelvic nerves and bladder sphincter. Indicated for cases with excess uric acid and
an irritable bladder. It will remove muco purulent conditions of the GUT.
Removes solids in the urine as a diuretic function. Reduces excess uric acid.

Preparations
Combines with Daucus in obstruction of micturition.

Dosage and mode of application
Dried fol Sig 2g
Tincturae Sig 4ml
Liquidum extractum Sig 4ml

References
43 p15. 111 p290. 176 p429. 188 p75. 224 p1731.

Bellis perennis [Daisy]

Constituents
Bitters. Mucilage. Saponins. Essential oil – around 20% polyacetylenes. Tannin.

Primary pharmacological action: Astringent and tonic.

Therapeutic classes
Allays inflammation. Demulcent. Discutient. Vasotonic alterative. Antifungal.
Antibacterial – Mycetes, gram +ve, gram – ve bacteria. Antiviral – HIV.
Cardiac tonic. Antisclerotic. Expectorant.
Hepatic. Leaves stimulate metabolism.
Diuretic. Diaphoretic. Antirheumatic.
Antispasmodic. Anodyne. Vulnerary. Antineoplastic [1]. Dermatological agent.
Medicinal indications [Venus]
Heart and peripheral circulatory stimulant.
Respiratory congestion. Coughs. Catarrh. Sinusitis. Wheezing.
Aphthous ulcers. Hepatitis. Diarrhoea. Jaundice. Colic. Ulcerations.
Gout. Rheumatic pain. Sciatica. Scrotal inflammation. Hernia. Vaginitis.
Depression. Irritability. Muscle spasm.
Bruises. Furunculosis. Ulcers. Wounds. Fibrocystic breast disease. Tumours
[resulting from injuries]. Pyrexia.
Tissue conditions
Root is an vasotonic alterative against toxins and uric acid – it clears the blood.
Circulatory tonic to the heart and arteries improving blood supply to the
periphery in chilblains. Inflammatory skin conditions.
Heals wounds and counteracts debility following such injuries.
External use
Eye disorders with pain and inflammation - Collyr infusium Bellis, Ung Bellis.
Breasts - *internal* and external use.
Wounds - new/hernia/muscular contractures - crushed [fresh] fol et flos.
Paralysis - use the medicated bath.
Sciatica or gout - with Agrimonia and Stachys palustris.
Hung about the house they drive out fleas.
Preparations
Myocarditis with Crataegus and Calendula.
Swelling as a result of injury with Artemesia vulgaris.
Dosage and mode of application
Dried flos/herba/rad Sig 5g
References
188 p140. 228 p114. 236 p48. 246 p450. 251 p63. 263, 1997, 63, p503.

Berberis aquifolium [Mahonia]

Constituents
Alkaloids - berberine and oxycanthine.
Whole bark extract and extracts of berberine, berbamine and oxycanthine all inhibit proliferation of HaCaT cells which are a line of rapidly proliferating human keratinocyte cells. Berberis vulgaris contains more berberine and is stronger than Berberis Aq.

Primary pharmacological action:
A slowly acting
gently stimulating tonic hepatic and vasotonic alterative.

Therapeutic classes
Vasotonic alterative. Antioxidant. Antifungal - Herpes. Expectorant.
Emetic. Cholagogue. Choleretic. Tonic - laxative.
Diuretic. Urinary calculi. Diaphoretic.
Dermatological agent. Glandular stimulant.
Medicinal indications [Mars]
Septicaemia. Bronchitis.
Bilious headaches. Gastritis. Stomatitis. Leucoplakia. Catarrhal states of the stomach, intestine and urinary organs. Cholecystitis. Hepatitis. Dyspepsia.
Constipation. Diarrhoea.
Dysuria. Oedema. Arthritis. Rheumatism. Pyrexia.
Acne. Boils. Dandruff. Eczema. Pruritus. Psoriasis. Syphilis. Vaginitis.
Tissue conditions
Chronic skin disease is its hallmark.
Influences the glandular secretions of the GIT in catarrhal conditions with dyspepsia. Stimulates assimilation, secretion and excretion. A slow acting remedy enhancing absorption. Biliary disorders with weakness.
Blood Vasotonic alterative and antiseptic in skin eruptions of the head, face and neck. Specific in scaly and pustular skin disorders from blood impurities.
Lipoxygenase [LO] products are a result of oxidation and are inflammation mediators they are involved in the pathogenesis of psoriasis. LO inhibitors can remove free radicles. Aquifoleum successfully inhibits lipid peroxidation and free radicles.
Preparations
More effective in combination.
Skin conditions with - Arctium or Rumex.
Syphilis with Trifolium, Zanthoxylum, Iris.

Dosage and mode of application
Dried rad/rhiz. Sig 2g
Decoctum Sig 2g
Tincturae Sig 4ml
Liquidum extractum Sig 2ml
References
43 p41. 126 p244. 176 p339. 192 p395. 246 p124. 263, 1994, 60, 421. 263, 61, 1995, p74.

Berberis vulgaris [Barberry]

Constituents
The root is yellow in colour, due to the presence of the alkaloids [up to 13%] berberine and hydrastine. Hydrastine stimulates the medulla and is a vasoconstrictor. Isoquinoline alkaloid - Berberine is choleretic, bactericidal and a smooth muscle tonic. Jatorrhizine – fungicidal, antiarrhythmic and hypotensive. Oxyacanthine – bactericidal. Palmitine – adrenocorticotrophic, analgesic, antiarrhythmic and bactericidal.

Primary pharmacological action: Hepato biliary bitter tonic.

Therapeutic classes
Ophthalmic. Vasotonic alterative. Allays inflammation. Astringent. Antiseptic. Antimicrobial – Chlamydia trachomatis, Entamoeba histolytica, Giardia lamblia, Leishmania donovani, Neisseria gonorrhoeae, Neisseria meningitidis, Rhizopus oryzae, Scopulariopsis, Streptomyces sp. Treponema pallidum, Vibrio cholerae. Antibacterial – Bacillus subtilis, Colpidum colpoda, Corynebacterium diptheria, Diplococcus pneumoniae, Escherichia coli, Helicobacter pylori, Mycobacterium tuberculosis, Pseudomonas sp, Salmonella typhi, Shigella dysenteriae, Staphylococcus sp.
Antifungal - Aspergillus flavus and fumigatus, Candida albicans, Trichomonas vaginalis.
Antiviral – A and B influenza virus.
Antiarrhythmic. Hypotensive. Antihaemorrhagic.
Cholagogue. Choleretic. Digestive/hepatic/pancreatic/splenic tonic. Laxative. Antidiarrhoeal. Amoebicidal. Antimalarial.
Renal tonic. Antipyretic. Diaphoretic.
Uterine stimulant. Oxytocic.
Sedative. Anticonvulsant.
Antineoplastic. Immunostimulant.

Medicinal indications [Mars]
Opthalmia – trachoma. Mydriatic. Haemorrhage.
Aphthous ulcers. Gastritis. Cholecystitis. Cholelithiasis. Hepatitis. Indigestion. Diarrhoea. Dysentery. Constipation. Anal itching. Pancreatic. Hypoglycaemic. Jaundice. Antispasmodic action upon smooth muscle of the stomach and intestine. Giardiasis – inhibits Giardia lamblia. Cholera.
Inflammatory and infective conditions of the urinary tract. Lithuria.
Gout/Arthritis/Rheumatism.
Malaria – inhibits Plasmodium berghei and falciparum. Leishmaniasis – sandfly parasite. Inhibits acetylcholinesterase. Pyrexia. Psoriasis.

Tissue conditions

Oral administration provides a long duration of activity up to 72 hours. Chlorides of berberine inhibit the elastolytic activity of human sputum elastase. Elastase can degrade elastin, collagen, protoglycan and fibronectin at neutral pH contributing to tissue damage in pulmonary and musculoskeletal disease. Stimulates and tones the liver & gall bladder, stomach, spleen and intestines. Increases splenic blood flow and reduces splenic enlargement. Increases gastric secretions and improves the appetite and the assimilation of food. Stimulates, tones and astringes the gastro intestinal mucous membranes. Inflammatory and infective conditions of the respiratory, gastro intestinal and urinary tracts. Useful for acidic individuals where rheumatic diathesis is prominent. Indicated in jaundice and diarrhoea as a tonic.

Cautions

Diarrhoea. Pregnancy.

External use

Oropharyngeal infections/ulcers – decoction.

Dosage and mode of application

Dried cort/bacc. Sig 2g

Decoctum 2g

Tincturae Sig 4ml

Liquidum extractum Sig 2ml

References

43 p40. 111 p294. 126 p245. 191. 230 p5. 231 p140. 246 p123. 262 p57. 263 1993, 59, p200.

Betula alba/pendula [Silver birch]

Constituents
Flavonoids hyperoside [diuretic], quercetin. Betulorentic acid. Saponins.
Essential oil. Tannin. Resin. Volatile oil.

Primary pharmacological action: Litholytic diuretic.

Therapeutic classes
Astringent. Demulcent. Allays inflammation. Antimicrobial.
Cardiac stimulant. Anticholesterolaemic.
Mild laxative.
Urinary antiseptic. Diuretic. Diaphoretic.
Antirheumatic. Dermatological agent. Vulnerary. Intermittent fever.
Nervine relaxant. Anodyne.
Medicinal indications [Venus]
Urinary tract infections. Renal and cardiac oedema. Renal calculi. Urinary calculi.
Albuminuria. Dysuria. Gout. Renal colic. Arthritic pain. Arthritis. Eczema.
Wounds.
Tissue conditions
Betula supports the elimination of uric acid and calculi. A prompt diuretic to
relieve oedema of cardiac and renal origin. Infected urinary tract.
External use
Eczema and psoriasis – ung.
Preparations
Calculi with Alchemilla arvensis.
Sap oil has been used in acne, eczema, herpes, pruritus,
psoriasis.
Dosage and mode of application
Fol and sap - diuretic. Cort - antiseptic. Inner cort - astringent. Buds - laxative.
Dried fol. Sig 2g
Tincturae fol. Sig 5ml
Succus Sig 10ml
References
111 p293. 176 p433. 189 p31. 192 p59. 246 p72.

Borago officinalis [Borage]

Constituents
Alkaloids. Mucilage. Saponins. Tannins. Essential oil with essential fatty acids.
Emollient when the plant is young.
Depurative and sudorific when the plant is mature and flowering.
Diuretic when fruiting. [Glycosidal mineral content changes].

Primary pharmacological action: Adrenal trophorestorative.

Therapeutic classes
Allays inflammation. Antiviral – herpes. Antifungal – Trichophyton.
Demulcent. Depurative. Refrigerant. Tonic.
Expectorant. Pectoral.
Aperient.
Diuretic. Diaphoretic. Adrenotonic.
Galactagogue. Antispasmodic. Nervine tonic. Antidepressant. Antipyretic.

Medicinal indications [Jupiter]
Cardiac disease. Cardiac nerve trouble.
Bronchitis. Coughs.
Acidosis. Hepatitis. Jaundice. Constipation - mild laxative.
Cystitis. Nephritis. Rheumatoid arthritis. Pyrexia.
Menopausal disturbances.
Debility. Depression. Adrenal dysfunction.

Tissue conditions
Comforts the heart when saddened by grief. GLA from the oil has been shown to
be more effective than Oenothera in healing gut mucosa that has been damaged
by inflammation.

External use
Ocular inflammation and oedema - Lotion or poultice.
Ringworm – apply succus.
Wound inflammation and skin infections.

Dosage and mode of application
Oleum Sem Sig 500mg
Infusium herba Sig 5g
Tincturae Sig 10ml

References
192 p85/86. 246 p355. 247 p120. 250 p117. 299, Jan 1993/20.

Borreria verticillata [Coffee family]

Constituents
Indole alkaloids mainly borreine and borreverine. Root bark contains iridoids. The leaves contain essential oil

Primary pharmacological action: Dermatological agent.

Therapeutic classes
Anti bacterial - E. Coli, Staphylococcus aureus.
Diuretic.
Abortifacient.
Medicinal indications
Infection. Eczema.
Preparations
The juice obtained from the herb is used topically against dermatitis and eczema. Borreria natalensis is used in leprosy.

Boscia senegalensis [Caper family]

Constituents
Alkyl glucosinolates. Alkaloids - stachydrine and hydroxystachydrine. Flavonoids.

Primary pharmacological action: Antimicrobial.

Therapeutic classes
Antinfective. Antifungal.
Stomachic.
Aphrodisiac. Parturient.
Medicinal indications
Stomachic fruct & rad. Jaundice. Malaria – fol. Fungal infections – fol. Sexually transmitted disease. Aphrodisiac. Parturient – fruct and rad.
External use
Wound dressing.

Boswellia serrata [Indian frankincense]

Constituents
The gum resin [called sallai guggal] contains triterpenoids - boswelic acids these allay inflammation by inhibiting the enzyme that stimulates leucotrine formation and is antineoplastic.
Essential oil up to 16% mostly cymene and thujone.

Primary pharmacological action: Astringent and tonic.

Therapeutic classes
Allays inflammation. Antimicrobial. Antiseptic.
Circulatory stimulant. Antihaemorrhagic. Hypocholesterolaemic.
Reduces leucotrine formation.
Expectorant.
Bitter. Ulcerogenic. Hepatic.
Diaphoretic. Diuretic. Antirheumatic.
Anodyne. Emmenagogue.
Fumigant. Dermatological agent. Vulnerary. Antineoplastic.

Medicinal indications
Catarrh. Lipid lowering – hypocholesterolaemic.
Asthma. Pulmonary affections.
Hepatic problems. Diarrhoea. Crohn's disease. Colitis. Ulcerative colitis. Colic.
Gout. Urinary disorders. Rheumatic pain and stiffness of the joints.
Sexually transmitted disease.
Suppurating wounds. Dermal ulcers.
Brain & Nasal tumours. Hepatic carcinoma. Colon tumours. Leukaemia.

Tissue conditions
The triterpenoids inhibit DNA, RNA and protein in human leukaemic cells. By acting upon the DNA molecule binding sites the triterpenoids inhibit topoisomerase 1 and 2. Topoisomerase is an enzyme that acts upon DNA strands. Resins quell leucotrine production. Leucotrines are released by leucocytes during an inflammatory process. More effective than NSAID's. Inhibits the enzyme 5-lypoxygenase. Boswellic acids are anti

External use
Fumigant action – burn the incense.
Wound dressing or spray.

Dosage and mode of application
Use small dosage initially.
Liquidum extractum Oleo gum resin Sig 4ml
References. 188 p318. 263, 2001, 67, [5], p391. 392 p1. 402.

Bryonia alba/cretica/dioica [White/red bryony]

Constituents
Cucurbitacin glycosides increase glucocorticoids at rest. While decreasing glucocorticoids during times of stress.
Curcurbitacins and trihydroxycotadecadienoic acid are immunomodulatory.

Primary pharmacological action: Hydragogue cathartic.

Therapeutic classes
Anti catarrhal.
Increases RBC count, haemoglobin, fibrinolytic activity, enhances T cell activity.
Anticholesterolaemic. Cardiac tonic.
Pulmonary agent.
Emetic in large dosage. Splenic pain. Vermifuge.
Diaphoretic. Antirheumatic.
Adaptogenic tonic. Rubefacient. Immunemodulator. Antineoplastic.

Medicinal indications [Mars]
Pyrexia. Controls the temperature and the fever processes when the indications are present without being suppressive. Glandular enlargements.
Acute inflammatory diseases, aggravated by movement. Acute lung and bronchial disorders. Sharp stabbing pain with serous involvement. Bronchitis. Pneumonia and Pleurisy. Pleurodynia. Pertussus. Tuberculosis.
Endocarditis. Pericarditis. Rheumatic fever.
Typhoid with pulmonary involvement. Peritonitis.
Appendicitis - an important remedy if given early. Splenic and hepatic disorders with deep seated pain. Pancreatitis. Constipation, hard dry stool, cracked lips and excessive thirst in protracted fevers.
Orchitis. Mastitis - acute stages with hard, hot, painful breasts.
Synovitis with sharp pain on motion.. Rheumatic conditions especially of the fingers. Spinal tenderness. Lumbago. Synovial inflammations. Polymyalgia rheumatica. Neuritis. Neuralgia.

Tissue conditions
Increases T cells. Improves heart function.
Distress with cutting or tearing pain in acute inflammatory diseases, aggravated by movement, or pressure. Elevated temperature with firm pulse and tachycardia.
Short, dry, harsh or hacking coughs with soreness increased by coughing. Absent expectorant.
Sedates the nervous system and promotes the elimination of excess heat and opposes the dryness of the mucous membranes induced by inflammation which suspends secretion. Acute pulmonary and bronchial inflammation. Chronic

soreness of the chest with deep pain. Bronchitis with frothy sputum give in small doses and persist with its use. Pneumonia is a positive indication for Bryonia. Cardiac tonic in weak and delicate patients. Rheumatic fever with cardiac involvement.

Acts upon serous membranes - pleura, pericardium and peritoneum. Peritonitis, enteritis and appendicitis.

Absorbs the products of inflammatory action of a serous nature. It opposes the breakdown of tissue and pus formation. Effusions require longer term treatment. Muscular rheumatism especially with feet and hand joint inflammation.

Cautions

Large doses cause delirium, vertigo, weak pulse, cold perspiration, dilated pupils and central depression of the brain. Pregnancy. May cause diarrhoea.

External use

Mastitis with Phytolacca.

Rubefacient in sciatica and lumbago - locally and orally.

Neuralgia, face - with Sticta.

Preparations

Pleurisy with Asclepias and Zingiber. Alternating the last two remedies may prove a more rapid response. Pneumonia - Tr Bryonia 1ml Ipecac 0.5m Aqua 60ml Sig 2.5ml hourly. Alternate with Asclepias and Zingiber.

Peritonitis and septicaemia with Echinacea.

Rheumatic pain with Cimicifuga and Gelsemium. Filipendula, Apium or Menyanthes.

Mastitis and orchitis with Phytolacca, Pulsatilla, Salix or Echinacea.

Facial neuralgia with Sticta 10gtt aa in Aqua 120ml Sig 5ml every half an hour.

Dosage and mode of application

The physiological dose is small. Given alone or alternate with other medicines. Preferable in a syrup form to aid the taste.

Liquidum extractum Sig 10gtt in 120ml aqua. Sig 5ml hourly in acutes.

Dried rad Sig 0.6g

Tincturae 1:10 Sig 0.6ml

Liquidum extractum Sig 0.7ml

References

BPC 1923. King 1528. 43 p167. 126 p250. 176 p510. 246 p259. 270 4, [1] p85. 390 p377.

Bupleurum falcatum [Hares ear root]

Constituents
Triterpenoid saponins – saikosaponin. Polysaccharides. Sterols.

Primary pharmacological action: Hepatoprotective.

Therapeutic classes
Allays inflammation.
Antitussive.
Anticholesterolaemic.
Cholagogue. Intestinal tonic. Hepatorestorative. Laxative.
Diuretic. Nephroprotective. Diaphoretic. Febrifuge.
Uterine tonic.
Antineoplastic. Immunemodulator.
Medicinal indications
Colds. Influenza. Infections with lung involvement.
Chronic inflammatory disorders.
Nausea. Dyspepsia. Peptic ulcers. Hepatitis B. Hepatoprotective in all types of
hepatic disease e.g. infectious hepatitis, chronic hepatitis with hepatomegaly and
chemically induced liver damage. Autoimmune disease of the liver or kidneys.
Rectal/intestinal prolapse.
Uterine prolapse. Irregular menstruation. Pyrexia.
Tissue conditions
Remedy activity was most pronounced within 2 hours. Protects against toxic
damage.
Preparations
Prolapsed tissue with Astragalus.
Dosage and mode of application
Dried rad Sig 2g
Liquidum extractum Sig 4ml
References
179 p316. 271 no 50 & 51.

Butyrospermum paradoxum [Shea butter tree]

Constituents
The seeds contain Shea butter this is a fat consisting mainly of linoleic, oleic, palmitic and steric acids.

Therapeutic classes
Carminative. Stimulant.
Medicinal indications
Headache
Parturient
External use
Eyebath – fol.
Ointment in rheumatic pain and furunculosis.

Caesalpinia bonducella [Caesalpina, Guilandia]

Constituents
Bitters - bonducin/guilandinin. Sterols. Protein. Resin.

Primary pharmacological action: Tonic. Antiperiodic.

Therapeutic classes
Diuretic. Febrifuge.
Medicinal indications
As a tonic in malaria. Tuberculosis. Asthma.
Tissue conditions
Used to help the reduction of fever associated with malaria. Roasted seeds have been effective in the treatment of diabetes when used as a drink.
Dosage and mode of application
Powdered kernals Sig 1.5g
References
176 p178. 300, Vol. XL, 1, 74-85

Cajunus cajun [Pigeon pea]

Constituents
Flavonoids. Saponins. Amino acids including vicilin a holoprotein.

Therapeutic classes
Antimicrobial. Haematological.
Hypoglycaemic. Hepatic.
Medicinal indications
Hepatitis
Measles
Sickle cell anaemia - phenylalanine in the seed extract.
References
47 p318. 52.

Calendula officinalis [Marigold]

Constituents
Flavonol glycosides [immunostimulant] – isoquercitrin, rutin. Glycosides – rutin. Triterpene glycosides – lupeol [allay inflammation, anti oedematous]. Essential oils – [vulnerary]. Bitters. Volatile oils. Polysaccharides.

Primary pharmacological action:
Antiseptic and stimulating to the skin and mucous membrane.

Therapeutic classes
Ophthalmic. Deobstruent. Vasotonic alterative. Allays inflammation.
Antibacterial. Antiseptic. Astringent.
Antifungal - Trichomonas.
Antiviral - Aids/HIV.
A mild diffusive stimulant. Anti haemorrhagic.
Periodontal inflammation. Anti ulcer. Choleretic. Hepatic.
Splenic.
Diuretic. Diaphoretic.
Emmenagogue. Oestrogenic.
Antispasmodic.
Antineoplastic. Immunostimulant.
Lymphatic deobstruent. Antiphlogistic. Dermatological agent. Styptic. Vulnerary.

Medicinal indications [Sun]
Conjuctivitis. Tympanic membrane damage. Epistaxis. Inflammatory conditions of the oropharynx. Toothache.
Atheroma. Phlebitis. Thrombophlebitis. Varicose veins. Limb fatigue. Frostbite.
Peptic and intestinal ulcers. Jaundice. Hepatic and splenic congestion/disease.
Hepatitis. Constipation. Anal eczema. Proctitis.
Amenorrhoea. Dysmenorrhoea. Cracked nipples. Mastitis. Breast carcinoma.
Panic. Convulsions.
Lymph node enlargement or inflammation. Acute lymphoedema. Lymphadenoma
Acne. Eczema. Inflamed/infected skin. Dermal ulcers. Sebaceous cysts.
Bee stings. Burns. Cuts. Furunculosis.
Bruises. Sprains. Verrucas. Wounds. Smallpox. Measles.

Tissue conditions
Stimulates the vasomotor function to heal skin and mucous membranes. Prevents suppurative, toxic and infective conditions. Supports the eliminative processes in eruptive disease. Assists healing while tissue granulation occurs and is a pain reliever when wounds are present. A gentle diaphoretic in warm infusion for measles and smallpox. Helps correct foetid discharge in skin carcinoma. As an

Pharmacopoeia

Vasotonic alterative in smallpox and measles. Spotty complexion, greasy skin, eczema and warts. Soothing antispasmodic nervine.

External use
External activity is enhanced by giving Calendula internally. Topically allays inflammation, vulnerary.
Conjunctivitis as an eye lotion with Hamamelis.
Promotes granulation tissue [enhanced with Symphytum] - wounds, ulcers [gangrenous], bruises, burns, and inflamed lesions, use a dilute infusion or one part LE to three parts aqua or ung.
Pruritus vulvae or ani, haemorrhoids - lotion or LE.
Chronic suppurative otitis media – instil drops.
Carcinomatous changes [early stage 1] of the cervix and cervicitis have been cleared by using an infusion douche twice daily. May also be used upon tampons and inserted in vaginitis and cervicitis.
Trichomonas - Ol Calendula.
Skin conditions, muscle and ligament injury use the lotion.

Preparations
Burns with Chondrus, Ulmus or Aloe vera.
Varicose veins with Dist Hamamelis.
Antiseptic with Commiphora, Echinacea or Hydrastis.

Dosage and mode of application
Dried florets Sig 2g
Infusium Sig Sig 2g
Tincturae Sig 10ml
Liquidum extractum Sig 4ml
Ung Calendula @ 10%.

References
43 p44. 111 p299. 126 p262. 192 p346. 189. 230 p 13. 246 p479. 251 p105. 394 p44.

Calluna vulgaris [Heather]

Constituents
Flavonoid glycosides - quercetin, myricitrin. Phenolic glycoside –Arbutin.
Alkaloid – ericodin. Tannin up to 7%.

Primary pharmacological action:
Urinary antiseptic and tonic diuretic.

Therapeutic classes
Ophthalmic. Allays inflammation. Astringent.
Bacteriostatic. Antiviral – Herpes zoster.
Cardiac tonic.
Expectorant.
Stomach tonic. Cholagogue - gentle.
Antilithic.
Antidepressant. Antirheumatic. Vulnerary.
Medicinal indications
Conjunctivitis. Anorexia.
Cystitis. Gout. Lithuria. Urinary infection. Renal disorders. Prostate - BPH.
Nervine tonic in depression. Debility. Insomnia.
Rheumatism. Wounds.
Tissue conditions
Tonic to the stomach [anorexia] and heart. Antiseptic and astringent action upon
the urinary tract and is diuretic this accounts for its antirheumatic action. It has a
soothing effect upon the nerves.
External use
Conjunctivitis - collyr
Wounds - fomentation
Shingles - an oil made from the flowers
Dosage and mode of application
Dried herba/flor Sig 2g
Tincturae Calluna Sig 4ml
Liquidum extractum Sig 2ml
References
43 p46. 147 p215. 188 p221. 246 p309.

Cannabis indica [Marijuana]

Constituents
Tetrahydrocannabinol [THC] compounds are sedative and antispasmodic. THC is found at around 8mg in 1g Cannabis herba and 0.5g hashish resin. Around 8mg is required to produce an effect. Schmidt in 1992 – 650f, explained that there have been no reported deaths. Oleum is rich in lignans. Alkaloids - Cannabamine A-D. Vitamin K. Piperidine. Trigonelline. Scented essential oil contains Syzygium, eugenol, farnesene, guaiacol, humulene, limonene, phellandrine, salinene.
Bud resin up to 40% THC
Dried buds resin up to 25% THC
Upper fol up to 10% THC
Sem - no THC.
Cannabis is often smoked to produce effects. Nicotine suppresses THC. THC potentiates nicotine.

Primary pharmacological action:
Anti convulsant, Antispasmodic, Muscle relaxant.

Therapeutic classes
Ophthalmic. Allays inflammation. Antiviral - Herpes. Hypotensive agent.
Antiasthmatic. Bronchodilator. Pectoral.
Antianoretic. Antiemetic.
Antidiuretic. Antirheumatic. Antipyretic.
Analgesic. Anodyne. Hypnotic. Sedative. Tranquillizer.
Antigalactagogue.
Medicinal indications [Saturn]
Glaucoma. Toothache. Earache.
Angina. Coronary sclerosis. Palpitations. Hypertension.
Asthma. Bronchitis. Dry irritating coughs. Pertussus.
Anorexia [can also depress appetite]. Nausea. Heartburn. Flatulence. Vomiting.
Peptic ulcer pain. Cholecystitis-pain. Jaundice. Colic. Enteritis. Constipation-spasmodic. Cholera. Worms.
Cystitis. Renal colic. Spermatorrhoea. Urethritis. Gout. Rheumatic pain. Sciatica.
Tinnitus. Muscle spasm/cramp/tetanus. Tremors. Malaria.
Anxiety. Epilepsy. Excitability. Insomnia. Meningitis. Migraine. Myalgic encephalomyelitis [ME]. Nervous tension. Neurasthenia. Panic. Restlessness. Spasmodic neuralgia.
Dysmenorrhoea. Endometritis. Metrorrhagia. Vomiting of pregnancy. Enhances uterine subinvolution. Weak uterine contractions. Puerpural fever. Mastitis.
Corns. Eczema. Hair loss. Warts. Alcohol abuse.

Tissue conditions
Mentions of Cannabis can be found on inscriptions of pyramids. One Berlin papyrus mentions glaucoma. Scientists from Munich found traces of hashish, cocaine and nicotine in mummies from 1070 – 395 BCE.
Reduces intraocular pressure in glaucoma. Relieves bronchospasm. Small doses stimulate the sensory nerves. Larger doses depress sensory and muscle function and cause delirium, numbness, relaxation and eventual sleep.
Primarily acts as an antispasmodic to the nervous and muscular systems. Depression with irritability with pain. Tends to dry mucous membranes. Irritable conditions of the genito urinary tract. Irritable hyperasthesiae. Cannabidiol and tetrahydrocannabinol behave like antioxidants and can help prevent brain damage which often follows a stroke.
Fankhauser 1996, says - prescribed by physicians in Britain, France, Germany & USA from 1845-1951.
Cautions
Restrictions apply. Dosage is determined by the relief of symptoms.
Sexual dysfunction in the male, impotence/sexual dysfunction, use with care.
May induce hallucinations in susceptible subjects. There is a tendency to make the patient slow, dull, lazy and lifeless. While not addictive it can be a cause of a dependence. It depends upon the personality of the patient. May induce hypothermia. Not advised in infections of mucous membranes as it tends to dry the membrane and aggravate the infective process.
External use
Ophthalmic disorders – poultice or collyr.
Haemorrhoids – poultice.
Orchitis – poultice. Mastitis – poultice.
Neuritis - a pain reliever in a suitable base @10%.
Ulcers, Smallpox ulcers – poultice, ung, emulsion of sem.
Antirheumatic/bruises/sprains – hot poultice or ung. [with Art. Absinth].
Uterus – administered intravaginally contracts the uterus [Ebers. Maniche 1993].
Dosage and mode of application
Dried herba Sig 1g
Sem Sig 10g
Resin Sig 1g
Tincturae Sig 1ml
References
BP 1932. 126 p270. 160. 170/1/3. 176 p105. 228 p269. 255 p5,34, 87, 113, 121. 256 p82. 257 p270. 302, 1997, 38, 44-8. 297, 11.7.1998, p16. 301, 1998, 3 [1]. 387.

Capsella bursa pastoris [Shepherds purse]

Constituents
Flavonoid glycosides - diosmetin, quercetin. Volatile oils up to 0.2% - camphor.
Carotenoids. Vitamin A, C, K. Potassium. Amino acids.

Primary pharmacological action: Astringent.

Therapeutic classes
Allays inflammation. Antibacterial activity against gram positive bacteria. Tonic.
Antihaemorrhagic. Hypotensive. Vasodilator.
Diuretic. Urinary antiseptic. Prostate tonic.
Uterine tonic.
Vulnerary. Intermittent fever.
Central nervous system depressant.
Antineoplastic.
Medicinal indications [Saturn]
Haematemesis. Hypotensive. Varicose veins.
Epistaxis. Peptic ulcerations. Intestinal haemorrhage - passive. Acute or chronic
diarrhoea. IBS. Haemorrhoids. Protozoal fever. Malaria.
Bladder abscess. Acute or chronic cystitis. Chyluria [fat in urine]. Haematuria.
Spermatorrhoea. Excess uric acid. Arthritis.
Menorrhagia including fibroid haemorrhage. Metrorrhagia. Post partum
haemorrhage.
Bruises. Strains.
Tissue conditions
Stimulates an increased coronary perfusion [vasodilator]. Stimulates smooth
muscle. It is indicated in haemorrhage from any site. Coagulation was accelerated
in one study. Astringent tonic to the nose, stomach and intestine. Tonic action
upon the kidneys and bladder in catarrh and atony. Urinary conditions caused by
excess phosphate loss, brick dust sediments, uric acid are relieved if persisted
with. In urethral irritation from prostate disease. Enuresis. Nervous irritability and
irritable spermatorrhoea. Capsella benefits the pelvic viscera and generally tones
the prostate and uterine musculature. Its tonic action will relieve an aching back.
Preparations
Epistaxis plug the nose with juice upon cotton wool.
Aching back with tonics.
Haemorrhage with more powerful astringents.
Rheumatic troubles - apply a lotion of the green herb.
Renal disorders with Agrimonia or Parietaria.
Cystitis with Barosma.

Enuresis with Agrimonia or Equisetum.
Menorrhagia with Hydrastis or Trillium.
External use
The taste may be covered if required.
The green herb or lotion can be used to heal wounds and skin ulcers.
Skin toner – compress for breast skin
Dosage and mode of application
Dried herba Sig 4g
Tincturae Sig 10ml
Liquidum extractum Sig 4ml

  Conc. Inf. Capsella. Concentrated Infusion of Capsella
  230g dried herba with 550 ml aqua. Sig 10ml
References
6 p102. 43 p 47. 126 p274. 176 p354. 246 p146. 251 p144. 263, 1993, 59, Suppl.
PA670. 394 350.

Capsicum spp. [Cayenne]

Constituents
Capsaicinoid alkaloids – up to 1.5%. Capsaicin up to 1%, a pungent ingredient.
Capsaicin acts upon the sensory neurons decreasing substance P and pain
transmitters. Capsaicin is also analgesic, antimicrobial, spasmolytic, vasodilatory,
rubefacient and stimulant. Capsaicin stimulates the hypothalamus to reduce
temperature. Salicylates. Steroidal saponins - some are antimicrobial. Volatile oil.
Stimulates prostaglandins. Vitamins A & C.

Primary pharmacological action:
A general vasostimulant to the heart, arteries and capillaries
[vasomotor system]. A pure stimulant.
A cardiovascular stimulant.

Therapeutic classes
Ophthalmic. Stimulant. Antiseptic. Antimicrobial. Antibacterial.
Antiviral – herpes zoster. Allays inflammation.
Haemostatic. Circulatory stimulant. Hypotensive. Antioxidant. Antiplatelet.
Anticholesterolaemic. Antisclerotic. Antithrombus. Expectorant.
Carminative. Gastrointestinal stimulant.
Diuretic. Diaphoretic.
Parturient. Remittent fever - typhoid, malaria.
Antispasmodic. Anodyne. Anti addictive.
Rubefacient [counter irritant] – increases dermal blood flow. Topical analgesic.
Medicinal indications [Mars]
Stimulant for colds and chills. Deficient circulatory action. Cold extremities.
Haemorrhage. Scarlatina. Atherosclerosis. Lowers cholesterol & triglycerides.
Gangrene.
Tonsillitis. Laryngitis. Diphtheria. Pneumonia. Pleurisy. Influenza - tardy
reaction. Emphysema.
Toothache. Atonic dyspepsia. Nausea and vomiting. Peptic ulcers. Flatulence.
Colic. Diarrhoea - infective. Dysentery. Spasm of the stomach and intestines.
Haemorrhoids. Typhoid.
Bruises. Sprains. Carpal tunnel syndrome. Rheumatism. Sciatica. Lumbago. Osteo
arthritis. Rheumatoid arthritis. Skeletal muscle spasm.
Herpes zoster. Neuralgia – post herpetic. Diabetic neuropathy. Paralysis. Pareses.
Shock. Depression. Collapse. Coma. Headaches. Migraine. Addictions – tobacco,
alcohol, opium. Surgical trauma.

Medicinal indications con't
Impotency. Spermatorrhoea. Gonorrhoea. Syphilis.
Ovarian congestion. Post partum haemorrhage.
Yellow fever. Pyrexia. Abscess. Psoriasis.
Tissue conditions
Capsicum stimulates prostaglandins produced by body defences.
Applied internally or externally it is warming. Used as a stimulant when heat is
required to encourage healing in the tissues. It stimulates all tissues of the body
and is effect is felt wherever required. Carried by the vital force to any area with
carrier remedies. It potentiates other remedies.
Erythrocyte membrane changes have been noted namely – decreased
phospholipids, cholesterol reduction, acetylcholine enzyme activity reduction etc.
Slowly increases arterial tone and blood flow, equalises the circulation and
increases pulse pressure. Prevents absorption of cholesterol and supports intestinal
elimination of free cholesterol. Increases fibrinolysis. Capsicum is used for neural
depression and atony especially where these are dependent upon organ feebleness
from either general or local circulation or loss of nerve power [hypotrophic
states]. Haemoptysis can be checked using Capsicum internally along with a
vapour bath.
Stimulates oropharyngeal mucous membranes. Restores tone to the stomach,
stimulates gastro intestinal mucous membranes. Constipation and diarrhoea due to
atony. Haemorrhoids from portal hypertension.
In prostrating fevers it will secure a reaction, it stimulates the sweat glands.
Antiseptic activity aids in removing the products of cellular decay e.g.
[gonorrhoea, syphilis, mercury poisoning, gangrene]. Parturition and preventive
of post partum haemorrhage.
Capsicum is advised in chronic parenchymatous nephritis and pyelonephritis.
Pain is controlled by capsaicin a neuropathic pain reliever.
Cautions
Acute inflammation. Acute gastritis. Urticaria.
Care with sensitive skin as it tends to burn.
External use
Stimulates the release of substance P from nerve terminals which after a few days
depletes the terminals leading to a loss of pain.
Quinsy and diphtheria apply with friction to the throat.
Cold extremities with cyanosis rub with Lobelia and Capsicum.
Stimulating in all liniments. An external liniment is useful for all internal
inflammatory conditions e.g. pneumonia, pleurisy.
Herpes zoster. Neuralgia, rheumatic pain, sprains. Unbroken chilblains.
Meningitis, phrenitis - apply to the feet.
Sprains and bruises with Lobelia or coconut oil.
External haemorrhage or wounds apply the powder.

Pharmacopoeia

Preparations
Capsicum is rendered more diffusive by the addition of Lobelia for congestions and chills. Lobelia is used in all spasmodic affections including tetanus.
Gargarisma - with Hydrastis, Myrica or Commiphora.
CVA - by enema with suitable diffusives.
Dosage and mode of application
Fructus Sig 120mg
Tincturae 1:5 Sig 1ml
Tincturae 1:20 Sig 2ml
External oleoresin up to 5%
   Compound Tincture of Capsicum et Lobelia.
   Capsicum 5 Lobelia 20 Symplocarpus 5
   Antispasmodic. Advised in spasm and tetanus. Sig 20gtt PRN
   Stimulating Linimentum 1
   Capsicum 4 parts. Camphor 3 parts. Guaiacum 4 parts
   Stimulating Linimentum 2
   Capsicum 40 Cypressus 1 Mentha piperita 1 Origanum 1 Pinus 1

   Diphtheria & Scarlatina gargle [It can be used in an atomiser].
   Capsicum 2 parts. Commiphora 2 parts. Hydrastis 2 parts. Solidago 4 parts
   Acetum qs to 32 parts
   Sig Gargle and paint on the tonsils every two hours.
   Sprains, bruises & neuralgia lotion
   Capsicum 3 parts. Lobelia 16 parts. Artemesia absinthium 1 part.
   Rosmarinus 1 part Mentha viridus 1 part
   Linimentum Capsicum
   Capsicum 30ml. Ol Lavandula 5 gtt
   Soft soap 60ml and add 1 litre alcohol. Add 30ml strong Capsicum tincture next add the oils while shaking the bottle.
   Painted on the skin or applied on lint in rheumatic conditions, sciatica, or chest affections.
   Unguentum Capsicum
   Capsicum 10% in a base of yellow paraffin molle 60%.
References
43 p47. 111 p303. 126 p275. 176 p163. 189 p67. 230 p17. 246 p399. 296, 1993, Vol 342, p1130. 394 p52.

Carica papaya [Papaw]

Constituents
Proteolytic enzymes chymopapain and papain. Vitamin A and C. The leaf and root yield the alkaloid carpain - it is active against Tuberculosis.

Primary pharmacological action: Vulnerary.

Therapeutic classes
Allays inflammation. Antifungal – Candida. Discutient. Anthelmintic.
Dermatological agent. Vulnerary. Contraceptive.
Medicinal indications
Enterobius and cestodes infestations.
Herniated vertebral disc.
Wound healer - infected or purulent wounds, following surgery with incomplete healing, necrotic damage. It arrests local inflammation and is a topical debriding agent. Dry scaly skin conditions.
Tissue conditions
Women in Sri Lanka eat papaya fruit as a natural contraceptive. Papain, a powerful protein breaking enzyme attacks progesterone, a hormone essential for conception. Papain becomes 24 times more active in the blood stream by interacting with a protein from the blood, and confirms papaya fruits ability as a natural contraceptive.
Dosage and mode of application
Fresh fruit may be consumed as a desert.
Wounds - apply strips over the wound and dress.
References
192 p399. 303, May 1994, p250

Carum carvi [Caraway]

Constituents
Volatile oil – a ketone known as Carvone from 47-62% and
Limonine from 34-50%.

Primary pharmacological action: Carminative.

Therapeutic classes
Stimulant. Antimicrobial. Expectorant.
Aromatic. Carminative. Stomachic. Antiflatulent.
Antispasmodic.
Emmenagogue. Galactagogue. Rubefacient.
Medicinal indications [Mercury]
Laryngitis – garg. Bronchitis.
Anorexia. Flatulent dyspepsia. Stomach ulcers. Hiatus hernia. Diarrhoea.
Intestinal colic/flatus/pain. Constipation.
Dysmenorrhoea. Bruises.
Tissue conditions
A gently stimulating carminative. Prevents fermentation in the stomach, disperses
flatulence and colic. As an aromatic carminative for children.
External use
Bruises - poultice.
Preparations
Used as a flavouring to medicine and added to seedcakes. An essence will
promote milk production.
Colic and flatulence with Acorus, Chamaemelum.
Diarrhoea with Quercus.
Bronchial disturbances with Marrubium.
Dosage and mode of application
Powdered fructus Sig 2g
Infusium Sig 2g
Tincturae Sig 4ml
Liquidum extractum Sig 2ml
    Oleum Cari Sig 0.2ml
    Aqua Cari distillata 1:10 Sig 30ml
    Aqua Cari concentrate Sig 1ml
References
43 p48. 111 p312. 192 p109. 224. 246 p296. 304, 1994, Vol. 2 [2] p81-4.

Cassia acutifolia/angustifolia [Senna]

Constituents
Hydroxyanthracine glycosides up to 3% in the leaf, 3.5% pod [fruit]. These are sennosides and cause an increase in peristalsis. Aloe emodin. Flavonoids. Glycosides. Saponins. Resin. Volatile oil. Minerals up to 12%. Mucilage up to 10%.

Primary pharmacological action: Laxative.

Therapeutic classes
Tonic. Anti fungal - Trichophyton.
Carminative. Anthelmintic. Antipyretic.
Medicinal indications [Mercury]
Diphtheria - small dosage every three hours. Tonsillitis - dose every three hours. Biliousness. Dyspepsia. Constipation.
Eruptive diseases. Fevers. Psoriasis.
Tissue conditions
A moderately stimulating and ganglionic vasorelaxant action upon the intestine. Indicated for the relief of constipation. It acts within 2-6 hours. Soft stools are produced. Prevents reabsorption of fluid from the intestine.
It is useful and accords to physiomedical principles to give a single dose of cassia when acute infections occur in the throat e.g. tonsillitis and diphtheria. This will help the elimination of toxins causing tonsillitis, which would otherwise be reabsorbed and add to or cause the problem. Suitable in the post partum, it may purge suckling infants.
Cautions
Haemorrhoids. Inflamed/irritable conditions of the intestine e.g. IBS.
Preparations
With aromatics Anethum, Foeniculum, Zingiber to prevent griping.
With lobelia to aid the cathartic action.
Dosage and mode of application
Use with aromatics or carminatives.
Give at night a full dose for relief of constipation.
Fol is stronger than the pods.
Dry extract 0.5g
Dried fol Sig 2g
Dried sem pods Sig 2g
Liquidum extractum fol Sig 2ml.
Liquidum extractum sem. Sig 4ml.

Pharmacopoeia

Composita carminative, laxative and tonic - Cassia. Rheum. Mentha piperita.
Antibilious physic - Cassia. Ipomaea. Zingiber.
Confection Cassia
Cassia 10%. Coriandrum. Figs. Prunes. Liquorice. Sucrose et aqua. Sig 10-15ml
Syrupus Cassia
Cassia 25ml. Ol Coriandrum 0.5ml. Sugar 74.5ml. aqua to 100ml. Sig 8ml
Infusium Cassia concentratum
Cassia 2. Zingiber 1. Sig 2-8ml
Tincturae Cassia composita
Cassia, Carum & Coriandrum. Sig 2-4ml
For stat dose Sig 8-16ml.
Mistura Cassia composita
Cassia 4, Gentiana 4, Compound tincturae Cardomom1 [aa Cardomom,
Foeniculum, Coriandrum sem, seville auranti rind], Glycyrrhiza 4 parts. Sig 60ml.
References
43 p49/51. 111 p314. 176 p306. 189 p249. 192 p504. 223 p1342. 394 p344.

Castanea sativa [Sweet chestnut]

Constituents
Tannin around 9%. Mucilage. Fatty acids.

Primary pharmacological action:
A mild stimulating astringent tonic.

Therapeutic classes
Antitussive.
Antirheumatic. Febrifuge.
Medicinal indications [Jupiter]
Nuts – nutritive.
Bronchial catarrh. Spasmodic coughs. Trachieitis. Laryngismus stridulus.
Pertussus.
Hiccoughs. Diarrhoea. Dysentery. Haemorrhoids.
Fibrositis. Muscular rheumatism. Polymyalgia. Menorrhagia. Dandruff.
Tissue conditions
A mild and gentle remedy. Suitable for irritable conditions of the respiratory tract
which cause violent coughs. Good for protracted cases of hiccoughs.
External use
Burns and scalds - poultice.
Dandruff – lotion.
Preparations
Pharyngitis - garg.
Coughs, pertussus - with Prunus serotina or acetous syrup of Lobelia.
Rheumatic conditions with Apium, Cimicifuga and Filipendula,
Dosage and mode of application
Infusium bacc/fol. Sig 4g
Liquidum extractum Sig 4ml
References
43 p52. 111 p318. 176 p262. 189 p73. 246.

Castanospermine australe

Constituents
An Australian plant. Polyhydroxyalkaloid - Castospermine, mimics sugar.
The seeds have a high saponin content.

Primary pharmacological action: Anti infective.

Therapeutic classes
Antiviral – AIDS.
References
Herbarium 25. 295, 1992, 305 [6868] 1583-5.

Catha edulis [Khat]

Constituents
Cathine [D – norpseudoephedrine], Cathionone. Celastrin. Choline. Tannin.

Primary pharmacological action: Stimulant.

Therapeutic class
Anti ulcer. Antiobesity.
Antidepressant. Dermatological agent.
Medicinal indications
Anorexia. Obesity. Dermal ulcers.
Depression. Fatigue.
Tissue conditions
Some 40%, D – norpseudoephedrine is recovered in the urine within 6 hours.
Can produce euphoria. Reduces gastric secretion.
Dosage and mode of application
Restrictions apply. Dosage is determined by the relief of symptoms.
Fresh/dried fol chewed or infused. Sig 200g
References
192 p317. 224 p1738.

Catharanthus roseus
See Vinca

Caulophyllum thalictroides [Blue cohosh]

Constituents
Alkaloids of the isoquinoline and quinolizidine types - methylcystine [caulophylline] stimulates respiration and raises blood pressure, magnoflorine, laburnine, cytisine, sparteine [oxytocic] and baptifoline. Glycosidal saponins – Caulosaponin [leolin and caulosaponin is oxytocic], anagyrine, Gum. Resin. Phytosterol.

Primary pharmacological action: Uterine tonic. Antispasmodic.

Therapeutic classes
Optic trophorestorative. Diffusive relaxant. Allays inflammation. Stimulant. Demulcent. Vermifuge.
Diuretic. Diaphoretic. Antirheumatic.
Emmenagogue. Parturient. Uterine tonic. Oxytocic.
Nervine.

Medicinal indications
Ophthalmic.
Pertussus. Hypertension. Palpitation.
Aphthous ulcers. Intestinal colic or cramp.
Amenorrhoea. Dysmenorrhoea. Threatened miscarriage. Metritis. Ovaritis. Vaginitis. Relieves false labour pain. Rigid Os cervix. Encourages uterine sub involution. Puerperal convulsions.
Cystitis. Prostate disease. Urethritis. Nephritis. Rheumatic pain [in the asthenic]. Articular pain.
Nervous weakness with irritability. Panic. Epilepsy. Migraine.

Tissue conditions
An equally diffusive, relaxing and stimulating remedy expending its power upon the sympathetic nerves and uterus. Spasmodic stomach or intestinal pain. Tones and gives vigour to the uterus. Indicated for dysmenorrhoea from spasm or nervous irritability.
Co ordinates and stimulates normal uterine contractions, it is indicated for deficient uterine contractions with fatigue. Relieves false labour or post partum pain associated with spasmodic contractions. Prevents premature delivery. Parturition - use to dilate the Os cervix. It will relieve cerebral unrest due to pregnancy and prevent premature delivery. Prolongs gestation until the foetus is fully developed.

Cautions
Non gravid uterine prescribing presents no problems. Gravid uterine prescribing requires precision and presents no difficulties if prescribed for the above

conditions where spasm or inadequate uterine contractions are encountered during the second/third stage of delivery.

Small doses if required are advised during the first trimester of pregnancy.

Preparations

Parturition with Composition essence or Capsicum.

To improve uterine tone with Mitchella or Uva ursi.

Puerpural convulsions with Dioscorea and Scutellaria.

Cervix spasm use with Scutellaria and Lobelia.

Amenorrhoea with Leonurus.

Scutellaria - antispasmodic in restlessness or irritability.

Spasmodic vomiting - infusion of berries.

External use

Vaginitis & Leucorrhoea.

Dosage and mode of application

As an antispasmodic it requires to be given in large doses.

Dried rad/rhiz. Sig 5g

Decoctum Sig 30ml

Tincturae Sig 2ml

Liquidum extractum Sig 2ml

Liquor Caulophyllum et Pulsatilla

Caulophyllum 25ml. Pulsatilla 5ml

For antispasmodic effect. Sig 4ml

Liquor Caulophyllum et Pulsatilla compositus

LE Aletris 10ml. LE Caulophyllum 15ml. LE Pulsatilla 5ml.

LE Viburnum prunifoleum 20ml

Prescribed as Antispasmodic and Uterotonic. Sig 4ml

References

43 p54. 111 p320. 127 p212. 176 p480. 252 p194. 254 p104. 262 p73.

Centaurium erythraea [Centuary]

Constituents
Bitter iridoid - amarogentin. Triterpenoids. Phenolic acid. Alkaloids. Flavonoids.

Primary pharmacological action: Stomach & Hepatic tonic.

Therapeutic classes
Allays inflammation. Vasotonic alterative. Antiseptic. Antimutagenic. Detergent.
Antibacterial – Salmonella typhimurium.
Enhances leucocytosis. Vasomotor tonic.
Aromatic. Bitter. Hepatic. Cholagogue. Taenifuge. Antiparasitic.
Renal calculi. Renal colic. Antimalarial.
Analgesic – mild. Antipyretic. Dermatological agent. Vulnerary. Antivenomous.
Medicinal indications [Sun]
Blood impurities.
Anorexia. Dyspepsia. Heartburn. Vomiting. Jaundice. Indigestion. Enlarged liver.
Gout.
Depression.
Eczema. Freckles. Wounds. Ulcers. Snake bite. Kills lice & fleas.
Tissue conditions
Stimulates the appetite, hydrochloric acid and motility. Stimulating and removes
obstructions of the stomach, liver and gall bladder. Chronic liver and gall bladder
complaints. Corrects an oversecretion of bile. Tonic action influences the
sympathetic nervous system when depression is associated with digestive
disturbance.
Preparations
Sore mouth/aphthous ulcers - infusium.
Catarrh - with Angelica archangelica, Filipendula or Marrubium.
Jaundice with Berberis.
Tonic for delicate patients with Rubus.
External use
Ulcers/sore mouth/inflamed gums - mouthwash.
Freckles – lotion.
Wounds - lotion.
Dosage and mode of application
Taste may be improved with Angelica or Mentha piperita AC.
Infusium Sig 60ml
Dried herba Sig 4g
Liquidum extractum Sig 4ml
References. 43 p55. 142 p39. 237. 238. 246 p325. 251 p42. 263 1991 57 [1] 34-
7. 263, 62, 1996, p561

Centella asiatica [Gotu kola/Hydrocotyle]

Constituents
Triterpine saponins - asiaticoside is a wound healer [skin ulcers] and stimulates the epidermis. Asiaticoside is antileprotic and antitubercular. Flavonoids - quercetin and other glycosides. Aglycones known as Centellagenin A-E. Alkaloid - hydrocotylin. Volatile oil - terpenoids. Bitter - vallerin. Fatty acids up to 8.9%. Sterols. Resin. Tannin up to 9%. Amino acids. Phenols, phenolic glycosides.

Primary pharmacological action: CNS tonic.

Therapeutic classes
Ophthalmic. Vasotonic alterative. Allays inflammation.
Antibacterial - Mycobacteria tuberculosis. Antifungal.
Anticholesterolaemic. Peripheral vasodilator. Circulatory stimulant. Venous tonic.
Bitter. Laxative.
Diuretic. Antirheumatic. Febrifuge.
Emmenagogue.
Adaptogenic. Cerebral tonic similar to Panax. Sedative.
Antineoplastic.
Dermatological agent.Vulnerary.

Medicinal indications
Retinal detachment.
Hypertension. Lupus erythematosus. Scleroderma. Varicose veins and ulcers.
Sinusitis. Influenza. Pleurisy. Tuberculosis.
Tonsillitis. Peptic ulcers. Diarrhoea. Hepatic disorders. Anal fissures.
Haemorrhoids.
Bladder ulceration. Oedema. Syphilis. Impotence/sexual dysfunction. Cervical carcinoma. Addisons disease.
Acne. Dermal ulcers. Eczema. Leprosy. Pemphigus. Psoriasis. Wounds. Keloids.
Pyrexia. Steam treatment of malaria. Cholera. Dermal tuberculosis.
Amnesia. Anxiety. Fatigue. Insomnia. Depression. Parkinsons disease.
Withdrawal from drugs.
Rheumatic conditions. Damaged ligaments and tendons - tendonitis.

Tissue conditions
Strengthens the tone of the vein walls, improving microcirculation, and capillary permeability. Fibrinolitic activity is improved. Improves cholesterol balance.
Venous tonic in venous insufficiency, varicose veins and venous hypertension.
Supports the reticuloendothelial system which destroys aged blood cells.
Reduces blood urea and blood acidity.

Helpful for senility, improves memory retention by stimulating neuro transmitters. Allays inflammation in the skin where infection is present. Rebuilds skin tissue through growth and repair as it stimulates collagen synthesis [aging, postoperative wounds]. Heals stasis leg ulcers. Scarring from burns and reduces scarring - seen especially in keloid scars. It inhibits fibroblasts. Centella is effective in destroying 100% of cultured tumour cells.

Cautions

Epilepsy. Pregnancy.

External use.

Ulcers, surgical wounds, fistulas, wounds - Aerosol preparation. Helps ease decay in leprous ulcers. Cicatrisation following surgery. Eczema and psoriasis. Varicose ulceration. Steam treatment in malaria.

Preparations

Filipendula enhances the activity of Centella.

Dosage and mode of application

Dried fol. Sig 0.6g

Liquidum extractum Sig 4ml

References

43 p56. 191. 192 p250. 194. 239 p170. 270, 7, [5], p427-448. 274 48, p53. 275 1994 no42. 276, 1994, 37 [3] p92.

Cephaelis [Ipecacuanha]

Constituents
Alkaloid - emetine. Saponins. Glycosides.

Primary pharmacological action: Expectorant.

Therapeutic classes
Emetic - large dose. Stimulating to the stomach and liver. Amoebicide.
Diaphoretic.
Antihaemorrhagic. Antispasmodic.
Medicinal indications
Asthma. Bronchitis. Laryngismus stridulus. Pertussus. Pneumonia - hepatization.
Broncho pulmonary congestion. Vocal cord congestion. Spasmodic coughs.
Gastro intestinal inflammation. Amoebic dysentery. Cholera. Nausea and
vomiting. Malaria. Typhoid. Febrile diseases.
Convulsions of children - use an emetic.
Tissue conditions
Relaxes the lungs, stomach and intestines to secure thin mucus discharges. Acute
irritative and inflammatory conditions of the stomach or lungs. A safe emetic [in
full dosage] producing its effects within 30 minutes. Expectorant action is of an
irritant nature to the stomach and produces reflex mucus secretion and vomiting.
Vomiting reflexly clears chest mucus. Persistent irritation of the mucous
membranes with deficient secretion demand small doses of Cephalis. Nausea and
vomiting with pale mucous membranes and a white coated broad tongue or
pointed tip – give small doses, repeated frequently.
Cautions
The rhizome and root are powerful relaxants and can induce nausea. Its relaxant
action produces a thin watery stool. Cephalis produces more mucus not advised in
congestive conditions with excess mucus production.
Preparations
Pertussus with Marrubium and Tussilago.
Amoebic dysentery with Echinacea and lower bowel enemas.
Dosage and mode of application
Full dosage will produce a free emesis Sig 2g
Dried rad Sig 120mg
Tincturae Sig 1ml
Liquidum extractum Sig 0.12ml. Alkaloidal content 0.1%
Elixir Cephaelis
Liquidum extractum 5% in a flavoured base [glycerine] Sig 2ml.
[Alkaloidal content 0.1%].

Mist Pertussus
Tincturae Atropa 0.3ml, Tincturae Cephalis 0.3ml, Syrup of Tolu 2ml
Aqua Cinnamomum to 5ml. Sig 5ml
Syrupus Cephalis
Liquidum extractum Cephalis 7ml qs Syrupus 100ml Sig 30ml.
Paediatric: under 1 year of age - Syrupus Cephalis Sig 10ml
References
43 p57. 111 p328. 176 p246. 189 p154. 191. 224 p601.

Cetraria islandica [Iceland moss]

Constituents
Mucilaginous polysaccharides up to 50% - lichenin. Fumaric acid. Lichenostearic acid [ulcer protective, anti carcinoma, anti Aids]. CHO. Terpenes.

Primary pharmacological action: Demulcent.

Therapeutic classes
Antimicrobial – Helicobacter pylori.
Oropharyngeal agent. Antitussive. Expectorant.
Bitter tonic. Gastro intestinal demulcent.
Nutritive. Antiemetic. Immunemodulator.

Medicinal indications
Oropharynx inflammation eg laryngitis. Chronic catarrh. Asthma. Chronic bronchitis. Dry coughs. Tuberculosis. Pertussus.
Anorexia. Nausea. Gastritis. Gastric ulcers. Diabetes. Dysentery. Diarrhoea.
Typhoid.
Nephritis.
Malnutrition. Rickets.

Tissue conditions
Protective and soothing effects for the mucosal surfaces of the respiratory, gastro intestinal and urinary tracts. It gives strength to infants, the aged and the chronically sick. It allays vomiting and is a nutritive tonic in debility and in chronic wasting disease. Pulmonary disease with chronic coughs.

Preparations
Vomiting with Ballota, Mentha piperita, Chamomilla.
Respiratory disease with Glycyrrhiza.

Dosage and mode of application
Decoctum thallus 1:20 Sig 120ml
Jelly is often employed.
Infusium Sig 6g
Tincturae Sig 30ml
Liquidum extractum Sig 6ml

References
43 p58. 111 p334. 142 p48. 188 p246. 192 p 285. 233 p571. 246 p571. 394 p212.

Chamaelirium luteum [False unicorn root]

Constituents
Steroidal saponin - Chamaelirin.
An oestrogen like action maintains the endometrium.

Primary pharmacological action:
Tonic to the ovaries and uterus. CNS trophorestorative.

Therapeutic classes
Stimulant. Mucous membrane tonic.
Sialagogue - fresh. Bitter. Emetic – large dose. Antiemetic – small dose. Hepatic.
Anthelmintic.
Diuretic.
Pelvic tonic. Uterine tonic. Aphrodisiac. Hormone enhancer.

Medicinal indications
Anorexia. Dyspepsia.
Enuresis. Impotence/sexual dysfunction. Spermatorrhoea. Prostatic hypertrophy.
Incontinence.
Amenorrhoea. Menorrhagia. Dysmenorrhoea. Vaginal discharge/leucorrhoea.
Sterility - male and female. Uterine prolapse. Vomiting of pregnancy.
Threatened miscarriage. Partus preparator. Hormonal deficiency. PMS.
Menopause.

Tissue conditions
Tonic activity improves the appetite and assists digestion. Sensitive stomach. A
urinary stimulant. Prostate enlargement from atony with heavy dragging
sensations in the bladder. Phosphates in the urine. Bladder irritability.
Used in relaxed, weak [atonic] conditions of the uterus and suspending ligaments
e.g. uterine prolapse, vaginal weakness from relaxed tissues. Dragging sensation
in the lower abdomen, pelvic engorgement [venous congestion]. Ovarian pain.
Congestive pain before periods. Reproductive tonic to both male and female. It
increases the chances of female conception. Suitable for those of a nervous
temperament and of feeble constitution.

Cautions
It is an endangered species in the wild.

Preparations
Menorrhagia - with Trillium.
Dysmenorrhoea with Viburnum prunifoleum.
Delayed menses with Seneco aureus.
Threatened miscarriage with Hydrastis.
Tonic action is enhanced with Trillium.

Pharmacopoeia

Uterine tonic with Avena, Caulophyllum, Dioscorea, Viburnum.
Useful preparations are made with –
Aletris, Cimicifuga, Mitchella, Pulsatilla, Viburnum.
Dosage and mode of application
Small doses often produce remarkable results.
Dried rad/rhizome Sig 2g
Tincturae Sig 4ml
Liquidium extractum Sig 2ml
References
43 p60. 176 p476. 188 p222. 189 p272. 254 p104.

Chamomilla recutita [German chamomile]

Constituents
Azulenes [Chamazulene up to 15%] are relaxant and antiallergenic.
Flavonoids up to 8% - Apigenin is spasmolytic to smooth muscle.
Sesquiterpene lactones – matricin.
Volatile oil - up to 2%, chamazuline is antipyretic, antiseptic, antispasmodic and inhibits histamine release, Bisobolol up to 50% is spasmolytic.
Mucilage up to 10% - polysaccharides; wound healing and immunostimulating.
Amino acids. Fatty acids. Coumarins up to 0.1% – umbelliferone.

Primary pharmacological action:
Gastro intestinal carminative and antispasmodic.

Therapeutic classes
Ophthalmic. Antiseptic. Antiallergic. Allays inflammation. Antiphlogistic. Anticatarrhal.
Antimicrobial. Antibacterial – staphylococcus. Antifungal - candida.
Aromatic. Antiemetic. Antipeptic/Antiulcerogenic. Inflamed or spasmodic conditions of the gastro intestinal tract.
Diuretic. Diaphoretic. Febrifuge.
Antispasmodic. Analgesic. Sedative. Musculotropic.
Galactogogue.
Deodorant. Dermatological agent. Vulnerary. Immunostimulant. Antiphlogistic.
Medicinal indications [Sun]
Conjunctivitis. Meibomian cyst. Spasmodic coughs. Asthma.
Aphthous ulcers. Gingivitis. Peptic ulcers. Flatulent and nervous dyspepsia.
Heartburn. Nausea. Vomiting. Colic. Infantile colic. Intestinal spasm. Diarrhoea.
IBS. Haemorrhoids. Anal fissure.
Enuresis.
Facial neuralgia. Headache. Nervousness. Neuralgia. Insomnia. Motion sickness.
Panic.
False labour pains. Amenorrhoea. Dysmenorrhoea. Vaginal inflammation. Breast disorders - mastitis, abscess.
Infantile convulsions with or without teething pain. Nervous irritability of children. Night terrors.
Analgesic action in bruising, cramp, rheumatism, gout and joint pains. Carpal tunnel syndrome.
Skin cleanser. Allays dermal irritation and swelling form any cause - infective, burns and inflammation.

Pharmacopoeia

Acne. Anal or genital dermatitis. Blisters. Dermatitis. Eczema. Heat stroke. Impetigo. Neurodermatitis. Psoriasis. Urticaria. Wound dermabrasion. Nappy rash. Insect bites. Radiation burns. Pyrexia. Varicella.

Tissue conditions

Soothing to inflamed mucous membranes of the gastro intestinal tract. Catarrhal conditions of the eye, ear or nose. Soothing effect upon the gums in toothache particularly suited to babies teething pains.

A smooth muscle relaxant for the gastro intestinal tract. Used as a sedative in irritability and restlessness. Acts upon the sensory and motor nerves to allay nervous sensitivity. Colic will respond as will night terrors from the use of an infusion - taken at night to calm and sedate. Restless, irritable and fretful, disorientated and impatient conditions of the adult or child. Subacute inflammation or congestion of the liver with green stool, soreness of the anus with colic. Sudden fits of temper pre or during menstruation.

External use

Externally allays inflammation of the skin and mucous membranes.

Applied to the face in neuralgia and inflammatory pain.

Eye disorders - conjunctivitis, meibomian cyst, use the collyr or fomentation. As a mouthwash to protect the gums. Dental abscesses - poultice. Toothache in babies frequently apply the infusion to the gums.

Steam inhalation in ear infections, nasal catarrh.

External oedema, sunburn, urticaria, haemorrhoids and bruising, inflamed wounds of the skin, toothache and earache – fomentation. Radiation burns.

Eczema and mastitis – lotion, compress or balneum.

Burns - it decreases the temperature. Infusium or Ol Chamomilla with Ol Vit E.

A wash to lighten hair colour.

Nappy rash Ol Chamomilla + Ol Olive.

Breast disorders - mastitis, abscess, suppression of milk with Phytolacca.

Dosage and mode of application

Dried flos Sig 8g

Tincturae Sig 15ml

Liquidum extractum Sig 4ml

Garg infusium. Sig 3g

Inhalation Sig Inhale steam from an aqueous infusion.

Ung Chamomilla @ 10%

Balneum 100g in muslin.

References

43 p139. 189 p70/71. 192. 232. 233 p154. 246 p463. 394 p57.

Chamaemelum nobile [Roman Chamomile]

Constituents
Sesquiterpine lactones - nobilin is present at around 0.6%. Dark coloured
glycoside anthemic acid is responsible for the bitter taste. Volatile oil up to
1.75%. Flavonoids – diuretic, antispasmodic. Flavonoids are Alpha - bisabolol is
anti peptic. Azulene is antiallergic through its liberation of antihistamine bodies.
Coumarins. Bitter - anthemic acid. Metabolic stimulant - it increases glucose - 6
phosphate in skin cells. Stimulates mitochondria in oxidative phosphorization.

Primary pharmacological action:
Gastro intestinal antispasmodic.

Therapeutic classes
Tonic. Antimicrobial. Antiseptic. Allays inflammation of the skin and mucous
membranes. Metabolic stimulant.
Aromatic bitter. Carminative. Stomachic. Antiemetic. Intestinal colic.
Anthelmintic. Cathartic. Vasodilator.
Diuretic. Diaphoretic.
Sedative - mild. Anodyne. Emmenagogue. Antipyretic. Vulnerary.
Antineoplastic.

Medicinal indications [Sun]
Ocular irritation from smoke or chlorine. Nasal catarrh. Hay fever. Otitis media.
Inflammation of the oral cavity/aphthous ulcers. Anorexia. Gastro intestinal
sedative in dyspepsia, gastritis, heartburn, flatulence, peptic ulcers, colic,
diarrhoea, nausea and vomiting – gastric. Jaundice. IBS. Spasmodic colitis.
Haemorrhoids.
Nausea of pregnancy. Amenorrhoea when due to a chill. Dysmenorrhoea.
Menstrual headache. False labour pain.
Childrens fever or convulsions. Hyperactivity. Alopecia.
Anger. Panic. Facial neuralgia. Nervous irritability. Exhaustion. Anxiety and
migraine. Insomnia. Meniers disease. Motion sickness. Remittent fever - typhoid,
malaria.
Burns. Rashes. Wounds.

Tissue conditions
Considered stronger than Chamomilla in its action. Relaxes the vasomotor nerves
of the ANS. Antispasmodic and relaxes the stomach, circulation, nerves and
uterus. Nausea, flatulence or abdominal spasm from emotional upsets. Sufferers
showing irritability of mood with impatience. Enhances oxidative
phosphorylation in skin damage.

Pharmacopoeia

Cautions
Large doses are bitter and nauseating.
External use
Zingiber is a useful addition.
Bruises, toothache, earache, neuralgia – poultice.
Aphthous ulcers – dect. is anodyne.
Hair loss and to lighten the hair - use a rinse.
Colon irritability - enema.
Colic with Carum carvi and Mentha piperita.
General muscular tension, insomnia with Lobelia and antispasmodic tincture.
Wound healer – poultice.
Preparations
Cold preparations are more tonic with effects more pronounced to the stomach and uterus.
Digestive disease with:
Althea, Filipendula, Humulus, Mentha piperita or Symphytum.
Vomiting of pregnancy with Chamaelirium.
Dosage and mode of application
Dried flos Sig 4g
Tincturae Sig 4ml
Liquidum extractum Sig 4ml
References
43 p60. 111 p250. 176 p154. 189 p70. 230 p23. 251 p45.

Chasmanthera dependens [Moonseed family]

Constituents
Bitters. Alkaloids.

Primary pharmacological action: Vasotonic alterative.

Therapeutic classes
Antirheumatic. Tonic.
Medicinal indications
Bone and joint injuries
Nervous enervation
Sexually transmitted disease – rad.
Tissue conditions
General tonic properties to support the nervous system in exhaustion.
External use
The bark and leaves are used as an anti rheumatic liniment in fractures, sprains and bruises. For fractures fresh leaves are applied.
References
53.

Chelidonium majus [Celandine]

Constituents
Isoquinoline alkaloids [antibacterial and antifungal] - chelidonine, sanguinarine - antitumour, chelidoxanthine - same as berberine. The alkaloid content decreases on drying. Harvest the plant when in full flower as the alkaloids highest content is in the flower. Seed contains alkaloids and proteolytic enzymes. Enzymes that digest proteins are of use against warts. The 12 alkaloids are bound to organic acids - mallic acid, citric acid and galidonic acid. Flavonoids. Phenolic acids. Hydroxycinnamic acid esters are cholagogue and are degraded by heat.

Primary pharmacological action:
Hepatic, choleretic and cholagogue.

Therapeutic classes
Ophthalmic. Vasotonic alterative. Demulcent. Allays inflammation.
Antifungal - Aspergillus fumigatus, Candida albicans, C. pseudotropicalis, Microsporum canis and Trichophyton.
Antiviral – Epstein barr, Herpes.
Antimicrobial - gram positive bacteria, E. floccosum vaginalis. T. glabrata, M. canis, M. gypseum, Staphylococcus aureus, Streptococcus, Trichomonas and T. mentagrophytes.
Coronary vasodilator. Bronchodilator. Expectorant. Antitussive.
Spasmolytic to the gastro intestinal tract, liver, gall bladder and bile ducts.
Splenic. Pancreatic stimulant. Cathartic.
Diuretic. Diaphoretic.
Analgesic. Antispasmodic.
Dermatological agent. Vulnerary.
Antineoplastic. Immune stimulant.
Medicinal indications [Sun]
Conjunctivitis, Gonorrhoeal opthalmia.
Angina - antispasmodic.
Gastritis. Biliary colic. Cholelithiasis. Cholecystitis. Stomach carcinoma.
Obstructive jaundice. Inflamed bile ducts - icteris cataralis. Hepatitis. Splenic enlargement. Spastic constipation. Intestinal polyposis.
Eczema. Psoriasis. Ringworm. Leukaemia.
Migraine, orbital neuralgia. Rheumatism and gout.
Dermal ulcers. Condylomas. Papillomas. Warts. Softens corns.

Tissue conditions
Green or pale tongue and mucous membranes. Vasotonic alterative - detoxifying the blood. Hepatic congestion, jaundice with pale stool. Hepatic congestion with fullness and throbbing pain in the right hypochondrium or right sub scapula area. Stimulates the portal circulation and relieves congestion of the liver, gall bladder and pancreas. Intestinal mucous membrane Stimulates and detoxifies the mucous membranes, lymphatics and mesentery. Clear biliousness. Smooth muscle antispasmodic.
Cautions
Restrictions apply. Dosage is determined by the relief of symptoms.
Early pregnancy.
External use
Conjunctivitis. Cataracts – collyr et aqua rosae or dist aqua.
Colonic polyposis - enema [requires around ten enemas] Mediherb newsletter.
Topically antimicrobial.
Bruises and abrasions apply the fresh succus.
Eczema, Tinea, Verrucae, Warts, Ringworm, Malignancy - apply the fresh yellow succus or tincture BD/PRN – for three weeks.
Dosage and mode of application
Collyr - Infusium Chelidonium in an eyebath aqua frig.
Dried herba 2g
Tincturae herba Sig 2ml
Liquidum extractum Sig 2ml
References
16 p127. 43 p62. 126 p285. 176 p315. 188 p104. 189 p68. 246 p130. 251 p39. 263, 1993, 59, 189. 263,62, 1996. 271 No. 49

Chelone glabra [Balmony]

Constituents
Bitters. Resins.

Primary pharmacological action:
Hepatic. Gastrointestinal vasostimulant.

Therapeutic classes
Detergent. Sialagogue. Antibilious. Cholagogue - mildly stimulating. Cathartic.
Anthelmintic.
Medicinal indications
Anorexia. Dypepsia. Jaundice. Constipation. Ascaris and enterobius.
Tissue conditions
A ganglionic vasostimulant to the liver, gall bladder and intestines. Stimulates
salivary secretions. Gently stimulates the appetite in atonic weakness of the
stomach. Mild hepatic in cases of colitis.
Preparations
Tonic action with Hydrastis, Populus.
Dosage and mode of application
Liquidum extractum Sig 4ml
References
43 p62. 111 p334. 126 p286. 189 p24. 254 p100.

Chenopodium olidum/vulvaria [Arrach]

Constituents
Ascaridol. Tannin. Triterpenes. Trimethylamine.

Primary pharmacological action: Anthelmintic.
Therapeutic classes
Emmenagogue.
Antispasmodic nervine.
Medicinal indications [Venus]
Nematodes. Menstrual disorders.
Tissue conditions
Roundworms. Hookworms.
Preparations
Administer with a purgative.
Dosage and mode of application
Powdered sem Sig 4g
Infusium herba Sig 30ml
Liquidum extractum Sig 4ml
References
176 p504. 189 p17.

Chenopodium ambrosioides [Wormseed]

Constituents
Volatile oil 0.6%. Ascaridol. Triterpenes.

Primary pharmacological action: Anthelmintic.

Therapeutic classes
Antifungal. Expectorant.
Diuretic. Diaphoretic.
Antispasmodic.
Uterine antispasmodic. Emmenagogue. Dermatological agent.
Medicinal indications
Asthma - herba.
Amoebic dysentery. Nematodes - roundworms, hookworms.
Panic.
Emmenagogue action following a chill. Dosed at the rate of two doses close
together and not repeated for 1 week.
External use
Fungal skin infections. Dermal ulcers.
Cautions
Restrictions apply. Dosage is determined by the relief of symptoms.
The oil is highly toxic causing dizzyness, vomiting, convulsions. Avoid in
pregnancy.
Dosage and mode of application
Oleum et sucrose/emulsion mane - adult dose Sig 16gtt. 6-8 years Sig 6gtt.
[Bartrum]. Dose for two days follow with cathartic each dose - Oleum Ricinus
15-30ml.
Weiss recommends only robust children be treated at 1 gtt for each year and
followed by a second dose two hours later. After the second dose Oleum Ricinus
15-30ml.
Powdered sem boiled in milk Sig 4g [390p143].
Liquidum extractum Sig 4ml
References
111 p336. 126 p286. 142 p120/122. 176 p377. 189 p287. 236. 262 p45.

Chimaphilla umbellata [Pipsissewa]

Constituents
Quinones - hydroquinone known as arbutin. Napthaquinones - Chimaphilin.
Gum resin. Flavonoids - quercetin. Triterpenes. Methyl salicylate. Tannin.

Primary pharmacological action: Astringent Tonic.

Therapeutic classes
Allays inflammation. Vasotonic alterative. Lymphatic and glandular remedy.
Renal tonic. Diuretic. Urinary antiseptic. Diaphoretic.
Muscle antispasmodic.
Dermatological agent. Antineoplastic. Immunostimulant.
Medicinal indications
Glandular enlargement. Inflamed cervical lymph nodes.
Heart tonic.
Parotitis. Hypoglycaemic. Diarrhoea. Typhoid.
Bladder and prostate cancer. Urinary antiseptic. Albuminuria. Cystitis. Prostatitis.
Antilithic. Pyelitis. Oedema. Gonorrhoea. Rheumatism.
Epilepsy. Dermal ulcers. Typhus.
Breast carcinoma.
Tissue conditions
Urinary vasotonic alterative and antiseptic. Removes inflammation and solids
from the urine in inflammatory disorders. Purulent and muco purulent mucus
discharges.. Removes irritation from the urinary tract. Oedema following
measles. Detoxifies the blood and encourages catabolism. Chronic rheumatism as
it reduces uric acid. Reduces glandular enlargement when due to inflammation in
acute or chronic conditions.
External use
Applied to the skin as a vesicant.
Dermal ulcers – lotion.
Dose and mode of application
Dried fol Sig 3g
Liquidum extractum Sig 5ml
References
111 p337. 126 p288. 176 p377. 188 p339. 189 p218. 192 p430.

Chionanthus virginicus [Fringetree]

Constituents
Saponin - chionanthin.

Primary pharmacological action:
Gentle hepatic and pancreatic medicine.

Therapeutic classes
Vasotonic alterative. Relaxing and stimulating hepatic. Pancreatic restorative.
Tonic.
Diuretic. Uric acid remover.
Medicinal indications
Bitter tonic. Stomach fullness after eating. Atonic digestion. Duodenitis.
Cholelithiasis. Hepatic congestion and engorgement. Hepatitis. Icterus. Pancreatic
disease. Pancreatitis. Hypo/hyperglycaemia. Glycosuria. Jaundice. Splenic
enlargement. Malaria. Migraine.
Tissue conditions
Stimulates biliary secretions. Acute congestion of the liver - duodenitis, hepatitis,
infections of the liver or blood with congestive contraction of the liver. Light clay
coloured or green stool. Hepatic pain, colic, nausea, vomiting, icterus and yellow
urine.
For headache consequent upon disturbed hepatic or pancreatic function. Primary
remedy for diseases of the pancreas.
External use
Skin ulcers with suppuration.
Preparations
Stomach and digestive disorders with Filipendula.
Cholelithiasis with Berberis vulgaris, Dioscorea.
Dosage and mode of application
Liquidum extractum rad/bacc Sig 2ml
References
43 p63. 111 p338. 126 p286. 176 p314. 189 p120. 254 p100.

Chlorophora excelsa [Iroko tree]

Constituents
Phenols are fungicidal. Calcium carbonate. Tannin.

Primary pharmacological action: Astringent.

Therapeutic classes
Antibacterial. Antifungal.
Purgative.
Antirheumatic.
Galactagogue.
Medicinal indications
Dental caries. Throat disorders. Bronchitis.
Haemorrhoids.
Leprosy.
External use
Haemorrhoids, dysentery - enema.
Latex is applied for dental caries and for tooth removal.
Topically antibacterial.
Venereal chancres or elephantiasis of the scrotum - use the sitz bath.
Dosage and mode of application
Decoctum cort Sig 2ml
References
53.

Chondrodendron tomentosum [Pareira]

Constituents
Alkaloids – d-tubocurarine, l-curarine, l-beebirine. Tubocurarine binds to motor end plate receptors and is an acetylcholine antagonist it is a muscle relaxant causing muscle paralysis.

Primary pharmacological action: Muscle relaxant.

Therapeutic class
Antiseptic. Tonic. Laxative.
Diuretic. Urinary tract inflammation. Antilithic.
Emmenagogue. Antivenomous.

Medicinal indications
Jaundice. Constipation.
Oedema. Gonorrhoea. Rheumatism. Snakebite. Vaginal discharge.

Tissue conditions
Used in surgery to paralyse muscles. Respiratory depressant. Curare is used to make poison arrows.

Dose and mode of application
Solid extract Sig 1.5g
Liquidum extractum fol/rad/stip. Sig 10ml

References
189 p208. 192 p401.

Chondrus crispus [Irish moss]

Constituents
Polysaccharides - carrageenan. Sulphates. Mucilage. Iodine.

Primary pharmacological action: Demulcent.

Therapeutic classes
Mucous membrane demulcent for all mucous surfaces.
Antitussive. Emollient. Nutritive.
Medicinal indications
Chronic coughs. Colds. Bronchitis. Pneumonia. Tuberculosis.
Dyspepsia. Gastritis. Peptic ulcers. Diarrhoea. Dysentery.
Bladder and renal disease.
A culinary remedy used to thicken foods. As a drink it may be flavoured.
Tissue conditions
Inflammatory/irritable conditions of the respiratory, gastro intestinal and urinary tract.
Preparations
Bronchitis with Glycyrrhiza.
External use
Dermatitis use the lotion.
Dosage and mode of application
Dried thalus Sig 10g
Infusium thalus Sig 10g
Decoctum Sig 120ml
Jelly - thalus 10g, aqua 500ml, sucrose as required. Sig drink freely.
References
BPC 1959. 43 p64. 111 p339. 192 p290. 224 p921. 246 p572.

Cichorium intybus [Chicory]

Constituents
Indole alkaloids – harman. Flavonoids – esculine. Sesquiterpene lactones.
Coumarins. Bitter glycosides - Intybin. Inulin. Folacin – forms red blood cells
and synthesizes DNA, potassium and Vitamin A.

Primary pharmacological action: Digestive tonic.

Therapeutic classes
Ophthalmic. Allays inflammation.
Antibacterial – E. Coli, Pseudomonas aeruginosa.
Stomachic. Hepatic. Cholagogue. Choleretic. Hypoglycaemic. Splenic. Laxative -
mild.
Diuretic.
Sedative - mild. Dermatological agent. Antipyretic. Galactagogue.

Medicinal indications [Jupiter]
Conjunctivitis. Anaemia.
Anorexia. Gastritis. Jaundice. Cholelithiasis. Constipation. Splenic disorders.
Oedema. Gout. Rheumatism. Tones and firms up the breasts.
Used as a beverage and coffee substitute.

Tissue conditions
Increases the elimination of uric acid. Digestive tonic and nervine. Tones the
gastro intestinal tract and liver. Removes liver obstructions.

External use
Inflammatory disease use the succus as a compress.

Dosage and mode of application
Decoctum rad Sig 30ml
Succus Sig 15ml

References
236 p38. 246 p490. 272, 1995, 7 [5] p28-9. 285, 9, 1995, p281-286.

Cimicifuga [Black cohosh]

Similar actions with species C. heraclifolia, C. Foetida, C. alba and C. dahurica.

Constituents

Tetracyclic triterpene glycosides [steroidal saponins] - acetin and cimigoside affect the hypothalamic – pituitary receptor sites. Isoflavone - formonocetin binds to oestrogen sites. Resin up to 20%, cimicifugin [oestrogenic]. Ferrulic acid – allays inflammation. Tannin. Volatile oil. Fatty acids. Salicylic acid. 27 deoxyacetein – an oestrogen like activity [388]. This means Cimicifuga has anti oestrogen and anti LH activity enhancing oestrogen, [388] perhaps as researchers are unable to agree upon the molecular activity it should be considered as amphoteric – balancing hormones.

Primary pharmacological action:
Meningeal vasorelaxant. Uterine antispasmodic.

Therapeutic classes

Allay inflammation. Astringent - mild. Antiviral. Antimicrobial.
Vasodilator. Antitussive.
Diuretic. Antirheumatic.
Emmenagogue. Hormonal balancer. Uterotonic. Galactagogue.
Antineoplastic. Immunostimulant. Vulnerary. Antivenomous.
Sedative to ANS. Meningeal relaxant. Endocrine activity - pituitary.

Medicinal indications

Sore throats. Asthma. Pertussus - removes excessive nerve irritation.
Tuberculosis. Respiratory congestion.
Rheumatic fever. Rheumatic pericarditis. Arrhythmia. Angina. Slows the pulse.
Hypertension – vasodilator.
Nerve and muscular pain – lumbago, myalgia, sciatica, intercostal and trigeminal neuralgia. Osteo and rheumatoid arthritis.
Prostate irritability. Spermatorrhoea. Orchitis. Testicular pain. Mastitis.
Stimulates and contracts the uterus. Partus preparator, strengthens uterine contractions, relaxes a rigid Os cervix. Encourages uterine sub involution post partum. Post partum pain. Gynaecological problems – amenorrhoea, dysmenorrhoea, uterine prolapse, ovaritis.
Amenorrhoea provoking epilepsy. PMS. Menopausal anxiety, depression, flushes, palpitations, rheumatic pain, and headaches, vaginal dryness.
Chorea. Tinnitus. Epilepsy. Meningitis. Smallpox - to abort. Snake bites.
Wounds.

Pharmacopoeia

Tissue conditions
Increases bronchial secretions. A stimulating diffusive acting upon the liver and kidneys.
Reduces the level of LH and hypothalamic receptors which decreases progesterone. Cimicifuga is an oestrogen inhibitor [SERM] selective oestrogen receptor modulator. It will block the action of oestrogen at receptor sites e.g. breast. Does not affect FSH or prolactin. Because cimicifuga has these agonist activities it is able to stimulate some receptor sites and not others. Thus it will inhibit the resorption of bone stimulating hormone and block the effects of oestrogen upon breasts and endometrium.
It has an effect on bone mineral deposition.
It acts upon unstriped muscles. Trusted for muscle aches from over strain.
Menopausal panic, flushes and restlessness are indications. Vaginal cells proliferant – reduces dryness.
Partus preparator - allays spasmodic and erratic pain.
Relaxant to serous membranes in acute and chronic inflammatory disturbances.
Relaxes sympathetic ganglia. It leaves behind a gently toned impression upon the mucous and serous tissues.

Cautions
Avoid in relaxed conditions of the mucous membranes or a tendency to coldness.

Preparations
Use Cimicifuga in smaller doses than the remedies it is prescribed with.
Efficacy is increased with Gelsemium or Humulus.
Cerebro vascular accident from embolus - with Stachys and Capsicum.
Neuralgia with Scutellaria.
Uterine contractions with Trillium.
Smallpox with Asclepias and Zingiber.
Rheumatism with Menyanthes, Apium, Zanthoxylum.
Tinnitus with Ginkgo or Zanthoxylum.

Dosage and mode of application
Dried rad/rhizome. Sig 2g
Standardised extract Sig 8mg.
Tincturae Sig 2ml
Liquidum extractum Sig 4ml

References
111 p341. 126 p466. 176 p480. 230 p9. 239 p91. 248 p29. 249 p420. 388 p78. 394 p22.

Cinchona species
[equal action varieties are C. calisaya, C. Succirubra, C. Ledgeriana]

Constituents
Catechins. Alkaloids - quinine also cinchonine. Resin. Triterpenes - quinovin.
Tannins. Volatile oil.

Primary pharmacological action: Vasotonic alterative.

Therapeutic classes
Bitter. Antiperiodic. Antimalarial.
Passive haemorrhage.
Orexigenic.
Stimulating astringent to nerve structure. Nerve tonic. Spasmolytic.
Medicinal indications [Mars]
Influenza. Malaria.
Aphthous ulcers. Anorexia. Atonic dyspepsia. Splenomegaly. Diarrhoea.
Cramp. Rheumatism.
Tissue conditions
Atony and relaxation of the tissues. Often prescribed in the malarial condition.
Cautions
Restrictions apply. Dosage is determined by the relief of symptoms.
Pregnancy. Nausea. Tinnitus. Pyrexia. Deficient secretions of the skin, stomach
or intestines. Typhoid.
External use
Aphthous ulcers. Ulcers.
Preparations
Prescribe with an aromatic to taste.
Dysentery with succus citrus limonum.
Dosage and mode of application
Powdered cort Sig 1g
Tincturae Sig 4ml
Liquidum extractum Sig 1ml
References
BPC 1949. 43 p66. 111 p346. 126 p303. 176 p171. 189 p76. 224 p254.

Cinnamomum zeylandicum [Cinnamon]

Inferior and often substituted for the above is Cinnamomum cassia [cassia or chinese cinnamon].

Constituents

Volatile oil [antifungal, antiviral, Antibacterial] up to 4% mainly composed of cinnamaldehyde up to 80% - spasmolytic, diffusive - improves peripheral circulation, anti-infective and sedative. Camphor. Monoterpenes. Sesquiterpenes. Phenols up to 10%, eugenol. Mucilage and resin. Condensed tannins. Coumarin.

Primary pharmacological action: Antimicrobial.

Therapeutic classes

Antiseptic. Astringent. Refrigerant.
Antibacterial – Botulism, E coli, Helicobacter pylori. Antifungal – candida.
Antiviral. Anti alfatoxin.
Expectorant.
Diffusive stimulant. Hypotensive. Haemostatic.
Aromatic. Carminative. Antiemetic. Hypoglycaemic. Antidiarrhoeal.
Anthelmintic
Renal tonic. Antirheumatic.
Uterine tonic.
Febrifuge. Dermatological agent.
Antispasmodic. Sedative.

Medicinal indications

Colds. Coughs. Epistaxis. Influenza. Haemoptysis. Hypertension. Cold limbs.
Anorexia. Dyspepsia. Flatulent colic. Hyperchlorhydria. Nausea. Vomiting.
Peptic ulcers. Diarrhoea. Dysentery. Worms. Destroys E. Coli infections which are a common source of enteritis and food poisoning.
Exhaustion. Debility.
Post partum haemorrhage. Uterine atony. Menorrhagia. Dysmenorrhoea.

Tissue conditions

Antispasmodic to the gastro intestinal tract. Stimulating astringent to the gastro intestinal tract. Stimulates circulation to the joints. Skin infections of a bacterial or viral origin.
Restores tone to the uterus. Atonic uterus post partum.

External use

Respiratory conditions – inhalation.
Rheumatics – rub with Oleum.
Pediculosis, Scabies – Oleum.

Dosage and mode of application
Dried bacc Sig 1.5g
Tincturae Sig 6ml
Liquidum extractum Sig 1.3ml
    Aqua Cinnamomum Sig 30ml
    Ol Cassia Sig 0.2ml
References
43 p68. 126 p304. 176 p353. 188. 189 p77. 306, 1999, 1 [3] 24-6. 307, 1998, XIV [3]. 394 p65-71.

Citrus aurantium/limon [Orange and lemon peel]

Constituents
Bitters. Flavones - allay inflammation. Vitamin C. Terpenes – pith.

Primary pharmacological action: Sedative and antispasmodic.

Therapeutic classes
Aromatic. Allays inflammation. Antiseptic. Antibacterial. Antifungal.
Anticholesterolaemic. Nutritive. Carminative. Stomachic. Cholelithiasis.
Anxiolytic. Antineoplastic. Immunostimulant.
Medicinal indications
Flavouring agent. Tachycardia. Palpitations.
Stress induced digestive spasm. Insomnia. Anxiety. Nervous restlessness.
Tissue conditions
Contrary to popular opinion oranges and lemons have antacid effects. Acting as
cellular detoxifiers, blood oxygenator and reducing infective processes.
External use
Insect bites – diluted Oleum.
Dosage and mode of application
Oleum Auranti/Citrus Sig 0.2ml
Tincturae Sig 4ml
Liquidum extractum Sig 2ml
Elixir simplex Simple elixir Sig 8ml
References. 111 p365/366. 189 p172/205. 394 p287.

Clutia abyssinica [Spurge family]

Constituents
Methylcoumarins. Flavonoids. Sesquiterpenes. Volatile oil.
Therapeutic classes
Vasotonic alterative. Anthelmintic. Antimalarial. Uterine tonic.
Medicinal indications
Influenza. Hepatitis. Splenomegaly. Ascaria. Malaria.
Threatened abortion. Miscarriage. Convulsions.
External use
Leaf sap wash for wounds and inflamed skin conditions.
Dosage and mode of application
Rad Sig 2g
References. 53.

Cnicus benedictus [Holy thistle]

[Carduus benedictus/Carbena benedicta]

Constituents
Bitter sesquiterpene lactones up to 0.7% - cnicin [anti microbial, bactericidal and stimulates taste receptors] and artemisiifolin. Flavonoids. Phytosterols. Tannin up to 8%. Volatile oils up to 0.3%. Lignan lactones [lignanolides] - Arctigenin. Mucilage. Nicotinaminde. Calcium. Manganese. Magnesium. Potassium.

Primary pharmacological action: Stimulant tonic.

Therapeutic classes
Antimicrobial. Antiseptic. Vasotonic alterative. Antibacterial - Brucella abortus, Brucella bronchoseptica, Escherichia coli, Proteus sp., Pseudomonas aeruginosa, Staphylococcus aureus, Streptococcus faecalis.
Antihaemorrhagic. Venous tonic. Heart tonic. Expectorant.
Carminative. Bitter stomachic [stomach tonic]. Cholagogue. Emetic - large dose. Antidiarrhoeal.
Diaphoretic – hot preparations. Antipyretic.
Emmenagogue. Galactogogue.
Cerebral tonic. Antineoplastic. Vulnerary.
Medicinal indications [Mars]
Colds. Chills. Bronchial catarrh.
Anorexia. Atonic flatulent dyspepsia. Flatulent colic. Depurative to the liver and gall bladder. Cholelithiasis. Diarrhoea.
Oedema.
Eruptive fever - chicken pox, measles. Remittent fever - typhoid, malaria.
Cerebral tonic [improves cerebral circulation] improves the memory. Depression. Headaches. Tinnitus.
Tissue conditions
Tonic action aids appetite and digestion as it stimulates the secretions of the mouth and stomach. A gentle active cholagogue. Reduces biliary cholesterol concentrations. Purifies the blood. Venous tonic when the venous drainage is obstructed from uterine, prostatic or a congested pelvis. Cerebral tonic – improves memory. Increases milk production. Tonic at menarche.
Cautions
Allergic reactions.
External use
Wounds. Ulcers gangrenous and indolent [slow healing].
Preparations
Cold infusion is less nauseating.

Vasotonic alterative or to stimulate secretions with Rumex, Arctium.
Tonic properties with Centaurea.
Dosage and mode of application
Dried herba Sig 3g
Infusium Sig 3g
Tincturae Sig 10ml
Liquidium Extractum Sig 4ml
References
43 p70. 111 p327. 142 p47. 176 p390. 192 p71. 233 p126. 246 p489. 251 p93.
394 p27.

Codonopsis pilusula [Bellflower]

Constituents
Alkaloids. Mucilage. Saponins. Glucose.

Primary pharmacological action:
Adaptogenic tonic similar to Panax.

Therapeutic classes
Gentle tonic to the lungs, increasing the tone and balancing the mucous
secretions.
Stomachic. Splenic.
Medicinal indications
Stomach ulcers. IBS.
Dosage and mode of application
Dried rad Sig 5g
Tincturae Sig 5ml
References
47 p228. 305, 1999, 21 [3] 149-59

Cola acuminata/nitida [Cola tree]

Constituents
Purines. Methylxanthine alkaloids - Theobromine up to 0.1% and Caffeine up to 2.5%. Phenols. Tannin. Vitamin A, B2. Potassium. Choline.

Primary pharmacological action:
CNS stimulant and trophorestorative.

Therapeutic classes
Relaxed conditions of the tissue – atony. Cardioactive.
Antidiarrhoeal. Diuretic.
An astringent tonic [in atony] to the CNS and peripheral nerves. Antidepressant.
Adrenal supportive. Thymoleptic.
Vulnerary. Alcohol habit.

Medicinal indications
Atony. Coronary vasodilator. Heart weakness. Valvular disorders. Arrhythmia.
Pre-term infant apnoea. Asthma. COAD
Breath freshener. Heartburn. Dysentery. Atonic diarrhoea. Cholera.
Oedema.
Motion sickness. Depression. Neurasthenia. Neuralgia. Exhaustion. Depression
[with asthenia - weak muscles]. Cerebral anaemia. Panic attacks. Mood changes.
Wounds.

Tissue conditions
Caffeine stimulates the nervous system [CNS] and is beneficial for restorative
action in chronic tiredness, weakness and depression. Stimulates heart action.
Bronchial smooth muscle relaxant. Stimulating to skeletal muscle.

Cautions
Hypertension. Peptic ulcers. Restlessness.

Preparations
Male sexual tonic with Turnera and Serenoa.
Tonic and Antispasmodic Px Avena, Cola and Scutellaria
Depression with Stachys or Ginkgo.
Neuralgia with Pulsatilla.

Dosage and mode of application
Dried sem Sig 3g
Dry extract Sig 0.75g
Tincturae Sig 10ml
Liquidum extractum Sig 2ml

References
BPC 1934. 43 p71. 176 p207. 189 p163. 192 p155. 394 p72.

Colchicum autumnale [Meadow saffron]

Constituents
Alkaloids - colchicine up to 0.25%. Colchicine is hepatic. Flavonoids. Sterols.

Primary pharmacological action: Antirheumatic.

Therapeutic classes
Allays inflammation. Cardiac.
Emetic. Cathartic.
Anodyne. Anti leukaemic.
Medicinal indications [Saturn]
Rheumatic carditis and pericarditis [in the athletic habitus only].
Gout.
Chronic myeloid leukaemia. Hodgkins disease. Behcet's syndrome.
Tissue conditions
Inhibits cellular division by arresting mitosis in the metaphase. Used for relief of acute pain in gout.
Cautions
Restrictions apply. Dosage is determined by the relief of symptoms. Vertigo.
Heart disease. Renal disease. Alkaloid poisoning can cause gastro intestinal disturbances - nausea, abdominal pain, diarrhoea.
Antidote – stimulation with Capsicum, emetic and laxative.
Preparations
Gout with Eupatorium purpureum, Filipendula, Zea.
Dosage and mode of application
Dried corm Sig 200 mg
Dry extract Sig 30mg
Tincturae corm Sig 2ml
Tincturae Colchicum [BP]
LE Colchicum 10ml Alcohol to 100ml. [390 p450]
It contains 0.03% w/v alkaloids [600mcg in 2ml].
Sig 2ml [Up to 6ml daily in divided doses].
References
BPC 1973. 126 p314. 142 p272. 176 p383. 239 p170. 246 p507.

Coleus forskohlii [Coleus]

Constituents
Diterpenes - Forskolin up to 0.3%. Essential oil.

Primary pharmacological action: Cardiotonic.

Therapeutic classes
Ophthalmic.
Antiplatelet. Hypotensive. Vasodilator.
Antiasmatic. Bronchodilator.
Medicinal indications
Glaucoma.
Cardiomyopathy.
Asthma. Chronic obstructive airways disease.
Tissue conditions
Reduces the aqueous humour and helps clear glaucoma. Reduces intraocular pressure [in glaucoma].
Myocardial function is improved by positive inotropic effects. It relaxes arterial smooth muscle.
Cautions
Contraindicated in CVA from haemorrhage.
External use
Glaucoma - topical use.
Dosage and mode of application
Collyr - 4 gtt and dilute with aqua in an eyebath QDS.
Dried rad Sig 4g
Liquidum extractum Sig 4ml
References
48 p103. 189 p85. 308, May 1992.

Collinsonia canadensis [Stone root]

Constituents
Glycosides. Volatile oil. Resin. Mucilage.

Primary pharmacological action: Renal and circulatory tonic.

Therapeutic classes
Astringent. Stimulant. Diffusive. Antihaemorrhagic - passive haemorrhage.
Cardiac tonic. Vaso contractant [astringent tonic 194 p52] to the portal veins.
Stomachic. Hepatic.
Antilithic.
Uterine tonic. Nerve diffusive.

Medicinal indications
Otitis media. Regulates cardiovascular activity. Pericarditis. Varicose veins.
Pharyngitis. Aphonia. Laryngitis. Trachieitis. Influenza. Chronic pleurisy.
Enteritis. Rectal disorders: proctitis, rectal fissures, haemorrhoids. Constipation.
Renal and urinary calculi. Cystitis. Genito urinary catarrh.
Metritis. Amenorrhoea. Dysmenorrhoea. Vaginal discharge/leucorrhoea.
Uterine prolapse.

Tissue conditions
Specific in venous congestion or stasis. Atony [relaxation] of veins resulting in
poor venous return or sluggish capillary flow resulting in throat or rectal
disorders. Chronic laryngitis, aphonia with relaxed larynx and dark fauces.
Improves heart tone and cardiac output. Debilitated heart from rheumatic disease
and overstrain e.g. athletes.
It tones vein walls in varicosity. Tones the portal system relieving congestion e.g.
haemorrhoids. Pain or rectal spasm. Rectal or varicose vein fullness and
heaviness. Dry intestinal mucous membranes from deficient capillary circulation
with hard and dry stool. Tones the intestinal mucous membranes.
Atonic uterine activity effecting blood loss – amenorrhoea, dysmenorrhoea,
menorrhagia, metritis with dark blood or vaginal discharge/leucorrhoea.

External use
Sprains and bruises use a poultice of fresh fol.

Preparations
Laryngitis with antiseptics - Calendula, Baptisia, Commiphora.
Heart disorders with Selenicerus.
Colitis with Geranium mac.
Haemorrhoids with Hamamelis oral and local.
Prostate enlargement with Hydrangea.
Varicocoele with Calendula.

Metritis with Uva ursi.
Vaginal discharge/leucorrhoea with Lamium, Trillium, oral and douche.
Dosage and mode of application
Dried rad Sig 4g
Tincturae Sig 4ml
Liquidum extractum Sig 4ml
Mist. Collinsonia et Hamamelis. [Mixture of Collinsonia and Hamamelis]
LE Sig 30gtt aa every 2 hours. Indications: Haemorrhoids and haemorrhages.
References
BPC 1934. 43 p72. 111 p371. 126 p315. 176 p264. 189 p259. 192 p526. 194 p52.
246 p363.

Combretum micranthum [Jungle weed]

Constituents
Polyphenolic compounds. Catechins. Tannin. Resin.

Primary pharmacological action:
Stimulant to the liver, gall bladder and kidney functions.

Therapeutic classes
Antiseptic. Vasotonic alterative.
Antimicrobial against Escherichia coli, Staphylococcus and Streptococcus.
Anthelmintic.
Antineoplastic. Drug withdrawal.
Medicinal indications
Blackwater fever.
Neoplastic solid tumours.
Morphine and opium habit.
External use
Wounds and abscesses with suppuration.
References
148 p148. 189 p87. 224 p1772.

Commiphora molmol [Myrrh]

Constituents
Around 60 gums have been isolated. Resins up to 60% which consist of alpha, beta and gamma commiphoric acids. Guggulsterols - lower cholesterol and triglycerides. Steroids. Volatile oil up to 8% as steroid guggulsterol. Terpenoids - alpha amytrin. Flavonoids – allay inflammation.

Primary pharmacological action:
ANS trophorestorative to the GI tract.

Therapeutic classes
Antiseptic. Astringent. Allays inflammation. Stimulant. Antimicrobial.
Antibacterial. Antifungal – Candida, Tinea and Scabies. Antiviral –Aids/HIV.
Stimulates the pulse. Anticholesterolaemic.
Expectorant.
Oropharyngeal agent. Carminative. Purgative.
Emmenagogue. Diaphoretic.
Antispasmodic. Analgesic. Local and systemic anaesthetic.
Dermatological agent. Vulnerary. Fumigant. Disinfectant.
Thyroactive. Antirheumatic. Antivenemous.

Medicinal indications [Sun]
Lowers serum lipids, cholesterol and triglycerides.
Rhinorrhoea. Pharyngitis. Excessive muco-purulent secretions.
Mercurial ptyalism. Aphthous ulcers. Receding gums. Gingivitis. Tonsillitis. Oral candidiasis. Laryngitis.
Chronic tonsillitis. Gastritis - full pale tongue. Flatulent dyspepsia. Intestinal ulceration. Intestinal antiseptic. Obesity.
Rheumatism.
Furunculosis. Dermal ulcers. Wounds. Abrasions.
Amenorrhoea. Dysmenorrhoea. Vaginal discharge/leucorrhoea. Gonorrhoea.
Pelvic congestion causing heaviness.
Mild thyroid stimulating activity.

Tissue conditions
Mucosal and dermal infection and inflammations. Used for healing ulcers both internally and externally due to its astringent nature. Stimulates polymorphs. Inflammatory or infected conditions of the oropharynx. Chronic tonsillar enlargement, sore spongy gums. Stimulating astringent to the GIT mucous membrane surfaces as it diminishes and restrains mucus discharges. Stimulates hydrochloric acid production and thus improves appetite and digestion.

Inflammatory or congested conditions of respiratory, urinary and pelvic organs associated with purulent, infected mucus.

A stimulating antiseptic in cases of decaying tissue. Stimulates leucocytosis. Used as an purifying incense.

External use

Vapour from the gum resin is used for ocular inflammation.

Aphthous ulcers, herpes, gingivitis, pharyngitis, tonsillitis - gargle and mouthwash 5% dilution.

Wound dressing use diluted and in small amounts, it may be combined with stimulation.

Scorpion bites - bark decoction.

Varicose veins and haemorrhoids 1% Commiphora et Hamamelis dist qs.

Fumigant action – burn the incense.

Caution

Cover the taste.

Care in acute gastric inflammation and irritability of the mucous membranes.

Dosage and mode of application

Give in small doses, you will often find that drop doses are sufficient.

Tincturae resin Sig 2.5ml

Liquidum extractum Sig 2ml

Gargle Sig 60gtt aq frig

Dental powder @ 10% strength

Thompsons No 6 Myrrh compound. [Capsicum 1 part and Myrrh 4 parts] Highly stimulating compound for asphyxia, drowning, electrocution, where a vital positive stimulant is required. Sig 2ml

References

43 p72. 111 p285. 176 p210. 233 p163. 239 p170. 394 p273.

Commiphora mukul [Guggul]

Constituents
Resin containing sterols are called guggulsterones and are anticholesterolaemic.

Primary pharmacological action: Anticholesterolaemic.

Therapeutic classes
Allays inflammation. Antiseptic. Astringent.
Antiplatelet. Antifibrotic. Antioxidant.
Antirheumatic.
Anti obesity.
Thyrostimulant.
Medicinal indications
Inflammatory conditions.
Cholesterolaemia. Hypertension.
Arthritis. Lumbago. Osteoarthritis. Rheumatism. Gout.
Acne.
Obesity.
Tissue conditions
Lowers LDL cholesterol and triglycerides. Increases HDL cholesterol.
Supports cytochrome P450 enzyme reactions - it aids detoxification.
Improvement is found with long term use 12 weeks plus. Antiseptic activity on
mucous membrane and skin injuries.
Cautions
Pregnancy.
Preparations
Laxative with Piper nigrum, Piper longum and Zingiber.
External use
Skin injury – antiseptic activity.
Dosage and mode of application
Tincturae Sig 2ml
References
187. 192 p375. 392 p1.

Conium maculatum [Hemlock]

Constituents
Contains the alkaloid Coniine around 0.2% fol and 2.5% rad, which sedates nerves. Volatile oil.

Primary pharmacological action: Anodyne. Sedative.

Therapeutic classes
Vasotonic alterative. Cardiac tonic.
Genito urinary activity. Rheumatic disorders.
Ovarian activity. Pelvic disorders.
Antispasmodic. Antineoplastic.
Medicinal indications [Saturn]
Laryngitis. Laryngismus stridulus. Asthma. Pertussus. Tuberculosis Palpitations.
Ulcer pain. Pain of hepatitis. Painful or itchy ano rectal conditions - fissures, haemorrhoids.
Torticollis. Sciatica. Rheumatic pain.
Testicular venous congestion. Prostate congestion. Uterine and ovarian congestion from poor venous return. Ovarian pain. Cervical ulceration. Eases the pain of cancer. Mastitis. Fibrocystic breast disease.
Acute mania. Panic. Chorea. Epilepsy. Tetany - muscular spasm.
Tissue conditions
Sedates the motor nerves and muscles by diminishing spinal irritability.
Excitability, nervousness or restlessness. Mania. Insomnia. Chorea.
Nervous irritability, restlessness and tension. Anodyne actions in carcinoma and neuralgia.
Cautions
Restrictions apply. Dosage is determined by the relief of symptoms.
Depresses motor nerves. Depresses the respiratory centre. Overdose - withdraw and give an emetic. Give stimulants.
External use
Rheumatism and neuralgia - compress fol.
Anal fissure, pruritus ani, haemorrhoids.
Dosage and mode of application
Powdered fol Sig 0.5g
Liquidum extractum Sig 0.4ml
Ung Conium fol/fruct 7%.
References
King p592. 126 p319. 142 p246/336. 176 p104. 246 p293.

Convallaria majalis [Lily of the valley]

Constituents
Cardioactive glycosides. Convallatoxol and convallatoxoloside comprise 24% of the total glycosides. Convallotoxin oxidises to form convalloside which has an inotropic action upon the myocardium.

Primary pharmacological action:
Cardiac trophorestorative and tonic.

Therapeutic classes
Allays inflammation. Cardiac nervine tonic. Antisclerotic. Diuretic.
Vermifuge - nematodes.
Spasmolytic. Cerebral tonic. Antiepileptic.
Vulnerary.
Medicinal indications [Mercury]
Inflammatory conditions.
Coronary insufficiency. Angina. Arteriosclerosis. Congestive cardiac failure [cardiac dilatation]. Hypotension. Acute heart failure with bradycardia and oedema. Heart hypertrophy. Valvular stenosis. Aortic stenosis. Auricular fibrillation. Palpitations. Tachycardia. Praecordial oppression. Oedema. Nematodes - thread and roundworms. Burns and scars.
Tissue conditions
Acts upon the cardiac nerve supply. Strengthens the myocardium. Slows and strengthens the heart rate. Cardiac insufficiency due to hypertension. Dyspnoea and oedema from a cardiac cause [cardiac asthma]. Tones the heart muscle. Small doses activate ATP in the myocardium. Taken for acute conditions - heart failure, palpitations. Increases diastole. Tachycardia with capillary obstruction.
Preparations
Hypotension or heart disorders with:
Capsicum, Crateagus, Leonurus, Phytolacca, Selenicerus.
Cautions
Restrictions apply. Dosage is determined by the relief of symptoms.
Ventricular tachycardia.
Dosage and mode of application
Acute conditions full dose.
Infusium flos/herba Sig 15ml
Injection IV in dilution over 4 minutes [390].
Tincturae 1:8 Sig 1.2ml
Liquidum extractum Sig 2ml
References. 126 p321. 176 p222. 251 p102. 254 p90. 390 p623.

Coptis trifolia/chinensis/teeta [Goldthread]

Constituents
Berberine group.

Primary pharmacological action:
Astringent and Tonic. [Similar activity to Berberis and Hydrastis]

Therapeutic classes
Allays inflammation. Antibacterial - Trichomonas vaginalis. Antimicrobial.
Antiviral – AIDS 94% effective. Blood cleansing vasotonic alterative.
Stomachic. Cholagogue. Antiprotozoal.
Dermatological agent.

Medicinal indications
Haemostatic – to gastro intestinal and genito urinary tracts. Septicaemia.
Infections. Epistaxis. Respiratory infections.
Halitosis. Flatulence. Hepatitis. Gastroenteritis. Colitis. Bacillary dysentery.
Typhoid.
Debility. Intermittent fevers.
Abscesses. Dermatitis. Eczema.

Tissue conditions
Inflamed and irritable infective conditions of gastro intestinal, respiratory and
genito urinary mucous membranes and skin.

Preparations
Bronchitis, Pneumonia, Pleurisy with Zingiber.
Peritonitis with Zingiber.
Nephritis with Zingiber.

External use
Aphthous ulcers – mouthwash.
Wound infections, ulcers – poultice or ung – astringent disinfectant.
Trichomonas vaginalis – douche.

Dosage and mode of application
Powdered rhiz Sig 1.2g
Tincturae Sig 3.5ml
Liquidum extractum Sig 4ml

References
111 p380. 126 p324. 239 p170. 278, 1991 54 [1] 143-54.

Corallorhiza odontorhiza [Crawley]

Constituents
Bitters.

Primary pharmacological action: Relaxing diaphoretic.

Therapeutic classes
Allays inflammation. Demulcent. Diffusive.
Febrifuge.
Sedative. Emmenagogue.
Medicinal indications
Bronchial irritation with wheezing and deficient secretions. Asthma.
Tuberculosis.
Flatulent and bilious colic. Typhoid.
Pyrexia [with] inflammatory conditions - Pneumonia. Pleurisy.
Meningitis. Phrenitis.
Amenorrhoea. Dysmenorrhoea. Post partum pain.
Erysipilas.
Tissue conditions
A diffusive and relaxing diaphoretic. Relieves arterial excitement and congestion
from pyrexia and inflammatory conditions. Similar in action to Asclepias.
Dosage and mode of application
Decoctum Sig 30ml
Liquidum extractum rad. Sig 2ml
References
111 p644. 126 p322. 176 p456. 188p134. 189 p95.

Corydalis ambigua/yanhunuo

[Pinyin/Chinese fumewort] similar actions.

Constituents
Alkaloids - cardiotonic and hypotensive. Bulbocapnine and Isocorydine -
stimulate contraction of skeletal muscle. THP - di tetrahydropalmatine is
analgesic and sedative.

Primary pharmacological action: Stimulant.

Therapeutic classes
Vasotonic alterative. Antiseptic.
Cardiac. Antiarrhythmic. Hypotensive. Diuretic.
Antitussive.
Bitter tonic.
Analgesic. Antispasmodic. Sedative. Hypnotic. Tranquilliser.
Uterine remedy. Antineoplastic.
Medicinal indications
Improves coronary blood flow. Myocardial supportive remedy following
myocardial infarction.
Gastralgia. Abdominal pain. Colic.
Dysmenorrhoea. Uteritis. Postpartum pain. Syphilis.
Anxiety. Headache. Insomnia. Meniers disease. Parkinsons disease - tremor.
Chorea. Nystagmus. Epilepsy.
Tissue conditions
Indicated where there is pain - it has a morphine like action.
Dosage and mode of application
Dried rad 3g
Liquidum extractum Sig 3.5ml
References
47 p472. 176 p376. 188 p130.

Crataeva nurvala [Varuna]

Constituents
Glucosinolates. Flavonoids. Saponins. Sterols. Tannins.

Primary pharmacological action: Antilithic.

Therapeutic classes
Bladder tonic. Prostatic hyperplasia. Eliminates sodium. Urinary antiseptic.
Medicinal indications
Cystitis. Kidney and bladder calculi. Urinary incontinence.
Tissue conditions
Allays inflammatory conditions of the genito urinary tract with infection or calculi. Bladder atony with consequent prostatic disturbance. An genito urinary trophorestorative.
Dosage and mode of application
Decoctum dried rad/cort Sig 10ml
Liquidum extractum Sig 3ml
References
48 p112.

Crataegus monogyna/oxacanthoides
[Hawthorn]

Constituents
Leaves, berries and blossoms contain flavonoids around 1% [when the buds are just showing white] – hyperoside [0.1%], quercetin and rutin. C. monogyna shows a higher level of flavonoid and hyperoside than in the leaves of C. laevigata. Oligomeric procyanidins around 3% – catechin, epicatechin, responsible for cardiovascular protection. Volatile oil in the flowers. Bioflavonoids are often found in the red colouring at the bottom of the extract - shaking up the bottle will disperse them. Amines. Tannins. Saponins.

Primary pharmacological action:
Cardiac muscle tonic [cardiotonic] and trophorestorative to the myocardium.

Therapeutic classes
Astringent. Antioxidant. Cardiomyopathy. Cardioactive tonic. Congestive heart failure. Antiarrhythmic. Beta blocker. Hypotensive. Thrombosis. Vasodilator. Coronary vasodilator. ACE inhibitor.
Inotropic. Chronotropic. Dromotropic. Bathmotropic [a]. Diuretic.
CNS depressant. Sedative. Spasmolytic.

Medicinal indications [Mars]
Angina. Buergers disease. Coronary artery disease. Carditis. Palpitations. Rheumatic fever. Extrasystoles. Ventricular fibrillation. Paroxysmal tachycardia. Valve insufficiency from sclerosis. Mitral regurgitation and stenosis. Hypertension. Arteriosclerosis. Myocardial disease. Endo, myo and pericarditis. CCF – congestive heart failure. Psychogenic cardiac disturbances.

Tissue conditions
Improves cardiac function by sustaining nutrition and vasoperfusion. Vasodilator to the coronary arteries increasing coronary circulation it will therefore improve dyspnoea and palpitations. Reduces peripheral resistance.
Inotropic action upon the myocardium, increasing the refractory [rest] period - slows and strengthens the beat through increased vagal stimulation. Increases myocardial contraction. Beta adrenergic blocking activity = antiarrhythmic in extra systoles and paroxysmal tachycardia. Enhances superoxide dismutase and scavenges free radicles. Suitable for ageing heart conditions.

Preparations
Nervous palpitations - with Melissa and Lavandula.
Hypertension with Tilia and Viscum.
Cardiac disease of the elderly - Capsicum, Leonurus, Selenicerus, Zanthoxylum.

Dosage and mode of application
Tell the patient to shake the mixture.
Dried fol Sig 3g
Infusium flos Sig 30ml
Tincturae fleur/bacc/fol Sig 10ml
Liquidum extractum Sig 2ml
References
6 p90. 43 p74. [a] 142 p167 quoted by Weiss from Ammon H. Planta medica
35/2/3/4 1981. 192 p265. 230 p59. 239 p123-4. 246 p187. 263 Dec, 1993. 265.
270, 1997, 4 [3] p267-271. 310 Vol 2, No 3, 1991/92. 394 p188.

Croton eleuteria [Cascarilla]

Constituents
Bitters – cascarillin. Lignan. Resin. Tannin. Volatile oil.

Primary pharmacological action: Bitter tonic.

Therapeutic classes
Hypotensive.
Aromatic. Expectorant.
Antispasmodic. Hypnotic. Sedative.
Medicinal indications
Chronic bronchitis.
Atonic dyspepsia. Flatulence. Diarrhoea. Dysentery.
Debility. Convalescence. Pyrexia. Intermittent fever.
Tissue conditions
Stimulating to mucous membranes. Enhances food absorption - increases weight.
Cautions
Restrictions apply. Dosage is determined by the relief of symptoms.
Preparations
Relieves Cinchona induced nausea and vomiting.
Dosage and mode of application
Dried bacc/fruct/sem Sig 2g
Infusium Sig 30ml
Tincturae fruct/sem. Sig 4ml
Liquidum extractum Sig 3ml
References
43 p62. 176 p334. 187p166.189 p62.

Curcuma longa [Turmeric]

Constituents

Diarylheptanoids called curcuminoids [antineoplastic, cholagogue] are found in the yellow pigment at around 6% and are antioxidant. Volatile oil [choleretic] up to 5% of which 60% are sesquiterpine ketones. Fixed oil. Vitamin C. Potassium.

Primary pharmacological action:
Cholagogue, Choleretic and hepatoprotective.

Therapeutic classes

Ophthalmic. Allays inflammation. Antioxidant. Astringent. Depurative. Stimulant. Tonic. Vasotonic alterative. Antiallergic.
Antibacterial – Salmonella, Staphylococcus aureus.
Antifungal – Trichophyton rubrum.
Antiviral - Herpes zoster, HIV.
Anticholesterolaemic. Antioxidant. Inhibits platelet aggregation. Hypolipidaemic.
Anorexia. Aromatic. Carminative. Stomach tonic. Laxative. Anthelmintic.
Antiprotozoal.
Diuretic. Antirheumatic. Anaphrodisiac.
Dermatological agent. Vulnerary. Insecticide.
Antineoplastic. Immunostimulant. Antimutagenic. Cytotoxic.
Analgesic. Antispasmodic. Adrenal supportive.

Medicinal indications

Conjunctivitis. Haemorrhage. Bronchitis.
Toothache. Gastritis. Reduces gastric acidity-Heartburn. Gastro-duodenal ulcers.
Nausea. Vomiting. Indigestion. Liver toxicity. Viral hepatitis. Flatulence.
Jaundice. Toxic to salmonella. Diarrhoea. Worms.
Musculoskeletal pain and inflammation in Rheumatoid and Osteo Arthritis.
Strengthens connective tissue.
Headache.
Amenorrhoea.
Dermal ulcers. Eczema. Inflammatory skin disorders. Psoriasis. Leprosy. Insect repellent. Leech bites.
Oral, breast, colon, prostate and skin carcinoma.

Tissue conditions

Half life is around 2 hours. Scavenges nitric oxide from the blood [anaphrodisiac]. Stimulates the reduction of cholesterol by cholagogue action.
Supports the inhibition of HIV virus.
Inhibits the growth rate of carcinoma cells. Interleukin – 8 receptor expresses itself upon the cell surface of neutrophils. Inhibits pro-inflammatory cytokines

and the production of interleukin – 8 by tumour cells. Blocks the growth of breast carcinoma, prostate carcinoma, colon carcinoma – where defective DNA is found. It is a lymphocyte DNA protective.
Used as a yellow colouring in food dishes.
Cautions
Can irritate the stomach.
External use
Scabies, wounds and fungal infections – topically antimicrobial.
Dosage and mode of application
Dried rhiz. Sig 4g
Infusium Sig 1.5g
Tincturae Sig 10ml
Liquidum extractum Sig 4ml
References
111 p391. 189 p271. 192 p552. 230 p99. 239 p170. 263, 91 57[1] 1-7. 272 1994, 7 [1] p41. 265 1998, 10 [2]. 309, 49:105-107. 389. 394 p397.

Cyamopsis tetragonolobus [Guar gum]

Constituents
Galactomannan. Protein. Saponins.

Primary pharmacological action: Hypoglycaemic.

Therapeutic classes
Hypercholesterolaemia. Antidiabetic. Antiobesic.
Medicinal indications
Lipid lowering.
Diabetes. Obesity and weight reduction.
Dosage and mode of application
Fibre from sem Sig 10g
References
239.

Cymbopogon citratus [Lemon grass]

Constituents
Volatile mainly citral, a terpine aldahyde. Aldehyde rich essential oils are effective against Aspergillosis and Tinea.

Primary pharmacological action: Hepatic and flavouring agent.

Therapeutic classes
Tonic. Carminative. Stomachic.
Antipyretic. Diaphoretic.
Diuretic. Antirheumatic.
Emmenagogue. Mosquito repellent.

Medicinal indications
Diarrhoea. Jaundice. Hypotensive. Diuretic. Refreshing herbal tea.
The essential oil is antibacterial, analgesic, and antipyretic.

Dosage and mode of application
Herba Sig 5g
Rad Sig 2g

References
270, 5 [4] 307-329. 275, 1995, No 44, p25-7.

Cynara scolymus [Artichoke]

Constituents

Phenolic acids up to 2%, Chlorogenic acid. Cynarin enhances and protects hepatic function. Volatile oil - Sesquiterpine lactones up to 6% - Cynaropicrin stimulates hepatic function. Inulin. Sterols.

Primary pharmacological action:
Hepatic trophorestorative [Hepatoprotective].

Therapeutic classes

Vasotonic alterative. Tonic. Antioxidant.
Hypocholesteraemic. Hypolipidaemic. Antisclerotic.
Antiemetic. Cholelithiasis. Choleretic. Cholagogue. Hepatostimulant. Impaired fat digestion. Laxative.
Diuretic. Uric acid diathesis. Lithuria.
Thyroactive.

Medicinal indications [Venus]

Cholesterol disturbances.
Appetite disorders. Nausea. Dyspepsia. Irritable Bowel Syndrome. Improves fat digestion. Flatulence. Hepatic atony. Jaundice. Bloating. Fat intolerance.
Nephrosclerosis. Rheumatism Gout. Renal calculi.
Itchy skin. Aids alcohol metabolism.

Tissue conditions

Reduces serum cholesterol and triglycerides, increases HDL and inhibits LDL. It may be used as a sugar substitute for diabetics. Hepatic protective and supportive. Gall bladder stimulant. Aids in the reduction of IBS - bloating, flatulence and abdominal discomfort/pain.

Dosage and mode of application

Dried fol Sig 3g
Dry extract 1:12 0.5g
Rad Sig 4g
Tincturae Sig 6ml
Liquidum extractum Sig 2ml

References

142 p88. 239 p87. 246 484. 270 Vol. 1, p107. 310, 1995/6, Vol. 4, No 1, p21-26. 394 p10.

Cypripedium pubescens [Ladies slipper]

Currently an endangered species.

Constituents
Glycosides. Volatile oil. Tannin. Resin.

Primary pharmacological action: Meningeal vasorelaxant.

Therapeutic classes
Nerve relaxant and antispasmodic. Hypnotic. Sedative.

Medicinal indications
Irritability of the nervous system. Manic depression psychosis. Insomnia.
Neuralgia. Tension of the nerves and muscles. Anxiety. Panic. Migraine.
Dysmenorrhoea. Sexual irritability.

Tissue conditions
A pure relaxant with no stimulating properties. Used in all cases of tension
within the nervous system. Relieves pain from spasm.

Preparations
Generally combined with a nervine - Scutellaria.
Manic depression - with Lobelia.
Prescribed with tonic medicines its power is increased.

Dosage and mode of application
Dried rad Sig 4g
Tincturae Sig 4ml
Liquidum extractum Sig 4ml

References
BPC 1923. 43 p76. 192 p324. 246 p557.

Cytisus scoparius [Sarothamnus, Broom]

Constituents
Quinolizidine alkaloids. Sarothamnine and genistein [vasoconstrictor] are alkaloids which inhibit conduction. The alkaloidal activity produce the main actions. Flavonoids have a beneficial effect upon the myocardium. Volatile oils.

Primary pharmacological action: Cardioactive and Diuretic.

Therapeutic classes
Anti haemorrhagic.
Emetic. Cathartic.
Oxytocic. Uterine astringent.
Antineoplastic.
Antivenomous.
Medicinal indications [Mars]
Arrhythmia. Heart disturbances. Oedema.
Jaundice.
Thyrotoxicosis.
Tissue conditions
Regulates heart rhythm by reducing the conductivity of cardiac muscle.
Extrasystoles and arrhythmias benefit from its use. Reduces atrial and ventricular fibrillation. It is tonic to the venous return. It depresses respiration and is a peripheral vasoconstrictor. Used for functional palpitation with hypotension.
Cardiac disturbances with oedema.
Preparations
With Convallaria, Selenicerus.
Diuretic with Taraxacum and Juniperus.
Phlebitis with Petroselinum, Daucus, Galium and Symphytum.
Cautions
Can cause bradycardia and hypertension. Pregnancy.
Dosage and mode of application
Dried herba/fol Sig 2g
Infusium 1:10 Sig 60ml
Decoctum 1:20 Sig 120ml
Tincturae Sig 2ml
Liquidum extractum Sig 4ml
References
Martindale quote BPC 1949. 43 p192. 111 p398. 176 p438. 189 p43. 246 p194. 262 p80.

Datura stramonium [Jimsonweed]

Constituents
Tropane alkaloids, around 0.5%, atropine, hyoscine and hyoscyamine are anticholinergic. Flavonol glycosides - quercetin. Coumarin. Tannin.

Primary pharmacological action:
Antispasmodic. Anticholinergic.

Therapeutic classes
Antiasmatic. Anodyne.
Muscle antispasmodic – respiratory, gastro intestinal and urinary tracts.
Medicinal indications [Jupiter]
Asthma. Pertussis.
Hyperchlorhydria. Enteritis. Diverticulitis. Colitis. Peritonitis.
Spasmodic urethral stricture.
Parkinsons disease. Delirium tremens. Panic. Mania. Meningitis. Neuralgia.
Muscle spasm. Epilepsy.
Dysmenorrhoea. Intermittent fever.
Tissue conditions
Nerve innervation. Cerebral irritation with red or bloated face. The smoke from burning the herb is inhaled for coughs and asthma. Tends to dry the mucous membranes.
Eases neuralgic and spasmodic pain of the gastro intestinal tract. Nervous skin irritation.
Delirium, rage, garrulous, fearful and restless, unable to rest, violent excitability, spasm with pain, bloating all confirm cerebral irritability. Parkinson tremor or salivation.
Cautions
Restrictions apply. Dosage is determined by the relief of symptoms.
Glaucoma. Arrhythmia.
High doses are sedative and cause red eyes, drowsiness, amnesia, and REM reduction during sleep.
External use
Opthalmia - collyr.
Inflamed glands, parotitis, orchitis, mastitis, rheumatic pain, painful haemorrhoids - apply the oleum, unguentum or crem.
Anal itching - use the unguentum.
Preparations
Asthma - inhale the smoke.
Crushed leaves and seeds are used to allay pain and to ease bites from insects.

Pharmacopoeia

Pre-med prior to operations to cause drowsiness.
It has been misused by law enforcement agencies.
Dosage and mode of application
Dry extract Sig 60mg. Up to 500mg in Parkinsonism.
Infusium fol/fleur Sig 200mg
Tincturae 1:10 Sig 2ml
Liquidum extractum Sig 0.2ml
Cigarettes de Datura. Stramonium cigarettes Each contains 1g Stramonium.
References
126 p657. 176 p185. 189 p300. 233 p209. 224 p248. 246 p400.

Daucus carota [Wild carrot]

Constituents
Alkaloid – daucin. Flavonoids – apignein, luteolin. Volatile oil up to 1.6%.
Tannin.

Primary pharmacological action: Stimulating diuretic.

Therapeutic classes
Ophthalmic. Deobstruent.
Carminative. Stomachic. Anthelmintic.
Antilithic. Antirheumatic.
Antineoplastic.
Vulnerary.
Medicinal indications [Mercury]
Night blindness.
Cystitis. Gout. Urinary gravel or calculi. Oedema. Urinary stricture. Gout.
Polymyalgia.
Amenorrhoea. Dysmenorrhoea. Menopausal flushes. Abscesses
Tissue conditions
The volatile oil has an irritant diuretic action upon the kidneys.
External use
Abscesses, cancer, ulcers, wounds – poultice.
Preparations
Diuretic tea – Agropyron, Barosma, Daucus, Medicago and Uva ursi.
Dosage and mode of application
Dried herba Sig 4g
Liquidum extractum Sig 4ml
References
43 p77/78. 111 p398. 127 p161-5. 188 p453. 192 p452. 233 p221/222.

Delphinium [Staphysagria/Larkspur]

Constituents
Diterpine alkaloids around 1% - Delphinine, Delphisine and Delphinoidene.
Volatile oil. Mucilage. Fixed oil.

Primary pharmacological action: Nervine tonic.

Therapeutic classes
Ophthalmic. Allays inflammation.
Emetic. Cathartic. Anthelmintic.
Genito urinary inflammation.
Nervine. Central nervous system stimulant. Insecticide. Parasiticide.
Medicinal indications
Hordeolum. Motion sickness. Vomiting of pregnancy.
Prostatic disease/enlargement. Cystitis. Spermatorrhoea. Prostorrhoea.
Impotency. Gonorrhoea.
Exhaustion. Neurasthenia. Panic. Depression. Facial and cervical neuralgia.
Pediculosis.
Tissue conditions
Panic or depression with outbursts of anger or moodiness sometimes associated
with altered fertility cycle and or pelvic congestion. Nervous irritability. Soothes
irritable, chronic inflammatory and atonic conditions of the urethra, prostate,
seminal vesicles and testes. Settles irritation of the lumbar, sacral and pelvic
nerves. Sexual irritability, panic, despondency or violent outbursts of passion.
Cautions
Restrictions apply. Dosage is determined by the relief of symptoms.
Acute inflammation. Can cause vomiting and purging. Depresses the medulla
oblongata. Death by asphyxia. Intensified by Hydrastis.
External use
Pediculosis - lotion of powdered sem for destroying hair lice.
Neuralgia, paralysis – lotion.
Scurf with Ung Rose.
Preparations
Impotence/sexual dysfunction or prostatic disease with Serenoa and Avena.
Antidote to strychnine.
Dosage and mode of application
Powder decoction sem Sig 150mg.
Tincturae 1:10 Sig 0.25ml.
Tr Delphinium 4ml aqua to 120ml. Sig 5ml TDS.

Unguentum Staphysagria. BPC 1949. Stavesacre ointment.
Mixture of bees wax and lard with Stavesacre 20%.
Lotion Staphysagria BPC 1949. Stavesacre lotion.
Staphysagria 10%, apple cider vinegar, alcohol, glycerine, aqua, perfumed with
oleum Lavandula 1gtt.
References
BPC 1949. 126 p653. 176 p455. 189 p258. 246 p115. 390 p950.

Desmodium ascendans

Primary pharmacological action:
Hepatic deficiency from
inflammation, viral, toxic or alcohol aetiology.

Dosage and mode of application
Tincturae herba Sig 5ml

Dicentra canadensis [Turkey corn]

Constituents
Alkaloids - Cularine, Cularidine. Resin. Fumaric acid.

Primary pharmacological action: General vaso stimulant.

Therapeutic classes
Vasotonic alterative. Diffusive tonic.
Gastro intestinal tonic.
Diuretic. Emmenagogue.

Medicinal indications
Dysentery. Diarrhoea. Jaundice.
Chronic skin conditions. Scrophularia. Syphilis - ulcers, nodes and bone pain.
Lymphadenopathy. Rheumatism.
Amenorrhoea. Dysmenorrhoea. Vaginal discharge/leucorrhoea.

Tissue conditions
Vasotonic alterative activity is unequalled in the above conditions as it supports
the elimination of toxins. Gastro intestinal conditions with furred tongue, halitosis
and sluggish digestion. It improves nutrition via its tonic effects for gastro
intestinal atony. Promotes lymphatic and blood waste removal and enhances
repair.

Preparations
Vasotonic alterative action with Arctium, Stillingia and Zanthoxylum.

Dosage and mode of application
Infusium rad Sig 30ml
Liquidum extractum Sig 4ml

References
111 p400. 126 p325. 188 p432. 189 p270.

Digitalis lanata/purpura [Foxglove]

Constituents
Cardio active glycosides up to 1.4%, known as cardenolides - unsaturated lactones. Digitalis purpura contains the cardioactive glycoside Digitoxin. Digitalis lanata contains the cardio active glycoside Digoxin and is less cumulative. Digoxin is excreted by the kidneys.

Primary pharmacological action: Cardioactive.

Therapeutic classes
Diuretic
Medicinal indications [Venus]
Dyspnoea. Cardiac failure. CCF. Jugular fullness. Arrhythmias. Heart failure with bradycardia. Cerebral arteriosclerosis. Hypotension. Mitral stenosis and regurgitation. Ascites. Oedema. Vulnerary.
Tissue conditions
Cardiac cells have an ATPase enzyme system binding site where Digitalis exerts it's effects. Binding of glycosides causes the inhibition of the sodium and potassium pump activity thereby increasing intracellular sodium and reducing potassium. Depolarisation of the cell membrane releases calcium to act as a muscle contractant. Myocardial ischaemia leads to calcium overload which causes arrhythmias. Regulates contractility, irritability, and impulses through the AV node, Hiss and bundle branches reducing conductivity.
Stimulates the vagus nerve [parasympathetic stimulation], this slows and strengthens the heart beat [prolongs diastole] - positive inotropic effects. Lengthening diastole increases coronary perfusion, improves coronary circulation and increases the force of myocardial contraction. It is indicated for acute or chronic heart failure. Prolongs diastole and Vaso contractant to the myocardium and arteries. Vasocontractant to the mesentery. Improves cerebral circulation. Increases renal blood flow with subsequent diuresis.
Therapeutic blood concentrations of cardioactive glycosides from D. lanata are achieved more quickly. D purpura cardioactive glycosides are excreted more slowly so there is an increased absorption and more chance of accumulation with toxic effects. While patients will have different levels of tolerability serum concentrations provide evidence of toxicity. Symptoms provide an instant referencing for any toxicity. Laurence gives the half life of Digoxin as 48 hours
Cautions
Restrictions apply. Dosage is determined by the relief of symptoms.
Digoxin toxicity appears at levels above 2.6mol/litre. Toxicity includes arrhythmia, fibrillation, respiratory effects, nausea and vomiting [centrally

induced], diarrhoea, sweating, seizures, syncope. Contra indicated in angina because digitalis increases the requirement for O2. Heart block. Right heart hypertrophy.

Toxicity can be increased in patients with thyroid disturbance, renal disturbance, blood acidosis, alterations in blood calcium, potassium and sodium.

External use

Breast milk depressor – fol

Dosage and mode of application

Treatment is determined by the glycoside requirement and level of tolerance.

In heart failure a small to very small dose is required.

Duration of use – short term.

Standardised powder

Infusium fol Sig 7ml [Ellingwood. p215]. Infusium fol Sig 15ml [174 p226].

Tincturae D. purpura 1:10 fol Sig 1 ml [174 p226].

Tincturae D. purpura 1:10 fol Sig 1.75ml [184 p49].

Tincturae D. purpura 1:10 fol Sig 1ml [188 p189].

Tincturae D. purpura Sig 1ml [BPC 1959].

References

BPC 1959. 126 p333. 175. 176 p215. 183 p6.38. 224 p487. 228 p122.

Dioscorea villosa [Wild yam]

Constituents
Steroidal sapogenins – dioscin. Dioscin is converted into diosgenin by the
removal of sugar in the gut. Starch. Prostglandin antagonist.

Primary pharmacological action: ANS antispasmodic.

Therapeutic classes
Allays inflammation.
Hypocholesterolaemic. Expectorant.
Carminative. Antibilious. Emetic. Cholagogue. Hypoglycaemic. Biliary
antispasmodic. Hepatic trophorestorative. Amoebicidal.
Diuretic. Diaphoretic. Antirheumatic. Antipyretic.
Parturient. Oestrogenic.
Anodyne. Analgesic. Antineoplastic.
Thyroactive.
Medicinal indications
Goitre. Intermittent claudication. Spasmodic asthma. Laryngitis stridulus.
Spasmodic stomach cramp/hiccoughs. Dyspepsia. Nausea. Vomiting. Hepatic
congestion. Cholecystitis. Jaundice. Biliary and intestinal colic, irritation or
spasm. Diverticulosis. Diarrhoea. Dysentery. Peritonitis. Appendicitis
Haemorrhoids.
Urinary tract infections. Gonorrhoea. Syphilis. Leprosy.
Muscle cramp. Neuralgia. Rheumatic pain. Arthritis. Rheumatoid arthritis.
Dysmenorrhoea. Nausea of pregnancy. Vaginal dryness. Mastitis. Hormonal
imbalance.
Furunculosis. Carcinoma – nerve tissue.
Tissue conditions
Smooth muscle relaxant for pain/spasm within the gastro intestinal, biliary,
urinary and generative organs. Dioscorea calms the Autonomic nervous system.
A frequent problem encountered in acute rheumatic conditions are irritated
intestinal nerves. This adds to the problem of removing the toxins and acids
creating the rheumatic condition. Dioscorea allays the irritation and relaxes the
nerves. It produces freedom from rheumatic pain. Intestinal bloating, bilious and
intestinal colic with pain are eased.
Cautions
Avoid in atonic [relaxed] conditions.
External use
Mastitis or vaginal dryness – lotion or gel applied BD.

Preparations
Viburnum species and Zingiber in restlessness and irritability [during pregnancy].
Colic, intestinal flatulence with Angelica, Nepeta or Zingiber.
Colic - use full dosage.
Dosage and mode of application
Full dose expected to work quickly, within 2 hours.
Dried rad/rhizome. Sig 4g
Tincturae Sig 5ml
Liquidum extractum Sig 4ml
References
43 p78. 176 p278. 188 p454. 192 p570. 194 p54. 230 p103. 246 p523. 271 No 24.

Dipsacus fullorum/sylvestris [Teazle]

Constituents
Bitters. Glucoside – scabioside. Inulin. Mineral salts.

Primary pharmacological action: Vasotonic alterative.

Therapeutic classes
Ophthalmic. Depuritive. Deobstruent.
Aperitif. Stomachic. Hepatic. Anthelmintic.
Dermatological agent. Antineoplastic.
Medicinal indications [Venus]
Hordeolum. Anorexia. Jaundice. Fistula.
Eases wrinkles on the face. Acne. Eczema. Impetigo. Psoriasis. Whitlow.
Tissue conditions
Cleansing and depurative to the blood.
External use
Ocular inflammation - collyr.
Warts - ung.
Fistulas - ung.
Skin wrinkles - dect.
Dosage and mode of application
Infusium flos/rad. Sig 5g.
References
127 p793. 160. 246 p434.

Dodonea viscosa [Hop bush]

Constituents
Coumarin – fraxetin is antioxidant and anodyne. Diterpenoids. Essential oil – 0.04%. Flavonoids. Phenols. Saponins – dodonoside. Tannins. Resin. Beta sitosterol.

Primary pharmacological action: Vasotonic alterative and tonic

Therapeutic classes
Allays inflammation. Discutient. Tonic. Antimicrobial – broad spectrum. Antiviral.
Antioxidant. Hypotensive.
Cathartic.
Anodyne - fol. Spasmolytic.
Dermatological agent. Antipruritic. Febrifuge. Antivenomous.
Medicinal indications
Hypertension.
Colds. Diptheria. Laryngismus stridulus. Pneumonia. Tuberculosis.
Haemorrhoids.
Gout. Rheumatism.
Burns. Scalds. Dermal ulcers. Pyrexia. Stings – stonefish, stingrays.
External use
Rheumatic pain – fol poultice is heating.
Burns, scalds, rashes and wounds – rad.
Stings apply succus and chew the fol.
Dosage and mode of application
Infusium Sig 30ml
Tincturae fol/rad. Sig 4ml
References.
265, 1999, 11 [1] p11-14.

Drima altissima [Squills] see Urgenia

Drosera rotundifolia [Sundew]

Constituents
Flavonoids. Napthaquinones - Plumbagin are antimicrobial. Tannin. Resin.
Carotenoids. Acids - Vitamin C.

Primary pharmacological action: Expectorant.

Therapeutic classes
Demulcent. Antibacterial - Gram positive Staphylococci, Streptococci and
pneumococcus and gram negative bacteria.
Anti viral - Influenza.
Antifungal - Microspori. Antiprotozoal.
Hypotensive. Expectorant.
Antirheumatic.
Antispasmodic.

Medicinal indications [Sun]
Upper respiratory tract infections. Sinusitis. Asthma. Bronchitis. Pertussus.
Trachieitis. Nervous coughs. Pneumonia. Tuberculosis.
Gastritis. Gastric ulcers. Muscular pain.

Tissue conditions
Soothing and tonic to respiratory mucous membranes. Cough from associated
pulmonary, cardiac or gastric disorders. Irritating, spasmodic coughs associated
with dryness of the mucous membranes.
Acts upon the muscular system in fibrositis and muscular pain.

Preparations
Asthma with Grindelia.

Dosage and mode of application
Dried herba Sig 2g
Tincturae Sig 1ml
Liquidium Extractum Sig 2ml

References
43 p80. 189 p262. 246 p158. 247 p61. 274 44, 1994, 35.

Dryopteris felix mas [Male fern]

Constituents
Filicine. Filmaron. Filicic acid. Oleo resin. Tannin.

Primary pharmacological action: Anthelmintic.

Therapeutic classes
Antiviral.
Cestodes and Ascaris. Vulnerary.
Medicinal indications [Saturn]
To expel tapeworm and round worm.
Tissue conditions
It is preferable to support intestinal elimination as fast as possible following ingestion. Give the remedy and follow with Castor oil. Follow with a meal of ground oats or Ulmus with soya milk. Inspect the evacuation to check for worm sections or parasites.
Cautions
Toxic remedy.
External use
Wounds – fronds.
Dosage and mode of application
Powdered rhiz/fronds. Sig 10g
Liquidum extractum Sig 6ml
Follow with Oleum Castor or saline to promote rapid expulsion of the remedy.
References
111 p280. 142 p118. 188 p283. 192 p342. 246 p565. 390 p150.

Echinacea species [angustifolia, pallida and purpura]

Constituents
Caffeic acid derivatives – Echinoside [up tp 1%] is antibacterial. Polysaccharides allay inflammation. Polyacetylines inhibit infections. Alkylamides stimulate lymphocyte production and Echinacin inhibits hyluronidase. Volatile oil. The root activates leucocytes and inactivates hyaluonidase [which assists the infection process].

Primary pharmacological action:
Vasotonic alterative and lymphatic vasotonic.

Therapeutic classes
Antiseptic. Antimicrobial. Allays inflammation. Antiallergic. Antioxidant - free radical scavenger. Antifungal.
Antibacterial - Escherichia, Proteus mirabilis, Pseudomonas aeruginosa, Staphylococcus aureus.
Antiviral – Aids/HIV, Candida, Coxsackie, Genital herpes, Influenza, Herpes, Listeria, Trichomonas, Vesicular pox virus.
Peripheral vasodilator. General blood cleanser. Immunostimulant. Adrenal stimulant.
Antineoplastic. Dermatological agent and dermal anaesthetic. Vulnerary. Antivenomous.

Medicinal indications
Allergies. Catarrh. Chronic respiratory infections. Diphtheria. Tuberculosis.
Scarlatina. Raynards disease. Gangrene. Varicose leg ulcers.
Gingivitis. Stomatitis. Toothache. Pyorrhoea. Aphthous ulcers. Peritonsillar abscess. Tonsillitis. Influenza. Eruptive fever in morbilla.
Mucous membrane ulcers.
Dyspepsia from fermentation. Intestinal disinfectant. Liver or Intestinal carcinoma. Typhoid. Malaria.
Urinary tract infections. Syphilis.
Acne. Abscess. Burns. Eczema. Erysipilas. Furunculosis.
Rodent ulcer. Mastitis. Mammary carcinoma. Meningitis.
Puerpural fever from [septicaemia]. Ulcerations both external and internal use.
Leukaemia. Insect stings. Snake bite.

Tissue conditions
Stimulates macrophages to produce interleukins and tumour necrosis factor.
Stimulating Vasotonic alterative for acute toxic conditions of the blood and lymph e.g. septicaemia. Stimulates cellular and hormonal immune defence mechanisms. Infections of the respiratory, gastro intestinal and urinary tracts.

E

Dirty tongue with deficient secretions. Frequent infections and feeling run down. Lowered immune response to illness. Abscesses and blood poisoning. Ill effects of vaccination jabs. Asthenia and delayed healing of tissue. Stimulates adrenal cortex.

Echinacea is an immunostimulant. Activates macrophages and interferon activity. Increases T cells. Stimulates phagocytosis.

Cautions

No significant differences between two groups were found in the rate of major or minor birth defects or pregnancy outcome, delivery method, maternal weight gain, infant birth weight or foetal distress. The first prospective study suggests that gestational use of Echinacea during organogenesis is not associated with an increased risk for major malformations. Archives of Internal Medicine 2000, 160, 3141-3

External use

Insect bites and stings. Snake bites. Ulcerations. Dermatological infections. Topically in ung, crem and pessaries.

Preparations

Echinacea can be used with any of the following formulas.

Furunculosis with Arctium, Baptisia and Iris.

Pharyngitis and tonsillitis with Baptisia and Commiphora.

Lymphatics and immune system [carcinoma] with Phytolacca, Galium.

Septicaemia with Baptisia and Commiphora.

Peripheral circulation with Zanthoxylum and Crataegus.

Dosage and mode of application

Dried rad/rhiz Sig 1.5g

Tincturae Sig 5ml

Liquidum Extractum Sig 2ml

Succus Echinacea Sig 3ml

References

69. 188 p132. 188 p161/162. 192 p189. 212. 213. 214/5. 230 p31. 263, 1993, 59, Suppl. PA671/2. 239 p103. 263 2000, 66, [3], p241. 394 p88.

Echium vulgare [Burgloss]

Constituents
Alkaloids of the pyrrolizidine type.

Primary pharmacological action: Pulmonary tonic.

Therapeutic classes
Allays inflammation. Demulcent. Tonic. Expectorant.
Diuretic. Diaphoretic. Febrifuge.
Antivenomous. Anti gonadotrophic.
Medicinal indications [Sun]
Feverish colds. Nervous disorders - depression. Headache. Epilepsy.
Tissue conditions
Acute pulmonary conditions with fever. Relieves inflammatory pains.
Dosage and mode of application
Infusium herba Sig 30ml
References
189 p48. 246 p348. 262 p309.

Eclipta alba [Huanguilla]

Constituents
Wadeloactone – allays inflammation and inhibits haemorrhage.

Primary pharmacological action: Deobstruent.

Therapeutic classes
Depurative. Tonic.
Antihaemorrhagic.
Anti catarrhal. Antiasmatic.
Splenic deobstruent.
Oestrogenic.
Dermatological agent. Insecticidal. Antivenomous.
Medicinal indications
Toothache.
Haemorrhage.
Catarrh. Cough.
Dyspepsia. Hepatitis. Marasmus. Jaundice. Splenitis.
Lumbago.
Headache. Vertigo. Elephantiasis. Snake bite.
Tissue conditions
The active ingredient wedelolactone inhibits the liberation of creatinine kinase induced by snake venom.
External use
Applied to the hair the leaves feed the hair roots.
Skin blemishes – lotion of dect.
Dosage and mode of application
Tincturae herba Sig 4ml
References
53. 338. 346.

Elaeis guineensis [Palm tree]

Constituents
Fruit mesocarp oil [coconut oil] contains carotines. Glycerides of fatty acids including oleic acid, palmitic acid, linoleic acid. Sterols.

Primary pharmacological action:
Cleansing Vasotonic alterative.

Therapeutic classes
Pectoral.
Uterine tonic.
Dermal remedy - antimicrobial.
Galactogogue - partially fermented palm wine.
Cephalgic.
Medicinal indications
Root decoction for: Bronchitis. Headache.
Gonorrhoea. Menorrhagia.
Tissue conditions
The oil from the palm kernel and fruit mesocarp are used as an antidote for poisoning.
External use
Fruit mesocarp and seeds are used in cooking, creams, soaps,
A soap made with palm fruit ash is used in skin disease and infections.
Fresh wounds - fol extract.
References
53.

Elettaria cardamomum [Cardamom]

Constituents
Volatile oil up to 4%. Fixed oil. Starch.

Primary pharmacological action: Digestive tonic. Carminative.

Therapeutic classes
Stimulant. Antiseptic. Antiviral.
Aromatic bitter. Stomachic. Cholagogue.
Antispasmodic.
Orexigenic. Aphrodisiac.

Medicinal indications
Sinus disturbances. Asthma. Colds.
Anorexia. Gastritis. Nausea. Vomiting. Food poisoning. Gastro enteritis. Flatulent dyspepsia. Colic. IBS. Coeliac disease.
Depression, nervous exhaustion or irritability associated with poor digestive function. Fatigue. Poor memory.

Preparations
Allays the griping of purgatives.
Stomach, intestinal infections, enteritis with Cinnamomum, Zingiber.

Dosage and mode of application
Dried sem Sig 2g
Tincturae Sig 4ml
Liquidum extractum Sig 4ml

Tincturae Composita Cardamomum [Compound Tincture of Cardamom]
Cardamomum Sem	7g
Carum sem	7g
Cinnamomum bach	7g
Raisins	60g
Alcohol	550ml

Prepare by maceration. Sig 4ml

References
BP 1973. 43 p81. 192 p111. 239 p170.

Eleutherococcus senticosus [Siberian ginseng]

Constituents
Eleutherosides,A - G up to 0.9%. Triterpenoid saponins. Volatile oils up to 0.8%.
Polysaccharides - blood sugar balancers.

Primary pharmacological action: Adaptogenic and Tonic.

Therapeutic classes
Allays inflammation. Antiviral – Candidiasis, HIV.
Antiplatelet. Improves capillary function. Circulatory tonic. Anti anaemic.
Antidiabetic. Hypoglycaemic. Hepatocyte supportive.
Renal tonic. Aphrodisiac. Gonadotrophic. Adrenal and thyroid trophorestoratives.
Anti stress. Sedative and stimulant. Antispasmodic.
Antirheumatic. Immunostimulant. Antineoplastic. Cytostatic.

Medicinal indications
Inhibits platelet aggregation. Atherosclerosis. Rheumatic heart disease. Improves
coronary blood supply. Normaliser blood pressure from hyper/hypotension.
Improves capillary function and resists hypoxia.
Anorexia. Flatulence.
Oedema. Renal pain/enhances renal function. Infertility.
Rheumatoid arthritis. Rheumatism. Joint pain. Muscle spasm.
Addictions. Debility. Chronic fatigue syndrome. Fatigue. Insomnia. ME.
Neuroses. Improves memory. Prolonged stress or anxiety. HIV. Leukaemia.

Tissue conditions
Improves vitality. A useful remedy in chronic fatigue syndrome. Adaptogenic
reducing fatigue, weakness and stress. Improves exercise performance and mental
ability during stress. Improves speed and quality of work. Improves general
health. One study showed a reduction in the number of days lost from work due
to illness. A favourable effect upon acute craniocerebral trauma.
Gonadotrophic activity. Improves reproductive capacity.
Immunomodulatory effects - increases resistance, interferon and T Lymphocytes.
Candida is destroyed by specific immune defending cells. Aids in the recovery
from addictions – drugs, alcohol. Counters chemo & radiotherapy/radiation effect

Cautions
Care in hypertension.

Dosage and mode of application
Dried rad/bacc. Sig 1.3g. Infusium Sig 3g
Tincturae Sig 15ml
Liquidum extractum Sig 3ml
References. 179 p535. 192 p 236. 230 p51. 239 p154.

Embelia schimperi [Ibinini]

Constituents
Embelin around 7% which is oestrogenic and progestrogenic. Naphthaquinones. Tannin. Resin.

Primary pharmacological action: Antispasmodic - stem bark.

Therapeutic classes
Vasotonic alterative. Antibacterial. Antitubercular.
Carminative. Anthelmintic - fruit. Antiparasitic.
Medicinal indications
Effective against: Ascarides, Dipylidium caninum, Mycobacterium tuberculosis.
Oesophagostomum columbianum, Paramphistomum cervi, Tanea, Trichuris ovis.
Tissue conditions
Effective within 30 minutes against the above parasites.
Antifertility agent as it prevents the implantation without being blastotoxic.
Cautions
Restrictions apply. Dosage is determined by the relief of symptoms.
Dosage and mode of application
Powdered fruct. Sig 4g. Embelia ribes/robusta fruct. Sig 16g.
Liquidum extractum Sig 4ml
References
390 p148.

Ephedra sinica/nevadensis [Ma huang]

Constituents
Alkaloids up to 3% - Levo ephedrine around 90%, is alpha adrenergic and minimally raises pulse and blood pressure. Flavonoid glycosides. Dextra-iso ephedrine is beta adrenergic [bronchodilator].

Primary pharmacological action: Bronchodilator.

Therapeutic classes
Cardiac stimulant. Hypertensive.
Antiallergic. Nasal decongestant. Antiasthmatic. Pertussus.
Bladder tonic. Febrifuge.
Cerebral stimulant. Nerve stimulant.
Dermatological agent. Antispasmodic.

Medicinal indications
Myocardial weakness.
Colds. Hay fever. Pertussus. Sinusitis/Rhinitis. Asthma. Bronchospasm. Influenza
Enuresis. Oedema. Pyrexia.
Narcolepsy. Myasthenia gravis. Headache/Migraine. Allergic rashes.

Tissue conditions
A sympathomimetic remedy. Spasm is reduced in frequency and intensity due to the beta receptors of sympathomimetic amines. Dyspnoea of emphysema is reduced. Inotropic cardiac stimulant. Sympathetic effects - increases the sphincter tone. Relaxes the detrusor muscle of the bladder wall. Stimulates the CNS - sleep is not so deep. Myasthenia gravis - adrenergic receptor agonist.

Cautions
Restrictions apply. Dosage is determined by the relief of symptoms.
Glaucoma. Hyperthyroidism. Coronary thrombosis. Hypertension. Prostate enlargement. Restlessness. Monoamine oxidase inhibitor.

External use
Hayfever - aqueous nebula spray - vasoconstrictor effect upon the nasal mucosa.

Preparations
Asthma with Grindelia, Lobelia, Symplocarpus.

Dosage and mode of application
Dried cut herba 23g provides 300mg of ephedrine.
Children Sig 40mg herba per kg of body weight.
Dried rad Sig 2.5g. Inf. Sig 2g. Tincturae Sig 10ml
Liquidum extractum Sig 3ml

References
BPC 1954. 43 p82. 224 p10. 239 p170. 246 p570. 394 p110.

Epilobium parvifoleum [Rose bay willow herb]

Constituents
Flavonoids – herba. Ellagitannins – Oenotherin A & B inhibit prostate enzymes aromatase and 5 alpha reductase. Tannin.

Primary pharmacological action: Astringent.

Therapeutic classes
Demulcent. Antimicrobial. Diffusive stimulant.
Haemostatic.
Antidiarrhoeal.
Diuretic - fol. Prostatic disturbances.
Emollient. Vulnerary.

Medicinal indications [Saturn]
Opthalmia.
Pharyngitis. Haemoptysis.
Aphthous ulcers. Gastroenteritis. Dysentery. Diverticulosis. Diarrhoea. Colitis.
Enteritis. Typhoid.
Cystitis. Prostatitis. Benign prostatic hyperplasia.
Menorrhagia. Eczema.

Tissue conditions
Diarrhoea [colicky] from relaxed or irritable conditions of the intestine.
Contracted tongue, dry mucous membranes, shrunken papillae. Diffusive stimulating astringent leaving behind a tonic effect.
Epilobium parviflorum inhibits 5-alpha-reductase i.e. inhibits benign prostatic hypertrophy.

Preparations
Haemorrhage with Myrica.
Pharyngitis use the gargle.

External use
Eczema – ung.

Dosage and mode of application
Decoctum Sig 15ml
Tincturae rhiz Sig 5ml
Ung @ 10% of fol

References
111 p410. 126 p353. 127 p847/848. 176 p344. 278, 59, 1996. 263, 1997, 63, p1771. 389.

Equisetum arvense [Horsetail]

Constituents
Silica around 7.5% and water soluble Silicic acid 14% are vulnerary to connective tissue, nails and teeth.
Saponins.
Flavonoids up to 1%, isoquercetinoside up to 0.12% is diuretic.
Phenolic acids up to 0.7%.
Calcium 1.3%. Manganese. Potassium 1.8%.

Primary pharmacological action: Astringent and tonic diuretic.

Therapeutic classes
Stimulant. Allays inflammation.
Antihaemorrhagic. Atherosclerosis. Stimulates WBC production.
Antilithic. Bladder tonic. Antipyretic.
Dermatological agent. Vulnerary.
Antineoplastic. Immune enhancer.

Medicinal indications [Saturn]
Induces leucocytosis. Antihaemorrhagic.
Epistaxis. Laryngitis. Tuberculosis.
Gastric haemorrhage. Indigestion. Intestinal ulcers. Haemorrhoids. Dysentery.
Obesity.
Acute cystitis. Enuresis. Haematuria. Oedema. Prostatitis. BPH. Incontinence.
Inguinal hernia. Nocturia. Urinary infections. Renal and bladder calculi.
Gonorrhoea with purulent discharge.
Rheumatic conditions. Gout.
Vaginitis. Menorrhagia. Uteritis. Uterine carcinoma.
Brittle nails. Hair loss. Fractures.
Burns. Dermatitis. Dermal ulcers. Frostbite. Wounds.

Tissue conditions
Nasal, pulmonary, gastric and genito urinary haemorrhage. Oedema of the mucous membranes of the genito urinary tract and pelvic tissue. Eliminates the urinary solids. Dissolves renal calculi and removes urates and uric acid. Clears acute inflammatory conditions of the Genito urinary system. Strengthens the hair, nails and teeth due to the silica it contains. Supports the removal of lead from the tissues.

External use
Earache, Epistaxis, Laryngitis - fomentation.
Infected or bleeding wounds, fractures - use a poultice or lotion.
Tumours – poultice.

Preparations
Give an infusion of the fresh leaf and stalk for acute conditions.
Genito urinary haemorrhage/inflammation/infective processes with Agropyron, Barosma, Betula, Calendula, Capsella, Hydrastis, Hydrangea, Rosa canina or Zea. Uterine fibroids with Pulsatilla.
Dosage and mode of application
Dried herba Sig 4g
Tincturae Sig 10ml
Liquidum extractum Sig 4ml
Lotion and poultice – steep 20g herba in 250ml aqua covered for 10 minutes.
Balneum 60g
References
43 p83. 188 p234. 192 p 280/1. 230 p61. 246 p562. 251 p96. 254 p102. 311 Vol 10 No 4. 394 p208.

Erigeron canadense [Fleabane]

Constituents
Flavonoids – apigenin. Volatile oil up to 0.6% containing dipentine, d-limonine, linalool and terpineol. Terpenes –sitosterol, alpha spinosterol. Tannin. Bitters.

Primary pharmacological action: Astringent tonic.

Therapeutic classes
Opthalmia. Allays inflammation. Antibacterial - mycoplasma tuberculosis. Antifungal. Phagocytic. Antihaemorrhagic. Antidiarrhoeal. Diuretic. Antilithic. Antirheumatic. Uterine tonic. Vulnerary.

Medicinal indications [Venus]
Conjunctivitis. Epistaxis. Haemoptysis. Tuberculosis. Chronic bronchitis. Haematemesis. Diarrhoea. Dysentery. Mucus colitis. Prolapsed rectum. Calculi. Cystitis. Haematuria. Albuminuria. Nephritis. Enuresis. Gonorrhoea. Dysmenorrhoea. Menorrhagia. Post partum haemorrhage. Uterine prolapse. Ecchymosis. Cholera. Typhus.

Tissue conditions
Controls haemorrhage of the gastro intestinal and genito urinary tracts by contracting involuntary muscle [astringent]. Indicated for relaxed mucous membranes with free mucus discharge.

External use
Rheumatism - use the liniment.
Repels fleas burn the herb.

Dosage and mode of application
Oleum as a haemostatic is more effectual.
Tincturae herba/sem Sig 10ml
Liquidum extractum herba/sem Sig 4ml

References
111 p411. 126 p360. 176 p351. 189 p117. 228 p122. 269, Autumn 1994.

Eryngium maritimum [Sea holly]

Constituents
Mucilage. Saponins. Acids. Resin. Potassium. Silica.

Primary pharmacological action: Astringent diuretic.

Therapeutic classes
Allays inflammation. Tonic.
Expectorant. Antitubercular.
Aromatic. Sialagogue. Hepatic.
Antilithic. Diaphoretic. Antirheumatic.
Uterine stimulant. Nervine.
Medicinal indications
Pharyngitis. Laryngitis. Bronchitis. Tuberculosis.
Glossitis with gastric irritation. Dyspepsia. Jaundice. Constipation.
Haemorrhoids. Prolapsus ani.
Oedema. Renal colic. Urinary calculi. Haematuria. Cystitis. Urethritis. Nephritis.
Rheumatism. Prostatic enlargement [BPH]. Prostatitis. Incontinence.
Impotence/sexual dysfunction. Gonorrhoea.
Menorrhagia. Partus preparator. Frigidity.
Paralysis.
Tissue conditions
Obstructions of the liver and spleen.
Preparations
Hepatic and uric acid dissolver – with Daucus.
Jaundice with Berberis vulgaris.
Calculi with Hydrangea, Althea, Eupatorium purpureum, Zea.
Cystitis with Gelsemium.
Dosage and mode of application
Dried rad Sig 4g
Tincturae Sig 5ml
Liquidum extractum Sig 4ml
References
43 p84. 246 p280. 252 p207.

Erythrina senegalensis [Coral flower]

Constituents
Thirty Erythrina alkaloids with a curariform activity. The main alkaloid up to
70% is erysodine. Glycosides. Isoflavonoids.

Primary pharmacological action:
Muscular relaxant. Anticonvulsant.

Therapeutic classes
Allays inflammation. Antibacterial.
Digestive relaxant.
Analgesic.
Parturient.
Dermatological agent.
Medicinal indications
Toothache. Ear pain. Pharyngitis. Bronchial disturbances. Coughs.
Abscesses. Wounds. Skin infections. Arthritis.
Infertility. Parturient - to ease pain. Post partum remedy.
Aphrodisiac. Sexually transmitted disease
Pre-med treatment.
Tissue conditions
The alkaloids are active when taken orally. Anticonvulsant activity occurs at the
muscle synapse. CNS is not involved in the activity.
External use
Ear pain – infusium fol. Sig guttae. Instill into ear.
Abscesses, Earache, Wounds – poultice.
Dosage and mode of application
Decoctum bacc Sig 1g

Erythroxylum catuaba [Catuaba]

Constituents
Alkaloids. Essential oils. Sterols. Tannins.

Primary pharmacological action:
Central nervous system stimulant.

Therapeutic classes
Effective against: HIV. Escherichia coli. Staphylococcus aureus.
Anxiolytic. Antidepressant. Nervine tonic. Aphrodisiac.
Medicinal indications
Impotence/sexual dysfunction. Agitation. Depression. Exhaustion. Fatigue.
Neurasthenia. Insomnia. Pain. Poor memory.
Dosage and mode of application
Infusium Sig 30ml
Tincturae Sig 1ml
References
44 p86.

Pharmacopoeia

Erythroxylum coca [Coca leaves]

Constituents
Tropane alkaloids up to 2.5% - Cocaine. Flavonoids. Volatile oil. Vitamin A.

Primary pharmacological action: Cerebral vasostimulant.

Therapeutic classes
Ophthalmic. Stimulant. Antifatigue. Anodyne. Anaesthetic.
Medicinal indications
Ophthalmic anaesthetic. Mydriatic.
Nausea. Vomiting. Neutralises hunger. Pain. Depression. Migraine. Insomnia.
Headache.
Tissue conditions
Central nervous system stimulant. It relieves hunger and fatigue. Anodyne for
intractable pain. Exhaustion with nervous depression, it elevates the mood.
Insomnia caused by gloom or worry. For use as a temporary remedy only.
Cautions
Restrictions apply. Dosage is determined by the relief of symptoms.
Used irrationally it causes dependence. Sensory paralysis. Hallucinations.
Restlessness. Tremors.
External use
Local anaesthetic and vasoconstrictor. May be used to anaesthetise the urethra
before bladder irrigation.
Dosage and mode of application
Liquidum extractum fol. Sig 2ml
References
126 p306. 176 p208. 188 p118. 189 p81.

Eschscholzia californica [Californean poppy]

Constituents
Isoquinoline alkaloids are sedative and hypnotic - Cryptoline, Protoline, Chelidonine. Bitters. Flavone glycosides - Rutoside.

Primary pharmacological action: Antispasmodic nervine.

Therapeutic classes
Analgesic. Anxiolytic. Soporific. Sedative. Hypnotic.
Medicinal indications [Moon]
Irritable bowel syndrome. Enuresis.
Anxiety. Depression. Insomnia. Restlessness. Migraine. Neuralgia. Neuropathy.
Tissue conditions
Has a significant effect upon the CNS neurotransmitters.
Preparations
Insomnia with Passiflora.
Dosage and mode of application
Dried herba Sig 3g
Infusium Sig 3g
Tincturae Sig 4ml
Liquidum extractum Sig 4ml
References
142 p289. 188 p82.

Eucalyptus globulus [Eucalyptus]

Constituents

Essential oil [3.5%] antimicrobial, composed mainly of Eucalyptol [cineol].
Terpenes. Tannins up to 11%. Volatile oils up to 3% of which 95% is cineole.
Bitters. Resin. Flavonoids – hyperoside, rutin.

Primary pharmacological action: Expectorant.

Therapeutic classes

Antibacterial – Enterobacter, Escherichia coli, Haemophillus influenzae,
Kleibsiella, Porphyromonas gingivalis, Proteus mirabilis, Pseudomonas,
Staphylococcus, Streptococcus mutans.
Antifungal – Aspergillus aeguptiacus, Tinea and Trichoderma Viride.
Antiviral.
Aromatic. Antiseptic. Astringent. Stimulant.
Cardiac. Circulatory stimulant.
Decongestant. Pulmonary antiseptic. Anti tubercular.
Nephritic. Diaphoretic. Febrifuge.
Antispasmodic. Rubefacient. Antimalarial. Insect repellent.
Uterine disorders and vaginal tonic.

Medicinal indications

Scarlatina. Sinusitis. [Supperative] otitis media. Asthma. Catarrh. Inflammatory
conditions of the respiratory tract with infection. Tonsillitis. Laryngismus
stridulus. Bronchial conditions with infection and dyspnoea. Bronchitis.
Pneumonia. Haemoptysis. Tuberculosis.
Cystitis. Nephritis. Pyelonephritis. Pyelitis. Amoebic dysentery – enema.
Remittent and eruptive fever - Typhoid. Malaria - Steam therapy.
Cervicitis. Cervical erosion. Vaginal discharge/leucorrhoea.

Tissue conditions

Indicated for relaxed mucous membranes with mucoid or purulent discharge.
Pale coated, dirty tongue with halitosis. Coldness of the extremities with cold
perspiration.

Cautions

Avoid concurrent use with Hydrastis.

External use

Respiratory conditions – inhalation.
Ulcers, abscesses, wounds, gangrene - use the fol and diluted oleum as a
emplastrum or compress.
Vaginal discharge/leucorrhoea, sexually transmitted disease –
douche with Ol Eucalyptus and saline.

Insect repellent - use the oil.

Preparations

An antiseptic and anaesthetic gargle which provides effects catarrh, sinusitis and diphtheria.

Inhalation of the essential oil is beneficial for pulmonary complaints.

Dosage and mode of application

Infusium fol. Sig 2g.

Tincturae Sig 10ml

Liquidum Extractum Sig 4ml

Inhalation Ol 5gtt diluted in water. Place a towel over the basin and inhale.

Ol Eucalyptus BPC 1973 Sig 0.2ml.

References

188 p174. 189 p110. 240. 274, 44, 1994, p35. 274, 1996, 59, 823.
285, 9, 1995 p281-286. 394 p119.

Eucalyptus interferes with mobile telephones.

An article in the Sydney Morning Herald newspaper [Jan/Feb 2003], stated that mobile phone performance is frequently far worse along the Murray River in New South Wales than in similar areas of Europe. Despite the area being relatively flat it is notorious for conversations breaking up or never starting. There are rows of Eucalyptus trees lining the Murray River and it is believed that Eucalyptus leaves are able to absorb mobile phone radio emissions.

Euonymous atropurpureus [Wahoo/Spindle bark].

Constituents
Sterols - Euonysterol, Atropurpurol, homoeuonysterol. Alkaloids - Asparagine.
Cardenolide glycosides – digitaloids. Tannin. Volatile oil.

Primary pharmacological action:
Tonic hepatic and cholagogue.

Therapeutic classes
Vasotonic alterative. Depurative.
Cardioactive – mild. Circulatory stimulant.
Tonic expectorant.
Bitter. Hepatic and biliary ganglionic vasostimulant for the liver with tonic
properties. Antiflatulent. Dyspepsia. Pancreatic tonic. Splenic tonic.
Anthelmintic. Laxative.
Diuretic. Antirheumatic. Antiperiodic.
Dermatological agent. Antiparasitic.

Medicinal indications
Tuberculosis. Chronic bronchitis.
Hepatic enlargement. Jaundice. Dyspepsia. Flatulence. Constipation.
Nutritive tonic in malarial anorexia. Acne. Psoriasis. Head lice.

Tissue conditions
Relaxing and stimulant, slow in action. Yellow tongue, anorexia, dyspepsia and
constipation. Tension of the liver, pancreas or gall bladder. Anorexia, indigestion
and constipation from hepatic congestion. Pyrexia associated with hepatic
disorders.

Cautions
Pregnancy. Lactation.

Preparations
With Hyoscyamnus, Pulsatilla and/or Rhamnus purshiana.

Dosage and mode of application
Dried rad/cort. Sig 1g
Tincturae Sig 2.5ml
Liquidum extractum Sig 1ml

References
43 p86. 111 p416. 126 p364. 176 p329. 188 p449. 192 p559. 224 p1337. 233
p95. 246 p230.

Eupatorium perfoliatum [Boneset]

Constituents
Flavonoids. Terpenoids. Volatile oil. Tannin.

Primary pharmacological action: Relaxing diaphoretic.

Therapeutic classes
Stimulant. Mild tonic. Allays inflammation.
Expectorant.
Laxative. Febrifuge.
Antispasmodic.
Dermatological agent.
Medicinal indications
Scarlatina.
Bronchitis. Catarrh. Colds. Influenza. Night sweats in Tuberculosis. Pneumonia.
Stomachic. Cholagogue. Choleretic. Taenifuge.
Gout. Rheumatism.
Pyrexia. Intermittent fever – malaria. Smallpox. Yellow fever.
Tissue conditions
Warm infusion in intermittent fevers. After four or five doses perspiration
results. Bone pain in pyrexia. Early stages of pneumonia. Excess respiratory
mucus with little power to expel it. Acts slowly and persistently. It relaxes the
mucous membranes of the stomach, liver and gall bladder also the intestines.
Thirst, dry mouth with dry faeces call for Eupatorium. The relaxing properties
are dissipated by the heat and the stimulating, antispasmodic and tonic properties
are left. It is a bitter and relaxant to the liver. Colds, catarrh and pneumonia
where there is biliousness and constipation give an enema, then a hot infusion till
free emesis takes place. The relaxation of mucous membranes will then take
place. Subsequent smaller doses may be continued. The production of a free
outward circulation relieves the hyperaemic condition. With eruptive fevers more
stimulation will be needed. It is valuable in the treatment of rheumatism
especially of the gouty and bilious types. It calms the nervous patient. Large
doses are emetic and purgative.
Preparations
Influenza with Achillea, Sambucus and Zingiber or Capsicum.
Dosage and mode of application
Dried herba Sig 2g
Tincturae Sig 4ml
Liquidum extractum Sig 2ml
References. 43 p86. 111 p420. 126 p364. 176 p269. 254 p86. 262 p77.

Eupatorium purpureum [Gravel root]

Constituents
Benzofuran compound - Euparin. Flavonoid - Eupatorin. Volatile oil. Resin.

Primary pharmacological action
Relaxing and mildly stimulating diuretic.

Therapeutic classes
Antilithic. Diuretic. Antirheumatic.
Emmenagogue. Tonic.
Medicinal indications
Chronic coughs.
Oedema. Strangury, stricture. For brick dust urine. Urinary phosphates. Oxalic
acid. Bloody and painful micturition. Urethritis. Prostatitis. Calculi. Cystitis.
Dysuria. Haematuria. Impotence/sexual dysfunction. Gout. Rheumatism.
Uterine tonic.
Strains or sprains.
Tissue conditions
Influences the kidneys, bladder and uterus. Improves the ability to eliminate more
urinary solids e.g. calculi. For irritable and inflamed conditions of the urinary
tract, a constant desire to urinate with mucus and haematuria. Tones the mucous
membrane and casts off sediments and urinary solids. Tonic to the uterus in
malposition or prolapsus occurring from chronic inflammatory conditions.
Musculoskeletal disorders - backpain, neuralgia, rheumatic pain, muscular strains.
Preparations
Aching back with Mitchella and Hydrastis.
Enhances vasotonic alterative prescriptions.
Dosage and mode of application
Dried rad Sig 4g
Tincturae Sig 2ml
Liquidum Extractum Sig 4ml
References
43 p87. 111 p423. 126 p366. 176 p438. 189 p133. 254 p84.

Euphorbia nerifolia [Milk spurge]

Constituents
Thuhar is a milky fluid which exudes from the sap.

Primary pharmacological action: Purgative.

Therapeutic classes
Diuretic. Antirheumatic.
Dermatological agent.
Medicinal indications
Earache. Asthma. Chronic coughs with phlegm.
Rheumatism.
Oedema. Paralysis.
Syphilis. Leprosy. Warts
External use
Toothache, ringworm, psoriasis, warts – apply fresh milk from stems.
References
191 p71.

Euphorbia capitata/hirta/pilulifera
[Pill-bearing spurge]

Constituents
Interestingly two components have been isolated one is spasmodic - choline and the other antispasmodic - schikimic acid. Flavonoids - Leucyandin, quercetin. Terpenoids - Sitosterol. Resin.

Primary pharmacological action: Bronchodilator.

Therapeutic classes
Ophthalmic. Antibacterial – Gram +ve and Gram -ve bacteria, Mycobacterium tuberculosis. Antifungal – candida.
Expectorant.
Hypoglycaemic. Amoebicidal.
Antispasmodic. Sedative. Galactagogue. Antivenomous.
Medicinal indications
Conjunctivitis
Asthma. Bronchitis. Hay fever. Catarrh. Laryngeal spasm. Emphysema.
Tuberculosis.
Enteritis. Amoebic dysentery - active against Entamoeba histolytica.
Gonorrhoea.
Tissue conditions
Antispasmodic to smooth muscle.
External use
Warts – apply milky juice.
Dosage and mode of application
Herba Sig 300mg
Tincturae Sig 2ml
Liquidum extractum Sig 0.5ml
References
BPC 1949. 43 p88. 53. 126 p368. 176 p287. 192 p 424. 262 p55.

Euphrasia officinalis [Eyebright]

Constituents
Iridoid glycosides - Aucubin. Flavonoids quercetin. Alkaloids. Phenethyl glycosides. Tannins. Volatile oils. Bitters. Sterols. Vitamin C.

Primary pharmacological action: Ophthalmic astringent tonic.

Therapeutic classes
Antihistamine. Allays inflammation. Astringent. Antimicrobial – Bacillus subtilis, Escherichia coli, Micrococcus aureus, Mycobacterium phlei. Antifungal – Penicillium italicum. Hepatoprotective.

Medicinal indications [Sun]
Inflammatory and congestive conditions of the eye. Blepharitis. Conjunctivitis. Arc eyes with watering. Hayfever. Allergies. Coryza. Eye fatigue. Hordeolum. Otitis media. Sinusitis. Upper respiratory catarrh.

Tissue conditions
Tonic to the eye and upper respiratory mucous membranes. Coryza, copious mucus discharges from the eyes, nasal, ear membranes and sinus's.

External use
As a wash or collyr with Chamomilla, Foeniculum, Hamamelis, Hydrastis, Sambucus or Solidago.

Dosage and mode of application
Dried herba Sig 4g
Tincturae Sig 4ml
Liquidum extractum Sig 4ml

References
43 p89. 111 p426. 126 p369. 176 p251. 246 p411. 251 p72.

Ferrula assa-foetida [Asafetida]

Constituents
Resin up to 60% assa - resino - tannols. Gums up to 25%. Volatile oils up to 17% - polysulphides are the main constituents. Coumarins.

Primary action: Antispasmodic.

Therapeutic classes
Antiseptic.
Hypotensive. Anticoagulant.
Expectorant.
Carminative. Vermifuge.
Anodyne. Sedative.
Medicinal indications
Hypertension. Palpitations. Asthma. Coughs. Bronchitis. Pertussus.
Anorexia. Flatulence. IBS. Nematodes.
Anxiety. Chorea. Depression. Dizzyness. Epilepsy. Hypochondria. Infantile convulsions. Neurosis. Neurasthenia. Panic.
Dysmenorrhoea. Galactagogue.
Tissue conditions
A diffusive and relaxant [antispasmodic] medicine. Influences the mucous membranes as an antiseptic. Dry bronchial coughs. Disorders of the stomach [anorexia] with headache. Gastro intestinal spasm.
External use
An injection against ascaris.
Enema in spasmodic conditions – nausea, vomiting, pain, intestinal spasm.
Dosage and mode of application
Powdered resin Sig 1g
Tincturae resin Sig 4ml
Emulsion Asafoetidae 1:25 of aqua dist. Average dose 15ml.
Enema Asafoetida tincturae 6-12% v/v in mucilage of starch. Sig 120ml.
Mistura Asafoetida composita.
Asafoetida 5g. LE Rhamnus purshiana 10ml. Infusion Valeriana to 30g. Sig 10ml.
Tablet Asafoetida. Each tablet to contain 1g. Sig 1-2 PRN
References
126 p286. 142 p250/288. 176 p123. 189 p18. 233 p24.

Filipendula ulmaria [Meadowsweet]

Constituents
Polyphenolic tannins up to 15%. Flavonoids up to 6% – rutin.
Phenolic glycosides – spiraein. The glycosides of salicylates hydrolyse in the
stomach; the A-glycones such as salicylic acid up to 0.2%, become freely
available. The alkaline environment of the intestine allows transformation of the
salicylic acid into its sodium salt - sodium salicylate which is absorbed into the
blood. Coumarin. Mucilage. Vitamin C.

Primary pharmacological action: Antacid.

Therapeutic classes
Astringent. Allays inflammation. Antibacterial – Bacillus subtilis, Escherichia
coli, Klebseillia pneumoniae, Proteus vulgaris, Pseudomonas aeruginosa, Shigella
flaxneri, Staphylococcus aureus, Staphylococcus aureus haemolyticus,
Staphylococcus epidermidis, Streptococcus pyogenes haemolyticus.
Aromatic stomachic and tonic. Anti ulcer.
Antilithic. Diuretic. Urinary antiseptic – mild. Diaphoretic. Antirheumatic.
Analgesic.
Antipyretic. Immunostimulant.
Medicinal indications [Venus]
Halitosis. Gastritis. Hyperchlorhydria. Dyspepsia. Regurgitation. Peptic ulcers.
Colitis. Diarrhoea.
Cystitis. Infections of the genito urinary passages. Prostatic enlargement. Calculi.
Uric acid eliminator. Pyrexia.
Menorrhagia. Vaginal discharge/leucorrhoea. Cervicitis. Vaginitis.
Antirheumatic - arthritis, gout, tendonitis and sciatica.
Tissue conditions
A pleasant and reliable tonic to the digestive system.
Use the root in relaxed [atonic] states of the intestine. Use the root [greater
astringency] in colitis, gastritis, enteritis, diarrhoea and dysentery. Filipendula
immunomodulatory effects are found to inhibit compliment activation and T cell
proliferation. Modulatory activity has been observed upon the cellular immune
system. The warm infusion is diaphoretic. The flowers are more active than the
leaves in rheumatic conditions.
External use
Wounds, insect stings – lotion.
Preparations
Combines with Rubus, Chelone, Berberis vulgaris, Erythraea, Pimpinella in the
above mentioned conditions.

Pharmacopoeia

Acidity and heartburn with Melissa or Althea.
Dosage and mode of application
Infusium herba/flos Sig 5g
Decoctum rad Sig 5g
Tincturae herba Sig 10ml
Liquidum extractum Sig 6ml
References
43 p91. 192 p357. 194p45. 233 p159. 246 p169. 263, 1993, 59 Suppl. pA674.
394 p254.

Foeniculum vulgare [Fennel]

Constituents
Volatile oil around 6% containing anethole [a phenol], limonene, pinene.
Flavonoids. Coumarins. Sterols. Fixed oil up to 20%.

Primary pharmacological action: Carminative.

Therapeutic classes
Ophthalmic. Aromatic. Allays inflammation. Vasotonic alterative.
Antibacterial – Aerobacter aerogenes, Bacillus subtilis, Escherichia coli, Listeria,
Mycobacterium avium, Proteus vulgaris, Pseudomonas aeruginosa, Salmonella
enteriditis, Staphylococcus albus and aureus, Streptococcus pyogenes.
Anticoagulant. Expectorant. Bronchodilator.
Aperitif. Carminative. Antiflatulent. Diuretic.
Orexigenic. Galactagogue. Oestrogenic. Aphrodisiac. Uterine stimulant.
Antispasmodic. Antipyretic. Antirheumatic. Antivenomous. Alcohol habit.
Medicinal indications [Mercury]
Conjunctivitis. Blepharitis. Pharyngitis. Chronic coughs.
Anorexia. Flatulent dyspepsia. Hiccups. Nausea. Jaundice. IBS. Colic.
Constipation. Colitis. Obesity.
Bladder pain. Pyrexia. Rheumatism. Suppressed or insufficient lactation.
Tissue conditions
More stimulating than Pimpinella. More relaxing than Anethum or Cummin.
Antispasmodic to smooth muscle of the gastrointestinal tract and sphincters. As a
general tonic for the brain - improves memory. Vasotonic alterative and antitoxic
to bites of dogs, scorpions, snakes.
Reduces the toxic effects of alcohol.
Preparations
Collyr with Euphrasia.
Oral and throat inflammation with Salvia.
Add to prevent griping of laxatives and allay flatulence.
Flatulent colic with Acorus or Alpinia.
Dosage and mode of application
Infusium crushed dried fruct Sig 3g
Tincturae Sig 15ml
Liquidum extractum Sig 3ml
Conc. Aqua Foenic. Concentrated Fennel water Sig 1ml
References
43 p93. 111 p428. 188 p181. 192 p206. 228 p345. 246 p291. 251 p75. 272, 7
[4] p26-33. 394 p126.

Fraxinus excelsior [Ash]

Constituents
Coumarins. Flavone glycosides - rutin, quercetin. Volatile oil. Resin. Tannin.

Primary pharmacological action: Voluntary muscle stimulant.

Therapeutic classes
Allays inflammation. Astringent. Tonic.
Circulatory stimulant.
Hepatic. Cholagogue. Splenic. Laxative.
Diuretic. Diaphoretic. Febrifuge. Antirheumatic.
Uterine tonic.
Antivenomous. Antiperiodic.
Medicinal indications [Sun]
Halitosis – chew fol. Oedema from hepatic disease.
Pyelonephritis. Gout. Rheumatism. Arthritis.
Uterine/prostate hypertrophy. Uterine tumours. Endometritis with oedema.
Enlarged cervix. Subinvolution following childbirth. Uterine prolapse.
Intermittent fevers.
Snake bite and snake repellent.
Tissue conditions
A slow and persistent remedy. Uric acid eliminator. Tones the uterus and
ligaments.
Preparations
Alchemilla vulg. Aletris, Cimicifuga, Harpagophytum, Mitchella, Viburnum
species.
Dosage and mode of application
Liquidum extractum fruct/fol/bacc. Sig 2ml
References
1 p130.189 p19. 246 p322.

Fucus vesiculosis [Kelp] also known as Laminaria

digitata/japonica/saccharina thallus is also from Macrocystis pyrifera].

Constituents
Iodine. Polysaccharides - anti HIV. Polyphenols – anti HIV. Tannin. Sterols. Vitamins and minerals.

Primary pharmacological action:
Lymphatic Vasotonic alterative. Thyroactive.

Therapeutic classes
Demulcent. Deobstruent.
Antifungal – Candida. Antibacterial – Escherichia coli and Neisseria meningitidis.
Antiviral – HIV.
Antihypertensive. Anticoagulant.
Diuretic. Renal disease. Antirheumatic.
Emmenagogue. Antiobesity.
Antineoplastic.

Medicinal indications
Blood thinner. Fatty degeneration of the heart. Hypothyroidism. Goitre. Obesity.
Cystitis. Rheumatism. Breast carcinoma.

Tissue conditions
When T4 levels are raised the thyroid is unlikely be controlled with Fucus.
Stimulating to the thyroid [underactivity], lymphatics, mucus and serous
membranes. Intestinal deobstruent. It influences basal metabolic rate and is tonic.
Plethoric, torpid obesity with cold clammy skin.
Compounds within Fucus can help the body in eliminating - strontium 90.
Individuals needing seaweed often prefer the dark, and feel better at night. For
children who move regularly and are unable to form bonding relationships.
Contains an abundance of vitamins, minerals and trace elements. It makes a useful
organic plant fertiliser if applied to the leaves. Contains calcium which can be
used for patients who complain of dreams where there is a strong anxiety element
from potential threats or intrusive people.
Laminaria tents [cervical in situ] have been used to dilate the cervix during
delivery [192 p311].

External use
Uterine atony producing menstrual irregularity. Rheumatic and arthritic pain -
liniment clears pain from the muscles and joints.

Preparations
Arctium, Galium, Glechoma, Medicago.

Dosage and mode of application
Both species of Fucus and Laminaria are interchangeable in treatment.
Start with small dosage and gradually increase. Check a thyroid function test.
Dried thallus Sig 10g
Tincturae Sig 10 ml
Liquidum extractum Sig 8ml
References
BPC 1949. 43 p94. 192 p311/324. 194. 246 p571. 251 p21. 278, 1993, 56,
no4 p478.

Fumaria officinalis [Fumitory]

Constituents
Alkaloids. Flavonoids. Bitters. Resin. Mucilage. Acids.

Primary pharmacological action: Dermatological agent.

Therapeutic classes
Ophthalmic. Antibacterial - Bacillus anthracis, Pseudomonas and Staphylococcus.
Stomachic. Hepatic. Cholagogue. Cholelithiasis. Laxative.
Diuretic.
Antispasmodic.
Dermatological agent.
Medicinal indications [Saturn]
Conjunctivitis. Deficient coronary circulation.
Vomiting. Hepatitis. Cirrhosis. Biliary colic. Jaundice. Constipation.
Oedema. Gout.
Eczema. Psoriasis.
Tissue conditions
Antispasmodic to smooth muscle in colic. Hepatic disorders with yawning and
excess tiredness. Specific in skin disorders with biliary involvement.
External use
Conjunctivitis - collyr.
Preparations
Skin diseases with Rumex or Arctium.
Dosage and mode of application
Dried herba Sig 4g
Tincturae Sig 4ml
Liquidum extractum Sig 4ml.
References. 43. 192 p217.

Galega officinalis [Goats rue]

Constituents
Alkaloid - Galegine. Flavonoids. Saponins.

Primary pharmacological action: Antidiabetic.

Therapeutic classes
Hypoglycaemic. Vermifuge.
Diuretic. Diaphoretic.
Galactagogue. Antipyrexial. Antivenomous.
Medicinal indications [Mercury]
Diabetes. Increases breast size. Stimulates milk production by 15% Tired, achy feet. Plague. Snakebite.
Combinations
Breast size with Foeniculum and Vitex.
External use
Achy feet – footbath.
Dosage and mode of application
Dried fol. Sig 2g
Tincturae Sig 5ml
Liquidum extractum Sig 2ml
References
43 p96. 127 p697. 188 p203. 189 p131. 192 p240.

Galeopsis ochroleuca [White hemp nettle]

Constituents
Silica around 0.8%, induces leucocytosis. Saponins. Tannin.

Primary pharmacological action: Pulmonary tonic.

Medicinal indications
Expectorant in pulmonary disease. Asthma.
Enuresis. Stress incontinence
Dosage and mode of application
Liquidum extractum Sig 4ml
References
246 p369.

Galium aparine [Clivers]

Constituents
Coumarins. Iridoid glycosides asperuloside is laxative. Phenols. Flavonoids.
Tannins. Sterols. Anthraquinones in the root. Silica.

Primary pharmacological action:
Relaxing, diffusive and soothing diuretic.

Therapeutic classes
Demulcent. Refrigerant. Aperient. Cholagogue. Choleretic.
Antilithic. Antirheumatic.
Lymphatic vasotonic alterative. Antineoplastic. Soporific.
Remittent fever - typhoid, malaria.
Medicinal indications [Moon]
Sore tongue. Infectious mononucleosis.
Obesity. Jaundice. Typhoid fever. Malaria.
Diuretic enabling best effects in acute complaints: dysuria, stricture, strangury and
inflammatory conditions. Cystitis and urinary gravel. Rheumatism. Arthritis.
Gonorrhoea. Benign prostatic hyperplasia. Ovarian cysts.
Lymphadenopathy. Tubercular lymphadenopathy.
Dandruff. Psoriasis. Lichen. Eczema. Erysipilas. Allergic rashes. Freckles.
Urticaria. Taken internally as a hair tonic. Insomnia.
Smallpox. Melanoma. Breast tumours use the juice internally and externally.
Tissue conditions
Influences the urinary tract. Galium is a powerful cleanser of the tissues. It aids
the elimination of solids in the urine. An infusion will help with weight loss.
Fresh plant preparations are best for effect.
External applications
Deodorant activity for axilla use.
Breast tumours, cysts, abscesses - mix Galium with Linseed and poultice breast.
Antihaemorrhagic in burns, wounds – lotion fresh succus.
Acne, Freckles, psoriasis - cold water infusion.
Preparations
Genito urinary cleanser – Barosma, Galium and Uva ursi.
Dosage and mode of application
Dried herba Sig 4g
Tincturae Sig 10ml
Liquidum extractum herba Sig 4ml
Succus Sig 10ml
References. 43 p97. 111 p439. 126 p382. 189 p79. 194. 246 p338. 251 p51.

Galium odoratum [Sweet woodruff]

Constituents
Coumarin. Iridoid alkaloids - asperuloside [allays inflammation, purgative].
Anthraquinones. Flavonoids. Tannin.

Primary pharmacological action: Tonic.

Therapeutic classes
Allays inflammation. Antibacterial. Anticoagulant. Venous stasis.
Aromatic. Digestive tonic. Stomachic. Hepatic. Cholagogue.
Diuretic. Antilithic. Antipyretic.
Galactogogue.
Antispasmodic. Sedative. Antidepressant. Vulnerary.

Medicinal indications [Mars]
Phlebitis. Thrombophlebitis. Varicose veins.
Heartburn. Jaundice. Hepatic pain. Biliary obstruction. Dysentery. Constipation.
Renal colic. Dysmenorrhoea. Menopause. Pruritus vulvae.
Frigidity. Panic. Insomnia. Migraine. Neuralgia. Paralysis. Restlessness.
Cuts. Tinea. Wounds.

External use
Hepatic and biliary disorders – poultice.
Aromatic activity - the flos are sweet smelling.
Paralysis - rub with dect. or oleum.
Wounds - apply fresh fol.
Pruritus vulvae – douche.

Dosage and mode of application
Galium verum has a very similar activity.
Dried herba Sig 5g
Infusium herba. Sig 30ml

References
142 p191. 149 p124. 188 p456. 228 p257. 246 p335. 272, 1996, 8, [4].

Ganoderma lucidem [Reishi mushroom]

Constituents
Polysaccharides – Lentenin, Triterpenes [antineoplastic].
Germanium – antineoplastic.

Primary pharmacological action: Anti infective.

Therapeutic classes
Allays inflammation. Astringent. Detoxifier. Tonic. Vasotonic alterative.
Antibacterial - Baccilus pneumoniae, Streptococci, Staphylococci.
Antiviral – candida, HIV.
Antioxidant. Hypotensive. Anticholesterolaemic. Cardiotonic. Increases WBC's
and haemoglobin. Leucopenia.
Antihistamine. Antiallergic. Antitussive. Expectorant. Nourishing.
Analgesic. Antidepressant.
Antineoplastic. Immunostimulant.
Medicinal indications
Hypertension. Hypercholesterolaemia.
Allergic asthma. Bronchitis.
Depression. Dizzyness. Insomnia. Weakness. Improves longevity. Myalgic
encephalomyelitis.
Hepatoma. Sarcoma. Anti radiation and chemotherapy agent.
Tissue conditions
Lowers serum cholesterol, thrombocytes and platelet aggregation, it enhances
myocardial activity. Antioxidant action is produced by eliminating hydroxyl free
radicles. Inhibits histamine release. Stimulates and enhances bone marrow
nucleated cell proliferation. Asthenics with weakness. The central depressant and
peripheral anticholinergic action relaxes muscles. Immune activity enhances
natural killer cell activity. Stabilises immunoglobulin levels and inhibits mediator
release. Anti HIV activity in vitro and in vivo [Kim et al]. Increases production of
Interleukin 1 and 2.
Dosage and mode of application
Dried mushroom Sig 10g
Powder Sig 0.5g
References
188 p368. 261 [includes citation on Kim et al 1994]. Health: State of the art,
January 1995. Asian Food Journal 1994, 9 [2] p69-72

Garcinia cambogia [Malabar tamarind]

Constituents
200 species of Garcinia are noted. The fruit rind contains [-] hydroxycitric acid [HCA], which inhibits the enzyme [ATP citratelyase] responsible for converting Carbohydrates into fat. Tamarind can help weight loss. Bioflavonoids. Resin. Gum. Tamarindus indicus – Tamarind is used in Senna confection. It is moist and stringy and very sweet.

Primary therapeutic class: Antihepatotoxic activity.

Therapeutic classes
Anticatarrhal. Antimicrobial. Antiviral.
Purgative. Taenifuge.
Antirheumatic.
Antineoplastic.
Antimalarial. Aphrodisiac.

Medicinal indications
Seeds for - headaches, bronchitis, coughs and pharyngitis. Also colic.
The fruit rind is used as a fat burning agent. The resin is purgative.
Powdered bacc is used for malignant tumours.
Sap - parasitic skin disease.
Latex gum - gonorrhoea internally.

Cautions
Inflammatory conditions of the Gastro intestinal tract. Haemorrhoids. Pregnancy.
Always combine with carminatives to lessen its strength. It is a potent hydragogue cathartic.

External use
Latex gum - wounds

Dosage and mode of application
Dried rind Sig 5g

References
189 p264. 393.

Gaultheria procumbens [Wintergreen]

Constituents
Phenols - gaultherin. Essential oil up to 1%, of which 98% is methyl salicylate. Arbutin – urinary disinfectant. Enzyme action releases bound gaultherin into methyl salicylate during maceration.

Primary pharmacological action: Antirheumatic.

Therapeutic classes
Stimulant. Tonic. Astringent. Allays inflammation.
Aromatic. Carminative. Antiflatulent.
Diuretic. Anaphrodisiac.
Emmenagogue. Galactagogue. Analgesic. Cephalgic. Antipyretic.

Medicinal indications [Saturn]
Chronic mucus discharges. Colds. Asthma. Bronchitis. Diphtheria. Persistent coughs.
Cholagogue. Colic. Diarrhoea. Haemorrhoids.
Dysuria. Haematuria. Urethritis. Cystitis. Prostatitis. Nephritis. Undue sexual excitement [male and female]. Spermatorrhoea. Amenorrhoea. Headache.
Articular inflammation. Rheumatoid arthritis. Intercostal neuralgia. Myalgia. Sciatica.

Tissue conditions
Stimulating and diffusive. Stimulates the portal circulation. An infusion allays inflammation and irritation of the bladder, prostate and urethra.. Oil is antiseptic. Chewing the fresh fol relieves tender gums.

Cautions
Pregnancy. Gastro intestinal irritability e.g. ulcers. Laxity of the tissues.

Preparations
Rheumatic conditions – Filipendula, Dioscorea, Menyanthes, Apium.
Diphtheria - use the spray.

External use
Rheumatic muscle pain and inflammation, lumbago, neuralgia, sciatica – liniment, poultice or dect.

Dosage and mode of application
Dried fol Sig 1g
Tincturae Sig 2ml
Liquidum extractum Sig 1ml

References
43 p97. 111 p440. 126 p383. 176 p401. 188 p455. 192 p575. 224 p1262. 311 Vol 10 No 4

Geijera parvifolia [Wilga]

Constituents
Coumarin, essential oil, tannin.

Primary pharmacological action: Nervine relaxant.

Therapeutic classes
Hypnotic. Tonic.
Medicinal indications
Restlessness. Sleep disturbances. Tension.
Dosage and mode of application
Tincturae 3ml

Gelsemium sempervirens [Yellow jasmine root]

Constituents
Indole alkaloids - Gelsemine, Gelseminine and Gelsemoidin.

Primary pharmacological action:
Sedative, antispasmodic - allays ANS & CNS irritability.

Therapeutic classes
Ophthalmic. Allays inflammation.
Cardiac sedative. Hypotensive. Vasodilator. Febrifuge.
Parturient.
Analgesic. Antispasmodic. Anaesthetic. Cephalgic.

Medicinal indications
Acute inflammatory conditions. Conjunctivitis. Iritis.
Pertussus. Laryngismus stridulus. Influenza.
Extrasystoles. Palpitations. Tachycardia. Hypertension. Cramp. Intermittent
claudication. Rheumatic fever.
Temporal arteritis. Pneumonia. Pleurisy.
Motion sickness. Vomiting of pregnancy. Appendicitis. Sphincter relaxant. Gastro
enteritis. Diarrhoea. Dysentery.
Acute nephritis. Spasmodic urethral stricture. Cystic tenesmus. Spermatorrhoea.
Acute rheumatism.
Acute malaria. Remittent fever - typhoid, malaria.
Facial neuralgia. Trigeminal neuralgia. Intercostal neuralgia. Sciatica. Chorea.
Acute cerebral hyperaemia - Meningitis. Cramp. Migraine. Panic. Epilepsy from
acute cerebral hyperaemia. Insomnia. Tetanus. Nervous irritability and sensitivity
in peritonitis, salpingitis, metritis, purpural fever. Coccydynia.
Premature labour pain. Dilates a rigid Os uteri. Dysmenorrhoea. Salpingitis.
Ovaritis.

Tissue conditions
Restlessness. Contracted pupils. Sthenic fevers of childhood [robust fevers]. CNS
depressant and sedative acting upon the central and motor nerves - it reduces the
cerebral blood flow. Cardiac and vascular sedative. As a sedative it will control
fever and act as a sedative. Quiets nervous irritability, equalises the circulation, is
diaphoretic and rebalances the secretions. Antispasmodic in nerve and gastro
intestinal conditions. Relaxes the splanchnic nerves. Sphincter relaxant.
Anaesthetic to sensory nerves.
During confinement it relaxes the pelvic nerves [anodyne] and allays nervous
excitement. Indicated for sharp, cutting pain. Rectifies ineffectual contractions
and allays pain.

Cautions
Restrictions apply. Dosage is determined by the relief of symptoms.
Asthenia give with care. Hypotension. Typhoid fever use carefully.
Overdosage from restriction of cerebral blood and paralysis of the motor nerves
includes diplopia, dizzyness, ptosis, dyspnoea.
Antidote - stop the remedy and give an emetic. Capsicum. Tannin.

Preparations
To increase its potency with Lobelia.
Arrhythmia with Crataegus.
Migraine with Piscidia.
Neuralgia with Passiflora.
Meningitis with Echinacea.
Antispasmodic with Lobelia.
Acute gonorrhoea as a bladder irrigation to allay pain.
Parturition/post partum pain and restlessness use with Pulsatilla.

Dosage and mode of application
Dried rad and rhizome Sig 60mg
Tincturae 1:10 Sig 1ml. 1ml contains 0.03 – 0.034 alkaloids.

Compound Gelsemium & Hyoscyamnus
Gelsemium 0.3ml Hyoscyamnus 1ml Preservative to 10ml. Prepare fresh.
Sig 1ml.

References
43 p98. 126 p385. 176 p72. 189 p125. 244 p1763. 225 p19.

Gentiana lutea [Gentian]

Constituents
Bitter glycoside – gentiopicroside up to 4%. Phytosterols. Tannin. Triterpenes.
Volatile oil.

Primary pharmacological action: Gastro Intestinal tonic.

Therapeutic classes
Antiseptic. Vasotonic alterative. Antibacterial – Salmonella, Shigella.
Sialagogue. Strong bitter tonic. Gastric stimulant. Antibilious. Cholagogue.
Anthelmintic. Febrifuge.
Emmenagogue. Antivenomous.
Medicinal indications [Mars]
Anorexia. Stomach atony/Atonic dyspepsia. Heartburn. Nausea. Vomiting.
Motion sickness. Flatulence. Flatus. Splenic affections. Intestinal atony.
Diarrhoea. Food poisoning. Jaundice. IBS. Nematodes.
Gout. Bites from scorpions, rabid dogs.
Amenorrhoea. Panic attacks. ME. Malaria.
Tissue conditions
Gentian is given to promote the appetite and hydrochloric acid. It is tonic to the
gastro intestinal tract. Tones the mucous membranes and is tonic to the portal
system. It may be given in states of nervous exhaustion and debility.
Cautions
Large doses irritate the stomach. Gastric irritability or inflammation. Ulcers.
Pregnancy. Polycythaemia.
External use
Ulcerations.
Preparations
With Agrimonia, Centaurium, Zingiber or other suitable tonics for the GIT.
Anorexia with Valeriana.
Exhaustion, irritability, panic with – Ferrula, Humulus, Scutellaria and Valeriana.
Dosage and mode of application
Combine with an aromatic or demulcent to make it more palatable.
Dried rad/rhiz Sig 2g
Tincturae Sig 10ml. Liquidum extractum Sig 4ml
Concentrated Compound Gentiana Infusium Concentrated Compound
Infusion Gentian. Px Gentiana, Auranti, Citrus aa [Tr 1:5] Sig 2ml [NBP].
Compound Gentiana Tincturae Compound Gentian tincture. Gentian 10g
Auranti 4g Elettaria sem 1.5g Alcohol 45% to 100ml Sig 5ml.
References 43. 111 p441. 126 p390. 176 p267. 188 p 197. 192 p225. 225. 251p84

Geranium maculatum [Cranesbill]

Constituents
Tannin. Gum. Pectin.

Primary pharmacological action: Astringent tonic.

Therapeutic classes
Vasotonic alterative. Allays inflammation. Styptic. Haemostatic.
Renal astringent. Uterine tonic.
Vulnerary.
Antineoplastic.
Medicinal indications [Mars]
Haemorrhage.
Oral and throat infections/inflammation. Tooth extraction - socket haemorrhage
and to aid healing.
Epistaxis. Haemoptysis. Tuberculosis.
Haematemesis. Gastritis. Peptic ulceration. Diarrhoea. Dysentery. Colitis.
Intestinal ulceration. Haemorrhoids. Cholera.
Bladder inflammation. Renal haemorrhage.
Haematuria.
Vaginal discharge/leucorrhoea. Menorrhagia. Metrorrhagia. Post partum
haemorrhage.
Burns. Plague.
Tissue conditions
Haemostatic in venous haemorrhage. Indicated for relaxed conditions of the
gastro intestinal tract. Excessive mucus discharge - tonic influence.
External use
Tooth extraction, socket haemorrhage - sprinkle with dried powdered rad.
Ulcers. Wounds. Haemorrhoids.
Preparations
Peptic ulceration with Symphytum, Althea, Agrimonia.
Dysentery with Hydrastis.
Dosage and mode of application
Dried rhiz Sig 2g
Tincturae Sig 4ml
Liquidum extractum Sig 4ml
References
43 p101. 111 p446. 126 p391. 176 p347. 189 p95. 192 p27. 254 p70.

Geum urbanum [Avens]

Constituents
Phenolic glycosides. Tannin. Essential oil.

Primary pharmacological action: Astringent tonic.

Therapeutic classes
Antiseptic. Allays inflammation. Tonic. Antihaemorrhagic.
Stomachic. Antidiarrhoeal. Hepatic. Splenic.
Styptic. Febrifuge. Vulnerary.
Medicinal indications [Jupiter]
Pharyngitis. Laryngitis. Haemoptysis. Tuberculosis.
Aphthous ulcerations. Gingivitis. Halitosis. Peptic ulcer. Dyspepsia. Colitis.
Gastro enteritis. Dysentery. Diarrhoea. Ulcerative colitis. Haemorrhoids.
Cystitis. Gonorrhoea.
Vaginal discharge/leucorrhoea. Menorrhagia.
Intermittent fever. Plague.
Insect bites.
Tissue conditions
Mild astringent, soothing and warming tonic to the stomach and intestinal
glands. Pain of a tearing or spasmodic nature aggravated by food or exercise.
Abdominal viscera congestion. Removes obstructions of the liver and spleen.
Soothing to mucous membranes. Strengthens the joints. Dissolves ecchymosis
from injury.
Preparations
Gargle in sore throat, inflamed gums.
Spots and freckles - bathe the skin.
Dosage and mode of application
Infusium herba Sig 4g
Liquidum extractum Sig 4ml
References
43 p102. 111 p448. 127 p73. 160 p21. 192 p34. 246 p178. 251 p10.

Ginkgo biloba [Maidenhair tree]

Constituents
Terpenoids [lactones] of the diterpine type - Ginkgolides A, B, C, J.
Bioflavonoids [antioxidants] protect against hypoxia. Ginkgobalide [B] inhibit
platelets [anti allergic] and thrombus formation. Antagonises broncho -
constriction. Inhibits lipid peroxidation. Sterols.

Primary pharmacological action:
Cerebral tonic and stimulant to the cerebral circulation.
Vasoprotective.

Therapeutic classes
Ophthalmic. Antiallergic. Allays inflammation. Antioxidant.
Circulatory stimulant. Vasodilator. Antisclerotic. Anti platelet aggravating factor.
Anticholesterolaemic. Antithrombotic. Anti-ischaemic.
Antiasmatic. Anti-oedematous.
Anti depressant.
Immunostimulant. Antineoplastic.
Dermatological agent.

Medicinal indications
Glaucoma and Macular degeneration are ischaemic eye diseases. Retinopathy.
Cochlear deafness.
Cerebral atherosclerosis. Cerebro vascular insufficiency. CVA due to embolus or
ischaemia. Coronary sclerosis. Angina. Arrhythmia. Arterial insufficiency.
Hypertension. Raynauds disease. Vascular spasm. Vascular fragility. Intermittent
claudication. Thrombosis. DVT. Temporal arteritis. Cramp. Acrocyanosis – cold
hands and/or feet.
Asthma - inhalation of fol. Antitussive and expectorant - seeds. Tuberculosis.
Oedema. Impotence/sexual dysfunction [erectile dysfunction]. PMS.
Tinnitus. Headaches. Vertigo. Neuralgia. Dementia. Infarct dementia. Depression.
Cognitive performance [memory or concentration loss] and social functioning,
psychosis and brain injury have responded using ginkgo. Alzheimers disease.
Parkinsons disease. Anxiety.
Sarcoma. Dermal ulcers.

Tissue conditions
Vasoprotective having an amphoteric action relaxing vasospasm of the arteries or
toning [vasocontracting] in arterial relaxation. Toning blood vessels protects
against capillary permeability. The flavonoids enhance catecholamines and
inhibit monoamine oxidase.

Pharmacopoeia

Improves ocular blood flow by increasing end diastolic velocity in the ophthalmic artery. Stabilises cellular membranes. Improves myocardial contraction and coronary flow. Protects against hypoxia and free radicles. The fact that flavonoids are poorly absorbed is of little significance says Morfort in Planta Medica. Improves cerebral perfusion to the hippocampus and corpus striatum - these areas are concerned with neurotransmitters and are deficient in CVA, aging, alzheimers, parkinsons etc. Prevents CVA. Improves acetylcholine receptors and cholinergic transmission of nerve impulses.

Ginkgo increases the amount of neural transmission and increases the number of receptor sites for nerve transmission, this improves brain function. For cerebrovascular deficiency. Cerebral disorders due to ageing - memory impairment, senility, senile dementia, alzheimers disease. Ginkgo is an antioxidant. It improves local circulation to reduce inflammation caused by platelet activating factors. Indicated in peripheral arterial insufficiency and chilblains. Aids recovery from CVA.

Studies reveal action against sarcoma.

Cautions

CVA due to haemorrhage.

External use

Phospholipids found in Ginkgo are lipophilic and are absorbed through the skin. These improve capillary cell function and are vasodilatory.

Dosage and mode of application

Dried fol/sem. Sig 3g

Dry extract Sig 50mg

Tincturae Sig 10ml

Liquidum extractum Sig 4ml

References

192 p231. 230 p45. 239 p116. 246 p570. Lancet 1992, 340, 1136. 263, 62, 1996, p289. 270 1997, 4, 1, p3-13. 270, 1996, 3 p265. 295, 2001, 322 [7278] 73-75. 298, 2000, Vol. 5, No. 3. 301, 1998, Vol. 3 [1]. 308, 1997, 278 [16] p1327-32. 310, 1995/6, Vol. 4, No. 1, 3-20. 389. 394 p160.

Glycyrrhiza glabra [Liquorice]

Constituents

Triterpenoid saponins up to 24% - Glycyrrhizin [antineoplastic and allays inflammation] and glycyrrhetinic acid have been shown to inhibit the enzyme 11b-hydroxysteroid dehydrogenase [HSD], it is found in the liver and kidneys. HSD is responsible for the conversion of the active adrenal hormones cortisol and corticosterone to inactive forms like cortisone and 1-dehydrocorticosterone. This suggests that taking Glycyrrhiza could result in greater levels of cortisol and corticosterone with improvement in trophic response to the adrenal tissue. Flavonoids up to 1%, known as flavonols and isoflavones. Coumarins. Amino acids. Sterols. Volatile oil. The sweet taste is due to a terpene - glycyrrhizin [6-8%]. Starch up to 30%. Volatile oil.

Primary pharmacological action:
Normaliser of the hypothalamic-pituitary-adrenocortical system Demulcent.

Therapeutic classes

Vasotonic alterative – detoxifier. Soothing and allays inflammation.
Antibacterial - Mycobacterium smegmatis, Mycobacterium tuberculosis, Staphylococcus aureus, Streptococcus mutans.
Antifungal - Candida albicans.
Antiviral - Hepatitis A, Herpes sp., Aids/HIV.
Antioxidant. Expectorant – relaxing. Antitussive.
Anti ulcer. Choleretic. Hepatoprotective. Laxative.
Adaptogen. Antidepressant. Anxiolytic. Antispasmodic. Anodyne.
Adrenal tonic trophorestorative. Adrenocortical insufficiency.
Ovarian activity. Infertility.
Antineoplastic. Immunostimulant. Antipyretic. Emollient.

Medicinal indications [Mercury]

Coughs. Cold sores. Asthma. Bronchitis. Infective conditions. Diphtheria.
Pulmonary tuberculosis. Pneumonia. Pleurisy.
Gastritis. Peptic ulcers. Colitis. Constipation. Colic. Viral hepatitis.
Irritation of the urinary organs. Rheumatism. Arthritis.
Adrenocortico insufficiency. Addisons disease. Polycystic ovarian syndrome.
Autoimmune conditions. Allergies. Eczema. Tetanus.

Tissue conditions

Maximum levels of serum activity within 4 hours. Soothing demulcent for irritated and inflamed tissue e.g. bronchitis. Gastritis, ulcers, colitis, constipation are relieved from discomfort and pain. Smooth muscle relaxant. Supportive of adrenal activity with mild cortisone [aldosterone] effects. Given to babies it helps cut teeth. Safe with diabetics as a form of sweetening. Rebalances testosterone. Anovulatory women with raised testerone levels fond that they were reduced by using Glycyrrhiza. Adaptogenic as it inhibits oestrogen when oestrogen levels are high and vice versa.

HIV cases show improvement in their liver and immunological function.

External use

Inflamed skin lesions.

Cautions

Hypertension. Hypokalaemia is unusual, Martindale's quotes a woman as suffering from hypokalaemia after ingesting *40 grams* of liquorice daily for 9 months. When remedy is discontinued symptoms clear. Acute renal disorders. Excessive ingestion of Glycyrrhiza can inhibit 11 beta-hydroxysteroid dehydrogenase which may result in sodium retention using over 20g daily.

Preparations

As a vehicle to disguise bitters.

Coughs with Prunus serotina.

Raised testosterone levels with Paeonia.

Dosage and mode of application

Dried rad/rhiz. Sig 4g

Dry extract Sig 600mg

Tincturae Sig 5ml

Liquidum extractum Sig 5ml

References

43 p233. 176 p261. 179 p472. 189. 192. 203. 224. 230 p71. 233. 239 p170. 246 p199. 263 1991 57 [1] p119. 311, Vol. 11, No. 3, 13-14. 394 p233.

Glycyrrhiza uralensis [Chinese liquorice]

Constituents
Glycyrrhetic acid inhibits tumours. Glycyrrhizin. Glucose. Starch.

Primary pharmacological action: Similar to Glabra.

Therapeutic classes
Detoxifier. Anti allergic.
Pectoral.
Cholagogue. Anti ulcer & reduces hydrochloric acid. Intestinal antispasmodic.
Antineoplastic.
Medicinal indications
Anti cholesterolaemic. Coughs. Bronchitis. Sore throats.
Anti diabetic. Jaundice. Inhibits hepatic fibrosis. Hepatitis B infection.
Counters poisons and toxins found in foods/plants/diphtheria and tetanus.
Tissue conditions
Supports the adrenal glands. It is nutritive and balances blood sugar levels. As a
demulcent similar to the above genus Glabra. Soothes mucous membranes.
Cautions
Contra indicated in hypertension
Dosage and mode of application
Dried rad Sig 2g
Tincturae Sig 3ml.
References
47 p327.

Gnaphalum ulignosum [Cudweed]

Constituents
Volatile oil. Tannin is antiseptic.

Primary pharmacological action: Antiseptic.

Therapeutic classes
Astringent. Demulcent. Allays inflammation.
Anticatarrhal. Antitussive.
Diaphoretic - mild.

Medicinal indications
Glossitis. Pharyngitis. Tonsillitis. Nasal catarrh. Relaxed sore throat.
Infectious mononucleosis. Laryngismus stridulus. Laryngitis. Pertussus.

Tissue conditions
The astringency reduces chronic inflammatory action.

Preparations
Pertussus with Mentha piperita.
Pharyngeal conditions – Baptisia, Capsicum, Commiphora, Echinacea.

Dosage and mode of application
Infusium herba Sig 4g
Tincturae Sig 4ml
Liquidum extractum Sig 4ml

References
43 p 221. 111 p455. 189 p98. 246 p452.

Gossypium hirsutum [Cotton]

Constituents
Fixed oil in the seed contains polyphenol bisquiterpine as gossypol up to 2%.
Catechol. Flavonoids.

Primary pharmacological action: Prostatic and uterine tonic.

Therapeutic classes
Antiviral. Antibacterial.
Prostatic. Contraceptive – male.
Emmenagogue – bacc. Oxytocic. Galactagogue – sem. Vaginal contraceptive.
Medicinal indications
Hypoglycaemic.
Lowers sperm count and degeneration of the germ cells in the seminiferous
tubules. Amenorrhoea. Dysmenorrhoea. Endometriosis. Fibroids. Metrorrhagia –
fibroids. Partus preparator.
Tissue conditions
Oral contraceptive in men, it may cause permanent sterility. Taken for up to 90
days checking the sperm count, then maintenance doses once a week. Increases
contractions during labour.
Cautions
Heart disturbances. Renal damage with high dosage. Hypokalaemia.
Preparations
Amenorrhoea – Leonurus, Sanguinaria.
Dysmenorrhoea – Pulsatilla.
Dosage and mode of application
Solid extract Sig 1.25g
Tincturae bacc. Sig 4ml
Liquidum extractum Sig 4ml
References
43 p105. 111 p456. 126 p395. 127 p228. 176 p483. 189 p93. 192 p248.

Grifola frondosa [Maitake]

Constituents
Maitake D-fraction.

Primary pharmacological action: Immune enhancer.

Therapeutic classes
Antiviral - HIV.
Hepatic.
Antineoplastic.
Medicinal indications
Hypertension.
Diabetes. Obesity.
Tissue conditions
Immune supporter in HIV. Potentiates natural killer [NK] cells. Activates macrophages through increased production of interferon. Grifolia is common to the UK.
Dosage and mode of application
Dried mushroom Sig 10g
References
310 Vol 4, [4] p168.175.

Grindelia camporum/robusta [Grindelia]

Constituents
Essential oil up to 0.12% contained mainly in flos - alpha pinene, borneol, camphene and limonene in the stem oil. Myricine in fol oil. Saponins. Resin.

Primary pharmacological action: Bronchial antispasmodic.

Therapeutic classes
Anticatarrhal. Allays inflammation. Antiasthmatic. Expectorant.
Cardiac depressant. Hypotensive.
Hepatic. Splenic.
Diuretic – mild.
Sedative. Vulnerary. Dermatological agent.

Medicinal indications
Catarrh. Sore throats. Hay fever. Asthma. Bronchitis. Pertussus. Pneumonia.
Emphysema.
Splenic enlargement. Cystitis. Malaria.
Dermal ulcers. Eczema. Dermatitis – from Rhus tox. Impetigo.
Sexually transmitted disease.

Tissue conditions
Specific for asthma with wheeze, a hard dry cough and tight chest. Use long term in chronic bronchitis. Hepatic and splenic congestion with dyspepsia.

Cautions
Large doses can cause renal irritation.

External use
Dermatitis from ivy use a lotion plus oral medication.
Eczema and vesicular eruptions.
Dermal ulcers.

Preparations
Asthma with Lobelia.
Asthma [child] Grindelia 1, Pulsatilla 2, Tilia 2, Glycyrrhiza 2.
Bronchitis add Glycyrrhiza 2 parts and Grindelia 1 part.

Dosage and mode of application
Dried herba Sig 3g
Tincturae Sig 1ml
Liquidum extractum Sig 1ml

References
BPC 1949. 43 p106. 126 p397. 176 p320. 188 p207. 194. 263, 1992, 57. 263,59, PA364.

Guaiacum officinale [Lignum vitae]

Constituents
Heartwood resin around 20%. Phenolic lignans [antimicrobial] from the resin - known as C-18 lignans. Beta sitosterol. Terpenoids - saponins. Gums.

Primary pharmacological action: Antirheumatic.

Therapeutic classes
Vasotonic alterative. Allays inflammation. Astringent.
Circulatory stimulant.
Expectorant – mild.
Laxative - mild.
Diuretic - mild. Diaphoretic. Antirheumatic.
Uterotonic.
Dermatological agent.

Medicinal indications
Pharyngitis. Lung congestion. Influenza. Tuberculosis. Tonsillitis. Dysentery.
Diarrhoea.
Ankylosing spondylitis. Rheumatoid and Osteo arthritis. Rheumatic pain. Gout.
Dupuytrens contracture [often associated with arthritis].
Chronic skin diseases – eczema, furunculosis, psoriasis. Syphilis. Mercurial poisoning – an antidote.
Amenorrhoea and dysmenorrhoea from uterine atony.

Tissue conditions
Stimulating to the stomach and secretory organs. Detoxifies the blood through the eliminatory channels. The bark cleanses the blood of uric acid and relieves inflammatory processes.

Cautions
Avoid in acute inflammatory conditions of the gastro intestinal tract.

Preparations
Use an emulgent when dispensing.
According to indications with Apium, Filipendula, Iris, Menyanthes, Smilax, Zingiber.

Dosage and mode of application
Dried bark/heartwood/resin Sig 2g
Tincturae Sig 4ml
Liquidium Extractum Sig 2ml

References.
BPC 1934. 43 p107. 111 p457. 126 p399. 176 p351. 188 p208.

Gymnema sylvestre [Gymnema, Asclepias germinata]

Constituents
Contains gymnemic acid as its saponin which is a triterpenic heteroside.
Gymnemic acid inhibits the stimulation of a gastro intestinal hormone [gastric
inhibitory peptide] which is found in the duodenal membrane and has action upon
the release of insulin.

Primary pharmacological action: Antidiabetic. Hypoglycaemic.

Therapeutic classes
Cardiac stimulant. Hypocholesterolaemic.
Pancreatic trophorestorative. Laxative.
Diuretic. Antiobesity.

Medicinal indications
Reduces cholesterol and triglyceride levels.
It is hypoglycaemic. It partially stops the uptake of sugar from the intestine.
Reactive hypoglycaemia. Sugar cravings. Weight loss associated with diabetes.

Tissue conditions
Chewing the leaves has a temporary paralysing effect upon the taste buds. It will
suppress the craving for anything with a sweet taste - small dose applied to the
tongue.
Anaesthetizes the sweet taste buds. Improves blood sugar control. Supports the
requirement for insulin or hypoglycaemic drugs. Supports the trophorestorative
effect to the pancreatic insulin secreting cells [restores damaged pancreatic
tissue]. Reduces insulin requirements by 50%.

Preparations
Diabetes with Azaderacta, Galega or Trigonella.

Dosage and mode of application
Dried fol Sig 5g
Infusium Sig 30ml
Liquidum extractum Sig 3ml

References
48 p115. 271 No75, April 2001. 392 p1.
Gupta. S. Journal of Medical research. 50:1, 1962.
Gupta. S. Journal of Medical research. 52, 200. 1964.

Hagenia abyssinica [Kousso]

Constituents
Volatile oil. Bitters. Tannin. Butyrophenones – protokosin and kosotoxin.

Primary pharmacological action: Anthelmintic.

Therapeutic classes
Purgative. Taenifuge.
Antispasmodic.
Antineoplastic.
Medicinal indications
Expels tapeworms.
Dosage and mode of application
Liquidum extractum flos Sig 4ml.
References
111 p298. 189 p164.

Hamamelis virginiana [Witch hazel]

Constituents
Kaempferol and quercetin as flavonols [flavonoids]. Quercetin binds to type 2 oestrogen binding sites and bind isoflavonoids thus preventing oestrogens and so enables the reduction of oestrogens to target tissue. Volatile oil up to 0.5%, some 40 are aliphatic alcohols.
Tannins up to 10% in the fol these are catechins, gallotannins, proanthocyanidins. Tannisn in bacc up to 12%. Essential oils. Resin. Saponins. Vitamin P.

Primary pharmacological action: Cleansing astringent.

Therapeutic classes
Ophthalmic. Antiseptic. Allays inflammation. Tonic - gentle. Refrigerant. Antioxidant. Antihaemorrhagic. Vasoconstrictor.
Oropharyngeal agent.
Prolactin depressor.
Analgesic.
Dermatological agent.

Medicinal indications
Purulent opthalmia. Conjunctivitis. Phlebitis. Varicose veins. Catarrh. Epistaxis. Pharyngitis. Haemoptysis. Tuberculosis. Gingivitis. Tonsillitis. Haematemesis. Diarrhoea. Mucous colitis. Dysentery-second stage. Cholera. Intestinal haemorrhage. Rectal prolapse. Haemorrhoids. Gonorrhoea - tuberculous. Gonorrhoeal urethritis. Varicocoele. Haematuria. Uterine prolapse. Cervix congestion. Os dilation. Post partum haemorrhage. Mastitis.
Dermal damage. Eczema. Inflammatory skin disease. Neurodermatitis. Wrinkles. Wounds.

Tissue conditions
Excessive mucus discharges with relaxed tissues. Chronic inflammatory conditions of the nasopharynx. Congested tissues with venous fullness affecting the pelvic organs, genitalia or rectum. Perineal pain. Pallid or deep red tissues with venous congestion. Indicated for internal and external haemorrhage. Tonic activity upon the veins, improves venous return in poor venous tone. Eases the pain of haemorrhoids. Internal burns resulting from the intake of poisons. Os cervix enlarged and open with relaxed condition of the tissue. Relaxation of the uterine and vaginal walls. Analgesia following episotomy.

External use
Inflamed eyes, blepharitis, conjunctivitis - collyr [with Hydrastis].
Sore throats and aphthous ulcers use garg.

Pharmacopoeia

Checks milk leakage from the breasts.
Mastitis - apply lotion.
Haemorrhoids with Ranunculus or Aesculus as a suppository or ointment. Diluted as an enema in haemorrhoids - with Tsuga.
Gonorrhoea - with Hydrastis as an injection to the bladder.
Localised inflammation - inflammatory swellings, furunculosis, insect bites, blisters, bruises, tumours, sprains, varicose veins - apply upon lint or poultice and keep moist.
Skin - inflammation, acne, freckles, dilated facial capillaries, blisters, bed sores. Used as a skin toner. Wrinkles, eczema – dist Hamamelis or crem.
Wounds - poultice or lotion. Often used as Distilled [Dist] Hamamelis.

Dosage and mode of application
Dried fol/bacc Sig 2g
Decoctum Sig 3g
Tincturae Sig 5ml
Liquidum extractum Sig 4ml
Garg. Sig 3g
Dist Hamamelis. Apply to affected area PRN.
Ung Hamamelis @ 10%
Suppository – 1g decoctum extract.
Compress @ 10 % decoctum.
Poultice @ 30%
Spray hydrosol dist hamamelis

References
43 p109/110. 111 p461. 179 p591. 188 p455. 189 p285. 263, 63, 1997, p106.
394 p413.

Harpagophytum procumbens [Devils claw]

Constituents
Iridoid glycosides up to 3% - harpagide, harpagoside [analgesic, allays inflammation] and procumbide. Phenols - Acetoside. Flavonoids - Kaempferol. Glucose around 50%. Amino acids. CHO. Sterols. Triterpenes. [233 p78].

Primary pharmacological action: Antirheumatic.

Therapeutic classes
Allays inflammation. Antifungal – weak. Hyperlipidaemia. Antiarrhythmic. Bitter tonic. Stomachic. Cholagogue. Hepatic. Diuretic. Lymphotonic. Tobacco habit. Analgesic. Sedative. Antineoplastic. Dermatological agent. Antipyretic.

Medicinal indications
Hypercholesterolaemia. Hyperlipidaemia. Antiarrhythmic – ventricular arrhythmias.. Arteriosclerosis.
Allergies. Pleurodynia.
Anorexia. Dyspepsia. Heartburn. Flatulence. Hepatic disease. Malaria [239 p101].
Arthritis. Fibrositis. Fibromyalgia. Gout. Lumbago. Low back ache. Neuralgia. Rheumatism. Sciatica. Tendonitis. Rheumatoid arthritis. Osteo arthritis. Headache. Degeneration of the locomotor system.
Menopause. Dysmenorrhoea.
Acne. Furunculosis. Psoriasis. Itchy skin. Adhesions from scar tissue.
Skin carcinoma. Nicotine poisoning.

Tissue conditions
Cleanser and detoxifier of the lymph and blood. Stimulates the lymphatic system. Chronic inflammation of the urinary tract or gastro intestinal tract - stomach, liver or gall bladder. Affects the duodenum and enterohepatic circulation. Regulates the amount of calcium entering the cell.

Cautions
Avoid in pregnancy. Peptic ulcerations. Allergic rash.

Preparations
Full dose in acute pain.
Fresh root applied to wounds. Pulverised dry root is applied to a clean wound.
Crem or ung - irritable skin conditions; furunculosis, sores, ulcers.

Dosage and mode of application
Dried rhiz/tub Sig 2g
Tincturae tub Sig 10ml
Liquidum extractum Sig 2ml
References. 43 p111. 189 p102. 192 p181. 239 p101. 270, 3, [1], 1996. 394 p84.

Hedera helix [Ivy]

Constituents

Saponins [as hederagenin glycosides] up to 6% – expectorant, antifungal, antineoplastic, antispasmodic, anti leishmania, mollusicidal. Sterols. Flavonoids. Alkaloids - emetine which is amoebicidal. Essential oil up to 0.1% contains beta-caryophyllene, germacrene, sabinene, alpha-and beta-pinene and limonene.

Primary pharmacological action: Anthelmintic.

Therapeutic classes

Secretolytic. Antifungal. Antibacterial. Anti protozoal – Trichomonas.
Cardiodepressant. Haemostatic. Pulmonary expectorant.
Cathartic. Anthelmintic. Amoebicidal. Mollusicidal.
Antirheumatic. Febrifuge.
Regulates glands. Anti Cellulite. Dermatological agent. Emollient.
Analgesic. Antispasmodic. Sedative.
Antineoplastic. Cytotoxic.

Medicinal indications [Saturn]

Corneal ulcers. Leishmania protozoa.
Catarrh. Otitis media. Sinusitis. Haemoptysis. Pertussus. Bronchitis.
Dysentery. Jaundice. Amoeba. Kills liver fluke. Leishmania.
Arthritis. Rheumatic pain.
Oedema. Syphilis. Lymphadenopathy. Cellulitis. Itchy skin.
Burns and scalds. Skin itch. Neuralgia. Neuritis.

Tissue conditions

Inflammatory conditions of the respiratory tract. Saponins stimulate gastric peptic glands and via parasympathetic effector cells stimulate expectoration.

Cautions

Contact dermatitis.

External use

Corneal ulcers use collyr. Otitis media apply auristillae. Sinusitis use an nebulae.
Sunburn-apply the fol infusion.
Muscles, ligaments and tendons - infusion or oleum.
Splenic pain apply a lotion.

Dosage and mode of application

Infusium fol Sig 2g
Tincturae Sig 5ml
Liquidum extractum Sig 1ml

References

127 p442. 189 p155. 246 p273. 293, 6, 1994, p187-188. 394 p216.

Helleborus niger [Black hellebore]

Constituents
Cardiac glycosides - helleborin. Helleborein – minimal absorption from the gastro intestinal tract. Steroidal saponins. Protoanemonin.

Primary pharmacological action: Cardiotonic.

Therapeutic classes
Heart failure.
Hepatic. Hydragogue cathartic. Purgative. Nematodes.
Diuretic.
Emmenagogue.
Anxiolytic. Antispasmodic. Anaesthetic. Antineoplastic. Counter irritant.

Medicinal indications [Saturn]
Pericarditis.
Hepatic disorders with oedema. Constipation.
Oedema.
Amenorrhoea. Eclampsia.
Meningitis. Cerebral haemorrhage. Delirium. Mania. Panic. Depression. Epilepsy.
Inflamed and irritated skin. Lice.

Tissue conditions
Acts similarly to Digitalis creating a positive inotropic effect. Increases the force and strength of the heart and slows the pulse. Small doses stimulate intestinal gland secretion and stimulate the liver. Abdominal disorders associated with emotional disturbances - panic, mania, depression.

Cautions
Restrictions apply. Dosage is determined by the relief of symptoms.
Avoid in any irritable or inflamed conditions. Inflammation of the stomach and intestines. Large doses cause vomiting. Avoid in bradycardia.

External use
Used externally as a counter irritant in rheumatic disorders.

Dosage and mode of application
Always use in small dosage
Liquidum extractum rhiz. Sig 0.6ml

References
126 p404. 176 p331. 189 p141. 192 p270. 262 p69.

Hemidismus indica [Indian sarsparilla].

Constituents
Coumarins. Spaonins. Volatile oil.

Primary pharmacological action: Vasotonic alterative.

Therapeutic classes
Allays inflammation. Astringent. Aromatic. Blood toxicity. Diuretic.
Anxiolytic. Irritability. Dermatological agent. Febrifuge.
Medicinal conditions
Suppurative conditions.
Urinary infections. Cystitis. Dysuria. Prostatitis. Urethritis. Renal infections.
Sexually transmitted disease.
Allays itching. Eczema. Erysipilas. Psoriasis. Urticaria.
Tissue conditions
Allays inflammation in mucous membranes. Purifying activity upon cellular
structure and the blood [Vasotonic alterative]. Anger and irritable nerves. Similar
in activity to Smilax.
Dosage and mode of application
Dried herba. Sig 3.5g
Tincturae Sig 5ml
References 234.

Heracleum mantegazzianum [Giant hogweed]

Constituents
Furanocoumarins - psoralin.

Primary pharmacological action: Dermatological agent.

Therapeutic classes
Hypotensive. Stomachic. Sedative.
Medicinal indications
Hypertension. Epilepsy. Vitiligo.
Cautions
Phototoxic. Can cause severe contact dermatitis.
Dosage and mode of application
Herba, Fruct, Rad.
References. 149 p126. 176 p128.

Hieracium pilosella [Mousear hawkweed]

Constituents
Coumarin. Flavonic glycoside luteolin. Caffeic acid.

Primary action: Broncho spasmolytic.

Therapeutic classes
Anticatarrhal. Antibacterial.
Expectorant.
Sialagogue.
Diuretic.
Vulnerary.
Medicinal indications [Saturn]
Asthma. Bronchitis. Pertussus. Haemoptysis.
Hernia. Fractures. Brucellosis.
Combinations
Respiratory conditions with:
Grindelia, Lobelia, Marrubium, Polygala, Tussilago, Verbascum.
External use
Fractures – compress.
Hernia – compress/lotion.
Dosage and mode of application
Dried herba Sig 4g.
Liquidum extractum Sig 4ml
Syrup Sig 20ml
References
43 p159. 189 p356. 246 p498.

Humulus lupulus [Hops]

Constituents
Volatile oil up to 3% which consists mainly of monoterpenes, sesquiterpenes, chalcones and flavonoids. Polyphenol condensed tannins, up to 4%. Oleo resin bitters, up to 30% - phenolic compounds, bitter acids are antimicrobial and consist of humulone, lupulone and derivatives. Amino acids.

Primary pharmacological action:
CNS trophorestorative and Sedative.

Therapeutic classes
Antibacterial. Antimicrobial. Bitter tonic. Cholagogue. Choleretic. Anthelmintic. Diuretic. Antirheumatic.
Galactagogue. Anaphrodisiac. Oestrogenic.
Analgesic. Anodyne. Antispasmodic [spasmolytic]. Hypnotic. Sedative. Antineoplastic

Medicinal indications [Mars]
Earache.
Toothache. Anorexia. Hyperchlordria. Indigestion or diarrhoea of nervous origin. Colic. Mucus colitis IBS. Intestinal spasm. Nematodes – Ascaris, Enterobius. Cestodes – Tanea.
Bladder irritability. Premature ejaculation. Priapism.
Amenorrhoea. Dysmenorrhoea. Mastitis. Menopause.
Delirium. Headache. Insomnia. Restlessness, tension or excitability. Mental strain or worry. Muscle spasm. Nervous tension. Neuralgia. Panic attacks.

Tissue conditions
Humulus gently relaxes conditions of spasm or pain in the CNS. Muscular relaxant. Active cerebral hyperaemia. Nervousness, excitability or irritability. Tendency to worry. It relieves painful intestinal spasm. Abnormal or excessive sexual excitability in male and female. Nervous irritability with spermatorrhoea.

Cautions
Avoid in severe depression.

External use
Hop pillow - insomnia.
Insomnia - balneum at 1ml LE. Added to 100 litres aqua.
Ulcers, inflammation, furunculosis use as an antiseptic and anodyne.
Facial neuralgia apply a fomentation.
Eczema - with Datura or Solanum dulcamera.

Preparations
Gall bladder disturbance with spasm and pain - Humulus with Dioscorea,
Cichorium, or Mentha piperita.
Dosage and mode of application
Small doses are advised in nervous anxiety while larger doses in insomnia and
where sedation are required.
Dried strobile Sig 1g
Dry extract Sig 80mg [0.08g].
Soft extract Sig 1g
Tincturae Sig 10ml
Liquidum extractum Sig 2ml
References
43. 176 p124. 192 p273. 233 p 129. 239 p126. 394 p193.

Hydrangea arborescens [Seven barks]

Constituents
Flavonoids - kaempferol. Saponins - hydrangin. Gum starch. Resin.

Primary pharmacological action: Demulcent diuretic.

Therapeutic classes
Pulmonary agent.
Hepatic pain. Cathartic.
Haematuria. Nephritic. Antilithic.
Anodyne.
Medicinal indications
Broncho pulmonary affections with irritation.
Prostatitis. Urethritis. Cystitis. Urinary calculi. Enlarged prostate. Acute nephritis.
Rheumatic complaints - joint stiffness.
Tissue conditions
Soothing and anodyne to the urinary tract. Bladder and renal calculi. Nutritive to urinary mucous membranes. Eases backache associated with renal disturbances.
Dosage and mode of application
Dried rhizome Sig 4g
Tincturae Sig 10ml
Liquidum extractum Sig 4ml
References
43 p113. 126 p408. 176 p444. 188 p236. 189 p149.

Hydrastis canadensis [Golden seal]

Constituents
Isoquinoline alkaloids primary pharmacological action - Hydrastine up to 4%, Berberine up to 4%, canadine. Resin. Tannin. Fatty acids. Volatile oil.

Primary pharmacological action:
Vasotonic alterative to all systems.

Therapeutic classes
Ophthalmic. Mucous membrane tonic [astringent]. Anticatarrhal. Vasotonic alterative. Antiseptic. Allays inflammation.

Anti bacterial - Chlamydia aureus and trachomatis, Corynebacterium diphtheriae, Diplococcus pneumoniae, Entamoeba histolytica, Escherichia coli, Neisseria gonorrhoeae, Neisseria meningitidis, Pseudomonas aeruginosa, Salmonella typhi and para typhi, Shigella dysenteriae, Staphylococcus, Streptococcus, Trichononas vaginalis.

Anti fungal: Candida, Trichophyton.

Anti Spirochaete - Treponema pallidum, Vibrio cholerae.

Antiprotozoal: Giarda lambia. Klebsiella. Leishmania donovani.

Antihaemorrhagic. Vasoconstrictor. Antihaemorrhagic.

Bitter. Stomachic. Cholagogue. Choleretic. Antiulcerogenic. Hypoglycaemic. Splenic tonic. Laxative.

Diuretic. Lymphadenopathy.

Immune enhancer. Antineoplastic. Sedative. Dermatological agent. Vulnerary. Oxytocic. Uterine tonic.

Medicinal indications
Conjunctivitis. Trachoma. Corneal ulceration. Blepharitis. Otorrhoea. Otitis media. Tinnitus.

Aphthous ulcers. Anorexia. Pyorrhoea. Stomatitis. Catarrh. Colds. Infections of the mucous membranes. Influenza. Tuberculosis.

Food sensitivity/allergy. Anorexia. Atonic dyspepsia. Cholecystitis. Gastritis. Nausea and vomiting. Peptic ulcerations. Potentiates insulin effect. Enteritis. Colitis. Diarrhoea. Hepatic disorders - atony. Haemorrhoids. Anal fissures. Typhoid fever.

Oedema. Infective conditions of the urinary system. Prostatic disorders. Gonorrhoea. Syphilis.

Meningitis. Dysmenorrhoea. Menorrhagia. Endometrial haemorrhage. Post partum haemorrhage. Nipple fissures.

Wounds. Dermal damage. Eczema. Ringworm. Erysipelas. Icterus.

Pharmacopoeia

Tissue conditions

Berberine has a maximum concentration after three hours. Equalises the circulation. Stimulant and astringent to involuntary and smooth muscle. Supports healing of peptic ulcerations. Improves assimilation of foods.

Hydrastis supports and tones the veins [including the portal circulation] and the right side of the heart. Tones [astringes] the mucous membranes of the entire body and allays inflammation. Indicated for acute and chronic inflammatory conditions of the respiratory, gastro intestinal, genito urinary and pelvic viscera.

Skin diseases dependent upon poor intestinal elimination - eczema, acne, furunculosis. Small doses allay the nausea of pregnancy.

Cautions

Pregnancy.

External use

Babies and infants oral candida - mix with maple syrup [[Jupiter] and apply.

Soothes and heals skin disorders - Acne. Eczema. Pruritus. Wounds. Sores. Tinea.

Eyes - dilute collyr and use in an eyebath or ung. Use sterile water.

Trachoma an infection of the eye which causes blindness - use the lotion, ung.

Skin – abscess, abrasion, furunculosis, laceration – lotion.

Anal irritation, fissures, anal eczema, rectal prolapse.

Vaginal disorders – candida, vaginal discharge/leucorrhoea use a douche/pessary.

Preparations

Hydrastis will be carried with the addition of the specific remedy for that site.

Aphthous ulcers, halitosis, pharyngitis, nasal catarrh, laryngitis -Garg/inf/collut.

Diphtheria and scarlatina with Myrica, Capsicum and Commiphora.

Heart tonic with Capsicum. Hypertension with Tilia and Valeriana.

Hepatic or stomach disorders with Bryonia, Chionanthus, Iris, Leptandra.

Peptic ulcers with Althea, Commiphora, Phytolacca, Geranium maculatum.

Renal disorders with diuretic or organ remedy.

Spinal nervine with Humulus and Scutellaria.

Uterine tonic with Viburnum prunifoleum.

Dosage and mode of application

Dried rad/rhizome. Sig 1g

Dry extract Sig 120mg

Tincturae Sig 2ml

Liquidum extractum Sig 1ml

Collyr Sig 2-3gtt in an eyebath with tepid aqua.

Ung – Hydrastis [1:5] 2ml. Hydrous wool fat to 60g. Melt under a gentle heat add the tincture and mix.

References

BPC 1949. 69 p198. 111 p472. 126 p417. 179 p292. 192 p244. 224 p1768.

Hyoscyamnus niger [Henbane]

Constituents
Tropane alkaloids principally hyoscine [Scopolamine]. Alkaloids are parasympatholytic with an action similar to Atropa. Flavonoid glycosides.

Primary pharmacological action:
Antispasmodic to the Gastointestinal and Genitourinary Tracts.

Therapeutic classes
Mydriatic. Allays inflammation.
Pectoral sedative.
Carminative. Antinausea.
Anodyne. Antispasmodic. Hypnotic. Sedative.
Medicinal indications [Saturn]
Earache. Pain of mumps. Palpitations.
Asthma. Pertussus. Irritable coughs. Bronchitis. Pneumonia.
Vomiting. Flatulent colic. Intestinal spasm. Colic. Abdominal pain. Sphincter spasm of the GIT and GUT.
Urinary antispasmodic. Gout. Aphrodisiac.
Headache. Neuralgia. Mania. Panic. Motion sickness. Excitability. Restlessness with irritability. Delirium tremens. Muscle spasms. Parkinsons disease.
Delirium of pyrexia.
Dysmenorrhoea. Herpes zoster pain.
Tissue conditions
Nervous tension with irritability, insomnia or exhaustion. Sedative and antispasmodic to the CNS and ANS. It inhibits actylcholine and is anticholinergic. Nervous irritability. Fear, night terrors, muttering, illusions. Restlessness, flushed face with dilated pupils. It relaxes smooth muscle within the gastro intestinal, biliary and genito urinary tract. Indicated for organ pain. Haemorrhoidal pain. Parasympatholytic - decreases secretions of the mouth, stomach, bronchus and skin. Sedative in the irritable coughs of bronchitis. Bladder nerve irritability. Pain in the bladder and kidney. Urethral irritation after the passing of catheters etc. Locomotor ataxia. Tremors. Headache from irritability. Paraplegia with restlessness. Talkativeness. Hallucinations. Delusions. Garrulousness. Tremor of Parkinsons disease.
Dysmenorrhoea and ovarian pain.
Cautions
Restrictions apply. Dosage is determined by the relief of symptoms.
Dilated pupils, dry throat, giddiness, limb weakness, paralysis, loss of speech, delirium, hallucinations, coma. Glaucoma. Arrhythmia. Prostatic disease.

Pharmacopoeia

External use
Ulcer, haemorrhoidal, tumour pain.
Earache - Instill 5gtt infusium.
Preparations
Potentiated by Gelsemium, Datura or Passiflora.
Pertussus with Syrup Prunus serotina.
With purgatives to prevent griping.
Dosage and mode of application
Small doses stimulate and large doses sedate.
Dried fol/flos Sig 1g
Tincturae Sig 1ml
Liquidum extractum Sig 0.25ml
References
BPC 1911. 126 p421. 176 p109. 228 p122. 233 p131. 246 p396.

Hypericum perforatum [St John's Wort]

Constituents
Naphthodianthrones – hypericin around 0.6% and pseudohypericin. Hypericin was isolated by Buchner in 1830. Hypericin and pseudohypericin, the main antiviral components of Hypericum, can cross the blood brain barrier. Melatonin. Polyphenolic glycoside - hyperforin up to 4%, affects serotonin levels. Maoi inhibition, catechol – O – methyl transferase inhibition. Selectively inhibits serotonin at post synaptic receptors. Flavonoids – hyperoside up to 2%, rutin up to 1.6% are antidepressant. Catechin tannins - up to 15%. Volatile oils. Acids. Sterols.
One study showed no differences between control groups when given standardised Hypericum this lack of dose-response effect provides support for the theory that hypericin is not the main active constituent [270, 1999].

Primary pharmacological action: Nervine tonic.

Therapeutic classes
Astringent. Antiseptic. Allays inflammation.
Antibacterial – gram negative and gram positive, Escherichia coli, Mycobacterium tuberculosis, Proteus vulgaris, Pseudomonas aeruginosa, Staphylococcus aureus and Streptococcus mutans.
Antiviral – Aids/HIV, Cytomegalovirus, Epstein barr virus, herpes simplex 1 & 2. herpes genitalis, Herpes zoster, Hepatitis C, Parainfluenza virus A and B, vesicular stomatitis virus. Antiretroviral.
Antihaemorrhagic.
Antiparasitic - nematodes - threadworms.
Diuretic. Renal disturbances. Venereal disease.
Nervine. Antidepressant. Anodyne. Prolactin depressor.
Dermatological agent. Vulnerary.
Antineoplastic. Antivenomous.

Medicinal indications [Sun]
Earache. Toothache. Herpes infections. Pertussus.
Anorexia. Gastritis. Diarrhoea. Dysentery. Jaundice. Gastro intestinal ulcerations. Colon carcinoma. Haemorrhoids. Malaria.
Enuresis. Incontinence. Nervous bladder. Sexually transmitted disease.
Anxiety. Depression. Excitability. Insomnia and hypersomnia. Insanity. Obsessive compulsive disorder. SAD syndrome.
Panic. Concussion. Headache. Pain. Disseminated sclerosis. Shock.
Menopausal neurosis.

Pharmacopoeia

Musculoskeletal disorders. Rheumatic and muscle pain – [Fibro] myalgia. Neuralgia. Sciatica. Neuromuscular inflammation - pain due to torn muscles. Pain of the toes and fingers from injury eg fractures, sprains. Spinal injury. Lacerated or puncture wounds. Burns – eases oedema. Tetany. Pruritus.

Tissue conditions

Maximum activity between 4-6 hours. More detailed information is available in the pharmacokinetic section of this chapter. Melatonin levels - Hypericum perforatum [flowers] 4.39. Hypericum perforatum [leaves] 1.75.

Increases the ability to detox [synthetic drugs] by increasing the activity of cytochrome p450 detoxification mechanisms. Dilates the coronary arteries. Antispasmodic to the gastro intestinal, renal tract, uterus and prostate. Increases helper T lymphocytes. Spinal irritability or pain from muscle spasm, injury, tender spinous processes. Shock or concussion. Reduces the levels of prolactin, thought to be due to enhanced dopamine output. Dopamine suppresses prolactin output. Prolactin dysregulation causes anxiety like syndromes.

Hypericum oleum macerated in sunlight produces a red colour and is due to the lipophilic break down products of hypericin it has around three months vulnerary life. Preparation by heat extraction produces a lower level of hyperforin with a shelf life of six months. 'As it does not meet regulatory criteria in EU guidelines it has not been accepted as a medicine for major depression !' [394 p360].

Cautions

Avoid sunbathing – photosensitisitivity/phototoxic.

External use

Vitiligo.

Wound healer - burns, blisters, ulcers, chronic mastitis, tumours, bruises, shingles - use the Ol or infusium.

Spinal injury, joint pain – Oleum or suppository.

Diverticular disease, fissure – suppository.

Topically - inflammation, pain, radiation burns, nerve tissue regenerator.

Preparations

Sedative aa Lavandula, Melissa & Passiflora or Artemesia, Melissa, Verbena.

Dosage and mode of application

Dried herba/flos Sig 4g

Dry extract Sig 300mg

Tincturae Sig 4ml

Liquidum extractum Sig 4ml

References

43 p115. 126 p424. 176 p152. 179 p 543. 194 p52. 239 p157. 246 p248. 263 1992 58, p351. 270, 1994, Vol 1, p9. 271, No. 44, April 1995. 269, Biol. Nauki. 1992 [4] 709. 270, 1999, 6, [3], p141. 295, 7052 [313] p253-7. 312, 2000, 61 [8] p575-8. 313, 2000, 142 [5] p979-84. Biol. Psychiatry 1999, 46 (4) 581-584. 394 p362.

Hyssopus officinalis [Hyssop]

Constituents
Flavonoid glycoside – diosmin [antioxidant, allays inflammation. Terpenoids - marrubin [expectorant]. Volatile oil mainly camphor. Saponin. Tannin around 8%.

Primary pharmacological action: Expectorant.

Therapeutic classes
Stimulant. Tonic. Antibacterial – Pseudomonas aeruginosa.
Antiviral – herpes simplex, herpes genitalis, HIV.
Hypotensive.
Anti catarrhal. Antitussive. Pectoral.
Aromatic. Carminative. Anthelmintic.
Diaphoretic. Antirheumatic.
Emmenagogue.
Antispasmodic. Sedative.
Dermatological agent. Vulnerary. External antiseptic.
Medicinal indications [Jupiter]
Hypertension.
Colds. Herpes. Chronic catarrh. Quinsy. Hoarseness. Bronchitis. Asthma.
Tuberculosis.
Dyspepsia. Flatulence. Flatus.
Lithuria. Genital herpes.
Anxiety. Epilepsy – petit mal. Panic. Tinnitus – steam treatment.
Eruptive disease – chicken pox, measles, smallpox. Burns. Bruises. Wounds.
Body lice.
Tissue conditions
Diffusive, aromatic and stimulating to mucous membranes from the bitter in the volatile oil. Sustains the capillary circulation and peripheral nerves by diffusive activity. An absorbent remedy which relieves the lungs of excess mucus.
Preparations
Bronchial conditions with Marrubium.
Childhood pyrexia with Calendula.
External use
Bruises, sprains, stings and bites use the infusion and poultice.
Measles rash: Calendula and Hyssopus will cool the skin.
Skin parasites - decoctum.
Preparations
Nerve tonic for anxiety, epilepsy and panic with Stachys.
Pertussus with Angelica archangelica, Hyssopus and Mentha pulegrum.

Dosage and mode of application
Dried herba Sig 4g
Tincturae Sig 4ml
Liquidum extractum Sig 4ml
References
43 p116. 111 p478. 188 p244. 189 p151. 192 p 283. 246 p380. 272 1995, 7 [4]
p24/5. 263 1998, 64 p181/2.

Ilex paraguariensis [Yerba Mate]

Constituents
Xanthine alkaloids theobromine up to 0.9% - stimulant to the CNS. Minerals.
Flavonoids – kaempferol, rutin. Caffeine up to 2%. Triterpenoid saponins.
Tannins up to 16%. Vitamin B2, B6, Niacin, pantothenic acid, C. Volatile oil.

Primary pharmacological action:
Central nervous stimulant and tonic.

Therapeutic classes
Antioxidant. Tonic. Cardiotonic. Inotropic. Chronotropic.
Diuretic. Diaphoretic. Antirheumatic.
Analgesic – mild. Antidepressant. Antispasmodic. Antiobesity. Lipolytic.
Medicinal indications
Asthenia. Reduces the appetite. Anti obesity producing fat oxidation.
Gout. Rheumatic pain.
Fatigue. Depression. Exhaustion from stress. Headache [from stress]. Epilepsy.
Tissue conditions
Caffeine is stimulant to the respiratory and cardiovascular system, a coronary
dilator. Smooth muscle relaxant. Stimulant and tonic to the central nervous system
preventing memory loss. Slows the aging process. Increases physical and mental
energy. Stimulates elimination of uric acid.
Cautions
Avoid at night due to the stimulating action upon the CNS.
Dosage and mode of application
Dried herba/fol Sig 4g
Infusium Sig 30ml. Tincturae Sig 10ml. Liquidum extractum Sig 4ml
References 192 p589. 224. 246 p228. 278 58, 3, 1995, p438-441. 394 p249.
278 Winter 2000, p24-5. 281 Winter 2001.

Inula helenium [Elecampane]

Constituents
Sesquiterpenes. Inulin around 44%. Terpenoids. Sterols. Volatile oils up to 4%.
Resin. Mucilage.

Primary pharmacological action: Pulmonary tonic.

Therapeutic classes
Antiseptic. Bactericidal. Vasotonic alterative. Stimulant.
Aromatic. Anticatarrhal. Antitussive. Expectorant.
Stomachic. Hepatic. Anthelmintic.
Diaphoretic. Diuretic.
Vulnerary. Dermatological agent. Antivenomous.
Medicinal indications [Mercury]
Diphtheria. Bronchitis. Bronchiectasis. Colds. Pulmonary tuberculosis and night
sweats. Locke discovered in 1895 that Inula would destroy the tubercle bacillus.
Irritable coughs. Pertussus. Asthma.
Anorexia. Atonic dyspepsia. Digestive tonic - aids assimilation. Malnutrition.
Oedema. Itchy skin. Dermal ulcers. Snakebite.
Vaginal discharge/leucorrhoea. Endometriosis.
Tissue conditions
Tones the pulmonary mucous membranes and reduces catarrh. Warming to the
respiratory tract. Atonic conditions where the lungs are weak and debilitated.
Persistent coughs with substernal pain. It restores sluggish and impeded capillary
circulation after chills and exposure. Atony of the abdominal viscera. Tones the
alimentary mucous membranes.
Preparations
Sinus disturbance with Echinacea, Solidago and/or Euphrasia.
Tuberculosis with Inula and Echinacea. When pain occurs use Bryonia, Sticta or
Cimicifuga.
Asthma: Angelica archangelica 2 Inula 2 Grindelia 1.
Vaginal discharge/leucorrhoea with Barosma or Uva ursi.
Dosage and mode of application
Dried rad Sig 4g
Tincturae Sig 5ml
Liquidium Extractum Sig 4ml
References
43 p118. 111 p480. 126 p426. 176 p276. 233 p87. 246 p454. 251 p69. 254 p92.

Iris versicolor [Blue flag]

Constituents
Triterpenoid acids - isophalthalic, salicylic. Volatile oil - furfural, is stimulating to the mucous membranes. Tannin. Sterols. Resin.

Primary pharmacological action:
Lymphatic vasotonic alterative.

Therapeutic classes
Stimulant. Allays inflammation. Cardiac.
Anti emetic - small dose. Hepatic and cholagogue. Laxative. Pancreatic agent.
Diuretic. Adrenal agent. Thyroactive.
Ovarian and prostate congestion. Dermatological agent. Antipyretic.
Medicinal indications [Moon]
Hydropericardium.
Vomiting of pregnancy. Vomiting. Waterbrash. Hepatic disorders. Chronic hepatitis. Jaundice. Pancreatic deficiency. Constipation with flatus. Bilious headache. Indigestion. Splenic enlargement. Ascites. Cholera.
Chronic renal disease. Oedema. Gonorrhoea. Syphilis. Spermatorrhoea. Prostatic discharge. Addisons disease. Rheumatic complaints.
Skin disease - acne, eczema, herpes, impetigo, pruritus, psoriasis.
Lymphadenopathy. Enlarged thyroid - goitre.
Enlarged ovaries. Uterine fibroids. Uterine hypertrophy. Ulcerated Os cervix.
Vaginal discharge/leucorrhoea.
Intermittent, bilious and remittent pyrexia. Mercury poisoning.
Tissue conditions
Stimulating vasotonic alterative affecting the liver, pancreas, intestines, kidneys and skin. It has a stimulating action in chronic conditions of the biliary system, thyroid, spleen, lymphatics, prostate and uterus with atony [sluggishness].
Arouses secretions of salivary glands, liver, pancreas, intestines, kidneys and skin. Corrects faulty metabolism. Hepatic disorders, pale stools with sluggish and enlarged thyroid gland aggravated by fatty foods or pastry. Often combined for blood conditions resulting in skin disease [greasy skin], abnormal dermal pigmentation or rheumatic affections. Facial neuralgia and muscular wasting.
Miasmic tendencies - lymphatic, tubercular, and syphilitic. Emetic and cathartic in large dose.
Cautions
Nausea. Pregnancy.
External use
Psoriasis, eczema, tinea, prurigo - ung.

Preparations
Use a carminative when prescribing.
Action is best enhanced with other remedies.
Blood, skin and rheumatic diseases with vasotonic alterative also with renal and hepatic remedies to improve prescription activity.
Lymphadenopathy with Phytolacca.
Fibroids - with Chelone, Hydrastis, Rubus or Zanthoxylum.
Dosage and mode of application
Cathartic - full dose
Dried rad/rhiz. Sig 2g
Tincturae Sig 10ml
Liquidum extractum Sig 2ml
References
40. 43 p120. 126 p435. 176 p510. 194. 246 p528. 254 p74. 262 p74.

Jateorhiza palmata [Calumba]

Constituents
Isoquinoline alkaloids - palmitine and jatorrhizine. Palmitine is hypotensive, antimalarial and uterine stimulant. Jatorrhizine is sedative and antifungal. Volatile oil containing thymol. Bitter terpenes. Sapogenins - diosgenin.

Primary pharmacological action:
Gastro intestinal bitter vasotonic.

Therapeutic classes
Antiseptic. Antifungal. Disinfectant.
Sialagogue. Carminative. Bitter stomachic. Antiemetic. Laxative. Anthelmintic.
Orexegenic. Uterine stimulant. Febrifuge.

Medicinal indications
Hypertension
Bronchial affections. Pulmonary tuberculosis.
Nausea of pregnancy. Antiemetic. Anorexia. Gastric irritation. Vomiting.
Dyspepsia. Hypochlorhydria. Flatulence. Hepatic atony. Intestinal flatus.
Diarrhoea. Amoebic dysentery. Cholera.
Enuresis. Impotence/sexual dysfunction.
Remittent [Malaria] and intermittent fever. Motion sickness.

Tissue conditions
A very bitter tonic to the gastro intestinal tract, in digestive weakness or anorexia. It has no astringency. Milder than Gentiana in its action. Similar effects to Hydrastis.

Preparations
Prescribe with aromatics Anethum or Foeniculum.

Dosage and mode of application
Powdered rad Sig 2g
Tincturae Sig 2ml
Liquidum extractum Sig 2ml

References
111 p368. 176 p267. 188p82. 189 p57. 262 p85.

Juglans cinera/regia [Butternut/Walnut]

Constituents

Bitters. Ellagitannin up to 10%. Naphthaquinones – Juglone [antiviral HSV 1]. Volatile oil. Flavonoids up to 3%.

Primary pharmacological action:
Vasocompressor [astringent] to the hepatic and portal system.

Therapeutic classes

Ophthalmic. Vasotonic alterative. Depurant. Astringent. Antibacterial.
Antifungal - Candida, Tinea, Trichophyton.
Antiviral – Herpes simplex/zoster.
Cholagogue. Hepatic stimulant. Pancreatic stimulant. Hypoglacaemic. Laxative.
Anthelmintic.
Lymphatic agent. Dermatological agent. Insect repellent. Antivenemous.
Antineoplastic.

Medicinal indications

Blepharitis. Anaemia – iron deficiency. Chilblains. Varicose veins and ulcers.
Tuberculosis.
Aphthous ulcers. Tonsillitis. Cholelithiasis. Dyspepsia. Jaundice. Torpid or
sluggish, congested liver. Constipation. Diarrhoea. Dysentery. IBS.
Haemorrhoids. Cestodes. Trematodes.
Muscle sprains and damage.
Dermal inflammation. Acne. Burns. Eczema. Hyperhydrosis – hands and feet.
Impetigo. Lichen. Pemphigus. Pruritus. Psoriasis. Syphilis. Ringworm.
Intermittent fever - malaria. Remittent fever – typhoid. Hair lice.
Head pain. Lymphadenopathy.

Tissue conditions

Vasocompression is the term used to describe the ability of a medicine to constrict
the tissue, thereby supporting improved muscle tone, mucous membrane and
blood vessel. Compressing tissue improves blood vessel tone and ultimately blood
supply to that organ. A cleansing blood tonic. Inflammatory conditions of the
mucus membranes and skin. Chronic inflammation of the throat from intestinal
toxaemia e.g. tonsillitis - when toxins are eliminated through the tonsils. Dry,
congested and irritated mucous membranes. Gently tones the intestinal wall if
given over time. Stimulates lower bowel clearance this encourages the portal
system to decongest. Chronic constipation, waterbrash and flatulence.
A slow acting cathartic. Gastro intestinal irritability, tenesmus, with flatulence
diarrhoea or constipation. Skin conditions of a pustular or vesicular nature.

Pharmacopoeia

External use
Blepharitis – collyr.
Feet odour – foot bath.
Vaginal discharge/leucorrhoea – douche.
Lymphadenitis – compress fol.
Herpes zoster – lotion.
Dermal disorders with Viola tricolor.
Scalp itching or dandruff – lotion wash.
Dermal burns – lotion.
Malignant sores – lotion.
Poison bites from dogs and snakes – poultice.

Preparations
Anaemia with Rumex, Urtica.
Haemorrhoids with Scrophularia.
Vermifuge with Artmesia absinthium.
Skin disorders with Arctium, Rumex.
Strained ligaments and tendons with Hypericum.

Dosage and mode of application
Dried fol Sig 3g
Liquidum extractum inner cort Sig 6ml

References
43 p122. 111 p488. 126 p438. 188 p449. 189 p53&278. 246. 254 p98. 394 p401.

Juniperus communis [Juniper]

Constituents
Volatile oils up to 3.4% consisting mainly of monoterpenes 58% - pinine, camphor, camphine, terpenen - 4 - ol, [diuretic]. Acids - diterpenes. Flavonoid – apigenin. Tannins. Resin. Vitamin K.

Primary pharmacological action: Stimulating diuretic.

Therapeutic classes
Allays inflammation. Antimicrobial. Antiseptic. Antifungal - Penicillium notatum. Antiviral - herpes simplex. Carminative. Stomachic.
Antirheumatic. Emmenagogue. Dermatological agent. Rubefacient.

Medicinal indications [Sun]
Headaches. Bronchitis. Coughs. Chest infections.
Anorexia. Gastric stimulant. Flatulence. Colic. Intestinal pain. Typhoid fever.
Acute and chronic cystitis. Uric acid diathesis. Pyelitis. Pyelonephritis. Oedema.
Lumbar backache. Gonorrhoea.
Vaginal discharge/leucorrhoea. Atonic amenorrhoea. Dysmenorrhoea.
Eczema. Herpes. Lichen. Wound infections.
Rheumatic pain. Musculoskeletal disorders with inflammation. Tendonitis.

Tissue conditions
Dilates the glomeruli. Used in chronic renal hyperaemia with congestion. Renal atony, backache with mucus discharges. Test urine with labstix.

Cautions
Avoid in acute inflammation, haematuria, proteinuria. Nephritis. Nephron damage. Pregnancy as it stimulates uterine contractions.

External use
Oral infection – diluted Tr. Headache – diluted oleum to the temples.
Cade oil is distilled from Juniper and is used in dermatological conditions - eczema, prurigo, psoriasis, tinea.
Respiratory infections with congested mucus – inhalation.
Musculoskeletal disorders - liniment.

Dosage and mode of application
Always use in small dosage and administer with a demulcent.
Dried bacc Sig 3g.
Tincturae Sig 10ml.
Liquidum extractum Sig 3ml. Oleum Juniperus Sig 0.2ml

References
BPC 1934. 43 p124. 111 p492. 126 p439. 188 p156. 192 p304. 246 p568. 272, 1996, 8 [3] p24. 314, 2000, 15 [2] p139-43. 394 p218.

Krameria triandra [Rhatany]

Constituents
Tannin up to 20% mainly condensed tannins known as oligomeric
proanthocyanidins.

Primary pharmacological action: Astringent and tonic.

Therapeutic classes
Antimicrobial. Antitubercular. Antihaemorrhagic.
Periodontal disease. Antidiarrhoeal.
Styptic. Dermatological agent. Vulnerary.
Medicinal indications
Pharyngitis. Sore throat. Chilblains. Tuberculosis.
Gingivitis. Diarrhoea. Dysentery. IBS. Colitis. Intestinal haemorrhage [passive].
Anal fissure. Anal prolapse. Haemorrhoids.
Urinary incontinence. Haematuria.
Menorrhagia.
Wounds.
Tissue conditions
Haemolytic medicine for haemorrhage of mucus surfaces.
External use
Dentifrice - use the powder. Astringent wash for the mucous membranes of the
eyes, nose and gums. Nasal polyps.
Gingivitis, pharyngitis, sore throat - mouthwash or gargle.
Chilblains and wounds - apply topically.
External use
Nasal polyps - snuff.
Anal fissure, anal prolapse - decoction. Haemorrhoids - suppository or ointment.
Dosage and mode of application
> Gargarisma - Tincturae diluted with 10 parts aqua. Sig gargle QDS
> Gargarisma - Infusium 2g aqua 150ml Sig gargle QDS
Dried rad Sig 2g
Decoctum Sig 30ml
Tincturae Sig 4ml
References. BPC 1949. BPC 1954. 188 p260/372. 189 p234. 192 p467.

Lactuca virosa [Wild lettuce]

Constituents
Sesquiterpine lactones. Coumarins. Acids. Alkaloids - hyoscyamine. Flavonoids.
Terpenoid bitters. Resin.

Primary pharmacological action: Anodyne and sedative.

Therapeutic classes
Antitussive. Expectorant.
Antirheumatic.
Analgesic. Antispasmodic. Hypnotic.
Medicinal indications [Moon]
Irritable coughs. Pertussus.
Inflamed prostate. Muscular and articular pain.
Excitability. Hyperactivity. Insomnia. Restlessness.
Priapism. Dysmenorrhoea. Nymphomania. Uteritis.
Tissue conditions
Antispasmodic action upon smooth and striated muscle. Excitability in children.
Very low [nanograms] amounts of morphine have been found in Lactuca. Because
of the tiny proportion it is not considered a primary responsive activity however
together with other fractions it would compliment the activity of the whole plant.
Dosage and mode of application
Dried fol Sig 3g
Tincturae Sig 4ml
Liquidum extractum Sig 4ml
References
BPC 1934. 142 p214. 188 p454. 192 p569. 246 p494.

Laminaria digitata [Seaweed] [See Fucus].

Lamium album [White deadnettle]

Constituents
Flavonol glycosides – isoquercetin. Mucilage. Saponins. Tannin. Volatile oil.

Primary pharmacological action: Astringent.

Therapeutic classes
Allays inflammation. Anticatarrhal. Antiviral - Candida, Trichomonas.
Demulcent. Refrigerant.
Haemostatic.
Expectorant.
Diuretic.
Antispasmodic. Sedative – mild.
Vulnerary.
Medicinal indications [Venus]
Anaemia.
Catarrh. Epistaxis. Pleurisy.
Intestinal haemorrhage. Splenomegaly.
Respiratory, vaginal and urinary catarrh.
Oliguria. Prostatitis. BPH.
Metritis. Dysmenorrhoea. Metrorrhagia. Menorrhagia. PMS. Vaginal
discharge/leucorrhoea. Insomnia.
Tissue conditions
Tonic to the urinary tract, uterus and prostate and reduces catarrh. Uterine and
prostate circulatory tonic.
External use
Arthritis, gout and sciatica – poultice.
Boils. Tumours. Varicose veins.
Douche in metrorrhagia.
Preparations
Prostatitis with Serenoa and Hydrangea.
Uterine disorders with Vinca.
Wounds mix with honey.
Dosage and mode of application
Infusium herba Sig 10ml
Tincturae Sig 5ml
References
127 p579. 189 p15. 192 p131. 246 p370.

Larrea tridentata [Chaparral]

Constituents
Resin 20% composed of lignan nordihydroguariaretic acid [NGDA] - parasiticide
and antioxidant. The resin inhibits histamine release in allergic conditions.
Flavonoids around 20 compounds isolated. Flavonoid methyl esters are antiviral.

Primary pharmacological action: Vasotonic alterative.

Therapeutic classes
Allays inflammation. Antimicrobial - Baccilus subtilis, Pencillium, Pseudomonas
aeruginosa, Salmonella sp., Staphylococcus aureus, Streptococcus species.
Antifungal – Tinea, Trichophyton.
Astringent. Depurative. Antioxidant.
Antiallergic. Respiratory antiseptic. Antitubercular.
Bitter. Choleretic. Amoebicidal against: Entamoeba histolytica. Haemorrhoids.
Diuretic. Urinary antiseptic.
Uterine tonic. Antirheumatic.
Antineoplastic.
Vulnerary. Dermatological agent.
Medicinal indications
Allergies. Asthma. Bronchitis. Tuberculosis.
Syphilis.
Atonic dysmenorrhoea. Amenorrhoea.
Rheumatism. Lumbago. Tetanus.
Breast carcinoma. Melanoma.
Impetigo. Psoriasis.
Tissue conditions
Lower bowel tonic in cases of haemorrhoids and constipation. The bladder,
prostate and uterine tonic.
Preparations
Infective conditions – with Echinacea, Hydrastis.
Impetigo – lotion.
Syphilis – with Smilax.
Dosage and mode of application
Infusium fol Sig 5g
References
188 p106. 192 p131. 262 p92. 310 Vol3 No 1 1993/94.

Lavandula angustifolia [Lavender]

Constituents
Volatile oils up to 5% - camphor, cineole, borneol, linalyl acetate, up to 55%, linalool, up to 38%. Flavonoids – luteolin. Hydroxycoumarins – herniarin, umbelliferone. Triterpenes - ursolic acid. Tannin up to 12%. Perillyl alcohol is antineoplastic it blocks cell division and fragmenting cells so that they can easily be devoured by immune cells.

Primary pharmacological action:
Carminative and antispasmodic.

Therapeutic classes
Fragrant. Astringent. Antibacterial – MRSI, Staphylococcus.
Diffusive stimulant.
Antiflatus. Cholagogue. Choleretic.
Anticonvulsant. Anodyne. Sedative. Tonic. Antidepressant.
Rubefacient. Dermatological agent. Antirheumatic.
Antineoplastic.
Medicinal indications [Mercury]
Palpitations.
Loose teeth. Anorexia. Halitosis. Nausea. Motion sickness. Indigestion. Vomiting.
Intestinal spasm. Flatulent colic. Bloating. IBS.
A compound from lavender has shown promise in the treatment of cancer of the breast, colon, ovarian, pancreas and prostate.
Anxiety. Depression. Insomnia. Restlessness. Fainting. Headache. Migraine.
Vertigo. Memory loss. Neuralgia. Paralysis. Weakness of the limbs.
Muscle strain. Burns. Bruises. Cuts. Episeotomy.
Tissue conditions
Diffusively stimulating and antispasmodic to the nervous peripheries – calms GABA a neurotransmitter. Allays headaches, fainting, tension, panic and neuroses generally. Depression and anxiety that may be associated with an irritable bowel. Intestinal conditions producing pain and discomfort, gas with bloating and spasm. Culpeper gives uses for diseases of the head, stomach and uterus.
External use
Loose teeth - mouthwash.
Paralysis - apply the diluted oleum for rubefacient action.
Anxiety, depression, headache, tension – inhalation for antispasmodic effects.
Balneum general or foot – diluted oleum 5gtt eases tension and allays rheumatic pain.
Disinfectant – use the spray.

Preparations
As an adjunct to other remedies.
Anxiety, tension, irritability with Rosmarinus.
Dosage and mode of application
Dried flos/fol Sig 2g
Tincturae Sig 10ml
Liquidum extractum Sig 4ml
    Oleum Sig 4gtt on a sugar cube [approximately 4gtt = 80mg].
    Spray Aqua Lavandula. Lavender spray. Ethyl alcohol 25 % Oleum
    Lavandula 20gtt shake then add aqua to 100ml.
References
43 p128. 111 p504. 127 p471. 150. 192 p326. 230 p67. 246 p391. 281 Winter
1998. 287 1998 Jan/Feb 17. 394 p226.

Ledum latifoleum [Labrador tea]

Primary pharmacological action: Tonic.

Therapeutic classes
Ophthalmic. Vasotonic alterative. Demulcent. Expectorant. Pectoral.
Diuretic. Vulnerary. Dermatological agent.
Medicinal indications
Ecchymosis of the orbit [black eye] - dect.
Irritations of the pulmonary mucous membranes. Pertussus.
Dyspepsia. Dysentery. Rectal fissure.
Frequent urination.
Itching skin, eruptive skin disease [dect.]. Leprosy.
Antidote for bites and stings of insects. Pediculosis destroyer.
Arthritis with calcification. Back stiffness. Inflammatory pain of the joints. Gouty
pains. Tender heels and soles when walking. Sprains. Muscle twitching.
Tissue conditions
Cleanser and purifier of the system. Indicated for lack of heat in the body, yet heat
of the bedclothes at night is intolerable. An indication is chilliness, aggravation by
warmth and motion. Twitching of the muscles.
External use
Acne. Wounds caused by sharp penetrating objects.
Rectal fissures. Sprained ankles.
Strong decoction - external as a compress for skin disease, destroys pediculosis.
Dosage and mode of application
Dried fol Sig 5g. Infusium Sig 60ml
References. 127 p460. 189 p165.

Leonurus cardiaca [Motherwort]

Constituents
Alkaloids – betonicine, leonurine, stachydrine. Flavonoids. Volatile oil. Tannin up to 8%. Bitter glycosides. Diterpene lactone. Phenolic glycoside.

Primary pharmacological action: Antispasmodic.

Therapeutic classes
Diffusively relaxant. Antioxidant. Antiarrhythmic. Cardiotonic. Hypotensive. Carminative. Hepatic. Antidiarrhoeal.
Diuretic - suppression from cold.
Uterine stimulant - emmenagogue. Uterotonic.
Nervine - sedative.

Medicinal indications [Venus]
Arrhythmia. Tachycardia [with neurosis]. Auricular fibrillation. Neurogenic cardiac disorders. Palpitations. Endocarditis. Pericarditis.
Flatulence. Diarrhoea. Typhoid.
Amenorrhoea. Dysmenorrhoea. Menopausal neurasthenia/flushes. PMS.
Anxiety. Cramp. Convulsions. Depression. Epilepsy. Insomnia. Panic.
Schizophrenia. Thyroid tachycardia. Goitre. Cerebral ischaemia.

Tissue conditions
Acts as a diffusive heart tonic. Relaxing and antispasmodic to heart activity. Autonomic imbalance causing functional and organic cardiac rhythmic disturbances. Slowly acting adjuvant in functional and neurogenic heart disease. Panic and hormonal disturbances causing palpitations. As a sedative in nervous patients it allays irritability. Nervous spasmodic pain of the stomach, gall bladder or intestines. Thyroid hypertonicity [hyperfunction].

Preparations
False labour pain with Ballota and Rubus.
Hypertension with Ballota, Crataegus, Phytolacca.
Cardio vascular disturbances - with Melissa, Convallaria, Crataegus.
Sedative acts well with Valeriana or Verbena.
Emmenagogue with Cimicifuga.
Dysmenorrhoea with Viburnum opulus, Viburnum prunifoleum.

Dosage and mode of application
Dried herba Sig 4g
Tincturae Sig 10ml
Liquidum extractum Sig 4ml

References
43 p130. 111 p505. 188 p297. 189 p192. 192 p367. 246 p372. 394 p267.

Leptandra virginica [Blackroot]

Constituents
Volatile oil. Saponins. Tannin.

Primary pharmacological action:
A mild relaxing hepatic to the ducts and gall bladder.

Therapeutic classes
Antiseptic.
Stomach tonic. Hepatic, choleretic and cholagogue. Cathartic.
Diaphoretic. Remittent fever - typhoid, malaria.
Medicinal indications
Acute hepatitis. Cholelithiasis. Duodenitis. Jaundice - non-obstructive. Intestinal ulceration. Hepatitis. Enteritis. Diarrhoea. Constipation associated with liver and gall bladder disease. Portal obstruction with oedema. Typhoid. Dysentery. Colic. Bilious remittent fever cholera, malaria, typhoid when the liver or spleen are congested or disordered.
Skin disease. Depression.
Tissue conditions
Local ganglionic vasorelaxant to the liver and gall bladder. Pain in the liver or gall bladder with sub scapular pain.
Leptandra frees bile from congested liver tubules and a constricted gall bladder. Bile flowing from a previously constricted gall bladder has a more sticky character and is darker. Leptandra removes morbid obstructions in a mild and natural manner promoting the flow of bile without causing intestinal irritation. Malaria with hepatic involvement. Hepatic soreness, constipation, inactivity of the intestinal secretions [dry stool], thirst, anorexia, headache. Pyrexia in the early stages are relieved. Acute conditions with pain or jaundice from acute obstruction, consequent depression, bitter taste, jaundice [hepatitis], pain, flatulent colic, clay coloured stools.
Preparations
Hepatic sluggishness, torpor, inactivity - with stimulating agents e.g. Capsicum, Gentiana, Jateorhiza.
Congenial with Chelidonium, Dioscorea, Podophyllum.
Rectal disorders with Astringents e.g. Collinsonia.
Skin disorders with alterative vasotonic e.g. Rumex, Iris or Smilax.
Dosage and mode of application
Tincturae rad Sig 4ml
Liquidum extractum Sig 4ml
References. 43 p229. 111 p507. 126 p443. 176 p312. 189 p37. 254 p100. 262

Leptospermum petersoni

[Lemon scented tea tree - not melaleuca].
Leptospermum scoparium [Manuka] is 20 times stronger than Ti Tree oil against gram positive organisms and against dermatophyte infections.

Constituents
Flavonoids

Primary pharmacological action: Antiseptic.

Therapeutic classes
Anti microbial. Antiviral.
Carminative.
Sedative.
Medicinal indications
Fungal infections. Bacterial infections.
Tissue conditions
Used as an anti microbial agent when infection attacks the respiratory mucous membrane. Calms the nerves when there is irritability.
Preparations
Tincturae Sig 1ml
References
275, 1995, No. 44, 25-7

Levisticum officinale [Lovage]

Constituents
Volatile oils - phthalides [sedative and antispasmodic]. Essential oil. Terpenes.
Bitters. furanocoumarins. Sterols. Resin.

Primary pharmacological action: Diuretic.

Therapeutic classes
Antimicrobial. Anticatarrhal. Expectorant.
Carminative. Stomachic. Cholagogue.
Diuretic. Antilithic. Diaphoretic.
Emmenagogue. Parturient.
Antispasmodic. Sedative.
Medicinal indications [Sun]
Catarrh. Aphthous ulcers. Tonsillitis.
Anorexia. Dyspepsia. Gastritis. Flatulence. Flatulent colic.
Oedema. Cystitis. Renal oedema. Urinary calculi. Gout. Enuresis.
Dysmenorrhoea. Muscle spasm.
Tissue conditions
Stimulates the kidneys and uterus. Urinary tract inflammation.
Cautions
Pregnancy. Renal disease with care.
External use
Aphthous ulcers, tonsillitis - mouthwash.
Preparations
Flatulence, colic, intestinal spasm with Chamaemelum nobile, Angelica.
Dosage and mode of application
Dried fruct/rad/rhiz. Sig 4g
Liquidum extractum Sig 2ml
References
42 p130. 188 p277. 189 p177. 192 p336. 246 p300.

Ligustrum lucidum [Privet]

Constituents
Glycoside - Ligustrin. Bitter - Ligustron, Syringopikrin. Essential fatty acids.

Primary pharmacological action:
CNS stimulant & trophorestorative.

Therapeutic classes
Astringent. Tonic. Antioxidant.
Oropharyngeal disorders.
Diuretic.
Uterine tonic.
Immunostimulant.
Medicinal indications [Moon]
Macular degeneration. Retinitis.
Aphthous ulcers. Ulceration of the ears, mouth, stomach, intestines or bladder.
Diarrhoea.
Metrorrhagia. Atrophic vulvo vaginitis. Menopause.
Dizzyness. Acute cerebral infarction. Dementia. Parkinsons disease.
Fatigue. Grey hair. Hyperactivity. Insomnia. Irritability.
Allergic reactions: hypersensitivity, asthma, angioedema, Urtica.
Tissue conditions
Similar effect to Ginkgo. Increases cerebral blood flow. Astringent tonic to the
mucous membranes in catarrhal or ulcerative conditions of the gastro intestinal
and genito urinary tracts.
External use
Oral conditions - decoct.
Ear ulceration with offensive discharge – guttae.
Candida - lotion, crem.
Vulvo-vaginitis with Althea.
Dosage and mode of application
Decoctum fol/bacc Sig 15ml
Tincturae fol/bacc Sig 4ml
References
126 p445. 188 p313. 246 p323. 253 p14.

Ligusticum porteri [Osha]

Constituents
Bitters. Glycosides. Essential oil. Resin. Silica.

Primary pharmacological action: Stimulating diaphoretic.

Therapeutic classes
Aromatic. Antiviral.
Expectorant. Carminative.
Analgesic. Immunostimulant. Antipyretic. Antiparasitic.
Medicinal indications
Coughs. Colds. Influenza. Sinusitis. Pharyngitis. Bronchitis. Emphysema.
Tuberculosis. Silicosis.
Gastroenteritis. Colitis.
Amenorrhoea. Dysmenorrhoea. Retained placenta. Pyrexia. Measles.
Tissue conditions
A general stimulating remedy to mucous surfaces. Stimulates natural interferons.
Cautions
Pregnancy.
External use
Ligusticum porteri topically kills ectoparasites.
Dosage and mode of application
Tincturae rad Sig 3ml

Lilium tigrinum [Tiger lily]

Primary pharmacological action: Antispasmodic.

Therapeutic classes
Antiemetic. Parturient. Vulnerary. Antivenomous.
Medicinal indications [Moon]
Vomiting of pregnancy. Dysmenorrhoea. Ovaritis. Uterine prolapse. Uterine carcinoma. Bites – Adder snake.
Tissue conditions
Encourages uterine subinvolution. Eases the pain of uterine prolapse.
Restores hair growth.
Dosage and mode of application
Tincturae herba Sig 0.5ml
References. 126 p445. 176 p484. 228 p267&339.

Linaria vulgaris [Yellow toadflax]

Constituents
Alkaloid – peganine. Choline. Flavonoid glycosides – linarin, pectolinarin.
Tannin. Mucilage.

Primary pharmacological action: Depurative.

Therapeutic classes
Ophthalmic. Astringent. Vasotonic alterative [blood tonic]. Detergent.
Hepatic. Splenic. Cathartic.
Diuretic. Lithuria.
Uterine tonic. Dermatological agent.
Medicinal indications [Mars]
Tuberculosis.
Jaundice. Cholecystitis. Liver obstructions. Jaundice. Spleen disorders.
Constipation. Haemorrhoids.
Oedema. Cystitis. Sciatica.
Lymphadenitis - Bubonic plague.
Expels placenta.
Dermal ulcers. Macules. Scrophula.
Tissue conditions
Dissolves obstructions within the tissues of the intestines, kidneys and bladder.
Improves tissue nutrition and blood condition.
External use
Dermal disorders – sores, ulcers, macules – compress/lotion.
Haemorrhoids – poultice.
Combinations
With Cinnamomum or Cinchona.
Dosage and mode of application
Infusium Sig 30ml
References
147 p417. 188 p425. 189 p303. 253 p14.

Linum usitatissimum [Linseed, Flaxseed]

Constituents
Fixed oil up to 45%. Omega 3 & 6 essential polyunsaturated fatty acids known as Alpha-linolenic acid is metabolised to prostaglandins. Prostglandins are chemical messengers; hormone substances, they regulate blood pressure and clotting, heart rate, vascular dilation and immune responses.
Resin. Phosphates. Phyto oestrogens. Lignans. Sterols. Triterpenes.
Cyanogenic glycoside – linamarin, linustatin. Mucilage up to 10%.

Primary pharmacological action: Demulcent.

Therapeutic classes
Vasotonic alterative. Allays inflammation. Atherosclerosis.
Hypercholesterolaemia.
Antitussive. Expectorant. Pectoral.
Bulk laxative.
Antispasmodic. Hormonal adaptogenic.
Emollient. Vulnerary. Dermatological agent.
Antineoplastic.
Medicinal indications [Mercury]
Hypertension.
Allergies. Coughs. Sore throat. Asthma. Bronchitis. Pneumonia. Pleurisy.
Gastritis. Diabetes. Enteritis. IBS. Diverticulitis. Dysentery. Diarrhoea. Colic.
Spasmodic colitis. Constipation. Laxative abuse.
Urinary inflammation. Nephritis. Gonorrhoea. Dysmenorrhoea.
Arthritis. Systemic lupus erythematosus.
Abscess. Dry or itchy skin. Furunculosis. Psoriasis.
Tissue conditions
It is antispasmodic and demulcent in inflammatory conditions the gastro intestinal, respiratory and urinary systems. Indicated for inflammation of the stomach or intestines through its action upon the mucous membranes it aids resolution of the inflammatory phase and hastens suppuration. Regulates the intestinal function and is a gentle laxative.
All forms of spasmodic bronchial coughs.
Flaxseed lignans are associated with luteal phase lengthening, fewer anovulatory cycles, and a decreased tendency to ovarian dysfunction.
External use
Poultice of crushed seed alone or combined with mustard for bronchitis, ulceration, superficial or deep inflammation. A poultice allays irritation and pain and promotes suppuration.

Furunculosis – drawing poultice.
Burns and scalds - the oil or crushed sem as a wound dressing.
Bruises, sprains, strains - poultice.

Preparations

Furunculosis or abscess with powdered Lobelia.
As an addition to add demulcent activity in cough medicines.

Dosage and mode of application

Unstable and destroyed by heat, light and air. Take with water.
Infusium sem Sig 30ml
Sem whole or crushed Sig 10g. Granulated gruel used for mucilaginous action.
Oleum Sig 30ml
Tincturae Sig 10ml
Liquidum extracum Sig 2ml
Fomentation Sig 60g Linum flour.

References

43 p132. 126 p446. 142 p112. 192 p215. 230 p39. 246 p216. 277 Vol. 77, No 5, p1215. 394 p134.

Liriosma ovata [Ptychopetalum olacoides/Muira puama]

Constituents
Alkaloid known as muirapuanine. Phytosterols.

Primary pharmacological action: Aphrodisiac.

Therapeutic classes
Astringent. Aromatic. Stomachic.
Nervine stimulant and tonic. Antirheumatic.
Medicinal indications
Nervous stomach. Diarrhoea.
Neuralgia. Polio. Rheumatism.
Impotency. Menstrual disturbance. PMS. Nervous exhaustion. Depression.
Tissue conditions
Muira acts upon the spinal nerves, stimulating these nerves to improved function.
Enhances the sex drive in impotence/sexual dysfunction, frigidity, performance anxiety.
Dosage and mode of application
Powder rad/stem Sig 2g
Liquidum extractum Sig 5ml
References
43 132. 44 p161. 189 p195.

Lobelia inflata [Lobelia]

Constituents
Up to 0.5% alkaloids - the most important is Lobeline, it is a piperidine alkaloid.
It stimulates the carotid sinus. Piperidine group chemoreceptors are
bronchodilatory and block dopamine receptors. Bitter glycosides - lobelacrine.
August and September is best time for gathering. Resin. Gum. Volatile oil.
Chelidonic acid.

Primary pharmacological action:
Relaxant to the complete vasomotor system –
neuromuscular and autonomic.

Therapeutic classes
Relaxant. Stimulant. Arterial sedative.
Antiasmatic. Expectorant. Respiratory stimulant.
Emetic [irritant]. Cholagogue. Hepatic.
Diaphoretic. Antipyretic.
Antispasmodic. Nicotine withdrawal.

Medicinal indications
Angina. Cardiac neurosis.
Respiratory stimulant. Diphtheria. Asthma. Bronchitis. Pleurisy. Pneumonia.
Pertussus. Laryngismus stridulus. Dry or persistent coughs. Influenza.
Nicotine habit.
Hiccough. Nausea and persistent vomiting. Cholelithiasis. Hepatitis. Strangulated
hernia. Obstructed gall stones. Biliary colic. Intestinal spasm.
Muscular spasm. Myositis. Cramps. Sprains and strains. Rheumatic nodules.
Panic. Epilepsy. Tetanus.
Convulsions from pyrexia or meningitis. Intermittent fevers. Pyrexia in the
sthenic [also known as athletic habitus].
Puerpural eclampsia. Os rigidity. Smallpox.

Tissue conditions
Equalises the circulation and relieves tension therein from inflammation or
pyrexia. Removes tension by relaxing smooth muscle in the arteries. Stimulates
the carotid chemoreceptors and causes bronchodilation in small dosage. Large
doses are depressant. As an all round relaxant it will remove any tension in the
nerves, muscles [spasm] and mucous membranes.
Any accumulation of mucus is instantly removed after a full dose of lobelia.
Acute inflammatory conditions can be aided by the addition of lobelia - pleurisy,
pneumonia, hepatitis. Lung conditions are best treated with a syrup of lobelia as
this is less nauseating. Children suffering from coughs where there is a danger of

suffocation a dose will remove obstruction. Spasm within the trachea and bronchial tree. Rebalances the secretions of the skin when encumbered by dryness or deficient secretions. Large doses can stimulate the respiratory centre in the medulla oblongata to induce vomiting. Parturition - it relaxes the perineum and Os cervix. The use of Lobelia will not cause abortion of a healthy foetus.

Cautions
Restrictions apply. Dosage is determined by the relief of symptoms.
Avoid in CVA, paralysis, tendency to haemorrhage, depleted vital force.
Lobelia will entirely relax the uterus with constant use.
The whole body becomes relaxed with full doses and persistent use.

External use
Furuncles - powder paste.
Sprains and acute injuries to the joints, rheumatic nodules, intercostal myalgia – emplastrum.
Tetanus, arthritic joint pain, inflammatory conditions - Liniment Ol Lobelia.
Strangulated hernia - fomentation.
Bites and stings - lotion.

Preparations
Best combined with a diffusive [Capsicum or Mentha piperita] and nervine remedy for better effects.
Asthma with Capsicum, Euphoria, Drosera, Grindelia, Symplocarpus.
Expectorant with Cephaelis, Sanguinaria, Polygala senega.
Antiemetic use a tiny dose.
Lobelia emetic will remove obstructions in the stomach and liver.
Intestinal obstruction/spasm - give an enema of Lobelia and or Nepeta.
Strangulated hernia, intussusception, faecal impaction - enema.
With Zingiber to stimulate the capillaries and so prevent congestion in pneumonia.
Os or perineal rigidity - use small doses.

Dosage and mode of application
Powdered herba Sig 2g [Ref 390]
Solid extract Sig 4g
Simple Lobelia tincturae [1:8] Sig 2ml
Tincturae herba 1:8 Sig 2ml
Liquidum extractum herba Sig 0.6ml
Syrupus Lobelia 1:4 Sig 2ml
Emulsion expectorant et Linum usitatissimum.
Acidum Tincturae Lobelia Acid tincture of Lobelia. 1:10 Sig 4ml
Topically as per above dosage.

References
BPC 1973. 43 p134. 111 p519. 126 p455. 176 235. 188 p299. 192 p334. 230 p75. 233 p149.

Lotus corniculus [Bird's foot trefoil]

Constituents
Hydrocyanic acid is antispasmodic.

Primary pharmacological action: Antispasmodic.

Medicinal indications
Nervous disorders - anxiety, palpitations, depression, insomnia, vertigo.
Tissue conditions
An antispasmodic nervine remedy.
Dosage and mode of application
Infusium Sig 10g
Liquidum extractum Sig 1ml

Lycium chinense [Chinese sour date]

Constituents
Sterols. Linoleic acid. Carotine. Vitamins C, B1, B2.

Primary pharmacological action: Hepatic and Nephritic.

Therapeutic classes
Ophthalmic. Anticholesterolaemic. Antisclerotic.
Hepatic regenerator.
Mild tonic to the kidneys. Antirheumatic. Insecticide.
Tissue conditions
Exerts a gentle tonic action upon the liver and kidneys. Eye weakness often
associated with organ weakness. Indicated in low backache and general rheumatic
conditions. Weakness of the legs.
Dosage and mode of application
Dried rad Sig 5g
Tincturae Sig 5ml
References
47 p607. Albert Y. Leung, PhD. Herbalgram no 32.

Lycopus europaeus [Gypsywort]

Constituents
Bitters. Tannin. Volatile oils. Flavone glucuronides up to 0.22% including luteolin glucuronide [antigonadotrophic].

Primary pharmacological action:
Astringent tonic to the lungs. Thyroactive.

Therapeutic classes
Ophthalmic. Aromatic. Stimulating tonic which influences the mucous membrane.
Allays inflammation.
Circulatory diffusive [balances the circulation]. Haemostatic. Cardiac sedative.
Pulmonary tuberculosis.
Gastric tonic.
Sedative - mild. Thyroactive. Intermittent fever. Febrifuge.

Medicinal indications
Retinal haemorrhage. Cardiac irritability or oppression. Endocarditis. Pericarditis.
Palpitation. Tachycardia. Myocardial hypertrophy.
Chronic debilitating coughs. Tuberculosis early stages. Haemoptysis. Acute pulmonary complaints e.g. Pneumonia.
Gastritis. Enteritis. Diarrhoea. Dysentery. Typhoid. Tubercular diarrhoea.
Thyrotoxicosis. Reduces breast milk.
It will relax peripheral nerves to ease nervous tension in the CNS.

Tissue conditions
Lycopus is given in thyrotoxic [hyperthyroid] states to counteract thyroxine. As a thyroid sedative it often requires reinforcement with other remedies.
Antihaemorrhagic [passive haemorrhage] to the lungs, intestine, kidneys and uterus.
Slows and strengthens the pulse by equalising the circulation and nerve activity.
It improves the tone of the heart, reducing irritability and irregularity. In tachycardia dependent upon irritation of the cardiac nerve centres or when arising from organic lesions. Cardiac hypertrophy [constricts cardiac non striated muscle fibres]. Heart disease with irritability, irregular beat, dyspnoea and praecordial oppression. Tachycardia in smokers. Palpitations with anxiety. Relieves gastro intestinal irritation. Acute pulmonary complaints where a sedative is required in tuberculosis, emphysema, acute bronchitis. Muco purulent sputum of chronic bronchitis, pneumonia or tuberculosis.

Cautions
Breast feeding.

Pharmacopoeia

External use
Fistula - use an injection to support healing.
Urethral ulceration – irrigation.
Preparations
Pulmonary haemorrhage with Capsicum, Stachys palustris and Cinnamomum or Cephalis and Cinnamomum.
Endo or pericarditis with Convallaria and Selenicerus.
In hot infusion it influences the capillaries, soothes arterial excitement and tones the veins.
Cold preparations influence the GUT.
Tonic cough syrup – combine with Inula, Symphytum or Prunus.
Dosage and mode of application
Dried herba Sig 3g
Infusium Sig 30ml
Tincturae Sig 5ml
Liquidum extractum Sig 2ml
References
43 p136. 111 p549. 126 p464. 192 p93. 246 p383. 263, 61, 1995, 373.

Malva sylvestris [Common mallow]

Constituents
Flavonoid glycosides. Mucilage.

Primary pharmacological action: Demulcent.

Therapeutic classes
Astringent. Expectorant. Pectoral. Allays inflammation. Nephritis.
Medicinal indications
Colds. Bronchitis. Asthma.
Laxative.
Tissue conditions
Demulcent and soothing action upon the mucous membranes similar to Althea.
External use
Sore throat - gargle.
Infected finger wounds, insect bites, bee stings, skin inflammation - fol poultice.
Dosage and mode of application
Infusium Sig 30ml
Liquidum extractum Sig 8ml
References
111 p555. 127 p509. 246 p240.

Marrubium vulgare [White hoarhound]

Constituents
Alkaloids – betonicine up to 0.3%, stachydrine up to 0.3%. Bitter diterpenes up to 1% marrubin. Volatile oils mainly monoterpenes. Flavonoids mainly apigenin, luteolin and quercetin. Sterols. Mucilage. Vitamin C.

Primary pharmacological action:
Expectorant and tonic to the respiratory mucous membranes.

Therapeutic classes
Stimulant. Astringent. Diffusive. Antibacterial – Pseudomonas aeruginosa.
Antifungal – Trichophyton. Cardiac. Pectoral.
Aromatic. Bitter tonic. Emetic and laxative in large doses. Hepatic. Choleretic.
Diuretic. Diaphoretic. Antipyretic.
Antispasmodic. Sedative. Dermatological agent. Antivenomous. Antiparasitic.
Medicinal indications [Mercury]
Catarrh. Colds. Sinusitis. Laryngitis. Laryngismus stridulus. Asthma. [Acute]
bronchitis. Non productive coughs. Pertussus. Tuberculosis.
Mercurial ptyalism. Anorexia. Dyspepsia. Flatulence. Hepatitis. Intestinal
parasites. Vermifuge. Oedema. Snake and dog bites. Dermal ulcers. Malaria.
Tissue conditions
Increases the secretions of the respiratory tract and skin. Indicated for dry, non
productive coughs and irritable states of the mucosa. Increases bronchial mucus
secretions where deficiency of mucus and congestion of bronchial mucous
membranes exist. Diaphoretic activity relieves hyperaemia of the lungs by
diffusive action upon the capillaries. Tyler says it is anti-arrhythmic in therapeutic
doses and pro-arrhythmic in large doses.
Preparations
Earache - instil infusium guttae.
Cough/Bronchitis/Pertussus with Althea/Glycyrrhiz/Hyssopus/Primula &/or Zing
Hoarhound candy
Infusium [1:1] 15ml. Sucrose 1k. Aqua 550ml
Reduce the marc to firm consistency. Test by dropping a small amount into water,
marc should set. At this point add the infusium and mix. Put into moulds to set.
Dosage and mode of application
Dried herba Sig 5g
Liquidium extractum Sig 4ml
Syrupus BPC 1949 Sig 4ml
References
43 p136. 188 p232. 246 p367. 272, 1993, 5 [3] 16. 285, 9, 1995, p281. 394 p197.

Marsdenia condurango [Condurango]

Constituents
Glycosides. Essential oil. Sterols. Starch.

Primary pharmacological action :
Stimulating Vasotonic alterative.

Therapeutic classes
Antihaemorrhagic.
Aperitif. Stomachic. Anti ulcer. Gastric sedative and anodyne.
Sexually transmitted disease.
Anodyne. Antineoplastic.
Medicinal indications
Anorexia. Nervous dyspepsia. Stimulates the appetite. Chronic ulceration and carcinoma of the stomach.
Oedema. Syphilis.
Tissue conditions
Anaesthetises the tongue and eases pain of gastric ulcers or vomiting.
Toner and corrector of stomach function.
Cautions
Use small doses in irritable stomach conditions.
Preparations
Anorexia – Acorus, Chamaemelum nobile, Humulus.
Dosage and mode of application
Powdered bacc Sig 4g
Liquidum extractum Sig 4ml
References
BPC 1923. 43 p138. 126 p319. 192 p160/161. 246 p333.

Maytenus buchanani [Gymnosporia buchananii]

Constituents
Some 200 species are used medicinally.
An ansa macrolide called maytanside which is antitumour and antileukaemic.
Spermidine alkaloids - celacinnine and celallocinine. Sesquiterpine alkaloids
maytoline. Tannin. Extensively studied at the national cancer institute in
Bethesda, Maryland, USA.

Primary pharmacological action:
Antineoplastic. Antileukaemic.

Therapeutic classes
Astringent. Anti infective.
Stomachic. Mild laxative.
Aphrodisiac. Contraceptive.
Anodyne.
Immunostimulant.
Vulnerary. Antivenomous.
Medicinal indications
Aphthous ulcers. Toothache. Earache.
Haemoptysis. Pneumonia. Tuberculosis.
Dysentery. Constipation.
Rheumatic pain.
Infertility. Epilepsy.
Furunculosis. Leukaemia.
External use
Furunculosis, aphthous ulcers – decoction lotion.
Ulcers and wounds - apply powdered bark.
Dosage and mode of application
Dried cort 1g
References
53.

Medicago sativa [Alfalfa]

Constituents
Minerals - chlorides, sulphur, phosphorus, potassium. 12 Amino acids. Alkaloids
– asparagine, trigonelline. Coumarins. Flavone – Tricin [antispasmodic] is poorly
absorbed form the GIT. Silica. Phytoestrogens.
Vitamin A, B1, B6, B12, C, E, K. Folic acid. Pantothenic acid. Chlorophyll.
Carotines.

Primary pharmacological action: Nutritive tonic.

Therapeutic classes
Antiscorbutic. Anti anaemic. Anti cholesterolaemic. Anti haemorrhagic.
Smooth muscle antispasmodic.
Vulnerary.
Medicinal indications
Blood purifier. Purpura.
Acute infections of the upper respiratory tract. Sore throat. Hay fever.
In chronic lung tuberculosis it supports the nutrition of the organism.
Alkalizer of the body. Peptic ulcers. Constipation
Tonic to the brain and spinal cord.
Dosage and mode of application
Infusium Sig 10g
Liquidum extractum Sig 10ml
References
43 p 140. 176 p136. 189 p177. 246 p204. 315, Vol 1 [1].

Melaleuca alternifolia [Tee tree]

Constituents
Sesquiterpenes – pinene. Monoterpenes – terpinen-4-ol, alpha-terpinol and alpha pinene. Volatile oil. There are 79 species of Melaleuca.

Primary pharmacological action: Immunostimulant.

Therapeutic classes
Antifungal – Tinea, Trichophyton.
Antibacterial – MRSI infection, Staphylococcus aureus, Staphylococcus epidermis and Propionibacterium acnes. Expectorant.
Dermatological agent. Vulnerary. Antiparasitic.
Medicinal indications
Sinusitis. Respiratory infections. Colds. Bronchitis.
Toxic shock syndrome.
Abscess. Acne. Intertrigo. Wounds.
Tinea – pedis. Trichophyton - ringworm. Pediculosis.
Cautions
Oleum at high strength may produce skin sensitivity.
External use
Oleum can be used up to 80% strength.
Oral candida – dilute oleum 5gtt with vehicle e.g. Chondrus.
Respiratory disturbances – inhalation 5gtt aqua frig.
Toxic shock syndrome/Staphylococcus aureus infection,
Vaginal candida – Pessaries.
Acne, dermal parasites, warts, wounds – crem, gel or oleum.
Dosage and mode of application.
Oleum Sig 5gtt. Inhalation.
Crem et Ung Sig 20gtt et 60ml base.
References
192 p538. 239 p158. 264, June 1994. 239 p158. 265, 1995, Vol. 7 [3] p57-62.
296, 2001, 358 [9289] 1245. 316, 2000, 45 (5) 639-43

Melia azederach [White cedar]

Constituents
Alkaloid - margosine. Terpenes. Steroids. Anthraquinones.

Primary pharmacological action: Anti infective.

Therapeutic classes
Astringent. Deobstruent. Allays inflammation. Tonic.
Emetic. Anthelmintic – bacc, fol.
Emmenagogue – bacc. Anodyne. Antipyretic. Insecticidal – fol.
Medicinal indications
Infections. Colds. Asthma. Influenza.
Constipation. Worms.
Leprosy. Tropical parasites. Pediculosis. Malaria.
Headaches. Pyrexia.
Tissue conditions
Worm fevers and infantile convulsions.
Cautions
Berries and seeds are very strong and used as an anthelmintic, they can cause
gastro intestinal haemorrhage. Pregnancy.
External use
Eczema and Pediculosis – infusion and decoction.
Spraying plants with the aqueous extract of the fol keeps away the locust.
Dosage and mode of application
Powdered fol/flos/rad/bacc Sig 0.5g
Tincturae fol/flos/rad Sig 1ml
References
189 p20. 262 p56.

Melilotus officinalis [Sweet melilot]

Constituents
Glycosides - coumarin [anticoagulant] up to 0.45%. Melitoside dries to form free coumarin. Flavonoids. Tannin. Mucilage.

Primary pharmacological action: Antispasmodic.

Therapeutic classes
Ophthalmic. Allays inflammatory oedema. Antimicrobial. Astringent – mild. Antithrombotic. Anticoagulant. Venous insufficiency.
Aromatic. Expectorant.
Diuretic. Urinary antiseptic. Antirheumatic.
Analgesic. Sedative. Immunomodulatory. Antineoplastic. Emollient.

Medicinal indications [Jupiter]
Blepharitis. Conjunctivitis. Hordeolum. Earache. Hypertension. Ischaemic heart disease. Varicose veins. Thrombophlebitis. Phlebitis.
Lymphoedema. Elephantiasis. Post traumatic inflammation.
Flatulence. Intestinal colic. Haemorrhoids. Filiarasis. Brucellosis. Mononucleosis. Mycoplasmosis. Toxoplasmosis. Quassa fever. Psittacosis.
Colic. Dysuria. Renal cell carcinoma. Prostatic carcinoma. Rheumatism. Sciatica. Neuralgic soreness of the head, stomach or ovary. Headache. Insomnia. Tension. Dysmenorrhoea. Melanoma. Burns.

Tissue conditions
Headache of a throbbing character with a feeling of fullness together with cold hands and feet indicate Melilotus. Supportive treatment in deep vein thrombosis and thrombophlebitis. Headache from a disordered stomach. Painful conditions of the abdominal viscera with coldness of the extremities and soreness or tenderness upon pressure. Smooth muscle relaxant. Recurring neuralgia from cold or fatigue. Colic with flatus or diarrhoea.

External use
Hordeolum – compress.
Painful joints, contusions, sprains and bruising – compress/poultice/oleum.
Neuralgia – compress.

Cautions
Antidote is Vitamin K.

Dosage and mode of application
Infusium herba Sig 30ml
Tincturae Sig 5ml

References
126 p477. 188 p290. 189 p189. 246 p202.

Melissa officinalis [Lemon balm]

Constituents
Volatile oil around 0.375% which contains monoterpenes e.g. citronella [up to 40%] - these are relaxant and sedative to the CNS. Volatile oil – geraniol is antiseptic. Phenol carboxyl acid. Flavonoids - rosmarinic acid up to 4%. Triterpenes – ursolic acid.

Primary pharmacological action: Antispasmodic.

Therapeutic classes
Antimicrobial. Antibacterial – mycobacterium phlei, Streptococcus hemolytica.
Antiviral – herpes virus 1 & 2, herpes labialis, HIV 1, Newcastle disease, mumps.
Hypotensive.
Aromatic bitter. Carminative. Stomachic.
Diaphoretic. Febrifuge.
Emmenagogue.
Dermatological agent. Antivenomous. Vulnerary.
Analgesic. Antidepressant. Hypnotic. Sedative. Tranquilliser.
Medicinal indications [Jupiter]
Catarrh. Influenza. Feverish colds. Herpes simplex. Allergy. Asthma.
Palpitations
Anorexia. Dyspepsia. Flatulence. Colic. Dysentery. IBS. Intestinal spasm.
Amenorrhoea. Dysmenorrhoea. Retained placenta. Fertility cycle emotional
disorders. Menopausal flushes. Impotence/sexual dysfunction.
Arthritis – pain.
Anxiety. Depression. Headaches. Insomnia. Restlessness. Fainting. Nervous
irritability. Senility. Chronic fatigue syndrome. Nightmares.
Eczema. Venomous bites.
Tissue conditions
Nervousness [anxiety or depression] affecting the gastro intestinal tract –
dyspepsia. Eases flatulent distension causing palpitations. Relaxes gastro
intestinal and uterine smooth muscle. Supports calmness. Cognitive function –
attention and memory span improvement.
Cautions
Hypothyroidism – it is suggested that Melissa is hypothyroid. Pregnancy.
Preparations
Flatulence with Mentha piperita.
External use
Herpes apply dilute oleum or succus from bruised leaves.
Wounds – spray dilute oleum.

Pharmacopoeia

Dosage and mode of application
Dried herba Sig 5g
Dry extract Sig 1g
Tincturae Sig 10ml
Liquidum extractum herba Sig 4ml

References
43 p141. 192 p364. 239 p170. 251 p13. 263, 57 2 p105. 281 1999, 15. 389. 394 p231.

Menispermum canadensis [Yellow parilla]

Constituents
Alkaloid - menispermum and berberine.

Primary pharmacological action: Vasotonic alterative.

Therapeutic classes
Stimulant. Expectorant.
Bitter aperitif. Cholagogue. Laxative. Tonic.
Diuretic.
Medicinal indications
Pulmonary affections.
Dyspepsia - atonic. Constipation.
Rheumatic disorders. Syphilis.
Dermatological agent. Lymphadenopathy.
Tissue conditions
Vasotonic alterative tonic for the mucous membranes and secretions. Stimulates the stomach [appetite], liver and gall bladder. For chronic congestive conditions of the viscera - congestive conditions. Tongue coated at the base or with a red tip, poor appetite and constipation are indications.
Cautions
Full doses cause purging and vomiting.
External use
Gout and skin disease.
Preparations
Arctium, Rumex, Fraxinus.
Dosage and mode of application
Powdered rad Sig 2g
Liquidum extractum Sig 4 ml
References
111 p560. 126 p478. 127 p610. 147 p416.

Mentha piperita [Peppermint]

Constituents
Essential oil up to 4%, mainly menthol [around 78%], menthone. Esters mainly methyl acetate. Triterpenes – dissolve gallstones, lower biliary cholesterol, raise biliary lecithin, diuretic. Flavonoids – luteolin, menthoside. Tannin. Resin. Gum. Acetic acid.

Primary pharmacological action:
Gastric normaliser. Diffusive stimulant.

Therapeutic classes
Antibacterial – Pseudomonas aeruginosa, Streptococcus pyogenes, Staphylococcus aureus.
Antifungal – Candida.
Antiviral – Herpes simplex, influenza, infectious mononucleosis.
Antiseptic. Antiparasitic. Astringent. Decongestant. Tonic. Refrigerant.
Antitussive.
Aromatic. Carminative. Antiemetic. Cholagogue. Choleretic.
Diaphoretic.
Emmenagogue. Anti galactogenic.
Externally - analgesic, anaesthetic, cooling and counterirritant. Antipruritic.
Sedative. Antispasmodic.

Medicinal indications [Venus]
Colds. Nasal and respiratory catarrh. Irritating coughs. Sinusitis. Paroxysmal rhinorrhoea. Influenza. Oral inflammation.
Hiccups. Gastritis. Nausea. Vomiting. Stomach/intestinal flatulence.
Cholelithiasis. Biliary colic. Diarrhoea. IBS. Mucous colitis. Constipation.
Cholera.
Dysmenorrhoea. Morning sickness. Impotence/sexual dysfunction.
Depression. Anxiety. Migraine. Panic. Insomnia. Motion sickness.
Myalgia. Sciatica. Neuralgia.
Convulsions and spasm in infants. Pyrexia.
Itchy skin. Poison ivy dermatitis. Urticaria.

Tissue conditions
Increases capillary blood flow. Antispasmodic [blocks muscle contraction created by serotonin]. A smooth muscle relaxant to the oesophagus and sphincter.
Indicated for reflex pain and vomiting. Anaesthetises gastric sensory nerve endings. Increases peristalsis. Headaches consequent upon gastric disorders.
Renders urine sterile. The oil is used for flavouring. Reduces breast milk.

External use
Pharyngitis, laryngitis, hayfever, sinusitis - inhalation or gargle [antiseptic] - Anodyne in neuralgia and toothache.
Wound dressing, pruritus - use as an ointment or lotion [antiseptic].
Rheumatism, neuralgia and headache - apply the dilute oleum.
Preparations
To prevent griping [carminative] it is added to purgatives.
Colds and influenza - Achillea, Eupatorium perfoliatum and Pimpinella.
Chest conditions - spray the room or inhale through a steamer.
Dosage and mode of application
Dried herba Sig 4g
Dry extract Sig 1g
Infusium herba Sig 30ml
Tincturae Sig 10ml
Liquidum extractum Sig 4ml
> **Conc Aqua Mentha piperita** Concentrated peppermint water
> Sig 0.25ml
> **Oleum** Mentha Sig 0.2ml
> **Essence Mentha piperita**
> Ol Mentha 100ml Alcohol 90% to 1000. Sig 2ml

References
43 p141/42. 111 p562. 233 p175. 251 p127. 394 p299.

Mentha pulegium [Pennyroyal]

Constituents
Volatile oil around 2% is the principle component is Pulegone. Tannin.

Primary pharmacological action: Antispasmodic.

Therapeutic classes
Diffusive stimulant. Detergent. Antiseptic. Anticatarrhal. Refrigerant - external.
Carminative. Diaphoretic.
Sedative.
Emmenagogue. Vulnerary. Antivenomous. Insect repellent.
Medicinal indications [Venus]
Cramp. Scarlatina.
Colds. Catarrh. Bronchitis. Influenza. Pneumonia. Pleurisy. Tuberculosis.
Toothache. Anorexia. Waterbrash. Flatulent colic. Nausea. Vomiting. Splenitis.
Urinary calculi. Genital itching.
Amenorrhoea. Cervical ulceration. PMS. Uterine fibroids.
Motion sickness.
Intermittent pyrexia – measles, smallpox. Repels fleas, gnats and mosquitoes.
Tissue conditions
Antispasmodic to the uterus, prostate and intestine.
Cautions
Pregnancy.
External use
Antiseptic.
Toothache or earache - mouthwash and gargle.
Oleum as a cooling antiseptic and insect repellent up to 5gtt topically.
Dosage and mode of application
Dried herba Sig 4g
Liquidum extractum Sig 4ml
References
43 p143. 111 p563. 188 p331. 228 p265. 251 p124.

Menyanthes trifoliata [Bogbean]

Constituents
Iridoid bitter glycosides loganin and foliamenthin. Pyridine alkaloids. Flavonol
glycosides. Steroids. Volatile oil. Phenolic acids. Coumarins. Triterpenoids.
Tannin. Vitamin C.

Primary pharmacological action: Bitter tonic.

Therapeutic classes
Astringent. Deobstruent.
Choleretic. Laxative.
Diuretic. Febrifuge. Antirheumatic.
Analgesic.
Dermatological agent.
Medicinal indications [Mercury]
Anorexia. Dyspepsia. Jaundice. Constipation.
Glomerulonephritis [rad]. Oedema.
Rheumatic pain, stiffness and swelling. Rheumatoid arthritis. Polymyalgia.
Intermittent and remittent fever - typhoid, malaria. Scurvy.
Tissue conditions
Stimulates the appetite. Menyanthes supports detoxification via the liver and
kidneys for the elimination of excess toxins and acids.
Cautions
Large doses are purgative. Colitis. Diarrhoea. Dysentery.
Preparations
Rheumatic disease – Achillea, Apium, Arctium, Capsicum, Filipendula.
Sciatica with Achillea, Capsicum, gaultheria and Parietaria.
Dosage and mode of application
Dried fol Sig 2g
Tincturae Sig 5ml
Liquidum extractum Sig 2ml
References
43 p144. 111 p565. 192 p80. 233 p41. 246 p327. 251 p24. 262 p75. 269 1998 Vol
19, [1] p23-25.

Mitchella repens [the use of the term squaw vine is not used as being derogatory to native American Indians]

Constituents
Alkaloids. Tannins. Mucilage.

Primary pharmacological action: Uterine tonic.

Therapeutic classes
Astringent.
Diuretic. Antilithic.
Parturient. Uterine vasotonic alterative.

Medicinal indications
Colitis. Diarrhoea.
Oedema. Suppression of urine. Gonorrhoea. Renal calculi. Dysuria.
Partus preparator. Nipple soreness. Dysmenorrhoea. Vaginitis. Spermatorrhoea.
Nervousness. Panic attacks. Neurasthenia.

Tissue conditions
Tonic to the stomach, intestines, pelvic viscera and nervous system.
Parturient action is enhanced when contractions are feeble. Irritable conditions
from weakness or exhaustion are an indication for Mitchella. Uterine tone and
neurovascular action is improved. Postpartum haemorrhage is controlled.
Emotional symptoms associated with uterine dysfunction: panic, prolapse,
amenorrhoea, dysmenorrhoea, parturition. Parturient action can be effected by
taking several weeks prior to confinement.

External use
Nipple soreness - infuse the herb and apply as cream.

Preparations
Pre partum - use for several weeks.
Avena accentuates the action of Mitchella.
Uterine atony with Aletris, Chamaelirium, Avena or Rubus.
Parturition with Caulophyllum as an antispasmodic to the uterus.

Dosage and mode of application
Dried herba Sig 4g
Liquidum extractum herba Sig 4ml

References
43 p146. 111 p566. 126 p480. 188 p402. 192 p522. 254 p66.

Morus alba/nigra [Mulberry]

Constituents
Deoxynojirimycin. Anthocyanins as cyanidin. Flavonoids as rutin, moracetin.
Glucose. Protein. Vitamin C.

Primary pharmacological action:
Hepatic autonomic trophorestorative.

Therapeutic classes
Antioxidant. Antiviral AIDS/HIV. Refrigerant.
Hypotensive.
Expectorant.
Nutritive. Hypoglycaemic. Laxative.
Diuretic. Antipyretic
Antispasmodic.
Immunostimulant.
Medicinal indications [Venus]
Hypertension. Oedema.
Colds. Coughs. Influenza. Asthma.
Rheumatic pain.
Dizzyness. Tinnitus.
Tissue conditions
Obstructions of the liver, gall bladder or spleen.
Dosage and mode of application
Succus Sig 5ml
Tincturae bacc/cort/fol/fruct Sig 4ml
References
BPC 1934. 189 p195. 297, 17/8/1991 p38.

Myrica cerifera [Bayberry/Wax myrtle]

Constituents
A flavonoid myricitrin - bactericidal and cholagogue. Tannin. Terpenoids.

Primary pharmacological action: Stimulating astringent. Vasostimulant to the involuntary muscles.

Therapeutic classes
Deobstruent. Circulatory stimulant.
Anti tubercular.
Hepatic tonic.
Uterine tonic. Antineoplastic.

Medicinal indications
Poor circulation: cold extremities. Scarlatina. Cardiac tonic. Venous tonic.
Nasal catarrh. Sinusitis. Chronic enlargement of the tonsils. Influenza.
Tuberculosis.
Pyorrhoea. Aphthous ulcers. Stomatitis. Gastritis. Jaundice. Diarrhoea. Relaxed
bowel-atonic diarrhoea. Cholera. Dysentery. Typhoid.
Menorrhagia. Parturition. Prolapse. Ulceration of the cervix.
Measles. Pyrexia.

Tissue conditions
Excessive mucus discharges. A diffusive stimulant to the circulation and for cold
extremities, chills and influenza. Stagnant capillary circulation. In large doses it
acts as an emetic. Ulcerative tendencies within the gastro intestinal tract.
Rebalances atonic the mucous membranes to aid normal mucus secretion. It
cleanses and repairs the tissues of the intestines in conditions of ulcers and
fistulas. A tonic the uterus [and prostate] and associated musculature. Improves
contractions during parturition. A constituent of composition essence [See
Chapter 33].

Cautions
Careful prescribing in acutes.

Preparations
A component of the famous composition essence.
Pyorrhoea, aphthous ulcers - decoction internally and locally for the gums.
Catarrh and nasal polyps - snuff.
Pyrexia with Capsicum for heat generation.
Influenza with Asclepias and Zingiber.
Dermal ulcers and wounds - an antiseptic powder is added to a poultice.
Vaginal discharge/leucorrhoea and menorrhagia use the decoction orally and as
an injection.

External use
Polyps use as a snuff - very small amounts only.
Gargarisma for sore throats, tonsillitis.
Dosage and mode of application
Diaphoretic effect Infusium Sig 15ml every 15 minutes until diaphoresis occurs.
Powdered bacc Sig 4g
Liquidum extractum Sig 2ml
References
43 p146. 111 p570. 254 p66. 262 p59. 269 1998, Vol XV111, No 3.

Myristica fragrans [Nutmeg]

Constituents
Volatile oil - around 10%, monoterpenes, the major volatiles are pinine and camphine. Fixed oil up to 40%. Phenolic ethers.

Primary pharmacological action: Antispasmodic.

Therapeutic classes
Aromatic. Stimulant. Tonic. Allays inflammation.
Circulatory stimulant. Hypolipidaemic.
Carminative. Antiemetic. Cholelithiasis. Digestive stimulant.
Diuretic. Diaphoretic. Aphrodisiac.
Orexigenic.
Analgesic. Sedative.
Antineoplastic. Thyroctive.
Medicinal indications
Toothache. Inhibits platelet aggregation.
Halitosis. Dyspepsia. Nausea. Flatulence. Dyspepsia. Vomiting. Diarrhoea.
Dysentery. Colic.
Premature ejaculation.
Rheumatic pain.
Anxiety. Depression. CNS stimulant.
Pyrexia. Intermittent fever. Thyroid carcinoma.
Tissue conditions
Tends to inhibit prostaglandins. Stimulates the circulation. Stimulates hydrochloric acid. Allays nervous tension, headache and palpitations.
Cautions
Pregnancy. Large doses may cause dizzyness and headaches.
External use
Toothache – apply Tr on cotton wool.
Pneumonia, cholera, vomiting - apply the poultice to the chest or abdomen.
Dosage and mode of application
Fructus Sig 2g
Oleum Sig 0.2ml
References
111 p578. 187 p225. 188 p313. 192 p384.

Myroxylon balsamum [Tolu balsam]
[See also Styrax benzoin]

Constituents
Resin. Triterpenoids - oleanolic acid. Cinnamic acid. Benzoic acid. Vanillin.

Primary pharmacological action: Expectorant tonic.

Therapeutic classes
Disinfectant. Stimulating antiseptic to the skin and mucous membranes.
Expectorant.
Anthelmintic - Cestodes. Nematodes.
Antineoplastic.
Dermatological agent. Vulnerary. Pediculosis.
Medicinal indications
Chronic catarrh. Pharyngitis. Laryngitis. Bronchial irritation from chronic
conditions. Pertussus.
Haemorrhoids. Tapeworms. Pinworms. Anal itching.
Dandruff. Sore nipples. Dermal sores.
Tissue conditions
Dry, hacking coughs. Relaxed mucous membranes creating excess mucus
production.
A constituent of friars balsam.
External use
Bronchitis - Inhalation of Friars Balsam.
Preparations
Pertussus use the syrup as a carrier for pulmonary antispasmodics.
Dosage and mode of application
Tincturae balsam [oleo resin]. Sig 2ml
Tolu Syrupus @ 10%. Sig 8ml
Tolu base for lozenges Acacia 10g. Tr Tolu 2ml. Sucrose 100g. Aqua to 100ml.
[makes 100 lozenges]
References
188 p425. 192 p 36.

Myrrhis odorata [Sweet cicely]

Constituents
Volatile oil containing Anethole. Essential oil.

Primary pharmacological action: Carminative.

Therapeutic classes
Anti - infective. Expectorant. Tuberculosis – rad decoction.
Aromatic. Stomachic tonic. Mild laxative.
Diuretic.
Emmenagogue. Galactogogue.
Nervine tonic. Antivenomous.
Medicinal conditions
Coughs.
Stomach weakness. Flatulence. Flatus.
Oedema. Gout.
Antiseptic against dog and snake bite.
Preparations
Essence is aphrodisiac.
External use
Wounds and ulcers - use the ointment.
Dosage and mode of application
Decoction herba/rad/sem Sig 30ml
References
127 p201. 192 p529. 246 p283.

Nardostachys jatamansi [Indian spikenard]

Constituents
Sesquiterpenes. Coumarin. Essential oil.

Primary pharmacological action: Anti convulsant.

Therapeutic classes
Antibacterial. Tonic.
Neurocardiac sedative.
Respiratory stimulant.
Carminative. Stomachic. Laxative.
Diuretic.
Antispasmodic.
Antimalarial. Emmenagogue.
Medicinal indications
Palpitations. Angina. Arrhythmia. Hypertension. Varicose veins.
Colic. Intestinal spasm e.g. IBS. Haemorrhoids.
Anxiety. Panic. Depression. Epilepsy. Headaches. Syncope.
Tissue conditions
Increases the CNS monoamines from 5HT.
Intestinal smooth muscle relaxant.
Dosage and mode of application
Decoctum rad/rhiz. Sig 3g
Tincturae Sig 2ml
References
191. 304, 1994, Vol. 2 [2] p39-47.

Narcissus pseudonarcissus [Daffodil]

Constituents
Contains Nivaline and known as galanthamine which inhibit cholinesterase activity, also found in Galanthus nivalis – snowdrop.

Primary pharmacological action: Antispasmodic.

Therapeutic classes
Mydriatic.
Emetic. Antidiarrhoeal. Anthelmintic. Cathartic.
Diuretic. Antipyretic.
Antispasmodic.
Dermatological agent. Vulnerary.

Medicinal indications
Asthma. Pertussus. Respiratory congestion.
Rheumatism. Joint pain. Muscle strain. Sprains
Alzheimers disease. Myasthenia gravis. Paralysis. Polio. Epilepsy. Chorea.
Dermal regenerator. Intermittent fever. Burns. Frostbite.

Tissue conditions
Anticholinesterase activity, reversing neuromuscular blockade and allays spasmodic muscular contractions in myasthenia gravis.

External use
Wounds and ulcers.
Frostbite – crushed bulb.

Dosage and mode of application
Emetic dose of pwd flos. Sig 8g
Tincturae bulb Sig 0.5ml

References
192 p173/221. 246 p521/2. 262 p281.

Nepeta cataria [Catnep]

Constituents
Essential oil – carvacrol and thymol.

Primary pharmacological action:
Relaxing and diffusive diaphoretic with antispasmodic nervine properties.

Therapeutic classes
Refrigerant. Aromatic. Carminative.
Emmenagogue.
Analgesic. Antipyretic. Antivenomous. Antineoplastic.
Medicinal indications [Venus]
Toothache. Scarlatina. Colds. Bronchitis. Influenza.
Stomach spasm. Hiccups. Dyspepsia. Flatulence. Colic. Intestinal spasm.
Diarrhoea.
Convulsions. Insomnia. Panic attacks. Restlessness. Headache.
Amenorrhoea. Dysmenorrhoea. PMS.
Muscle spasm. Restlessness. Headache.
Pyrexia. Measles. Smallpox. Bites – Adder. Urticaria. Cancer.
Tissue conditions
Nepeta is a powerful yet gentle diaphoretic. It does not overstimulate pyrexia.
Effective remedy for fretful babies and children's complaints - cough, bronchitis, pyrexia.
When administered it gently soothes the nervous system and aids restful sleep.
Pain relief associated with digestive spasm. Nervous headaches associated with panic attacks. Eases amenorrhoea and dysmenorrhoea from an over excitable nervous system.
Preparations
Enema infusium equal parts of Nepeta and Dioscorea for intestinal spasm, invagination - volvulus, intestinal obstruction.
Nervous irritation, tension and headache with Chamomilla.
Bruising - use the lotion or fol poultice.
Pyrexia with Zingiber succus.
Dosage and mode of application
Frequent dosing in acute cases.
Infusion herba Sig 30ml
Liquidum extractum Sig 4ml
References
43 p148. 111 p585. 126 p281. 228 p108. 228 p265. 246 p375. 251 p36

Nepeta hederacea [Ground ivy]

Constituents
Saponins. Bitters. Flavonoid glycosides – hyperoside and rutin are astringent.
Triterpenoids - alpha and beta ursolic acid is ulcer protective and antiviral against
Epstein Barr virus. Ursolic acid is cytotoxic in colon, mammary and Lymphocytic
leukaemia. Polyphenols. Sitosterol. Volatile oils. Tannin Wax.

Primary pharmacological action: Astringent.

Therapeutic classes
Ophthalmic. General tonic. Stimulant. Allays inflammation. Antiviral – Epstein
barr virus. Anticatarrhal.
Antiallergic. Expectorant - mild. Antitussive. Pectoral. Antiasmatic.
Stomachic. Antiulcer. Splenic tonic.
Diuretic.
Dermatological agent. Vulnerary. Antineoplastic.

Medicinal indications [Venus]
Ocular inflammation. Toothache. Earache. Glandular enlargements. Tinnitus.
Abscesses. Coughs. Nasopharyngeal catarrh. Sinusitis. Asthma. Bronchitis.
Nervous coughs. Pertussis. Tuberculosis.
Gastritis. Dyspepsia. Gastrointestinal ulcers. Obstructive Jaundice. Diarrhoea/IBS
Haemorrhoids. Fistula.
Bladder carcinoma. Cystitis. Renal inflammation. Sciatica. Arthritis.
Tinnitus. Tension headaches.

Tissue conditions
Inflamed or infected mucous membranes of the eyes, ears, nose and throat.
Reduces mucus and infected catarrh.

External use
Nasal and ear infections, Scalp lice, Indolent ulcers, Abscesses, Itchy skin,
Eczema – use the lotion.

Preparations
Bronchial disorders with Glycyrrhiza, Hyssopus, Inula, Marrubium or Tussilago.
IBS with Agrimonia.
Mastitis – poultice.

Dosage and mode of application
Dried herba Sig 4g
Tincturae Sig 10ml
Liquidum extractum Sig 4ml

References
43 p149. 111 p586. 246 p377. 251 p88. 188 p208. 189 p135. 233 p121. 236 p68.

Nymphaea odorata [White water lily]

Constituents
Alkaloids – nupharine. Cardenolide – nymphaline. Gallic acid. Mucilage. Resin.
Tannin.

Primary pharmacological action: Tonic to the pelvic viscera.

Therapeutic classes
Ophthalmic. Anticatarrhal. Astringent. Antiseptic. Antimicrobial. Antiviral –
tinea. Demulcent. Vasotonic alterative. Deobstruent. Haemostatic. Periodontal
disease.
Prostatic. Renal disorders. Uterine tonic.
Anodyne. Antineoplastic. Sedative. Vulnerary.
Medicinal indications [Moon]
Healing demulcent to mucous membranes. Oral candida. Dysentery. Diarrhoea.
Pelvic organ disturbances - menorrhagia, metrorrhagia. Cervical ulceration.
Relaxed vaginal walls. Vaginal discharge/leucorrhoea. Prostate enlargement.
Gonorrhoea. Uterine carcinoma.
Soothes rashes and sunburn.
Tissue conditions
A mild and soothing astringent to the mucous membranes of the eye, oral cavity,
intestine, bladder, vagina, and prostate. Cleansing and deobstruent.
Parasympathetic relaxant – allaying sexual activity.
External use
Conjunctivitis – collyr.
Pharyngitis, laryngitis, aphthous ulcers - garg.
Furunculosis, skin ulcers, dermatitis. Uterine carcinoma - injection and oral
medication. Vaginal discharge/leucorrhoea. Cervical ulcerations. Prostatitis.
Preparations
Collyr - conjunctivitis.
Aphthous ulcers use the mouthwash.
Uterine carcinoma - with Trillium.
Cervical ulceration use a douche or pessary.
Dermatitis - use the fol poultice with Ulmus or Linum decoction.
Dosage and mode of application
Dried rad/rhiz. Sig 5g
Liquidum extractum Sig 4ml
References
12. 111 p587. 188 p451. 246 p109. 254 p104. 311, Vol. 11, No. 3, p6-7.

Ocimum basilicum/sanctum [Sweet basil]

Constituents
Flavonoids. Polyphenolic acids. Triterpine. Ursolic acid. Volatile oil. Mucilage.
Vitamins A and C.

Primary pharmacological action: Adaptogenic tonic to the Autonomic nervous system and Cardio vascular system.

Therapeutic classes
Allays inflammation. Mucilaginous. Stimulant. Antibacterial – salmonella.
Antifungal – Tinea.
Hypotensive. Anti catarrhal. Expectorant.
Aromatic bitter. Carminative. Antiemetic. Antiflatulent. Digestive tonic.
Vermifuge.
Diuretic. Diaphoretic.
Analgesic. Antidepressant. Anxiolytic. Antispasmodic. Adrenal stimulant.
Dermatological agent. Antiperiodic. Antivenomous. Insecticidal – oleum.
Immunoregulatory. Galactagogue.

Medicinal indications [Mars]
Hypertension
Sinus congestion. Earache. Pertussus. Asthma.
Aphthous ulcers. Indigestion. Nausea. Flatulent colic. Flatulence. Constipation.
Diarrhoea.
Impotence/sexual dysfunction. Sterility - increases sperm count. Malaria – rad
dect.
Anxiety. Tension. Depression. Exhaustion. Headaches. Insomnia. Irritability.
Motion sickness. Migraine. Neuralgia. Withdrawal from marijuana.

Tissue conditions
Relaxes smooth muscle spasm and allays tension through the gastro intestinal
tract as it relieves irritable intestinal conditions E.g. IBS. Enhances the production
of breast milk.

Cautions
Pregnancy

External use
Ringworm, fungal and bacterial infections of the skin – oleum.

Dosage and mode of application
Dried herba Sig 3g
Infusium herba Sig 30ml
Tincturae Sig 4ml
References. 192 p40. 262 p58. 399. 400. 401.

Ocimum tenuiflorum [Holy basil]

Constituents
Essential oil - monoterpenes. Flavonoids. Polyphenols.

Primary pharmacological action: Immunostimulant.

Therapeutic classes
Tonic. Vasotonic alterative.
Antihaemorrhagic.
Anticatarrhal. Expectorant.
Hepatic. Antimalarial.
Adaptogenic.
Antipyretic. Dermatological agent.

Medicinal indications
Blood impurities. Haemorrhage.
Upper respiratory tract infections. Catarrh. Sinusitis. Coughs. Bronchitis.
Influenza.
Gastric disorders. Peptic ulcer. Acute hepatitis.
Haemorrhage. Tropical Oesinophilia.
Fever. Skin disease. Malaria.

Tissue conditions
Enhances endurance as an adaptogenic tonic.
Used for infective conditions of the upper respiratory tract.

Preparations
Immune enhancer with Andrographis or Echinacea.

Dosage and mode of application
Dried herba Sig 3g

References
271, April 2001.

Oenothera biennis [Evening primrose]

Constituents
The fixed oil yields essential fatty acids - Gamolenic acid around 9% and Linoleic acid around 70% which are precursors of Prostaglandins [PG]. Oleic acid around 16%. Amino acid - tryptophan.

Primary pharmacological action:
Hormonal balancer. Nervine trophorestorative.

Therapeutic classes
Allays inflammation. Astringent. Demulcent. Antiallergic.
Anticoagulant. Vasodilator. Hypotensive. Inhibits platelet aggregation.
Nutritive. Gastro intestinal disorders.
Anodyne. Sedative.
Dermatological agent. Vulnerary.
Immunemodulator. Antineoplastic.

Medicinal indications
Hypertension. Raynauds disease. Hypercholesterolaemia. Platelet aggregation.
Corrects Omega 6 deficiency. Asthma. Pertussus.
Diabetes. IBS.
Rheumatoid arthritis. Sjogrens syndrome. Chronic fatigue syndrome. Multiple sclerosis. Diabetic neuropathy. Carcinoma.
Anodyne for pain. Schizophrenia. Dementia. Depression. Hyperactivity.
Neuralgia. Memory loss. Alzheimers disease.
Hormonal disturbance. Endometriosis. PMS. Mastalgia. Menopause.
Acne. Dermatitis. Eczema. Scaly skin. Psoriasis. Wounds. Brittle nails. Radiation damage.

Tissue conditions
Gamolenic acid and DGLA are precursors of Prostaglandins [PG], they enhance levels of prostaglandins within the tissues. PG is immunoregulatory, vasodilatory, inhibitor of platelet cholesterol synthesis. It inhibits inflammatory prostaglandins. Supports the regeneration of the myelin sheath [neurone membrane structure] in degenerative conditions. Supports the secretions of the exocrine glands of the lacrimal and salivary ducts. Atrophy of the exocrine glands suggests EFA deficiency. EFA decrease cholesterol and other platelet aggregations. EFA also improve renal blood flow. Endometriosis has improved in a number of patients. EFA's are known to support the immune system. In-vitro studies inhibit the growth of human cancer cell lines. Dermal hydrator in cases of skin dryness.

Cautions
Contraindicated for patients using epileptic drugs. Epilepsy. While it is suggested that EPO could cause epilepsy is it possible that as the medicine is used it could bring about a cure for such a condition. The law of cure states symptoms arise as part of the healing process.
External use
Bruises. Wound healer. Eczema. Dermal dryness.
Dosage and mode of application
Oleum expressed from the seed.
Ol Oenothera Sig 1-8g daily. Approximately 100mg GLA per 1g Oleum.
References
230 p35. 239 p105. 246 p266.

Olea europaea [Olive]

Constituents
Fol - Calcium elenoate is a potent antimicrobial. Fol contain quinine.
Triterpenoids. Tannins. Oleum is high in unsaturated fatty acids – oleic and
linoleic. Oleuropein – anti infective. Antioxidants – luteolin, quercetin and rutin.

Primary pharmacological action: Antinfective.

Therapeutic classes
Antiviral - candida, herpes simplex, herpes genitalis, Epstein bar virus, HIV..
Arrhythmia. Anticholesterolaemic. Circulatory diffusive. Spasmolytic.
Cholerctic. Stomachic. Effective against helicobacter pylori. Nutritive.
Medicinal indications
Toothache. Sinus and mouth infections. Influenza.
Hypotensive and circulatory diffusive. Inhibits LDL cholesterol.
Haemorrhoidal pain. Appendicitis - oral and fomentation. Laxative.
Urinary infections. Antiarthritic
Vulvovaginitis. Bladder infections. Improves energy in fatigue, ME. Psoriasis.
Tissue conditions
Soothes the mucous membranes of the stomach and gall bladder.
Spasmolytic upon smooth muscle of the bronchi and blood vessel walls. Dilates
the coronary arteries.
Preparations
Leaf decoction is antipyretic in malaria. Quoted by Hanbury in 1854 in the
Pharmaceutical journal of Provincial transactions the leaves are more effective
than quinine in reducing pyrexia.
Oleum Olive and lemon juice - cholelithiasis. Used as a condiment. Olives in oil
are eaten for their nutritive value. Organic olives are best as some non organic
varieties have been sprayed with mosquito insecticide. Mosquitoes congregate
around olive trees.
External use
Inspissated ear wax – warm oleum drops into the meatus.
Dandruff, dry, scaly dermatological conditions – oleum.
The oleum can be used to prepare medicinal oils.
Dosage and mode of application
Dried fol Sig 500mg
Liquidum extractum fol Sig 2ml
Oleum can be freely used.
References. 142 p161. 189 p204. 246 p323. 281, 1997 Vol. 13 [4]. 317, 13, 231-
7. 318, 1993, 74, p253-9. 319p 1975, 194-9, p421-5. 320, 1995, Vol.15, No 1.

Ononis spinosa [Restharrow]

Constituents
Flavonic glycoside - ononine. Triterpenes – beta sitosterol. Volatile oil. Tannin.

Primary pharmacological action: Diuretic.

Therapeutic classes
Allays inflammation. Expectorant.
Antilithic. Mild antiseptic diuretic.
Dermatological agent. Vulnerary.
Medicinal indications [Mars]
Aphthous ulcers.
Cystitis. Urinary calculi. Arthritis. Gout.
Tissue conditions
Ononis detoxifies the blood through it's diuretic power. It will increase urinary output by up to 20%. Soothes inflammatory conditions of the genito urinary tract.
External use
Infusion applied in aphthous ulcers and haemorrhoids.
Ulcers/wounds – fol.
Dosage and mode of application
Infusium is to be preferred Sig 30ml
References
188 p370. 189 p234. 246 p200. 247 p 79.

Opuntia vulgaris [Cactus flowers]

Constituents
Flavonoids. Mucilage. Tannin. Mallic acid.

Primary pharmacological action: Astringent.

Therapeutic classes
Allays inflammation.
Antihaemorrhagic.
Diuretic.
Vulnerary.
Medicinal indications
Pertussus.
Peptic ulcers. Amoebic dysentery. Diarrhoea. Colitis.
Prostatic hypertrophy.
Mastitis.
Haematomas and wounds.
Preparations
Mastitis with Phytolacca.
External use
Crushed fol and fruct.
Wounds with Arnica.
Dosage and mode of application
Dried flos Sig 1g
Liquidum extractum Sig 1ml
References
43 p151.

Origanum vulgare [Oregano/marjoram]

Constituents
Flavonoids - antioxidant, antiviral. Rosmarinic acid. Volatile oil around 3%
containing aldehydes are effective against Aspergillosis. Triterpenoids - ursolic
acid. Vitamin A, C.

Primary pharmacological action: Anti-infective.

Therapeutic classes
Ophthalmic. Stimulant. Tonic. Antifungal - Candida & Aspergillosis.
Antibacterial - 30 different organisms can be neutralised including: Bacillus
cereus, E.Coli, Giardia, Pseudomonas aeruginosa, Salmonella & Staphylococcus.
Antiviral - Herpes simplex, Herpes Zoster, genital herpes. Antioxidant.
Expectorant. Aromatic. Stomachic. Diaphoretic.
Emmenagogue. Antispasmodic. Antivenomous. Antineoplastic.
Medicinal indications [Mercury]
Viruses disintegrate with the oleum.
Conjunctivitis. Colds. Flu. Laryngitis. Lung infections. Asthma. Bronchitis.
Pertussus.
Oral infection. Halitosis. Nausea. Heartburn. Waterbrash. Colic. Intestinal pain.
Enuresis. Rheumatic pain.
Nausea of pregnancy. Amenorrhoea. Dysmenorrhoea. Pyrexia.
Headache. Depression. Fear. Insomnia. Panic. Motion sickness.
Tissue conditions
Most of the available evidence is from research upon the wild Mediterranean oil.
At one drop per thousand of wild oregano oil, water became sterile. Greek
researchers [University of Thessoloniki] in 1995 found that one in 4000 dilution
sterilised infected water. Stimulating to the immune system and increases the
levels of interferon. Eases intestinal spasmodic pain.
External use
Ear wax, eases pain in the ears - dect. or Oleum.
Preparations
Wounds - internal and local action.
Rheumatic pain use the oleum.
Neuritis use the liniment.
Dosage and mode of application
Dried herba Sig 3g
Infusium Sig 30ml
References. 111 p600. 129. 192 p349. 192 p394. 246 p381. 281, 1999, Vol. 15,
No. 4. 285, 9, 1995, p281-286.

Paeonia lactiflora [White peony]

Constituents
Monoterpine glycoside – Paeoniflorin up to 2%.

Primary pharmacological action: Antispasmodic.

Therapeutic classes
Ophthalmic. Allays inflammation. Antibacterial. Astringent.
Anticholesterolaemic.
Bitter. Hepatoprotective. Choleretic.
Febrifuge.
Emmenagogue.
Muscle relaxant.
Medicinal indications [Sun]
Blurred vision. Eyelid twitching.
Angina. Anticholesterolaemic.
Antiallergic. Pertussus.
Dysentery. Muscle cramps/twitching. Anal or rectal spasm.
Dysmenorrhoea. Polycystic ovaries.
Dizzyness. Epilepsy. Migraine.
Immune enhancer.
Tissue conditions
Keeps the blood thin by reducing cholesterol and platelets. It prolongs
prothrombin time.
Preparations
Menopause or fibroids with Cinnamomum cassia and Prunus persica.
Congenial combination with Glycyrrhiza.
Dosage and mode of application
Dried rad Sig 2g
Liquidum extractum Sig 4ml
References
111 p605. 239 p170. 246 p121.

Panax ginseng

and other related species quinquefolium, notogenseng.
[Synonyms: P. Schinseng, P. Pseudoginseng, P. Sanchi, P tienchi].
Red ginseng is unpeeled. White ginseng is peeled.

Constituents

Ginseng increases intracellular ATP. It has a corticosteroid like action. It has been of benefit in diabetes. Triterpine saponins [Terpenoids] which are complex ginsenosides and panaxosides [saponins] are the main active elements. Saponins are free radical scavengers. Volatile oil. Rich in steroidal compounds. Polysaccharides [glycans] are antineoplastic. Vitamins B1, B2, B12, Pantothenic acid.

Primary pharmacological action: Adaptogenic tonic [trophorestorative] via adrenal and pituitary action.

Therapeutic classes

Demulcent. Stimulant. Tonic. Antioxidant.
Cardiotonic. Antiarrhythmic. Vasodilator. Hypotensive. Antisclerotic.
Anticholesterolaemic. Pulmonary.
Stomachic. Antiulcerogenic. Hypoglycaemic. Hepatoprotective. Anti radiation.
Diuretic. Low sperm count. Aphrodisiac.
Antifatigue. Nervine. Sedative. Thymoleptic.
Antineoplastic. Immunostimulant. Alcohol habit.

Medicinal indications [Jupiter]

Heart failure. Palpitations. Hypercholesterolaemia. Reduces triglycerides.
Asthma. Colds. Infections. Tuberculosis.
Anorexia. Stomach tension with inability to digest food, stomach fullness. Peptic ulcers. Diabetes. Supports blood alcohol detoxification.
Enuresis. Oedema. Impaired renal activity. Gonadotrophic activity. Infertility.
Impotence/sexual dysfunction.
Addictions. Anxiety. Convulsions. Depression. Exhaustion. Insomnia. ME.
Inadequate memory. Neurasthenia. Neuralgia. Overactive thymus gland.
Radiation sickness.

Tissue conditions

Ginsenosides Rb1 and Rg1 have amphoteric action and either stimulate or relax the neurones of the central nervous system. This is another example of how unbalanced standarised extracts produced on a marker of an isolated constituent fail to represent the whole effect of the remedy.

Pharmacopoeia

Improves cardiac performance - inotropic effects and coronary vasodilator. Vasoconstrictor of femoral, mesenteric and renal arteries. Reduces blood coagulation. Reduces HDL cholesterol and triglycerides. Normalises blood pressure if given around 45 minutes before food. Regulates adrenocorticotrophic hormone. Induces production of interferon. Augments T cell lymphocytes and antiviral activity. Inhibits tumour angiogenesis by enhancing NK activity. Improves resistance to infections. Has anti compliment activity and is an immune modulator.

Adapts the nervous system against stress. Known as a longevity herb. It improves ones stamina in physical endurance, it improves muscular O2 utilisation. Mental ability from tonic effects are enhanced. Mood improver as it balances the mood. Depression with sexual inadequacy/impotence/sexual dysfunction. Improves psychomotor performance e.g. attention span, concentration and cognitive performance. It delays cellular necrosis. For improving ones well being, for all age groups during convalescence, debility and degenerative diseases. Enhances nitric oxide which increases cyclic GMP [see also Zizyphus]. Soothes internally inflamed organ tissue. Aids in the withdrawal from drug addictions. Moderates the ill effects of chemotherapy and radiotherapy [radiation].

Cautions
Hypertension.
Preparations
Antineoplastic effects are improved when preparations are used.
External use
Wound healing.
Dosage and mode of application
Large doses are required in neoplasm.
Dried fol/rad Sig 1g
Decocturm Sig 2g
Tincturae Sig 10ml
Liquidum extractum Sig 2ml
References
192 p234. 230 p47. 239 p89. 263 1991 57 [2] 132. 263, 63, 1997, p389-392. 285, 1994, 8 [8] p445-51. 394 p170.

Papaver somniferum [Opium]

Constituents
Alkaloids - some 25 have been isolated - morphine is the main one and present up to 17%. Codeine - depresses cough reflex, sedative, analgesic activity. Tannin. Starch.

Primary pharmacological action: Analgesic.

Therapeutic classes
Astringent. Allays inflammation. Antihaemorrhagic.
Antitussive.
Diaphoretic.
Anaesthetic. Anodyne. Antispasmodic. Sedative. Hypnotic.
Medicinal indications [Moon]
Inflammatory conditions. Toothache. Earache.
Angina. Myocardial infarction. Dyspnoea.
Excessive mucus secretions. Suppresses irritable coughs. Biliary colic. Diarrhoea [with] Peptic ulcer pain, IBS or intestinal spasm. Peritonitis. Appendicitis.
Renal colic. Articular rheumatic pain.
Pain. Shock. Nervous irritability. Depression - endogenous.
Climacteric depression associated with dissatisfaction and ill temperedness.
Hypochondriasis. Guilt feelings. Anxiety. Neuralgia. Convulsions. Meningitis.
Cholera. Tetanus.
Tissue conditions
Long duration of activity - up to three days. Allays pain, quiets nervous activity and sedates the patient allowing recovery. Post operatively relieves pain. Sedates troublesome coughs. Eases pain in advanced cancer.
Cautions
Restrictions apply. Dosage is determined by the relief of symptoms.
Addictive remedy. Acute irritated conditions with dry mucous membranes.
Nausea. Loss of appetite. Constipation.
Overdose is treated with Capsicum and stimulants.
External use
Opthalmia – pain.
Articular inflammation. Contusions, bruises, sprains – pain.
Dosage and mode of application
Powder Sig 200mg. Maximum 500mg in 24 hours.
Dry extract Sig 60mg
Tincturae 1:10 unripe capsules Sig 1ml [equivalent to 10mg morphine per ml].
Liquidum extractum Sig 2ml

Pharmacopoeia

Papaver Syrupus Syrup of Papaver [BPC 1949] LE Papaver 0.5ml
syrup to 5ml. Sig 4ml
Enema Papaver 6% in starch mucilage.
Lin. Papaver. Papaver liniment.
Equal volume of soft soap & Tincture Papaver.
It contains Morphia 0.5%.
Ung @ 7.5%

References
BPC 1954. 126 p501. 224 p974. 390 p1127.

Parietaria diffusa [Pellitory of the wall]

Constituents
Flavonoids - Quercetin, Quercetin binds to type 2 oestrogen binding sites and binds isoflavonoids thus preventing oestrogen activity and the reduction of oestrogens to target tissue. Kaempferol.

Primary pharmacological action: Demulcent diuretic.

Therapeutic classes
Depurative – fol. Antilithic.
Vulnerary.
Medicinal indications [Mercury]
Haemorrhoids.
Oedema. Cystitis. Pyelitis. Renal and bladder calculi.
Burns.
Cautions
Sensitivity to the herb with some individuals.
External use
Shingles – use an ointment.
Preparations
Genito urinary conditions – Althea, Taraxacum, Zea.
Dosage and mode of application
Dried herba Sig 5g
Tincturae Sig 5ml
Liquidum extractum Sig 4ml
References
43 p153. 189 p211. 246 p84.

Passiflora incarnata [Passionflower]

Constituents
Indole alkaloids up to 0.9% - harmene is the primary alkaloid. Flavonoids -
Vitexin and C-glycosylflavones, apigenin up to 2.5%, luteolin, rutin. Fatty acids.
Sterols. Passicol is a polyacetylene and is antimicrobial. Volatile oil. Vitamin K.

Primary pharmacological action: CNS sedative.

Therapeutic classes
Antibacterial. Group A haemolytic streptococci, Staphylococcus.
Anti fungal – Candida. Cardiotonic. Hypotensive. Vasodilator.
Antispasmodic. Anodyne. Analgesic. Anxiolytic. Hypnotic. Alcohol & drug habit
Medicinal indications
Hypertension. Tachycardia. Palpitations.
Spasmodic asthma. Pertussus [with convulsions].
Stomachic. Antiflatulent. Intestinal spasm. Diarrhoea. Dysentery. Haemorrhoids.
Dysmenorrhoea. Anxiety. Chorea. Epilepsy. Headache with exhaustion.
Neurasthenia. Insomnia. Neuralgia. Panic. Nervousness/Restlessness. Tetany.
Tissue conditions
A stomach sedative and antiflatulent, useful in easing gastro intestinal tract
disorders with anxiety.
Generally relaxes the brain and removes cerebral irritability, wakefulness and
over excited states. It is sedative to the CNS. Insomnia from overwork or stress.
It relaxes and settles psychomotor activity and spasmodic muscular convulsions
[epilepsy] and from meningitis. It is indicated for acute mania, nervousness and
neuralgic pain. For nervous headache and panic. It inhibits MAOI. Palpitations
from shock or nervous excitability.
Preparations
Insomnia with Humulus.
Pain with Gelsemium or Pulsatilla.
Drug addiction with Hyoscyamnus and Cannabis or with Avena, Humulus and
Valeriana.
Dosage and mode of application
Dried herba Sig 2g
Dry extract Sig 0.4g
Tincturae Sig 10ml
Liquidum extractum Sig 2ml
References
43 p153. 176 p107. 188 p330. 189 p209. 192 p408. 239 p141. 314, 2000, 15 [2]
p139-43. 394 p293.

Paullinia cupana [Guarana]

Constituents
Rich in guaranine, a natural xanthine and assimilated slowly. Saponins. Caffeine up to 5%. Tannin - large quantities up to 12%.

Primary pharmacological action:
Vitality stimulant [tonic]. Adaptogenic.

Therapeutic classes
Astringent. Stimulant. Antibacterial - Eschericha coli.
Cardiotonic. Antisclerotic. Antithrombotic. Inhibits platelet aggregation.
Diuretic. Antirheumatic.
Analgesic. Aphrodisiac. Nervine tonic. Antidepressant. Adrenal tonic.
Dermatological agent. Febrifuge. Immunostimulant. Alcohol habit.

Medicinal indications
Reduces appetite. Dysentery. Diarrhoea.
Rheumatism. Lumbago. Helps to prevent malaria.
Dysmenorrhoea. Headaches. Migraine. Muscle cramp. Relieves alcohol intoxication.
Jet lag. Depression. Pyrexia. Icterus. Supports weight loss.

Tissue conditions
Caffeine stimulates the nervous system. Atonic conditions with feeble pulse and expressionless eyes. Headaches occurring during menstruation. Headaches with pallor. Depression around menstruation. Mental exhaustion, depression or fatigue. Motor nerve paralysis. Advised as a nervine tonic in convalescence and debility. Revitalises the mind and body. Will combat hunger and provide energy. Combats intense heat and high humidity - heat fatigue.

Cautions
Pregnancy.

External use
Hair loss.

Dosage and mode of application
Powdered sem Sig 4g
Tincturae Sig 6ml
Liquidum extractum Sig 4ml

References
44 p123. 126 p400. 192 p260.

Pausinystalia yohimbe [Yohimbe]

Constituents
Indole alkaloids up to 6%, yohimbine up to 15% an alpha 2 adrenergic blocker.
Blocking the adrenergic neurones causes sympathetic stimulation by increasing
noradrenaline release in the adrenergic nuclei [postganglionic sympathetic]
[causing vasoconstriction] within the CNS – hypothalamus, thalamus and spinal
cord.

Primary pharmacological action: Aphrodisiac.

Therapeutic classes
Mydriatic. Sialagogue. Anti obesity.
Uterine antispasmodic. Prostate antispasmodic.
Medicinal indications
Impotence/sexual dysfunction. Spermatorrhoea. Low sperm count.
Dysmenorrhoea.
Exhaustion.
Tissue conditions
An alpha adrenergic blocker of short duration. Acts upon the pelvic nerves
reducing excitability and tension. Dilates the blood vessels to the skin, kidney,
intestines and genitalia. Enhances arousal and orgasm. Stimulates athletic
performance.
External use
Anaesthetic.
Cautions
Restrictions apply. Dosage is determined by the relief of symptoms.
Serious adverse reactions are rare and reversible [394].
Cardiovascular, renal or hepatic disease. Nervousness. Insomnia. Pregnancy.
Prostate disorders.
Preparations
Sexual tonic – Avena, Panax or Smilax.
Dosage and mode of application
Liquidum extractum bacc. Sig 4ml
References
176 p471. 188 p460. 192 p599. 224. 394 p431.

Petasites hybridus [Butterbur]

Constituents
Pyrrolizidine alkaloids - max intake 1mcg daily [German health department].
Sesquiterpine lactones - Petasin. Mucilage. Resin. Inulin. Essential oil.

Primary pharmacological action:
Antispasmodic to smooth muscle.

Therapeutic classes
Allays inflammation. Astringent. Demulcent.
Antitussive. Expectorant.
Heart tonic. Diuretic – mild.
Cholagogue. Gastro intestinal disorders.
Neurosedative. Anodyne.
Antineoplastic. Dermatological agent. Vulnerary.

Medicinal indications [Sun]
Colds. Pharyngitis. Laryngitis. Influenza. Asthma. Bronchitis. Pertussus.
Heart weakness.
Gastric ulcers. Gastritis. Gastroduodenitis. Biliary spasm. Intestinal spasm.
Urinary tract inflammation or spasm. Oedema. Spasm of the ureters and urethra.
Calculi.
Migraine. Cervical thoracic syndrome and lumbosacral pain. Arthritis.
Pyrexia. Antineoplastic.

Tissue conditions
Influences prostaglandin synthesis. Acts upon acachidonic acid metabolism and
inhibits leukotrines in the inflammatory effort. Demulcent activity for the
respiratory system – spasmodic coughs. Regulatory effect upon ANS tone
[antispasmodic] in acute spasm of the gastro intestinal, biliary and genito urinary
tracts. Migraineous headache associated with biliary disorder.

Dosage and mode of application
Decoctum flos/rad/rhiz. Sig 9g
Tincturae Sig 3ml

References
142 p90. 192 p100. 246 p475. 247 p166. 321, 2000, 38 [9] p430-435.

Petroselinum crispum [Parsley]

Constituents
Flavonoid glycosides - apigenin [allays inflammation, inhibits histamine, anti free radical], luteolin. Furanocoumarins. Volatile oils up to 7% Sem and 0.05% herba containing apiol and myristin. Coumarins. Fixed oil. Vitamins A & C.

Primary pharmacological action: Diuretic.

Therapeutic classes
Ophthalmic. Antiseptic. Antimicrobial. Mild tonic.
Hypotensive.
Expectorant
Carminative. Stomachic. Hepatic. Laxative.
Antilithic. Diuretic. Antirheumatic. Antipyretic. Antivenomous.
Antispasmodic. Sedative. Adrenal supportive.
Antigalactagogue. Emmenagogue - sem. Aphrodisiac.
Dermatological agent. Antineoplastic.
Thyrotonic.
Medicinal indications [Mercury]
Optic nerve tonic. Anaemia. Hypertension.
Cough. Asthma. Bronchial disorders. Tubercular night sweats.
Breath freshener in halitosis. Flatulent dyspepsia. Cholelithiasis. Jaundice.
Intestinal colic
Urinary retention. Dysuria. Oedema. Cystitis. BPH. Lithuria. Gonorrhoea.
Plague [192]. Amenorrhoea. Dysmenorrhoea. Mastitis. Menopausal flushes.
Stimulates the ovaries. Stops breast milk. Breast tumours.
Myalgia. Musculoskeletal conditions.
Skin - fissures, itching, soreness.
Cautions
Acute renal inflammation. Pregnancy.
Tissue conditions
Allays itching of the skin. Tonic effects upon the intestinal smooth muscles.
Antiseptic to the intestine. Removes obstructions of the liver and spleen. Indicated for sub acute conditions of the kidneys. Sympathetic nervine antispasmodic.
Eliminates garlic and onion breath.
External use
Conjunctivitis – poultice or collyr.
Mastitis, enlarged glands - fomentation with fol.
Bites [Adder snake bite] and insect stings - fomentation/lotion.
Baldness and dandruff - lotion sem/fol.

P

Preparations
Dermal tumours, breast tumours – poultice with Chelidonium, Symphytum, Trifolium and Viola odorata.
Oedema with Carum carvi, Foeniculum, Pimpinella anisum and Saxifraga.
Dosage and mode of application
Full dosage to allay skin irritation.
Dried herba/rad/sem Sig 4g
Tincturae Sig 10ml
Liquidum extractum herba/rad/sem Sig 4ml
References
43 p154. 188 p329. 192 p402/404. 228 p147/345. 246 p295.

Peumus boldus [Boldo]

Constituents
Isoquinoline alkaloids in fol. up to 0.1% – boldine [hepatoprotective].
Aromatic essential oil up to 3% composed of monoterpenoids – ascaridole.
Flavonol glycosides. Resin. Tannin.

Primary pharmacological action:
Stimulating Cholagogue and Choleretic.

Therapeutic classes
Allays inflammation. Antioxidant.
Antiobesity. Cholelithiasis. Hepatoprotective. Anthelmintic.
Urinary antiseptic and demulcent diuretic.
Mild sedative. Weak local anaesthetic.

Medicinal indications
Earache. Colds.
Dyspepsia. Flatulence. Stomach cramp. Hepatic congestion and enlargement.
Hepatitis. Cholelithiasis. Cholecystitis. Jaundice. Constipation. Ascarides.
Cestodes.
Gout. Rheumatism. Oedema. Cystitis. Prostate disorders. Gonorrhoea. Syphilis.
Headache. Dysmenorrhoea.

Tissue conditions
As a stomach tonic it increases gastric secretions. Hepatic and gall bladder
disorders. Pain present in the stomach or gall bladder are indications for use.
Relaxes smooth muscle of the intestine.

Cautions
Care in biliary disorders – it is a stimulating medicine.

Dosage and mode of application
Start with a small dose as large doses can be too stimulating in sensitive
individuals.
Dried fol Sig 1g
Infusium Sig 3g
Tincturae Sig 5ml
Liquidum extractum Sig 1.5ml

References
176 p319. 192 p81/82. 262 p76. 263 57 [2] 110. 394 p29.

Pfaffia paniculata [Paratudo/Brazilian ginseng]

Constituents
Beta – ecdysone, a vegetable hormone that revitalises cells. Sitosterol – helps maintain normal levels of cholesterol. Stigmasterol a natural precursor to oestrogen. Also saponins up to 11%. Pfaffic acid is antineoplastic. Cobalt. Amino acids. Germanium. Silica. Zinc.

Primary pharmacological action:
Adaptogenic tonic similar to Ginseng.

Therapeutic classes
Allays inflammation.
Hypocholesterolaemic.
Aphrodisiac. Hormonal imbalance.
Analgesic. Sedative.
Antimutagenic. Immunostimulant Antineoplastic.

Medicinal indications
Arteriosclerosis. Mononucleosis. Leukaemia.
Raised blood uric acid. Osteomyelitis.
Hormonal disorders – infertility, sterility. Menopause. Impotence/sexual dysfunction.
Pain. Exhaustion. Chronic fatigue syndrome.
Carcinoma. Melanoma.

Tissue conditions
Beta-disterone sterols have an enhancing effect upon the organism increasing muscle bulk and endurance. Pfaffic acid and the associated Pfaffosides inhibit the growth of tumours and melanomas. Restores acid base blood balance.

Cautions
Pregnancy

Dosage and mode of application
Dried rad Sig 2g

References
44 p214. 188 p335.

Phyllanthus amarus/niruri [Bahupatra]

There are around 600 different species of Phyllanthus.

Constituents
Lignans - phyllanthin and hypophyllanthin. Bitters. Alkaloids. Flavonoids.
Tannin - geraniin [anti viral].

Primary pharmacological action: Astringent and diuretic.

Therapeutic classes
Allays inflammation. Antiviral - HIV, Hepatitis B. Antibacterial.
Hypotensive.
Choleretic. Hypoglycaemic. Hepatic tonic. Hepatoprotective. Laxative. Tonic.
Antilithic. Prostatic disease. Urinary antiseptic. Febrifuge.
Uterine tonic.
Anodyne. Antispasmodic.
Immunostimulant.
Medicinal indications
Hypertension. Influenza.
Cholelithiasis. Dyspepsia. Jaundice. Colic. Diarrhoea. Hepatocarcinoma.
Urinary calculi. Oedema. Gonorrhoea.
Menorrhagia.
Bruises. Ulcers. Wounds.
Tissue conditions
Alkaloids are antispasmodic to the urinary and biliary tracts. It acts by
suppressing the antigen reaction of hepatocytes. Reduces antibodies to hepatitis
B. Research conducted in India showed that the virus was eliminated from the
body in 59% of cases.
Dosage and mode of application
Dried herba infusium Sig 30ml
Dried powder Sig 200mg
Liquidum extractum fol Sig 2ml
References
44 p89. 48 p122. 296, 1988, 2. 764. 265, 2000, 12 [4] p117-9.

Phyllanthus emblica [Emblica/Myrobalan]

Constituents
Tannins. A rich source of vitamin C.

Primary pharmacological action: Astringent and tonic.

Therapeutic classes
Ophthalmic. Anticatarrhal. Antibacterial. Refrigerant. Immunemodulator.
Antioxidant. Antihaemorrhagic. Cardiovascular disease.
Antiulcerogenic. Hepatic tonic. Laxative.
Diuretic.
Medicinal indications
Conjunctivitis. Anaemia. Antisclerotic. Anticholesterolaemic.
Colds. Bronchitis.
Hyperacidity. Dyspepsia. Jaundice. Peptic ulcers. Diarrhoea.
Urinary infections.
Vaginal discharge/leucorrhoea.
Myalgia. Scurvy.
Tissue conditions
Heals ulcerations in any part of the gastro intestinal tract.
External use
Applied to the scalp it will promote hair growth.
Dosage and mode of application
Tincturae herba/flos/rad/fruct Sig 4ml
References
191 p64.

Phyllitis scolopendrium [Heart's tongue fern]

Constituents
Aromatic bitter. Flavonoids – lucodelphidin. Mucilage. Tannin. Amino acids.

Primary pharmacological action: Splenic tonic.

Therapeutic classes
Astringent. Demulcent.
Expectorant. Pectoral.
Hepatic. Cholagogue. Laxative.
Diuretic. Antilithic.
Vulnerary.
Medicinal indications [Jupiter]
Bleeding gums. Hiccups. Enlarged spleen. Congestion of the liver. Mucus colitis.
Diarrhoea. Dysentery. Haemorrhoids.
Burns. Scalds. Scalp wash for oily hair.
Preparations
Splenic disorders with Chionanthus.
Dosage and mode of application
Dried fol/fronds Sig 4g
Tincturae Sig 6ml
Liquidum extractum Sig 4ml
References
43 p191. 127 p304. 160 p125. 188 p214. 246 p564.

Phytolacca americana [Pokeroot]

Constituents
Alkaloids - phytolaccine is antiviral. It affects gram +ve organisms. Pokeroot antiviral protein – [PAP]. Phytolaccins – Pap 2 and Pap 3. Tannin. Resin. Lectins. Triterpenoid saponins – phytolaccosides allay inflammation and are mollusicidal. Vitamin A, C.

Primary pharmacological action:
Lympho vasotonic alterative. Cerebral and cardiac vasodilator.

Therapeutic classes
Ophthalmic. Allays inflammation. Relaxant. Anticatarrhal. Depurative.
Antibacterial - gram +ve organisms. Antifungal.
Antiviral – Candida, influenza, polio, Herpes simplex 1 & 2, Tinea. Expectorant.
Emetic. Cathartic. Parasiticide. Antirheumatic.
Anodyne.
Antineoplastic. Immunostimulant.
Thyroactive.

Medicinal indications
Conjunctivitis. Gonorrhoeal and syphilitic opthalmia.
Angina. Endocarditis. Infected conditions of mucous membranes.
Chronic respiratory catarrh. Pharyngitis. Laryngismus stridulus. Trachieitis.
Laryngitis. Diphtheria. Influenza.
Aphthous ulcerations. Syphilitic faucial ulcerations. Mercurial poisoning.
Stomatitis. Tonsillitis. Adenitis. Emetic. Peptic ulcers. Diverticulitis. Ulcerative colitis. Haemorrhoid itch. Enhances weight loss.
Thyroid enlargement.
Breast abscess. Breast dysplasia. Fibrocystic breast disease. Nipple fissures.
Mastitis. Carcinoma of the breast and uterus. Ovaritis.
Gout. Syphilis. Gonorrhoea. Orchitis. Genital itching. Sciatica. Arthritis. Chronic rheumatism. Polymyalgia.
Dermal ulcers. Abscess. Acne. Eczema. Infectious mononucleosis. ME.
Lupus erythematosus. Pityriasis. Psoriasis. Ringworm. Scabies. Scrophula.
Sycosis. Tinea.
Helminthic infection - Schistomiasis. Bilharzia.
Lipoma. Lymphadenopathy. Leukaemia. Lymphoma. Osteosarcoma.

Tissue conditions
Optic trophorestorative [Thurston]. General vasotonic alterative to the system.
Local ganglionic vasorelaxant for cardiac troubles - vasodilator to the coronary arteries. Thyroid, axillary, parotid, and sub maxillary action. It breaks down

adipose tissue and helps to remove the fat from the system. Stimulates the intestinal lymphatics.

Stimulating influence upon the skin, mucous membranes, serous membrane. Hyperaemia of the gastro intestinal tract, spleen, uterus, testes and prostate. Deep cleanser of bone and muscle tissue. Rheumatic disorders - arthritis, gout, neuralgia, rheumatism. Indicated for pain in the feet, heels, hips and spine. Inflammation of the testicle or ovary.

Skin - eczema, scaly disorders, pustules, psoriasis, ringworm, tubercular eruptions, sycosis, scabies. Fissures, fistulas, abscesses, dermal ulcers.

Cautions

Pregnancy. Lactation. Avoid fresh plant tinctures and berries.

External use

Breast disorders; mastitis, sore nipples - oral and local applications.

Ulcers, parasitic affections, scabies – ung.

Burns - used internally and externally.

Preparations

Tonsillitis with Commiphora and Echinacea.

Lymphadenitis/lymphadenopathy – Commiphora, Echinacea, Galium, Iris.

Rheumatic conditions with Cimicifuga, Guaiacum and Zanthoxylum.

Dermal malignancy, epithelioma with Chelidonium, Thuja.

Dosage and mode of application

Emetic dose Sig 1g

Dried rad Sig 0.3g

Tincturae 1:5 Sig 0.3ml [390 p2032]

Liquidum extractum Sig 1ml

References

111 p607. 126 p535. 188 p344. 192 p436. 224 p1796. 246 p101. 254 p173.

Phytostigma venenosum [Calabar bean]

Constituents
Alkaloid up to 0.5% - calabatine, eseridine, eseramine, geneserine, physostigmine and physovenine. Volatile oil. Steroids.

Primary pharmacological action:
Sedative action upon the spinal cord.

Therapeutic classes
Ophthalmic. Myotic. Allays inflammation.
Antispasmodic.
Medicinal indications
Conjunctivitis. Glaucoma. Paralysis of the ciliary muscle. Retinitis. Granular lids.
Corneal ulceration. Prolapse of the iris. Scleritis. Strabismus. Ocular muscle
spasm. Eye pain.
Emphysema. Asthma. Tubercular night sweats.
Gastralgia. Intestinal relaxation causing constipation.
Impotence/sexual dysfunction. Premature ejaculation.
Myasthenia gravis. Meningitis. Tetanus. Epilepsy. Locomotor ataxia. Chorea.
Reflex paralysis. Puerpural convulsions.
Tissue conditions
Antidote to anticholinergics - atropine, curare, nicotine and strychnine.
Cholinesterase inhibitor of acetylcholine [anticholinesterase]. Dilates the blood
vessels and causes bradycardia. Catarrhal conditions of the mucous membranes in
atonic states of the gastro intestinal, pulmonary and genito urinary tracts. Allays
inflammation in meningitis.
Cautions
Restrictions apply. Dosage is determined by the relief of symptoms.
Boiling the seed will reduce its toxicity. Stomach inflammation. Vomiting.
Paralysis of the limbs. Death by asphyxia. Depresses the medulla.
External use
Ocular remedy for injuries and inflammation. Contracts the pupil. Iris prolapse.
Preparations
Ophthalmic use occasions watering and smarting when applied to the
conjunctiva. Induction of mydriasis lasts several hours.
Combines with Zanthoxylum, Capsicum.
Dosage and mode of application
Tincturae Sig 0.6ml
References
176 p187. 224 p998. 262 p84.

Picrasma excelsa [Quassia]

Constituents
Indole alkaloids. Bitter terpenoids - quassinoids. Coumarins. Sterols.

Primary pharmacological action: Anthelmintic.

Therapeutic classes
Tonic. Gastric stimulant. Bitter. Sialagogue. Choleretic.
Orexigenic. Pediculosis.
Medicinal indications
Anorexia. Atonic dyspepsia.
Nematode infestations – Ascarides, Entamoeba histolytica. Strongyloides
[Threadworms]. Pediculosis.
Debility. Intermittent and remittent fever - typhoid, malaria.
Tissue conditions
Used as an enema to expel threadworms. A bitter with no tannins.
External use
Pediculosis – use tincture 5-10ml diluted as a scalp lotion.
Injection for Ascarides etc.
Dosage and mode of application
Dried lignum Sig 0.6g.
Concentrated Quassia infusium 1:2. Sig 4ml
Tincturae Sig 4ml
Enemata 1:20 Sig 150ml PR each day for three days with suitable anthelmintic
per oram E.g. Tanacetum.
References
43 p157. 111 p609. 126 p588. 189 p229. 224 p256.

Picrorrhiza kurroa [Lomatum disectum]

Constituents
Iridoid glycosides - picrosides.

Primary pharmacological action: Bitter tonic, hepatoprotective.

Therapeutic classes
Antioxidant. Antiviral. Antiallergic.
Stomachic. Choleretic. Purgative.
Antimalarial. Antiparasitic - Leishmania donovani and Macrofilariids parasite inhibition. Antiprotozoal. Antifilarial.
Febrifuge. Dermatological agent.
Immunostimulant.
Medicinal indications
Free radicle scavenger. Increases phagocytes.
Asthma.
Dyspepsia. Hepatitis. Jaundice.
Pyrexia. Immunostimulant in respiratory disorders e.g. asthma.
Vitiligo. Chronic fatigue.
Tissue conditions
A very bitter remedy. Hepatoprotective comparable with that of Silybum.
Dosage and mode of application
Dried rhiz Sig 4g. [390]
Liquidum extractum dried rad Sig 1.5ml
References
48 p126. 263, 1991 57, [1] p25-8. 322, Vol 1, No 1. 390 p327.

Pilocarpus
jaborandi/microphyllus/pinnatifolius
[Jaborandi]

Constituents
Pilocarpine, around 0.4%, an Imidazole alkaloid. Pilocarpine is a
sympathomimetic it causes salivation and perspiration. Physostigmine.

Primary pharmacological action: Stimulating diaphoretic

Therapeutic classes
Ophthalmic. Miotic. Stimulant. Allays inflammation.
Sialogogue. Expectorant.
Cardiac sedative. Hepatic.
Diuretic. Antirheumatic.
Galactogogue.
Antispasmodic.
Dermatological agent - dry skin. Antipyretic.
Antivenomous. Antidote to poisons.

Medicinal indications
Conjunctivitis. Choroiditis. Glaucoma. Floaters. Iritis. Detached retina. Optic
neuritis. Optic nerve atrophy. Retinal haemorrhage. Iritis. Iridocyclitis [iris &
ciliary body]. Keratitis. Weak ocular muscles. Scleritis.
Otitis media - acute. Deafness - nerve. Auditory eczema.
Angina. Relaxes vascular tension. Serous effusions - ascites, pleurisy.
Stimulates salivary production. Stomatitis. Tonsillitis - acute. Laryngitis.
Laryngismus stridulus. Laryngeal oedema. Asthma. Diphtheria. Rhinitis.
Pharyngitis. Colds. Influenza. Bronchitis. Pleurisy. Pneumonia – congestive
stage.
Diabetes. Jaundice. Typhoid and malarial fever. Renal disease. Nephritis.
Gonorrhoea. Acute mastitis. Increases breast milk. Orchitis. Ovaritis. Metritis.
Rigid Os. Puerpural eclampsia.
Inflammatory arthritis. Articular inflammation. Muscular pain or spasm.
Lumbago.
Alopecia. Eczema. Pruritus. Psoriasis. Rhus poisoning.
Hydrocephalus. Meningitis.

Tissue conditions
Lowers intraocular pressure in glaucoma. Contracts the pupil after atropine use.
Dilates capillaries when directly applied to the scalp [in baldness]. Ptyalism.
Acute febrile inflammatory action with deficient secretions of the skin and

mucous membranes. Pulse full and hard. Pyrexia with dry skin. Athletic pyrexia with restlessness. Subacute rheumatic pain and inflammation. Promotes salivation, perspiration and all glandular secretions by opening the capillaries. Uraemic poisoning with convulsions. Enhances diastole. Suppression of urine with a hard and sharp pulse. Rigid Os with pain and a sharp hard [contracted] pulse.

Cautions

Restrictions apply. Dosage is determined by the relief of symptoms.

Antidote is Atropa, Capsicum or Zingiber.

Cardiac conditions.

External use

Raised intraocular tension – collyr.

Baldness, hair loss or grey hair - apply the lotion @ 5%.

Erysipelas, eczema, mastitis, orchitis, epididymitis, articular inflammation-lotion.

Preparations

Pulmonary disease with Asclepias, Bryonia or Lobelia.

Dosage and mode of application

Minute doses relieve excessive perspiration.

Dried fol Sig 500mg

Tincturae 1:5 Sig 2ml [BPC 1949]

Lotion 5%.

References

BPC 1949. 126 p539. 176 p462. 192 p291-293. 224 p997. 282 No. 35, p24-31.

Pilosella officinarum [Mousear, hawkweed]

Constituents
Coumarin. Flavonoids.

Primary pharmacological action: Sedative expectorant.

Therapeutic classes
Tonic. Astringent. Antifungal.
Antihaemorrhagic.
Sialagogue. Anticatarrhal. Antitussive.
Diuretic.
Antispasmodic.
Vulnerary. Antivenomous.
Medicinal indications [Saturn]
Nasal polyps. Asthma. Pertussus. Bronchitis. Haemoptysis.
Aphthous ulcers. Haematemesis. Diarrhoea.
Oedema. Uterine prolapse.
Tissue conditions
Pertussus involves the mucous membranes of the stomach, lungs and nervous
system. Acts in cases of troublesome and distressing pertussus.
External use
Hernia - poultice.
Fractures - poultice.
Preparations
Pertussus – Verbascum, Tussilago.
Asthma - Grindelia.
Dosage and mode of application
Syrupus Sig 10ml
Infusium herba Sig 30ml
Liquidum extractum Sig 4ml
References
43 p158. 188 p299. 189 p194.

Pimento dioica [Allspice]

Constituents
Galloylglucosides. Vitamins A, B1, B2, C. Minerals. Protein. Volatile oil mainly eugenol.

Primary pharmacological action: Stimulating astringent, Tonic.

Therapeutic classes
Aromatic. Diffusive. Antioxidant. Carminative. Stomachic.
Medicinal indications
Colds.
Nausea and vomiting. Dyspepsia. Flatulence. Diabetes. Diarrhoea. Colic.
Musculoskeletal pain.
Panic. Fatigue.
Dysmenorrhoea.
Tissue conditions
A good addition to other medicines in the treatment of flatulence, diarrhoea and dysentery. Strengthens the stomach and relieves nausea. Enhances nutrient absorption.
As a vehicle for cathartics and bitter tonics.
In hot infusion it promotes circulatory diffusion and relieves irritation of the nervous system.
External use
Anaesthetic and antiseptic when used locally.
Chilblains.
Dosage and mode of application
Powdered fructus Sig 2g
Liquidum extractum Sig 4ml
Oleum Pimento Sig 0.2ml
References
111 p580. 126 p546. 189 p7.

Pimpinella saxifrage [Burnet saxifrage]

Constituents
Coumarin. Saponin. Volatile oil. Resin.

Primary pharmacological action: Stomachic.

Therapeutic classes
Resolvent. Antiseptic.
Anticatarrhal. Expectorant.
Aromatic. Aperitif. Carminative. Stomachic.
Diuretic. Diaphoretic.
Galactogogue.
Medicinal indications [Moon]
Toothache. Laryngitis. Hoarseness. Upper respiratory tract infections. Asthma.
Warming carminative; removes flatulence and indigestion. Cholecystitis.
Calculi. Oedema. Rheumatism. Gout.
Increases the milk flow.
External use
Throat affections, hoarseness – garg.
Toothache - chew on the fresh root.
Freckles on the skin - bathe with decoction.
Dosage and mode of application
Infusium rad. Sig 30ml
Tincturae Sig 1ml
References
142 p203. 228 p 155. 246 p285. 251 p30. 262 p81.

Pimpinella anisum [Aniseed]

Constituents
Flavonoid - quercetin. Glycosides - rutin. Volatile oil - trans anethole. Coumarins.
Oestrogenic like action.

Primary pharmacological action: Carminative. Antispasmodic.

Therapeutic classes
Antimicrobial. Expectorant.
Carminative. Parasiticide.
Spasmolytic.
Galactogogue. Emmenagogue.
Medicinal indications
Bronchial catarrh. Pertussus. Spasmodic cough. Trachieitis.
Flatulent colic.
Encourages the production of milk. Vaginal discharge/leucorrhoea. Increases
libido.
Chewed seeds make the breath sweet.
Quenches thirst. Diuretic.
Epilepsy in infants and children.
External use
Pediculosis and scabies.
Preparations
Added to purgatives to prevent griping.
Dosage and mode of application
Infusium dried fructus Sig 1g
Tincturae Sig 5ml
Syrupus Anisi [Syrup of Anise]. Concentrated Anise water 1:8. Sig 4ml
Aqua Anisi Conc BPC Concentrated Anise water. Oleum Anise 2ml, Ethanol
70ml, aqua to 100ml. Sig 1ml.
References
43 p160. 111 p610. 239 p170. 262 p47.

Pinellia ternata [Banxia]

Constituents
Alkaloids - Ephedrine. Polysaccharides. Phytosterols. Glycoside. Essential oil.

Primary pharmacological action: Anticatarrhal.

Therapeutic classes
Antiallergic. Haemostatic. Lympho vasotonic alterative.
Expectorant.
Antiemetic.
Analgesic. Anxiolytic. Antidepressant.
Immunostimulant.
Antineoplastic.
Anti venomous.

Medicinal indications
Bronchitis.
Gastric carcinoma. Gastritis. Vomiting from any cause.
Gonorrhoea.
Auto immune disorders. Lymphadenitis [TB]. Furunculosis.
Lymphoma. Mammary carcinoma.

Cautions
Avoid with Aconitum rad.

Dosage and mode of application
Tincturae rhiz/rad Sig 4ml

References
48 p170.

Pinus sylvestris [Scots pine]

Constituents
Flavonols – [OPC's] oligomeric proanthocyanidins support collagen synthesis.
Essential oil – mainly monoterpene hydrocarbons up to 97%, pinene and limonene. Resin. Bitters.

Primary pharmacological action: Antiseptic.

Therapeutic classes
Antibacterial. Antiviral. Vasotonic alterative.
Antioxidant.
Anticatarrhal. Expectorant.
Antirheumatic.
Antipruritic. Dermatological agent.
Medicinal indications [Mars]
Used as a flavouring for cough mixtures.
Sinusitis. Coughs. Chest infections. Bronchitis. Asthma. Pneumonia.
Tuberculosis.
Dyspepsia. Colitis.
Gout. Neuralgia. Rheumatism. Sciatica.
Eczema. Psoriasis.
External use
Antiseptic expectorant used as an inhalation.
Balneum indications - Rheumatic pain and muscular tension - as it diffuses the capillary circulation to the joints.
Skin disorders & hair loss – oleum/crem
Massage the dilute oleum for the relief of rheumatic pain.
Dosage and mode of application
Powdered needles/tur Sig 400mg
Tincturae 1:20 Sig 0.5ml
    Inhalation composita
    Ol Eucalyptus 4.5ml Ol Pumillo pine 4.5ml Ol Mentha piperita 1ml.
    Sig 20gtt aqua frig.
    Balneum Pinus. Pine oil bath.
    Add Oleum Pinus 5gtt to a warm bath.
References
188 p339. 189 p259/216. 394 p304.

Piper cubeba [Cubeb]

Constituents
Lignans. Volatile oil up to 20%. Resins. Gums.

Primary pharmacological action:
Stimulant to mucous membranes.

Therapeutic classes
Aromatic. Antiviral. Antibacterial. Allays inflammation.
Expectorant.
Carminative.
Diuretic.
Medicinal indications
Nasal catarrh. Laryngitis - chronic. Coughs. Bronchitis. Hay fever.
Atonic dyspepsia. Amoebic dysentery.
Urinary infections. Urethritis. Cystitis. Nocturia. Prostatic abscess.
Spermatorrhoea - seminal fluid discharge from atonic tissues. Gonorrhoea.
Syphilis. Vaginal discharge/leucorrhoea.
Tissue conditions
Stimulates the pulse. Stimulates the genito urinary mucous membranes. Atonic
conditions of the genito urinary tract. Debility with atony and excessive mucus
discharge from urinary mucous membranes. Preferable for chronic conditions.
Cautions
Avoid in acute inflammatory conditions.
Dosage and mode of application
Powdered fruct Sig 4g
Tincturae Sig 2ml
Liquidum extractum Sig 4ml
References
BPC 1934. 111 p612. 188 p136. 176 p460.

P

Piper methysticum [Kava kava]

Constituents
Alkaloid pipermethystine found in stem peelings and leaves is toxic.
Rhizome contains kavalactones [kavapyrones] - kavain and methysticin, acting upon the CNS and mediate neuronal effects on GABA receptor in the hippocampus and amygdala they are analgesic, anticonvulsant, antidepressant, muscle relaxant and sedative. Flavonoids.

Primary pharmacological action:
Nervine antispasmodic. Anxiolytic.

Therapeutic classes
Ophthalmic. Special sense organ remedy EENT. Local anaesthetic oral. Allays inflammation. Anticatarrhal. Antiseptic. Antifungal. Antibacterial.
Gentle stomach tonic.
Antiseptic diuretic.
Analgesic. Anticonvulsant. Antidepressant. Anxiolytic. Sedative. Hypnotic.
Muscle relaxant.
Vulnerary.

Medicinal indications
Ocular pain. Earache.
Palpitations. Chest pain. Hypotensive. Cerebral hyperaemia.
Asthma. Bronchitis.
Toothache. Oral anaesthetic. Anorexia. Gastric irritation. Atonic dyspepsia.
Intestinal spasm. Anal pruritus.
Cystitis [with spasm]. Dysuria. Urethritis. Prostatic enlargement. Prostatitis.
Bladder atony. Gonorrhoea. Syphilis. Enuresis. Oedema. Filariasis.
Gout. Rheumatism. Skeletal muscle relaxant – pain and stiffness. Leprosy.
Pain. Anxiety. Depression. Dizzyness. Headaches. Insomnia. Restlessness.
Neuralgia. Parkinsons disease with tremor. Epilepsy. Jet lag.
Ovaritis, endometritis and vaginitis. Dysmenorrhoea. Flushes.
Menarche/menopause - mood swings/anxiety. Vaginal pruritus. Weight reduction.

Tissue conditions
Stroke from ischaemic aetiology benefits from the use of Kava. Clears anxiety, nervousness and depression. Its aids sleep, clearer thinking and memory.
Diminishes spinal nerve reflex activity. Stimulates the vagus nerve, heart rate and lowers arterial pressure. Acts upon the genito urinary mucus membranes in irritation and inflammation [particularly in acute inflammation]. Antimicrobial in urinary and genital infections soothing inflamed and irritated tissues of the bladder [cystitis], urethra and testes. Neuralgia – ocular and aural, gastro

Pharmacopoeia

intestinal or genito urinary tracts. Skeletal muscle spasm – neck tension, neuralgia.

Cautions
Restrictions apply. Dizzyness. Headache. Skin rash. Pregnancy. Lactation.

External use
Toothache, vaginitis.
Tinea, Trichophyton – ung, crem, lotion.

Dosage and mode of application
Dried rad/rhiz. Sig 1g. Dry extract Sig 400mg [0.4g]. Tincturae Sig 10ml.
Liquidum extractum Sig 4ml [Martindale p2020]

References
BPC 1934. 126 p546. 176 p441. 179. p456. 192 p309. 224 p1772. 230 p65. 239 p130. 390 p2020. 394 p223.

Hawaii scientists explain mystery of Kava toxicity.
Reports in CAM May 2003 sheds light upon the claims made of Kava toxicity.

Professor C.S. Tang of the University of Hawaii explains his findings.
For 2000 years Kava has been used as a herbal medicine with no reports of fatalities. Supplements of tablets and capsules are highly concentrated – with the alkaloid present it was a disaster waiting to happen.
Stem bark peelings were used to make herbal supplements. Traditional Kava drinkers discard the stem bark peelings relying upon the root and rhizome as a tea. An alkaloid pipermethystine has been found in stem peelings and leaves, a lower level in the bark of the stump. Pipermethystine is not found in the root or rhizome. Pipermethystine has a strong negative effect on liver cell cultures. Stem peelings and leaves made into supplements containing pipermethystine cause hepatic damage and death. Stem peelings contain high levels of kavalactones and these are responsible for the calming effects.
Pharmaceutical companies took the waste stems and leaves and extracted a cheap source of kavalactones, however they also extracted the alkaloid pipermethystine. Either they did not detect the alkaloid or did not look for it with disastrous consequences.
It takes 3-5 years for the root to reach maturity.

Dr Tang analysed plants from several countries and found that there are three alkaloids in the stems and leaves. These alkaloids are not found in the root or rhizome.

Further testing of liver function through blood tests will be carried out at the Hawaii Tropical and subtropical Agriculture Research programme. University of Hawaii, Manoa. [396].

Piscidia erythrina [Jamaica dogwood]

Constituents

Glycoside - piscidin. Isoflavones [antispasmodic] - Icthynone, jamaicin, piscidone, rotenoids. Rotenoids are antineoplastic, and destroy lice and fleas. Piscidic acid. Sterols. Tannin. Resin.

Primary pharmacological action: Antispasmodic.

Therapeutic classes

Ophthalmic. Allays inflammation. Astringent. Oropharyngeal agent.
Cardiotonic.
Antitussive.
Diuretic. Diaphoretic.
Parturient.
Dermatological agent. Vulnerary.
Analgesic. Anodyne. Hypnotic. Sedative.
Antineoplastic.

Medicinal indications

Inflammatory and painful conditions of the eyes e.g. orbital neuralgia. Pain of otitis media.
Tachycardia.
Spasmodic coughs. Pertussus. Asthma. Tuberculosis.
Infections/gum bleeding. Toothache. Colic. Diarrhoea. Dysentery. Intestinal pain.
Renal pain. Sciatica. Lumbar pain. Inflammatory pyrexia.
Delivery labour pain. Ovarian neuralgia. Amenorrhoea. Dysmenorrhoea. Rashes.
Anxiety. Cerebral excitability – hyperactivity. Delirium tremens. Headache.
Insomnia. Migraine. Neuralgia. Panic.
Wounds.

Tissue conditions

A quarter of the dose is eliminated in 24 hours indicating long duration of activity
Increases the secretions of the mouth and skin. Slows the pulse. Eases colic due to cholelithiasis, renal calculi and flatulence.
Overcomes nervous excitement and reflex irritability. Insomnia from worry or anxiety [neurasthenia]. Useful as a muscle relaxant/anodyne for striated and smooth muscle. Pain reliever in excitable nervousness. Controls night cough of tuberculosis. Parturient controlling erratic or spasmodic pain.
Reduction of dislocations causing pain.

External use

Rashes, wounds – infusium lotion.

Pharmacopoeia

Preparations
Anodyne:
with Pulsatilla and Dioscorea. Nervine-Capsicum, Scutellaria and Valeriana
Dosage and mode of application
Dried rad/cort Sig 4g
Tincturae Sig 5ml
Liquidum extractum Sig 8ml
References
BPC 1934. 126 p548. 176 p110. 179 p460. 188 p256. 192.

Plantago lanceolata/major [Plantain]

Constituents
Tannins as iridoid glycoside up to 2.5% aucubin has antiseptic effects on gastro intestinal infections. Alkaloids. Flavonoids. Acids - benzoic, caffeic. Allantoin. Resin. Saponins - antimicrobial. Amino acids. 5 phenylethanoid allays inflammation. Polysaccharide fractionsup to 6.5% are immunostimulatory. Potassium. Zinc.

Primary pharmacological action: Astringent.

Therapeutic classes
Ophthalmic. Antimicrobial against - Bacillus subtilis, Micrococcus flavus, Staphylococcus aureus. Antifungal – candida. Demulcent. Antiseptic. Allays inflammation.
Antihaemorrhagic. Vasotonic alterative [blood tonic]. Hypercholesterolaemia.
Antihistamine. Antiallergic. Pulmonary tonic. Expectorant. Antitussive.
Oropharyngeal conditions. Antacid. Antiulcer. Hepatoprotective.
Gently laxative [bulk laxative].
Diuretic. Uric acid diathesis. Antipyretic.
Antineoplastic. Immune stimulant. Lymphatic.
Dermatological agent. Emollient. Vulnerary. Antivenomous.
Analgesic.

Medicinal indications [Venus]
Blepharitis. Conjunctivitis.
Sinusitis. Coughs. Bronchitis. Haemoptysis. Tuberculosis.
Mercurial poisoning. Oropharyngeal ulcers. Gingivitis. Pyorrhoea. Toothache
Hyperchlorhydria. Gastroenteritis. Colic. Colitis. Gastro intestinal haemorrhage
[ulcers]. IBS. Diverticulitis. Constipation. Haemorrhoids. Intermittent fever -
Cholera. Amoebic and Bacillary dysentery.
Enuresis. Cystitis. Haematuria. Oedema. Gonorrhoea. Syphilis.
Menorrhagia. Vaginal discharge/leucorrhoea – candida.
Abscesses. Acne. Burns. Bites. Eczema. Erysipelas. Measles. Scalds. Stings.
Wounds. Dermal ulcers. Malignant dermal ulcers. Plague.

Tissue conditions
Diffuse and stimulating vasotonic alterative. Its chief spheres of action are the head, chest and intestines. Symptoms indicating its use are haemorrhage and exhaustion. Inflammatory respiratory conditions.
Toothache and earache chew the leaves. Cleansing the intestine of toxins.
Lubricates and stimulates in sluggish and atonic intestines. For chronic constipation. Dysentery.

Pharmacopoeia

Used in epidemics, in famine, in diseases where infection is conveyed in the faeces or contaminated water supply it is a natural cleanser. Inflammation, burning and itching conditions of the skin and mucous membranes.

External use

Eye disorders – collyr or oleum.

Earache use guttae.

Diverticulitis – enema.

Bites of insects, dogs, snakes, the leaf bruised and laid over the affected area.

First aid measure - use in place of dock leaves for nettle stings.

Heals cuts, leg ulcers and open wounds – fresh fol, rank it as a haemostatic comparable to Calendula and Achillea.

Malignant dermal ulcers - wash and poultice.

Earache, facial neuralgia - sedative poultice.

Preparations

Meniers disease with Pulsatilla, Zanthoxylum.

Dosage and mode of application

Plantago major [broad leaf] is to be preferred in treatment.

Infusium Sig 30ml

Tincturae rad/fol Sig 7ml

Liquidum extractum Sig 4ml

> **Gargle** infusium 1.5g
>
> **Poultice** – dampen herb and use the macerate.
>
> **Unguentum** @ 10%
>
> Method ung - Vegetarian cooking fat and add as many plantain leaves as it will absorb. Simmer for about 20 minutes, run into small jars.

References

43 p163. 188 p341. 192 p433. 251 p133. 271, No.15. 272, 1996, 8 [5] 67-9. 274 2000, 71, [1-2], p1-21. 394 p307.

Plantago ovata/psyllium

Ispaghula-pale seed, Psyllium-dark seed – a similar activity to both types.

Constituents
Mucilage up to 15% [30% in ovata] with the main polysaccharide d-xylose.
Triterpenes. Alkaloids - monoterpenes. Sterols. Fatty acids. Sugars. Protein up to 20%.

Primary pharmacological action: Demulcent bulk laxative.

Therapeutic classes
Allays inflammation. Anticholesterolaemic.
Antidiarrhoeal.
Diuretic.
Medicinal indications
Diverticulosis. Diarrhoea. Constipation. IBS. Colitis. Anal fissures. Bacillary dysentery.
Cystitis.
Furunculosis.
Tissue conditions
Reduces blood sugar levels by delaying sugar absorption in the intestine. Lowers cholesterol - LDL levels, this has been established using 5g BD. Regulates intestinal peristalsis. A bulk laxative it absorbs water from the intestine and increases the volume of the faeces. Used as a soothing demulcent for irritable conditions of the intestine. Inflammatory and spastic conditions respond to the demulcent activity. When haemorrhoids and fissures are present it provides a useful adjunct to treatment. It is noted that diabetics may be able to reduce their insulin dosage when the seeds are taken.
External use
Furunculosis – poultice.
Dosage and mode of application
Semen Sig 10g Soak the seeds in boiling water for two hours before ingestion. Take with plenty of fluid.
Liquidum extractum Sig 5ml
References
43 p164/5. 191p117. 192 p433. 204. 272, 1996, 8 [5] 67. 272, 1995, 7 [4] p67. 323, 2000, Vol. 120, No. 2, p107-111. 394 p314.

Podophyllum peltatum/emodi [Mandrake]

Constituents
Lignans - podophyllotoxin. Flavonoids. Glycosides. Resin.

Primary pharmacological action:
Choleretic. Cholagogue. Purgative.

Therapeutic classes
It has a very caustic taste and is a nauseant.
Stimulant. Vasotonic alterative. Antiviral.
Venous congestion.
Sialagogue. Hepatic. Hydragogue cathartic. Anthelmintic.
Antirheumatic. Antipyretic.
Dermatological agent.
Antineoplastic.
Medicinal indications [Mercury]
Ear pain.
Dyspepsia. Biliary colic. Emetic. Cholecystitis. Cholelithiasis. Jaundice.
Constipation. Haemorrhoids. Anal prolapse. Cholera. Typhoid. Anal warts.
Strongyloides
Remittent and intermittent fever - Malaria.
Eczema. Pustular or fissured skin reactions. Plantar warts.
Syphilis. Gonorrhoeal epididymitis. Genital warts. Ovarian carcinoma.
Headache. Insomnia.
Tissue conditions
Intestinal irritant activity. Used in sluggish conditions of the abdominal viscera.
Liquefies the bile and breaks down calculi. Hepatic enlargement or biliary
congestion, liver soreness with pain under the scapula. Stimulates secretions of
the salivary glands, mucous membranes, gallbladder, liver and intestines.
Dizzyness, headaches and anorexia associated with dyspepsia. Dirty, flabby
tongue with general plethoric fullness [congestion]. Full superficial veins. Gastric
disturbances with hepatic congestion. Portal and hepatic congestion.
Cautions
Restrictions apply. Dosage is determined by the relief of symptoms.
Gastro intestinal inflammation. Contracted skin. Dryness of the tongue.
Pregnancy.
External use
Ear pain - guttae succus with Aralia.
Venereal warts, Verrucae - apply the LE direct to the wart and protect with
paraffin molle to prevent excoriation of the surrounding skin.

Preparations
To allay griping use Atropa, Hyoscyamnus or Leptandra.
To render a milder action use with Lobelia and above Medicines.
Stomach disorders with Hydrastis.
Chronic hepatitis with Chelidonium, Chionanthus or Iris.
Emeto-cathartic action with Zingiber in pyrexia.
Malaria with Cinchona.
Syphilis with Phytolacca, Rumex, Sassafras, Iris, Sambucus and Carum carvi.
Dosage and mode of application
Always give in small doses as large doses produce watery stools and griping.
Resin Sig 0.06g
Tincturae rad/rhiz Sig 0.25ml
Liquidum extractum Sig 0.3ml
References
111 p617. 126 p555. 142 p324. 176 p310. 188 p283. 224 p1340. 228 p347. 390 p1633.

Polygala senega [Senega, Polygala tenuifolia/sibirica]

[Chinese senega is very similar]

Constituents
Saponins - Senegin A, B, C, D. Senegin is irritant to the gasto intestinal mucosa and excites reflex action upon the bronchial mucosa. Salicylic acid. Fats. Resin. Sterols.

Primary pharmacological action:
Pulmonary vasocompressor - pulmonary tissue astringent.

Therapeutic classes
Ophthalmic. Vasotonic alterative. Allays inflammation. Expectorant.
Sialagogue. Emetic.
Diuretic. Diaphoretic.
Emmenagogue.
Sedative. Antivenomous.

Medicinal indications
Blepharitis. Iritis. Palpitations.
Pharyngitis. Catarrh. Asthma. Bronchitis. Respiratory tract infections.
Laryngismus stridulus. Pneumonia - later stages.
Typhoid. Oedema. Syphilis. Pyrexia.
Multiple sclerosis. Amenorrhoea.
Anxiety. Restlessness. Insomnia. Eczema. Psoriasis. Snake bite.

Tissue conditions
Stimulant and cleansing to respiratory mucous membranes and skin. A useful remedy for chronic bronchial conditions with atony and loss of tone to the bronchial tubes. The saponins are not absorbed but irritate the gastric mucosa and by reflex action stimulate the bronchioles to expel mucus.

Cautions
A strong medicine use smaller doses to start with as it can cause gastric irritation.

Dosage and mode of application
Dried rad Sig 3g
Infusium 1:2 Sig 5ml
Tincturae Sig 4ml
Liquidum extractum Sig 4ml

Syrupus Senega.
Senega 4g, alcohol 10% to 50ml. Sucrose 78g, aqua to 100ml. Macerate in dilute alcohol then add sucrose. Strain & filter Sig 5ml

References
43 p196. 111 p623. 126 p626. 192 p502. 5224 p604. 246 p223. 271 [76].

Polygonum bistorta [Bistort]

Similar activity is found with P. aviculare/hydropiper.

Constituents
Tannin. Gallic acid. Gum. Mucilage.

Primary pharmacological action: Astringent and Tonic.

Therapeutic classes
Demulcent. Allays inflammation. Haemostatic. Anticatarrhal. Expectorant.
Antidiarrhoeal. Anthelmintic - Cestodes. Nematodes.
Diuretic.
Styptic. Dermatological agent. Antivenomous.
Medicinal indications [Saturn]
Catarrh. Laryngitis. Lung complaints. Respiratory haemorrhage.
Varicose veins and phlebitis.
Aphthous ulcers. Stomatitis. Peptic ulcers. Dysentery. Diarrhoea. IBS. Ulcerative
colitis. Cholera. Jaundice. Internal ulcerations. Haemorrhoids. Anal fissure.
Tapeworm, pinworm & threadworm.
Cystitis. Urinary tract haemorrhage. Hernia.
Menorrhagia. Leucorrhoea. Vaginal haemorrhage.
Malaria. Plague. Smallpox. Measles. Snakebite. Insect bites. Ext-Hae., & wounds
Tissue conditions
A powerful astringent, cleansing to the gastro intestinal mucous membranes.
Preparations
Malaria with Acorus.
Pyrexia with malaria, smallpox, plague and measles. Plague with Iris.
Skin conditions - Polygonum, Althea, Chamomilla, Sanicula, Stachys.
External use
Ulcerated tonsils - use the gargle.
Skin ulcers, varicose veins and phlebitis - lotion.
It has a powerful faculty to resist poisons used as a wash.
Efficacious astringent lotion made from pwd. Quercus and pwd. Polygonum rad
is invaluable for open wounds and haemorrhage, it has enormous cleansing
power.
Snake bites – poultice decoction and internal dose.
Dosage and mode of application
Powdered rad Sig 2g
Tincturae Sig 5ml
Liquidum extractum Sig 2ml
References. 43 p167. 176 p482. 192 p61. 247 p49-51. 251 p17. 262 p63.

Polygonum multiflorum [Flowery knotweed]

Constituents
Bitters. Tannins. Anthraquinones. Phospholipids. Emodin - immunostimulant.

Primary pharmacological action: Nervine tonic.

Therapeutic classes
Astringent. Anti-infective. Demulcent.
Anticholesterolaemic. Antioxidant. Hypotensive.
Aperient. Bitter. Hepatic tonic. Laxative.
Diuretic. Renal tonic. Antirheumatic.
Antispasmodic. Antimalarial.
Medicinal indications
Tinnitus.
Aphrodisiac. Menopause.
Ageing. Greying hair.
Insomnia. Neurasthenia.
Tissue conditions
A tonic for increasing vitality, and vital force to the liver and kidneys. Soothes
mucous membranes and diminishes excessive mucus production. Encourages
virility. For infertility in men [increases sperm count] and women. For pain in the
low back, knee, tendons and bones.
It helps premature greying of the hair.
Cautions
IBS.
Dosage and mode of application
Dried rad Sig 5g
Tincturae Sig 5ml
Liquidum extractum Sig 4ml
References
48 p49-51. 188 p216.

Polymnia uvedalia [Bearsfoot]

Primary pharmacological action:
Stimulating Vasotonic alterative.

Therapeutic classes
Discutient. Hepatic. Laxative.
Lympho vasotonic alterative.
Anodyne.
Medicinal indications
Pulmonary congestion. Pneumonia.
Abscesses. Chronic gastritis. Atonic dyspepsia. Hepatic enlargement. Splenitis.
Splenic enlargement.
Rheumatism. Myalgia. Intermittent fever.
Mastitis. Lymphadenitis - sub acute. Glandular tumours.
Uterine subinvolution and cervical hypertrophy. Metritis.
Tissue conditions
A stimulating glandular vasotonic alterative for the spleen and liver. Dyspepsia,
heartburn from sluggishness of the gastric and splenic circulation. Flabby relaxed
tissues of the abdomen with burning [chronic inflammation, congestion] of the
liver, spleen or stomach. Indicated for glandular hypertrophy.
External use
Hair tonic use the diluted tincturae with Bay Rum.
Mastitis and lymphoedema - plaster.
Spinal irritation with congestion of the spleen, liver, lymphatics or uterus.
Dosage and mode of application
Liquidum extractum Sig 3ml
References
126 p560. 176 p327. 189 p27.

Populus candicans/giliadensis/nigra
[Balm of Gilead]

Constituents
Flavones. Volatile oil around 2%. Phenolic glycosides - salicin, populin. Resins.

Primary pharmacological action
Pulmonary vasostimulant [Stimulating expectorant]

Therapeutic classes
Antiseptic. Allays inflammation. Antibacterial. Antiviral - Tinea. Antimicrobial.
Demulcent. Expectorant. Counter irritant.
Diuretic. Antirheumatic. Antipyretic.
Analgesic.
Immunostimulant.
Vulnerary. Dermatological agent.
Medicinal indications
Pharyngitis. Catarrh. Colds. Sinusitis. Aphonia. Laryngitis. Bronchitis.
Haemorrhoids. Rheumatic aches and pains. Arthritis.
Burns. Cuts. Dermal injury. Frostbite. Sunburn.
Tissue conditions
A stimulating expectorant - antiseptic and counter irritant. Influences the mucous
membranes. Inflamed or ulcerated gastro intestinal mucous membranes.
Cautions
Care in irritable conditions of the mucous membranes.
External use
Counter irritant in muscular rheumatism, myalgia – ung.
Preparations
Larnygitis – garg.
Pertussus with Pimpinella/Prunus serotina and Lobelia.
Rheumatic pain - liniment.
To avoid griping use with Zingiber.
Dosage and mode of application
Preferable to mix with a demulcent [Gum Arabic] or a syrup to cover the
disagreeable taste.
Syrupus Sig 5ml. Dried gem Sig 4g
Infusium gem Sig 4g. Tincturae Sig 8ml
Liquidum extractum Sig 8ml.
Ung 30%
References
43 p103. 224. 233. 394 p312.

Populus tremuloides [Quaking aspen]

Constituents
Phenolic glycosides populin, and around 2.4% salicin. Various benzoate
derivatives. Resin. Tannin. Triterpenes.

Primary pharmacological action: Tonic.

Therapeutic classes
Ophthalmic. Stimulant. Astringent. Allays inflammation. Antibacterial.
Stomachic. Cholagogue. Hepatic. Anthelmintic.
Diuretic. Antirheumatic. Antipyretic.
Uterine congestion.
Anodyne. Antiperiodic.
Vulnerary. Dermatological agent.
Medicinal indications [Saturn]
Purulent opthalmia. Colds.
Anorexia. Diarrhoea. Dysentery. Cholera. Jaundice. Ascarides.
Cystitis. Prostatic hypertrophy. Gonorrhoea. Pyrexia.
Rheumatic disorders: rheumatic pain, sciatica, rheumatoid arthritis. Articular
swelling.
Eczema. Intermittent fever - Malaria. Ulcers. Infected wounds.
Tissue conditions
Constitutional tonic to the mucous membranes of the gastro intestinal and genito
urinary tracts.
Preparations
Rheumatoid arthritis with Cimicifuga.
Dosage and mode of application
Dried bacc/fol Sig 4g
Tincturae Sig 4ml
Liquidum extractum Sig 4ml
References
43 p168. 111 p631. 126 p561. 176 p17. 188 p451. 192 p439. 246 p65.

Poria cocos [Hoelen - Chinese mushroom]

Constituents
Contains Poria up to 30%. Pinella. Polysaccharides. Amino acids. Phytosterols.
Glucose.

Primary pharmacological action: Cerebral tonic.

Therapeutic classes
Antidiarrhoeal.
Diuretic.
Antidepressant. Anxiolytic. Sedative.
Immunostimulant. Antineoplastic.
Medicinal indications
Palpitations.
Antacid. Diarrhoea.
Dementia and disease of old age.
Tissue conditions
Sedative to the nervous system.
Cautions
Avoid in relaxed conditions of the genito urinary system.
Dosage and mode of application
Decoctum fungus Sig 5g
Tincturae Sig 4ml
References
261.

Potentilla erecta [Tormentil]

Constituents
Condensed tannins form 70% of tannins - elagitannin laevigatins [hydrolysable]
B & F up to 3.5%, tormentol. Phlobaphene - red colouring matter.

Primary pharmacological action: Astringent.

Therapeutic classes
Deobstruent. Tonic. Antibacterial.
Antihaemorrhagic.
Vulnerary. Styptic.
Immunostimulant. Antineoplastic.
Medicinal indications [Sun]
Conjunctivitis. Epistaxis.
Aphthous ulcers. Gingivitis. Pyorrhoea. Tonsillitis. Peptic ulcer. Diarrhoea.
Colitis. Ulcerative colitis. Colic. Haemorrhoids. Cholera.
Hernia. Prostatic enlargement.
Smallpox. Wounds.
Tissue conditions
Powerful astringent which tones the intestine and mucous membranes.
Potentilla anserina [Silverweed] is very similar – LE dose 3ml.
Preparations
Conjunctivitis – collyr.
Mouth and throat disorders – garg. or with Acacia.
Intestinal conditions with acacia, Plantago or Polygonum.
Haemorrhoids with Hamamelis.
External use
Skin sores and ulcers – to ease pain use the poultice.
Vaginal discharge/leucorrhoea – douche.
Dosage and mode of application
Tincturae rad/rhiz Sig 4ml
Liquidum extractum rad/rhiz Sig 4ml
References
43 p170. 228 p341. 246 p180. 251 p147. 263, 1994, 60 p384. 274, 44, 1994, p35.

Potentilla reptans [Cinquefoil]

Constituents
Tannin.

Primary pharmacological action: Astringent.

Therapeutic classes
Allays inflammation. Antirheumatic. Antipyretic.
Nerve sedative. Antispasmodic.
Vulnerary. Dermatological agent.
Antineoplastic. Antivenomous.
Medicinal indications [Jupiter]
Conjunctivitis. Epistaxis. Peritonsillar abscess. Laryngitis. Coughs. Haemoptysis.
Aphthous ulcers. Peritonsillar abscess. Toothache. Diarrhoea. Dysentery.
Jaundice. Hernia.
Gout. Arthritis. Pyrexia.
Infected or bleeding wounds. Shingles.
Epilepsy. Panic. Cramp. Intermittent fevers.
Tissue conditions
Cooling to the blood in pyrexial conditions from infection.
External use
Sore, inflamed gums or aphthous ulcers - garg.
Gums - mouthwash .
Toothache - apply dect. upon cotton wool to the affected area.
Sinus infections and catarrh - spray into the nose.
Fistulas, wounds, tumours, shingles, nodes.
Rheumatic swelling of tendons and ligaments, sciatica, hernia - apply lotion or
poultice.
Dosage and mode of application
Infusium Sig 30ml
Liquidum extractum herba/rad. Sig 4ml
References
111 p638. 127 p316. 160 p69. 228 p249. 246 p181.

Primula veris [Cowslip]

Constituents
Condensed tannins. Flavonoids in flos allay inflammation and are antioxidant –
Apigenin - antispasmodic. Phenolic glycosides - primulaveroside. Quinones -
Primin compounds. Triterpenoid saponins – mainly in the root. Silicic acid.
Volatile oil up to 0.25%. CHO.

Primary pharmacological action: Sedative and antispasmodic.

Therapeutic classes
Astringent. Allays inflammation. Demulcent. Sternutatory.
Antioxidant. Anticoagulant.
Anticatarrhal. Irritant expectorant.
Antacid. Cholelithiasis.
Mild diuretic. Antirheumatic. Antipyretic.
Anodyne. Hypnotic. Sedative. Anaesthetic.
Medicinal indications [Venus]
Toothache. Hypertension. Temporal arteritis. Varicose veins. Intermittent
claudication.
Catarrh. Colds. Asthma. Bronchitis. Influenza. Pertussus. Trachieitis.
Lithuria. Gout. Muscular rheumatism. Lumbago. Sciatica.
Migraine. Nervous excitability - hyperactivity/restlessness. Irritability. Headache.
Panic attacks. Anxiety. Insomnia. Epilepsy. Chorea. Paralysis. Tremor.
Burns. Scalds. Measles.
Tissue conditions
Sensitivity and pain - a useful calming antispasmodic nervine. Rad is more
expectorant than the flower. Saponins stimulate expectorant action via irritant
action upon the GI tract as this leads to stimulation of the cough reflex.
Cautions
Excessive dosage causes vomiting.
Preparations
Respiratory conditions with Echinacea, Inula, Prunus, Sambucus or Thymus.
Nervous conditions – Escholtzia, Humulus, Passiflora, Scutellaria, Valeriana,
Verbena, Zizyphus.
Dosage and mode of application
Primula vulgaris [Primrose] has similar activity though not as strong.
Dried flos/rad/rhiz Sig 3g
Tincturae Sig 6ml
Liquidium extractum Sig 2ml
References. 43 p170. 188p132. 192 p169. 246 p315. 251 p60.

Propolis [Flower pollen]

Constituents
Propolis is a resin from shrubs and trees [poplar]. Composed of essential oils, pollen, resin and wax. Containing amino acids, vitamins – B complex, minerals. Hydroxycinnamic acid. Flavonoid aglycones. The Propolis is mixed with bees own saliva.

Primary pharmacological action: Constitutional tonic.

Therapeutic classes
Nutritive. Allays inflammation. Antibacterial. Antifungal. Antiviral. Antiallergic. Arteriosclerosis. Hyper/hypotension.
Oropharyngeal agent. Peptic ulcers. Cholelithiasis. Intestinal dysbiosis.
Diuretic. Antilithic. Prostatic enlargement.
Nervous disorders.
Antineoplastic.
Vulnerary. Dermatological agent.
Immunostimulant.

Medicinal indications
Coronary disease. Hyper/hypotension. Stimulates leucocytosis.
Laryngitis. Asthma.
Gingivitis. Tonsillitis. Halitosis. Anorexia. Duodenal ulcer.
Impotence/sexual dysfunction. Infertility.
Fatigue. Senility. Retarded mental development. Depression. Insomnia.
Endocrine insufficiency. Hormonal deficiency.
Abscesses. Acne. Allergies. Burns. Cellulite. Dermatitis. Herpes. Ulcers.
Prevents ulcer and abscess formation. Tinnitus. Chelates heavy metals.

Tissue conditions
An adaptogenic and supportive medication and tonic.

External use
Swab the area with Tr: Acne, Allergics, Herpes, Ulcers, Burns and Abscesses.
Vaginal infections and sores.
Soreness of the lips and mouth, use as a mouthwash.
Tinnitus - plug the ear with gauze soaked in emulsion.

Dosage and mode of application
5g per day in capsule form.
Asthma and bronchitis - alcoholic Tr Sig 20gtt TDS
Garg. Sig 5gtt PRN.
Emulsion 1:4 with sunflower ol.
References. 112 p108. 188 p357. 192 p440/609/625. 239 p147.

Prunella vulgaris [Self heal]

Constituents
Pentacylic triterpenes – betulinic acid, oleanolic acid and ursolic acid [diuretic and antineoplastic]. Rutin. Vitamins A, B, C, K.

Primary action: Astringent

Therapeutic classes
Ophthalmic. Vasotonic alterative. Antibacterial. Antifungal – Candida. Antiviral
Antioxidant. Hypotensive. Vasodilator. Haemostatic.
Bitter tonic. Vermifuge.
Diuretic. Antipyretic.
Antispasmodic.
Antineoplastic. Cytotoxic. Lymphatic. Vulnerary.
Medicinal indications [Venus]
Ophthalmic inflammation – blepharitis, conjunctivitis. Eye strain.
Hypertension.
Pharyngitis. Pulmonary inflammation. Tuberculosis.
Sore throats. Aphthous ulcerations. Stomatitis. Hepatitis. Jaundice. Flatus.
Diarrhoea. Dysentery. Colonic pain. Helminths.
Renal disorders. Haematuria.
Mastitis.
Epilepsy. Headache. Vertigo.
Glandular fever. Mumps.
Furunculosis. Wounds.
External use
Headache – succus applied to forehead.
Vulnerary action with Ajuga.
Wounds – infusion lotion.
Dosage and mode of application
Infusium herba Sig 30ml
References
127 p732. 147 p499. 160 p239/331. 189 p248. 192 p500. 272 1993, 6 [1] p18-19.

Prunus serotina [Wild cherry]

Constituents
Benzaldehyde. Cyanogenic glycosides – prunacin. Prunacin is converted into hydrocyanic acid. Volatile oil. Resin. Tannin.

Primary pharmacological action:
Demulcent and astringent tonic.

Therapeutic classes
Tonic to the respiratory and gastro intestinal tract. Antitussive. Expectorant.
Mild sedative to the circulatory and nervous systems. Nervine tonic.

Medicinal indications
Opthalmia. Weakness of the pulse. Nervous palpitations.
Irritable cough. Nervous coughs with palpitations. Chronic bronchitis. Pertussus.
Tuberculosis. Dyspnoea.
Anorexia. Nervous dyspepsia. Diarrhoea. IBS.
Nerve tonic in debility. Pyrexia.

Tissue conditions
Sedative effect upon irritable respiratory, gastro intestinal and urinary mucosal
surfaces. Clears irritating phlegm in the throat. Continuous irritable coughs.
Soothes the digestive tract. Useful for convalescence from acute inflammatory
conditions. Lessens vascular excitement.

Preparations
In a syrup form which tastes more agreeable.
Tuberculosis - use the syrup.
Opthalmia - use collyr.

Dosage and mode of application
Powdered cort Sig 2g
Tincturae Sig 4ml
Liquidum extractum Sig 4ml
Syrupus Prunus Syrup of Prunus
Infuse Prunus 60g in Aqua 550ml Cover and leave for three hours. Strain and add
glycerine or honey. Syrup Prunus Sig 10ml.

References
43 p172. 111 p639. 188 p453. 189 p 281. 192 p563. 224 p616. 246 p190.

Pueraria lobata [Kudzu]

Constituents
Isoflavonoids - diadzin and daidzein which suppress the desire for alcohol.

Primary pharmacological action: Vasodilator.

Therapeutic classes
Demulcent. Relaxant. Hypoglycaemic.
Antiemetic. Spasmolytic. Hypotensive.
Antipyretic. Antivenomous.
Medicinal indications
Gastritis. Headache.
Angina. Myocardial ischaemia. Cerebral ischaemia. Peripheral circulatory
insufficiency. Hypertension.
Dysentery. Gastroenteritis.
Pyrexia. Dehydration. Eruptive diseases. Increases breast size.
Dosage and mode of application
Tincturae rad Sig 4ml
References
Herbarium Dec 1993.

Pulmonaria officinalis [Lungwort]

Constituents
Tannin. Saponins. Allantoin.

Primary pharmacological action: Expectorant

Therapeutic classes
Astringent. Demulcent.
Antihaemorrhagic.
Diaphoretic.
Emollient. Vulnerary.
Medicinal indications [Jupiter]
Nasal catarrh. Coughs. Laryngitis. Bronchitis. Influenza. Tuberculosis.
Diarrhoea. Gastro intestinal haemorrhage. Haemorrhoids.
Menorrhagia. Wounds.
Tissue conditions
Inflammatory conditions of the respiratory tract.
Preparations
Taken hot it is diaphoretic.
Chronic pulmonary conditions with Plantago and Tussilago.
Dosage and mode of application
Dried herba Sig 4g
Tincturae Sig 4ml
Liquidum extractum Sig 4ml
References
43 p173. 189 p179. 192 p338. 246 p349.

Pulsatilla vulgaris [Pasque flower]

Constituents
Pulsatilla should not be used fresh. The glycoside ranunculin is converted to an acrid volatile oil – protoanemonin this occurs when the plant is crushed and in turn is converted to safer solid Anemonin in the dried plant. Flavonoids. Saponins.

Primary pharmacological action:
An antispasmodic nervine having special influence to the 5 special sense organs, genitourinary tract, uterus and prostate.

Therapeutic classes
Ophthalmic. Allays inflammation. Stimulant. Vasotonic alterative. Antiseptic. Bactericidal. Expectorant.
Diuretic. Diaphoretic.
Emmenagogue. Galactagogue.
Analgesic. Sedative. Drug habit.

Medicinal indications [Mars]
Hordeolum. Profuse lacrymation. Conjunctivitis. Eye tics. Cataract. Glaucoma. Opthalmia neonatorum. Scleritis.
Otitis media. Earache. Hearing loss.
Cardiac hypertrophy [right heart dilation]. Venous congestion.
Toothache. Gum abscess. Tongue with thick, creamy coating. Hiccough.
Stomach disorders with white coated tongue, inability to digest fat.
Asthma induced by pregnancy or amenorrhoea. Acute and chronic catarrh with infection. Bronchial and pulmonary inflammation. Pertussus. Tobacco addiction.
Skin eruptions with bacterial infection. Eruptive fevers – chicken pox, measles. Furunculosis.
Amenorrhoea from emotional aetiology. Dysmenorrhoea. Vaginal discharge/leucorrhoea. Ovaritis. Ovaralgia. Pelvic organ nerve irritation [pain]. PMS. Weak labour pain. Mastitis. Flushes.
Epididymitis. Orchitis. Spermatorrhoea. Prostatorrhoea. Varicocoele.
Anxiety. Depression. Insomnia. Headaches. Hyperactivity. Neuralgia. Over sensitivity. Panic. Schizophrenia. Senile dementia. Adrenal exhaustion.

Tissue conditions
The herb has a stimulating and relaxing influence to the mucous membranes of the respiratory and digestive organs. It is indicated for catarrh of the eyes, nose, ears and stomach. Excessive mucus discharges. Pulsatilla clears otitis media, catarrh of the nose and ears, catarrhal opthalmia. Headache with gastric disturbances. Pulsatilla helps to remove mental fear and apprehension. Used in

Pharmacopoeia

stomach catarrh with coated tongue. Nervous eye tics of children [frequent blinking].
Spasmodic cough of asthma, bronchitis and pertussus. Acute inflammatory conditions of the upper respiratory tract. Muco or muco purulent nasal mucus.
Measles - coughs and mucous membrane irritability.
Inflamed conditions of the genito urinary tract.
Nervous irritation in varicocoele, orchitis, phlebitis. Full doses depress heart activity and lower blood pressure.
Painful conditions of the male or female reproductive tract.
Enlarged prostate gland, sensitive urethra, spermatorrhoea with fear.
Impotence/sexual dysfunction from anxiety or fear. Nervous irritability with varicocoele. Over excitable sexual desire - masturbation in males and females.
Balances the ANS which it leaves toned and strengthened. As an antispasmodic and sedative to the nervous system it quietens hyperactivity, tension provoking headaches, neuralgia, spinal nerve irritation, tachycardia, insomnia and panic attacks. Neuralgia in anaemic patients.
It is a valued remedy for nerve exhaustion or nervousness in women with feeble pulse, deficient capillary circulation, amenorrhoea of the anaemic type, cold extremities and a general relaxed physical condition. Dysmenorrhoea from emotional aetiology. Ovaritis with pain. It relieves undue sensitivity of the vagina. Mastitis with fear or depression [see dose]. Depression or fear with painful agalactia breasts. Recommended for fair, blue eyed people. Weepy and nervous types with unsettled minds. Rheumatic joint aches of the hands and feet. Supports benzodiazepine withdrawal.

External use
Conjunctivitis use a dilute preparation. Neuralgia, rheumatism – fol poultice.
Preparations
Facilitates tonics and trophorestoratives e.g. Scutellaria.
Hearing loss with Crataegus.
Headache with excitability - Passiflora. Hyperactivity – Passiflora and Piscidia.
Insomnia/Orchitis with Piscidia. Dysmenorrhoea with Chamaelirium.
Skin diseases/septicaemia with Baptisia or Echinacea.
Cautions
The fresh plant should not be used. Gastritis.
Dosage and mode of application
Infusium herba Sig 0.3g
Tincturae Pulsatilla herba Sig 1.5ml
Liquidum extractum Sig 1ml
References
43. 126 p583. 176 p149. 188 p360. 189 p227. 192 p445. 233 p179. 246 p117. 394 p394.

Pygeum africana

Constituents
Amygdalin. Ferrulic acid esters. Phytosterols. Triterpenes.

Primary pharmacological action: Allays inflammation.

Therapeutic classes
Anti androgenic.
Medicinal indications
Prostatic enlargement. BPH. Impotence/sexual dysfunction. Infertility.
Dosage and mode of application
Tincturae stem/bacc Sig 5ml
References
403. 404. 405. 406.

Quercus robur [Oak]

Constituents
Saponins up to 10%. Tannin up to 15% - ellagitannin, phlobatannin. Gallic acid.

Primary pharmacological action: Astringent.

Therapeutic classes
Ophthalmic. Antiseptic. Antibacterial. Allays inflammation.
Antioxidant. Haemostatic. Venous tonic.
Oropharyngeal agent. Hepatoprotective.
Vulnerary. Dermatological agent.
Antineoplastic. Immunostimulant.
Medicinal indications [Jupiter]
Conjunctivitis. Varicose veins. Chilblains.
Nasal polyps. Laryngitis. Tuberculosis. Night sweats.
Aphthous ulcers. Chronic sore throats. Gingivitis. Tonsillitis. Diarrhoea.
Dysentery. Cholera. Prolapsus ani. Haemorrhoids. Anal fissures. Haemorrhage.
Urinary inflammation. Renal inflammation. Vaginal discharge/leucorrhoea.
Gangrenous wounds. Burns. Foot odour. Dermal inflammation – weeping
eczema. Tones the nipples – breast feeding.
Alcoholism. Intermittent fever.
Tissue conditions
Mucous membrane astringent for relaxed mucous membranes. Mucus discharges.
Ulcerations of the gastro intestinal tract. Malarial fever.
Preparations
Malaria with Chamomilla.
External use
Balneum for an astringent effect – use powdered Quercus 100g in muslin.
Bleeding gums, sore throats, tonsillitis - gargle.
Nasal polyps – snuff with Potentilla.
Haemorrhoids apply dilute liquid extract or enema.
Skin ulceration, burns – lotion @ 2g per 100ml
Skin abrasions/damage with Sambucus.
Vaginal discharge/leucorrhoea – douche.
Dosage and mode of application
Infusium Sig 3g
Liquidum extractum cort Sig 5ml
References
43 p175. 111 p649. 188 p315. 189 p203. 192 p388. 246 p75. 247 p43. 274, 44,
1994, p35-40. 394 p278.

Ranunculus ficaria [Pilewort]

Constituents
Anemonin and protoanemonin are lactones which are antibacterial. Tannin.
Triterpenoids. Vitamin C.

Primary pharmacological action: Astringent.

Therapeutic classes
Demulcent. Anodyne.
Medicinal indications [Mars]
Haemorrhoids.
Tissue conditions
Locally astringent to the rectal veins. Haemorrhoids can be very painful so early
use can be very relieving for the pain the patient suffers.
External use
Haemorrhoids use as an ointment and suppository.
Dosage and mode of application
Dried herba Sig 5g
Liquidum extractum Sig 5ml
Ung @ 5%
References
43 p177. 246 p119. 251 p131.

Rauwolfia serpentina [Indian snakeroot]

Constituents
Indole alkaloids around 0.15% related to reserpine [major alkaloid] is
hypotensive. Dihydroindole alkaloids - Ajmaline - antiarrhythmic. Alseroxylone.
Roxinil. Rescinamine – hypotensive.

Primary pharmacological action: Hypotensive.

Therapeutic classes
Ophthalmic. Thyroactive.
Peripheral vasodilator. Antiarrhythmic. Sedative.
Medicinal indications
Miosis. Hypertension. Cardiac arrhythmia. Paroxysmal tachycardia. Angina.
LVF. Raynauds disease.
Anthelmintic.
Anxiety. Mania. Chorea. Schizophrenia. Alcoholism. Migraine.
Pyrexia. Antivenomous.
Tissue conditions
Depletes norepinephrine through the inhibition of catecholamine storage in
postganglionic adrenergic nerve endings. Rauwolfia has cardiovascular and CNS
effects. CNS depressant and sedative achieving its activity as a psychomotor
relaxor. It inhibits the carotid sinus reflex. Depresses the myocardium and AV
conduction.
Where hypertension is found anxiety is a frequent accompaniment. Rauwolfia
calms the anxiety and corrects tachycardia and arrhythmia. Contracts pupils and
stimulates peristalsis.
Reduces anxiety. Schizophrenia - obsessive thoughts and compulsive behaviour.
Nymphomaniac tendencies. Fear.
Settles the irritability of hyperthyroidism. Snake bite.
Cautions
Restrictions apply. Dosage is determined by the relief of symptoms.
May cause impotence/sexual dysfunction. Depression. Where depression
intervenes during treatment reduce or stop the dose. Dry mouth/nose. Drowsiness.
Antidote – withdraw the medicine and give Capsicum.
Dosage and mode of application
Reduction of hypertension may take six weeks.
Dried extract Sig 60mg. Rad has been used in doses up to 2g. [224 p674. 390].
Dry extract Sig 60mg.
Tincturae 1:10 alcohol 60%. Sig 0.5ml
References. 192 p461. 224 p674. 254 p153/280/297/303. 390 p 808.

Rehmannia glutinosa [Diahuang/chinese foxglove]

Constituents
Iridoid glycosides – aucubin, rehmanniosides.

Primary pharmacological action: Tonic.

Therapeutic classes
Allays inflammation. Anti allergic.
Anticholesterolaemic. Circulatory stimulant [hypotensive]. Antihaemorrhagic.
Hepatic. Hypoglycaemic. Laxative.
Renal tonic. Diuretic. Antirheumatic. Adrenal trophorestorative.
Immunostimulant. Antipyretic.
Menstrual disorders [scanty flow]. Amenorrhoea. Metrorrhagia.
Medicinal indications
Anaemia. Hypertension. Circulatory tonic. Haemorrhage. Asthma.
Nephritis. Haematuria. Adrenal disturbance.
Dizzyness. Rheumatoid arthritis. Pyrexia with dry mouth. Urticaria.
Tissue conditions
Supports the adrenal cortex. Used in skin disease for its cooling nature.
Cautions
Indigestion and diarrhoea.
Dosage and mode of application
Dried rad Sig 3g
Decoctum Sig 10g
Tincturae Sig 5ml
Liquidum extractum Sig 4ml
References
48 p52. 239 p170.

Rhamnus frangula/cathartica
[Alder buckthorn/Buckthorn]

Constituents
Anthaquinone glycoside A and B [antineoplastic] – frangula emodin up to 7%.
Flavonoids. Glycosides. Tannin. Vitamin C.

Primary pharmacological action: Stimulant laxative.

Therapeutic classes
Antihaemorrhoidal. Astringent.
Diuretic.
Dermatological agent.
Antineoplastic.
Medicinal indications [Saturn]
Constipation.
Tissue conditions
Promotes water and electrolyte elimination by stimulating intestinal contractions,
increasing transit time and reducing fluid absorption. Cytotoxic to cancer cell
lines.
Cautions
Care in pregnancy. Use two year old bark as younger bark causes griping and is
emetic. Inflammatory bowel disorders.
Dosage and mode of application
Dried cort Sig 3g
Dry extract Sig 30mg
Decoctum Sig 2.5g
Liquidium extractum Sig 4ml
References
43 p94. 111 p654. 149 p140. 189 p46. 246 p234. 394 p36. 394 p36.

Rhamnus purshiana [Cascara]

Constituents
Anthraquinones also known as anthranoids up to 10%, mainly aloe-emodin.
Resin. Tannin.

Primary pharmacological action: Stimulant laxative.

Therapeutic classes
Gastro intestinal vasotonic. Tonic to the stomach, biliary tract and intestine.
Medicinal indications
Cholelithiasis. Dyspepsia. Jaundice. Constipation. Haemorrhoids.
Tissue conditions
Constipation from nervous tension or atonic intestinal muscles [Intestinal atony].
Rhamnus is severe and prompt in its action. It stimulates peristaltic activity.
When spasmodic activity is present in the intestine it is preferable to use milder
agents. Older bark becomes more gentle in its activity.
Cautions
Give small doses and usually with an aromatic or carminative to prevent griping.
Care in pregnancy. Fresh bark causes vomiting and tenesmus. Avoid in acute
irritable or spasmodic intestinal disorders. Haematuria. Electrolyte imbalance.
Potassium loss.
Dosage and mode of application
For a prompt cathartic action give a full dose at night.
Dried cort Sig 1g
Dry extract 300mg
Infusium Sig 2g
Elixir Sig 2ml in syrup
Tincturae cort Sig 5ml
Liquidum extractum Sig 4ml
References
224 p1335. 262 p87. 394 p47.

Rheum palmatum/officinale [rhubarb]

Constituents
Rhein inhibits the growth of bacteria in the intestine. Bitter. Emodin inhibits the growth of Trichomonas vaginalis. Anthraquinones - sennosides. Phenols. Tannins counters the effect of anthraquinones.

Primary pharmacological action: Laxative & antidiarrhoeal.

Therapeutic classes
Ophthalmic. Allays inflammation. Astringent. Tonic. Antiseptic. Antimicrobial.
Antibacterial - Helicobacter pylori, trichomonas vaginalis.
Antiviral - Herpes simplex.
Hypocholesterolaemic. Antihaemorrhagic.
Stimulating gastric bitter. Stomachic. Cholagogue - stimulating. Splenic.
Antiparasitic.
Antiuraemic. Renal tonic. Antirheumatic. Antipyretic.
Emmenagogue.
Analgesic.
Antineoplastic.

Medicinal indications [Mars]
Eye inflammation. Hyperlipidaemia. Hypertension.
Anorexia. Ulcers. Nausea. Vomiting. Gastro enteritis. Indigestion. Hepatitis.
Pancreatitis. Jaundice. Enteritis. Crohn's disease. Atonic constipation. Diarrhoea.
Dysentery. Gastro-intestinal haemorrhage. Anal fissures. Cholera.
Lowers uraemia. Increases glomerular filtration. Gout. Rheum may help
nephropathy by lowering cholesterol and triglyceride levels. Thus helping to
prevent glomerulosclerosis.
Amenorrhoea. Burns. Injuries. Pyrexia.

Tissue conditions
Acts upon the duodenum and stimulates peristalsis in the large intestine it tones
the stomach and intestine. Increases paracellular permeability. A red tip and side,
and elongated tongue is an indication for its use.
Sour faecal discharges. Gastro intestinal irritation with nervous irritability or
restlessness and light coloured faeces.
Rheum improves glomerular filtration. Rheum has helped control hypertension in
some pregnant women.

Cautions
Ileus. Intestinal spasm with crampy pain.

External use
Ulcers - use a dressing.

Preparations
Astringent and intestinal effect of Rheum is dependent upon the level of dose.
Large doses are laxative, small doses are used for diarrhoea.
Dysentery with Hydrastis.
Dosage and mode of application
Suitable for children.
Dried rad/rhizome Sig 4g as a laxative.
Dried rad/rhizome Sig 1g astringent/antidiarrhoeal.
Dry extract Sig 500mg
Tincturae Sig 5ml
Liquidum extractum Sig 4ml
References
111 p655. 126 p599. 188 p373. 192 p143. 224 p1341. 239 p170.254 p98.

Rhodiola rosea [Roseroot]

Constituents
Phenols including glycosides rhodioloside and salidroside - phenylpropanolide, rosavidine. Rosarin, rosavin, rosin, rosiridin, tyrosol, daucosterol and lotaustralin. Bioflavonoids. Beta-vicianosides. Sucrose.

Primary pharmacological action: Adaptogenic tonic.

Therapeutic classes
Stimulant. Anti anoxaemic.
Hepatoregenerator [hepatic trophorestorative].
Sexual stimulant - male. Asthenia [weakness].
Nervine tonic. Antifatigue. Antidepressant. Tranquilliser. Anti hypnotic.
Antineoplastic. Antitoxin.
Medicinal indications
Anoxaemia. Prevents stress induced cardiac damage.
Impotence/sexual dysfunction, erection weakness and premature ejaculation.
Amenorrhoea.
Anxiety. Depression. Fatigue. Poor memory. Radiation illness.
Tissue conditions
Significant effects are produced after 1-2 hours. Supports the cardiovascular system, adrenal glands and immune system. Enhances dopamine and serotonin [up some 30%] levels by enhancing the activity of serotonin precursors tryptophan and 5 hydroxytryptophan. Increases beta endorphin levels. Beta endorphins are analgesics. Stimulates mitochondrial energy known as creatinine phosphatase. Activates lipase in athletes and improves motor function. Reduces chromosomal damage and aids in the repair of DNA. Increases ones physical endurance, tolerance to anoxia, resistance to microwave radiation. Poisoning by toxins. Improves concentration and memory, reduces fatigue, increases attention span and alertness. Sexual impotence/sexual dysfunction and premature ejaculation with associated depression.
Dosage and mode of application
Liquidum extractum rad Sig 2ml
References
270, 2000, 7, [2], 85 & [5] 365. 281, 2001, 17 [1] 3. 389. 407. 408.

Rhus aromatica/glabra [Sumach]

Constituents
Gallic acid. Tannins. Essential oil. Resin.

Primary pharmacological action:
Stimulating, astringent, tonic diuretic.

Therapeutic classes
Astringent. Tonic. Antiseptic. Antihaemorrhagic. Hypoglycaemic. Styptic.
Medicinal indications
Haemoptysis.
Aphthous ulcerations. Stomatitis. Pharyngeal ulceration. Haematemesis.
Diarrhoea. Dysentery. Tubercular diarrhoea with night sweats. IBS. Colitis.
Divertiulosis. Diabetes. Cholera infantum.
Bladder atony. Bladder catarrh. Enuresis - sphincter weakness. Haematuria.
Prostatic hypertrophy. Nephritis. Incontinence. Gonorrhoea.
Menorrhagia. Purpura.
Tissue conditions
Tonic to the urinary and gastro intestinal mucous membrane in relaxed, catarrhal
or ulcerated conditions. Tongue pale and trembly. Purpura appearing at the
menopause. Trembling of the lower limbs. Small feeble pulse. Lassitude.
External use
Toothache – sap into cavity/gum.
Aphthous ulcers – LE.
Inflammation – poultice sem.
Otitis media – instil fresh succus.
Skin irritation – bacc.
Ulcers – lotion of LE.
Burns – gel.
Preparations
To improve the tone to the GUT and GIT with Geranium maculatum.
Stimulants enhance the prescription.
Vaginal discharge/leucorrhoea as a douche.
Aphthous ulcers, diphtheria - collutor.
Dosage and mode of application
Pulv bacc Sig 2g
Liquidum extractum rad/rhiz/bacc Sig 4ml
References
32 p179. 111 p662. 126 p608. 142 p250. 188 p409. 254 p102.

Ribes nigrum and rubrum
[blackcurrant/redcurrant]

Constituents
Anthocyanidins. Essential oil. Vitamin C. Tannin.

Primary pharmacological action: Astringent tonic.

Therapeutic classes
Refrigerant. Allays inflammation.
Hepatic. Laxative. Vermifuge.
Diuretic - fol. Diaphoretic.
Nervine. Immunostimulant.
Medicinal indications
Anaemic. Capillary fragility. Hypertension. Vasculitis. Sinusitis. Pharyngitis.
Aphthous ulcers. Gum strengthener. Tonsillitis. Sore throat. Jaundice.
Gout. Rheumatism. Pyrexia. Eruptive fever – rad.
Tissue conditions
Tonic to the mucous membranes and capillaries. Used in inflammatory conditions
of the mouth and throat.
Preparations
A Currant 'Rob' is made by adding currant juice to sugar.
Succus is diuretic and diaphoretic.
Haemorrhoids - bacc dect.
Calculi - bacc dect.
Dosage and mode of application
Succus fructus Sig 20ml
References
189 p36. 224 p1671. 246 p165.

Ricinus communis [Castor oil]

Constituents
Fixed oil - glyceride known as ricinoleic acid. Lectins. Alkaloid - ricinine.

Primary pharmacological action: Laxative and purgative.

Therapeutic classes
Ophthalmic. Antifungal – external against candida, trichophyton.
Anthelmintic.
Galactagogue.
Dermatological agent. Emollient.
Medicinal indications
Otitis media. Bronchitis. Constipation. Diarrhoea. Enteritis.
Fungal infections. Warts. Ulcers. Cysts. Softens bunions and corns.
Stimulates hair growth.
Tissue conditions
Acts upon the large intestine. Promotes mucus secretions. Light coloured stool
with burning at evacuation and colicky pain. Soothing in gastro intestinal
inflammation.
External use
Used as a vehicle to carry eye drops.
Eyes - irritation or inflammation.
Otitis – oleum.
Bronchitis apply a castor oil pack and cover with a warm towel to facilitate
absorption and elimination.
Galactogogue - fol application to breasts.
Apply to the navel of a new-born infant if for any reason it showed difficulty in
healing.
Cuts, abrasions, sores and ulcers - apply a poultice of leaves or Oleum.
Gangrene – with Commiphora molmol.
Improves hair growth. Apply oleum at bedtime twice a week wash out in the
morning.
Dosage and mode of application
Ol Ricinus expressed from the sem Sig 20 ml. With fruit juice to cover the taste.
References
188 p101. 189 p64.

Rosa damascena [Rose]

Constituents
Kaempherol selectively inhibiting the protein-splitting enzyme protease.
Quercetin and kaempherol inhibit HIV infection and allays inflammation.
Volatile oil.

Primary pharmacological action: Astringent.

Therapeutic classes
Ophthalmic. Antiviral – HIV. Has 9 anti viral compounds. Disinfectant.
Cardioactive. Hypolipidaemic. Anticholesterolaemic.
Cholagogue. Hepatoprotective. Laxative.
Emmenagogue. Antipyretic.
Antidepressant. Anxiolytic. Sedative. Aphrodisiac.
Dermatological agent. Local anaesthetic. Radiation damage.

Medicinal indications
Conjunctivitis. Aphthous ulcers. Gingivitis.
Uterine fibroids. Menorrhagia. Metrorrhagia. Infertility. Vaginal dryness.
Menopausal neurosis or depression.
Anxiety associated with depression. Insect bites. Eczema. Dermatitis. Anti
radiation burns/dermatitis.

Tissue conditions
Has anti HIV activity as it prevents the virus from maturing. Calms and tones the
nervous system.

External use
Conjunctivitis – aromatic water as a cooling astringent.
Collyr - conjunctivitis.
Skin toner - Aqua Rosae.

Dosage and mode of application
Tincturae flos Sig 4ml
Aqua Rosae [BPC1949]

References
284, No. 73, Feb. 2002, p19-21. 188 p376. 324, 1996, 229 [1] p73-9.

Rosmarinus officinalis [Rosemary]

Constituents

Volatile oil up to 1.5% consisting mainly of monoterpine hydrocarbons known as camphene, limonene, camphor up to 25%. Terpenoid bitters up to 4.6% – [diterpenoids] picrosalvin, oleanolic acid [10%], ursolic acid [5%] is antioxidant. Flavonoids – diosmetin, diosmin, hesperidin, apigenin. Phenols [phenolic acids] up to 3% as caffeic acid derivatives – rosmarinic acid is anticompliment and antioxidant. Tannin - oligomeric proanthocyanidins [15%]. Carnosol and Carnosic acid prevents DNA damage in cells damaged by alfatoxin. Rosmarinus oleum has activity against Cryptococci.

Primary pharmacological action: Tonic.

Therapeutic classes

Antimicrobial against Gram positive and Gram negative bacteria – Cryptococci, Corynebacteria, Escherichia coli, Kluyveromyces bulgaricus, Lactobacillus brevis, Pseudomonas fluorescens, Rhodotorula glutinis, Staphylococcus albus & aureus, Vibrio cholerae.
Ophthalmic. Antifungal. Stimulant. Astringent.
Cardiac tonic. Circulatory diffusive. Hypotensive.
Oropharyngeal agent. Carminative. Stomachic. Cholagogue. Choleretic. Hepatoprotective.
Diuretic. Diaphoretic. Antirheumatic.
Analgesic. Antispasmodic. Nervine. Tonic. Thymoleptic. Sedative.
Vulnerary. Rubefacient. Parasiticidal.
Emmenagogue.
Antineoplastic.

Medicinal indications [Sun]

Palpitations. Cerebro vascular accident. Chronic circulatory insufficiency with hypotension. Capillary fragility.
Colds. Influenza. Sinusitis. Bronchitis. Bronchial carcinoma.
Anorexia. Stomach atony. Jaundice. Hepatic tonic. Biliary atony. Cholecystitis. Cirrhosis. Flatulent dyspepsia. Gastro enteritis. Colitis. Parasites.
Oedema. Impotence/sexual dysfunction. Rheumatic disease.
Infertility. Disturbance of foetal implantation. Mammary tumours.
Amnesia or blindness from CVA. Depression. Fatigue. Headache. Giddiness. Syncope. Hyperactivity. Migraine. ME.
Eczema. Wounds.
Intercostal neuralgia. Joint pain. Myalgia. Sciatica.

Pharmacopoeia

Tissue conditions
Strengthens the eyes. Stimulates the vascular nerves. A diffusive, stimulant tonic for the brain, intestine and stomach. Improves the tone of the brain [improves memory and concentration] and stomach. Headaches which are due to stomach disorders e.g. over indulgence, are relieved. Antispasmodic to smooth muscle of the gall bladder and intestine. Infusion is used for colic. Chronic tiredness and depression are improved. Recovery from CVA and paraplegia is more likely when Rosmarinus is used. It calms, soothes and sedates the nervous system.

External use
Oleum is added to external prescriptions for liniments.
Oropharyngeal - Sore gums, halitosis and sore throat - mouthwash.
Analgesic and Rubefacient - Oleum in myalgia, sciatica and intercostal myalgia.
Scalp tonic to make the hair grow - use a lotion.
Balneum with extract, oleum, or infusium for a body tonic effect. Sig 10gtt.
Essential oil repels aphids.

Preparations
Tonic and antispasmodic effects use Lavandula and Rosmarinus.
Antiseptic tea, powerful - Artemesia absinthium, Verbena, Salvia and Lavandula.

Dosage and mode of application
Dried fol/herba Sig 4g
Dry extract Sig 0.5g
Tincturae Sig 10ml
Liquidum extractum Sig 4ml
> **Balneum** Put 60g herba into muslin create an closed infusion, cool and then add to the bath water. Immerse immediatly.
> **Essential oleum** Sig 4gtt.
> **Ung** @10%
> **Liniment** with 10% oleum

References
6 p98. 43 p181. 111 p665. 188 p376. 246 p171. 275 1995, No 44, p25-7. 287, 1998, Jan/Feb. 62. 394 p326.

Rubus idaeus [Raspberry]

Constituents
Polypeptides. Tannin. Rutin.

Primary pharmacological action: Astringent, Tonic.

Therapeutic classes
Ophthalmic. Antifungal – Candida.
A gentle tonic to the stomach and uterus. Stimulant. Mucous membrane tonic.
Antihaemorrhagic.
Oropharyngeal agent. Laxative Antidiarrhoeal – large doses.
Diuretic. Antipyretic.
Uterine tonic. Galactogogue. Parturient.
Dermatological agent.
Medicinal indications
Conjunctivitis. Sore or tired eyes. Coughs.
Aphthous ulcers. Stomatitis. Tonsillitis. Nausea. Vomiting. Diarrhoea. Cholera.
Relaxed intestine with diarrhoea. Dysentery. Gastro intestinal haemorrhage.
Haemorrhoids.
Gonorrhoea. Vaginal discharge/leucorrhoea. Candida. Pyrexia.
Pregnancy - last trimester. Uterine haemorrhage. Uterine prolapse. Depression.
Tissue conditions
Tonic to the gastro intestinal tract. Used as a partus preparator when it is only
used providing there has not been a history of precipitate labour. Care if early
labour pain is invoked; discontinue the remedy. Suitable for children with gastro
intestinal disorders.
Preparations
Conjunctivitis - lotion.
Tonsillitis - garg.
Diverticular disease, ulcerative conditions with Agrimonia, Althea.
Threatened miscarriage with Leonurus.
Vaginal and uterine inflammation with Santalum, Chondrus and glycerine or
Trillium and Commiphora.
Tuberculosis formula – [after Dr Coffin] Rubus, Agrimonia, Berberis vulgaris,
Galium aparine, Glechoma hederacea, Erythraea, Marrubium, Capsicum,
Glycyrrhiza.
Cautions
Avoid in the athletic typology pregnancies.
External use
Sore throats, tonsillitis – garg.

Haemorrhoids – poultice.
Sunburn – infusium lotion.
Dosage and mode of application
Dried fol Sig 8g
Liquidum extractum Sig 8ml
References
6 p70. 43 p182. 188 p366. 246 p170.

Rubus parvifolius [Australian raspberry]

Constituents
Essential oil. Diterpine lactones. Tannin

Primary pharmacological action: Astringent diuretic.

Therapeutic classes
Antilithic. Antipyretic.
Medicinal indications
Rheumatoid conditions. Nephritis. Urinary lithiasis.
Dosage and mode of application
Tincturae Sig 5ml

R

External use
Skin eruptions.
Mastitis.
Dosage and mode of application
Dried rad Sig 4g
Tincturae Sig 2ml
Liquidum extractum Sig 4ml
References
43. 111 p670. 192 p588. 236 p58. 246 p97. 251 p166.

Ruscus aculeatus [Butchers broom]

Constituents
Steroidal saponins up to 6% – ruscin, ruscogenin, ruscoside. Flavonoids. Sterols.

Primary pharmacological action:
Venous tonic, vasoconstrictor.

Therapeutic classes
Allays inflammation. Deobstruent. Ophthalmic.
Haemostatic. Reduces capillary fragility and permeability.
Laxative.
Diuretic. Diaphoretic.
Antispasmodic.
Emmenagogue.
Medicinal indications [Mars]
Diabetic retinopathy.
Deficient venous return - venous insufficiency, heavy legs. Haemorrhoids.
Varicose veins. Phlebitis. Limb oedema. Cramp.
Jaundice. Constipation. Anal fissures. Haemorrhoids.
Oedema. Arthritis.
Tissue conditions
Diminishes vascular permeability. Stimulates alpha adrenergic receptors in
smooth muscle veins. Vasocontractant to the veins in venous insufficiency, it also
reduces ankle circumference.
External use
Haemorrhoids – suppository, ung.
Fractures – poultice of Bacc.
Dosage and mode of application
Decoction fol/rhix/rad Sig 7.5ml
Liquidum extractum Sig 1ml
References
189 p52. 192 p98. 194. 246 p520. 325, 1999, 18 [4] p255-261. 394 p40.

Ruta graveolens [Rue]

Constituents
Coumarin. Lignans. Glycoside - Rutin strengthens the blood vessel walls.
Quercetin. Volatile oil up to 0.1%.

Primary pharmacological action: Antispasmodic.

Therapeutic classes
Ophthalmic. Stimulant. Disinfectant. Antiseptic. Antifungal - Tinea.
Hypotensive. Venous tonic.
Antitussive.
Carminative. Stomachic. Antiflatulent. Hepatic. Anthelmintic.
Emmenagogue. Uterine and ovarian tonic. Galactagogue.
Antiparasitic – pediculosis. Antivenomous.
Dermatological agent. Vulnerary. Rubefacient.

Medicinal indications [Sun]
Conjunctivitis. Ocular muscle strengthener. Cataract. Earache.
Arterial tension. Palpitations. Varicose veins. Cramp.
Pertussus. Laryngismus stridulus.
Nervous dyspepsia. Intestinal colic. Cestodes. Nematodes.
Gout. Rheumatism. Sciatica. Lymphadenopathy.
Panic. Epilepsy. Headaches with eye strain. Schizophrenia.
Atonic amenorrhoea from cold or shock. Dysmenorrhoea. Partum pain.
Breast pain.
Expels poisons. Insect bites. Lice. Rabies. Snakebite. Scaly skin.
Ganglion. Sprains Strains. Multiple sclerosis.

Tissue conditions
Strengthens and restores tone to ocular muscles and sharpens acuity.
Action on periosteum to facilitate formation of a callus in fracture cases. Articular
rheumatism of the wrists or feet Ruta brings a greater freedom of movement.
Chewing the leaves relieves headache, panic and palpitations.

Cautions
Pregnancy and menorrhagia.

External use
Eye wash for cataract, fatigued eyes.
Parasitical skin affections such as Tinea, pediculosis - use a powder.
Venom - suck out poison, then use internally and externally.
Ganglion/Cartilage damage/Sciatica - rubefacient liniment.

Preparations
Vertigo, palpitations and headache with Scutellaria and Valeriana.

Pharmacopoeia

Dosage and mode of application
Powdered herba Sig 1g
Liquidum extractum Sig 2ml
Ung @ 15%.
References
43 p184. 188 p378. 192 p473. 228 p341. 246 p221. 247 p87. 251p138

Fagopyrum esculentum contains bioflavonoids and rutin, it is used as a venous tonic in peripheral vascular disorders.

Salix alba [White european willow]

Constituents
Phenolic glycoside esters up to 11% – salicin up to 10%. Salicin is metabolised by intestinal micro organisms saligenin, this is oxidised in the liver and blood to salicylic acid. Salicylic acid inhibits prostaglandins in the sensory nerves thereby easing pain. Tannin up to 20% - as catechin, condensed tannin [procyanidin], gallotannin. Flavonoids up to 4%. Leaf and bark are similar.

Primary pharmacological action: Antirheumatic and tonic.

Therapeutic classes
Allays inflammation. Antiseptic. Astringent. Tonic. Antiplatelet.
Antirheumatic. Analgesic.
Antipyretic. Febrifuge. Antiperiodic.
Medicinal indications [Moon]
Toothache. Colds. Influenza. Respiratory catarrh.
Indigestion. Diarrhoea. Dysentery.
Ankylosing spondylitis. Articular pain. Gout. Rheumatic pain with inflammation.
Rheumatoid arthritis. Systemic inflammatory connective tissue disorders. Lumbar pain. Collagen disorders. Neuralgia.
Recurrent malarial fever. Fever.
Pain. Headache. Dysmenorrhoea.
Tissue conditions
Salicin is metabolised to saligenin in the gastrointestinal tract. After absorption from the gut it becomes salicylic acid. Indicated for general laxity of the tissues. Antiplatelet activity supports blood thinning.
External use
Indolent ulcers, aphthous ulcers, vaginal discharge/leucorrhoea.
Scalp tonic encourages hair growth - equal parts of Salix fol and Adiantum.
Preparations
Use with stimulating medicines to support the removal of the acids provoking an inflammatory condition.
Antirheumatic – Apium, Guaiacum, Menyanthes, Salix alba.
Head pain with Rosmarinus.
Dosage and mode of application
Dried cort Sig 3g [3g dried bacc = 30mg salicin].
Tincturae Sig 8ml
Liquidum extractum Sig 3ml
References
43 p184. 111 p674. 176 p457.188 p454. 246 p63. 272, 1977, 9, 6 p20 394 p408

Salix nigra [Black willow]

Constituents
Glucoside Salinigrin. Tannin.

Primary pharmacological action: Genito urinary antispasmodic

Therapeutic classes
Anaphrodisiac.
Antispasmodic. Sedative. Vulnerary.
Medicinal indications
Proctitis.
Gout. Cystitis. Spermatorrhoea, nocturnal emissions, uncontrollable lascivious
thoughts. Undue sexual excitement - masturbation. Nymphomania. Prostatitis.
Vaginitis. Ovaritis.
Tissue conditions
An Antispasmodic for pelvic disorders, when the pelvic nerves are irritable and
overexcitable. Strengthening to the sexual organs in sexual debility when used to
sedate over excitability. Used in excess excitability of the sexual organs
[masturbation] in male and female. Calms the sexual passions in both sexes and
relieves mental irritability leading to lascivious dreams.
Preparations
Sexual debility, impotence/sexual dysfunction or disinterest in sex - with
Chamaelirium luteum and Avena.
Vaginitis - douche.
Proctitis - injection.
Nerve sedative prescription
LE Passiflora   1ml
LE Pulsatilla   0.5ml
LE Salix nigra 3.5ml Sig Full dose to effect.
External use
Indolent ulcers. Gangrene. Rhus tox poisoning.
Dosage and mode of application
Liquidum extractum Sig 4ml
References
126 p613. 127 p846. 176 p456. 188 p454. 254 p106.

Salvia miltiorrhiza [Red root sage]

Constituents
Bitter. Diterpene danshinones are anti allergic.

Primary pharmacological action: Cardiovascular stimulant.

Therapeutic classes
Antibacterial. Antioxidant.
Angina. Hypotensive. Ischaemic heart disease. Antifibrinolytic activity.
Anticoagulant.
Pulmonary agent. Hepatic.
Renal tonic. Osteophytic.
Antineoplastic. Immunostimulant. Cytotoxic.
Mild sedative. Endocrine agent. Vulnerary.
Medicinal indications [Jupiter]
Angina. Palpitations. Myocardial ischaemia. Anticoagulant. Fibrinolytic.
Peripheral vasodilator. Cerebral vasodilator.
Pulmonary fibrosis.
Hepatic disease - fibrosis. Hepatitis - acute and chronic.
Menstrual disturbances.
Acne. Scleroderma. Lymphoma.
Insomnia.
Tissue conditions
Improves coronary blood flow and supports ATP. It can be used during and post
MI to improve myocardial function and tissue oxygenation from hypoxic damage.
It is vasodilatory. It does not increase cardiac output. It inhibits platelet activity.
Reduces thrombus formation. Supports pulmonary tissue. Increases RNA in
hepatocytes. Reduces the uraemic, phosphates and nitrogenous build up in renal
disturbance and chronic renal failure.
Supports the formation of osteoblasts after fracture.
Cautions
Pregnancy. Haemorrhage.
Preparations
Supports the action of Astragalus when cardiotonic action is required.
Hepatitis with Hypericum, Crataegus or Curcuma.
Dosage and mode of application
Dried rad Sig 2g
Liquidum extractum Sig 4ml
References. 48 p62. 263 1999, 65, p654. Cancer letters, 2000, 153 [1-2] p85-93.

Salvia officinalis [Sage]

Constituents
Volatile oils up to 2.8% composed of monoterpenoids mainly of alpha and beta thujone up to 10% [antimicrobial], camphor. Phenolic acids - rosmarinic. Condensed cattechin tannins up to 8%, salviatannin. Falvonoids up to 3%. Potassium. Calcium. Magnesium.

Primary pharmacological action: Antispasmodic.

Therapeutic classes
Stimulant. Tonic. Antibacterial - Bacillus subtilis, Escherichia coli, Kleibsiella ozanae, Salmonella species and Shigella sonnei.
Antifungal - Candida albicans, Candida krusei, Candida neoformans, Candida pseudotropicalis, Cryptococcus neoformans and Torulopsis glabrata.
Antiviral. Antiseptic. Astringent. Allays inflammation.
Antioxidant. Soothing diffusive. Secretory stimulant.
Aromatic. Carminative. Vermifuge.
Prostatic tonic. Adrenal trophorestorative.
Emmenagogue. Prolactin depressor. Oestrogenic. Ovarian infertility.
CNS stimulant.
Antihydrotic. Dermatological agent. Vulnerary.
Antineoplastic.

Medicinal indications [Jupiter]
Uvulitis. Gingivitis. Glossitis. Stomatitis. Tonsillitis. Pharyngitis.
Laryngitis. Tuberculosis. Pneumonia.
Teeth cleanser. Aphthous ulcers. Allays nausea. Flatulent dyspepsia.
Hyperhydrosis. Galactorrhoea. Breast carcinoma. Nymphomania.
Spermatorrhoea. Impotence/sexual dysfunction. Prostate cancer.
Dermal ulcers. Measles. Pressure sores. Wounds.
Menopause.
Amnesia. Depression. Panic. Paralysis.

Tissue conditions
Oropharyngeal inflammation. Strengthens both sides of the ANS. Tonic to the CNS. Reduces prolactin levels to reduce milk production. Relieves flushes and sweats associated with nervous exhaustion and hormonal disturbances. It may increase hormonal flushes in some through stimulation of the sympathetic nerves. Settles excessive sexual desire.

Cautions
Pregnancy. Breast feeding.

External use
Antiseptic gargle/mouthwash and for all oropharyngeal disturbances - ulcers especially. Can be used with apple cider vinegar in oral conditions.
Teeth – rub a leaf upon the gum and teeth to cleanse, refresh and strengthen the gums.
Dermal ulcers, wounds – fomentation infusium.
Hair - stimulates hair growth and removes dandruff.
Preparations
Oropharyngeal disorders with Honey, Plantago and Rosmarinus,
Dosage and mode of application
Dried/fresh fol Sig 4g
Dry extract Sig 0.36g
Essential oil Sig 0.3ml
Tincturae Sig 10ml
Liquidum extractum Sig 4ml
       Infusium Salvia et Acetum Sage vinegar
       Take Salvia 100g and macerate with 500ml acetic acid for 10 days. Press and filter.
       Sig 5ml Aqua cal PRN. Garg & mouthwash for aphthous ulcers, lichen planus, stomatitis, gingivitis, uvulitis.
References
BPC 1934. 111 p676. 224 p1026. 254 p70. 326, May 1995, Vol 13, No 5, p24-6.
Biologica [Bratislava] 1994, 49 [3] p359-64. 394 p330.

Salvia triloba [Greek sage]

Constituents
Volatile oil composed mainly of 1,8-cineole

Primary pharmacological action: Similar to Salvia officinalis.

Therapeutic classes
Antibacterial against gram +ve and gram -ve organisms. Antifungal - candida.
Carminative.
Antispasmodic
Medicinal indications [Jupiter]
Gingivitis. Sore throat. Oral monilia.
Vaginal monilia.
Dosage and mode of application
Less potent than S. officinalis. Liquidum extractum Sig 4ml
References 127 p703.

Salvia sclarea [Clary sage]

Constituents
Volatile up to 0.1%. Diterpenes. Mucilage.

Primary pharmacological action: Antispasmodic.

Therapeutic classes
Ophthalmic. Allays inflammation. Astringent. Tonic. Antifungal.
Aromatic. Stomachic. Carminative.
Renal activity. Aphrodisiac.
Oestrogenic.
Sedative.
Medicinal indications [Moon]
Ophthalmic - sem dect.
Sore throat. Dyspepsia. Colitis. IBS.
Dysmenorrhoea. Metrorrhagia. Menopause. PMS. Aphrodisiac – male and
female.
Anxiety. Depression. Fatigue. Insomnia. Muscle spasm – cramp.
Tissue conditions
Smooth muscle antipsasmodic to the gastro intestinal tract – colitis, IBA.
External use
Ophthalmic disturbances e.g. Conjunctivitis; watering, inflammation, foreign
bodies [dust] – soak sem in aqua for a few minutes to produce a mucilage.
Dosage and mode of application
Liquidum extractum herba Sig 4ml
References
189 p78. 192 p147. 228 p110.

Sambucus nigra [Elder]

Constituents
Flavonoids mainly flavonolic glycosides up to 3% - astragalin, hyperoside are
diuretic. Phenols up to 3%. Triterpenes up to 1%. Volatile oils up to 0.3%.
Tannin. Mucilage. Sterols.

Primary pharmacological action:
Relaxing vasotonic alterative and diaphoretic.

Therapeutic classes
Ophthalmic. Anticatarrhal. Allays inflammation.
Antibacterial – Pseudomonas aeruginosa. Antiviral – Epstein Barr, influenza.
Antiallergic.
Antioxidant. Vasotonic alterative.
Hepatic disease. Laxative. Bark is purgative, in large doses emetic.
Diuretic. Diaphoretic - bacc/flos.
Nerve relaxant. Anxiolytic.
Antineoplastic.
Dermatological agent. Vulnerary.
Medicinal indications [Venus]
Conjunctivitis. Toothache. Anaemia. Flos - blood purifier.
Colds. Nasal catarrh. Asthma. Rhinitis. Sinusitis. Pharyngitis. Laryngitis.
Trachieitis. Bronchitis. Influenza.
Adenitis.
Colic and diarrhoea - dried berries. Hepatic disorders of children.
Skin disease – burns, dermatitis, eczema, erysipelas, measles, psoriasis, sore
skin, wounds. Pyrexia.
Dermal carcinoma.
Lymphadenopathy - rad succus.
Epilepsy.
Tissue conditions
Various parts of Sambucus are used in treatments. ye ailments and injuries to the
eye nerves, respiratory conditions and skin disorders - flos. Cleansing to the
mucous membranes with detergent and vasotonic properties. Relaxes the
eliminative organs. Detoxifies the blood and skin.
Sore throats and coughs, epilepsy - baccus.
Antineoplastic to skin carcinoma.
External use
Inflamed eye conditions - Collyr Aqua Sambucus.
Wounds, pain and to abate inflammation - fomentation.

Pharmacopoeia

Sambucus flos are added to the water for washing the hands and face it will both whiten and soften the skin.

Dermatitis, eczema, burns, scalds - skin lotion.

It may be added to the bath water for its refreshing qualities.

Preparations

With Achillea and Mentha piperita in fevers or influenza.

Sinusitis with Pulsatilla.

Syrupus Sambucus. Syrup of elder berries.

Pick the berries when thoroughly ripe, remove the stalks. Simmer with a little water in a pan. After straining, add ginger root 30g and 10 cloves, to taste. Simmer one hour. Strain again. Add some sugar if desired and bottle. Sig 30 ml et aqua frig. An excellent remedy for coughs and colds.

Elderberry Rob

Stalked elderberries 2.5k sugar 500g simmer to a thick consistency. Cool, strain and bottle. Soothes coughs and bronchitis and is diaphoretic.

Dosage and mode of application

Dried flos Sig 5g

Infusium Sig 4g

Tincturae flos/fol Sig 10ml

Liquidum Extractum Sig 4ml

References

43 p186. 111 p677. 189 p106. 192 p193. 211. 233 p84. 246 p426. 282 No. 50, p55-57. 285 9, 1995, p281-286. 394 p103.

Sanguinaria canadensis [Bloodroot]

Constituents
Isoquinoline alkaloids - sanguinarine is antimicrobial to gram positive and gram negative bacteria, candida and fungi, also trichomonas. Alkaloid berberine. Resin.

Primary pharmacological action: Stimulating expectorant.

Therapeutic classes
Allays chronic inflammation. Tonic. Antiseptic. Antimicrobial – gram positive and gram negative. Antifungal – Candida, trichomonas, trichophyton. Antiviral. Cholagogue. Emetic and cathartic.
Antispasmodic.
Dermatological agent.
Antineoplastic.

Medicinal indications
Nasal catarrh and polyps. Sinusitis - chronic. Laryngismus stridulus. Laryngitis. Pharyngitis. Pertussis. Bronchitis. Asthma.
Oral plaque. Nausea from stomach disorders. Atonic dyspepsia. Jaundice. Hepatic congestion. Dysentery. Rectal carcinoma.
Rheumatism.
Amenorrhoea. Dysmenorrhoea. Impotence/sexual dysfunction.
Tinea. Eczema. Warts. Ringworm.
Skin malignancy. Sarcoma.

Tissue conditions
Chlorides of sanguinarine inhibit the elastolytic activity of human sputum elastase. Elastase can degrade elastin, collagen, protoglycan and fibronectin at neutral pH contributing to tissue damage in pulmonary disease and musculoskeletal disease. Mucous membranes are stimulated to increased mucus production. Respiratory irritation, inflammation or itching with red mucous membranes. Use for hard and dry coughs with irritation. It will relieve irritation of the bronchial tubes. Atony of the bronchi.
Stimulates the heart and circulation to the eliminative organs. The liver and uterus are influenced through stimulation. Stimulates the glandular system.
Impotence/sexual dysfunction from relaxed tissue. Feeble circulation with cold extremities.

Cautions
In acute inflammation of the respiratory tract. Tuberculosis. Care with chronic bronchial conditions.

Pharmacopoeia

External use
Oral plaque – collutoria.
Frostbite and chilblains – poultice with Ulmus.
Ringworm, warts – ung/poultice.

Preparations
Nasal polyps - snuff, always in very small dosage.
Cough remedy with Inula, Symphytum, Verbascum.
Amenorrhoea with emmenagogues.

Dosage and mode of application
Always give in very small doses and well diluted as its taste is very strong.
Dried rad Sig 0.5g
Tincturae Sig 1ml [Emetic Sig 2-5ml]
Liquidum extractum Sig 0.3ml [Emetic Sig 1ml]

References
43 p187. 111 p678. 126 p615. 176 p242. 192 p74. 262 p72. 263 1993, 59, p200.

Sanguisorba officinalis [Greater burnet]

Constituents of rad
Flavonoids [flavones]. Saponins. Tannins. Volatile oil. Vitamin C.

Primary pharmacological action: Astringent tonic.

Therapeutic classes
Antimicrobial. Antifungal – tinea.
Antihaemorrhagic.
Periodontal agent. Anti emetic.
Dermatological agent. Styptic. Vulnerary.
Medicinal indications [Sun]
Gum disease. Diarrhoea – acute or chronic. Ulcerative colitis. IBS.
Bacillary dysentery. Haemorrhoids. Anal disorders.
Metrorrhagia. Cervical erosion.
Sunburn. Eczema. Wound healer.
Tissue conditions
Astringent to the respiratory, gastro intestinal and genito urinary mucous
membranes. Decreases oedema in burns and reduces dermal infection.
External use
Throat infections – garg.
Wounds - poultice.
Eczema, anal irritation - lotion.
Preparations
Diarrhoea – with Acacia or Potentilla.
Dosage and mode of application
Dried herba 5g
Tincturae Sig 8ml
Liquidum extractum Sig 6ml
References
43 p189. 189 p50. 246 p176.

Sanicula europaea [Sanicle]

Constituents
Bitter. Allantoin. Saponins. Tannin. Essential oil. Vitamin C.

Primary pharmacological action: Astringent.

Therapeutic classes
Vasotonic alterative. Allays inflammation.
Haemostatic. Antitussive. Expectorant.
Oropharyngeal agent. Carminative.
Uterine tonic.
Dermatological agent. Vulnerary.
Antispasmodic - weak. Anodyne - weak.
Medicinal indications [Mars]
Varicose veins.
Catarrh. Coughs. Chronic bronchitis. Haemoptysis. Pneumonia. Tuberculosis.
Tonsillitis. Aphthous ulcers. Gingivitis. Flatulence. Gastro enteritis. Dysentery.
Diarrhoea. Haemorrhoids.
Chorea. Intermittent fevers.
Bruises. Dermal ulcers. Burns. Cuts. Erysipelas. Rashes. Wounds.
Metritis. Menorrhagia. Vaginal discharge/leucorrhoea.
Tissue conditions
Allays inflammation of mucous surfaces. Utilised in catarrhal conditions of the
respiratory passages. Inflamed or ulcerated gastro intestinal tract.
External use
Aphthous ulcers – collutoria.
Wounds.
Preparations
Blood disorder with vasotonic alteratives.
Scalp inflammation of children - decoction.
Dosage and mode of application
Liquidum extractum fol/rhiz Sig 4ml
References
127 p712. 189 p242. 246 p279.

Santalum album [Sandalwood]

Constituents
Hydrocarbons – santalenes. Santanol. Volatile oil.

Primary pharmacological action: Bacteriostatic.

Therapeutic classes
Antiseptic. Astringent. Disinfectant. Stimulant. Allays inflammation.
Antibacterial - gram positive bacteria – staphylococcus aureus.
Antiviral – herpes simplex.
Aromatic. Expectorant.
Urinary antiseptic. Diuretic. Genito urinary tonic.
Dermatological agent.
Analgesic. Antispasmodic
Medicinal indications
Varicose veins.
Herpes simplex [HSV 1 & 2]. Respiratory infections.
Dyspepsia. Tuberculosis of the gall bladder.
Urinary infections. Cystitis. Gonorrhoea. Impotence/sexual dysfunction.
Pyrexia. Anxiety. Tension.
Tissue conditions
Mucous membrane disturbances with inflammation or infective processes. Allays inflamed genito urinary conditions with pain.
Dosage and mode of application
Oleum Sig 5gtt in a maple syrup vehicle.
Liquidum extractum heartwood Sig 4ml
References
176 p461. 188 p381. 191p127.

Saponaria officinalis [Soapwort]

Constituents
Saponins are dermatological.

Primary pharmacological action:
Vasotonic alterative [Blood cleanser].

Therapeutic classes
Deobstruent.
Expectorant.
Hepatic. Cholagogue. Choleretic. Laxative.
Diuretic. Diaphoretic. Antirheumatic.
Dermatological agent. Anti leprotic.
Medicinal indications [Venus]
Catarrh. Asthma. Bronchitis. Jaundice. Hepatic infections.
Gout. Rheumatism.
Vaginal discharge/leucorrhoea. Gonorrhoea.
Acne. Dandruff. Eczema. Erysipelas. Poison ivy dermatitis. Psoriasis. Leprosy.
External use
Dermatitis, pruritus, furunculosis - succus.
Rheumatic pain - use a lotion.
Leprosy – poultice.
Fol and rad produce juice that can be used as soap and shampoo.
Dosage and mode of application
Dried rad/rhiz Sig 5g
Decoctum Sig 30ml
Liquidum extractum Sig 4ml
References
189 p254. 192 p514. 228 p157. 236 p20. 246 p107.

Saracena purpura [Pitcher plant]

Constituents
Alkaloids. Glycosides.

Primary pharmacological action: Astringent.

Therapeutic classes
Vasotonic alterative. Stimulant.
Stomachic. Laxative.
Diuretic.
Dermatological agent.
Tonic nervine.
Medicinal indications
Scarlet fever.
A laxative in chronic constipation.
Measles. Smallpox.
A stimulant and tonic nervine. Fears, inferiority complex, nightmares.
Tissue conditions
Stimulates and tones in relaxed conditions of the liver, intestinal glands and
kidneys. Allays indigestion and constipation.
Preparations
Suitable mixture - Asperula, Cassia and Fraxinus ornus manna.
Nervine effects are promoted with Scutellaria and Verbena.
Vasotonic alterative and stomachic properties are supported with Marsdenia,
Symphytum and Geranium maculatum.
Nightmares and fears with Althea and a relaxing nervine.
Dosage and mode of application
Powdered rad Sig 2g
Liquidum extractum Sig 4ml
References
127 p240. 176 p398. 189 p218.

Sassafras officinale [Sassafras]

Constituents
Isoquinoline alkaloids – boldine. Volatile oils - up to 9% saffrole - stimulates cytochrome P-450 enzyme. Mucilage. Gum resin. Lignans. Sterols. Tannins.

Primary pharmacological action: Vasotonic alterative.

Therapeutic classes
Ophthalmic. Antiseptic. Depurative. Stimulant. Vasotonic alterative.
Aromatic. Carminative.
Diuretic. Diaphoretic. Antilithic. Antipyretic. Antirheumatic.
Emmenagogue.
Dermatological agent. Vulnerary.
Analgesic.
Medicinal indications
Conjunctivitis. Sinusitis.
Diarrhoea.
Nephritis. Oedema. Syphilis. Uric acid complaints – lithiasis, lithuria.
Rheumatism. Gout. Arthritis. Pyrexia.
Skin diseases and eruptions. Remittent fever - typhoid, malaria.
Pediculosis. Lice. Fleas.
Tissue conditions
Cook explains its use in promoting the absorption of effusions. Used as a flavouring agent.
Cautions
Acute inflammation.
External use
The oil is used as a local anaesthetic.
Pith mucilage in opthalmia.
Cysts upon the scalp - apply an ointment.
Destroys pediculosis – use only 1-2% strength. Test an area on the scalp first.
Preparations
For more stimulation use with Arctium, Rumex, Smilax, Urtica.
Dosage and mode of application
Dried cort/bacc Sig 4g
Tincturae Sig 2ml
Liquidum extractum Sig 2ml
> **Essence Oleum Sassafras** Essence of Sassafras 1% alcohol to 1000ml.
> **Lotion** – max 2% strength.
References. 43 p190. 111 p684. 126 p621. 188 p382. 192 p490.

Schizandra chinensis [Chinese magnolia vine]

Constituents
Lignans - Schisandrin is a detoxifier it increases cytochrome P450 Gomisin A is hepatoprotective. Triterpine lactones. Resin. Essential oil. Vitamins C, E.

Primary pharmacological action:
Stimulating CNS nervine trophorestorative - Adaptogenic tonic.

Therapeutic classes
Allays inflammation. Antiviral – Hepatitis C.
Antioxidant.
Antitussive.
Cholagogue. Hepatoprotective. Antihepatotoxic.
Renal stimulant tonic. Antihydrotic.
Parturient.
Analgesic. Anxiolytic. Hypnotic. Sedative.

Medicinal indications
Indicated in chronic coughs and wheezing. Colds.
Hepatitis. Chemical liver damage. Diarrhoea.
Insomnia and weak memory. Pain. Fatigue.
Night sweats. Allergic skin disorders.

Tissue conditions
Hepatoprotective in hepatitis and detoxifier of the liver when due to chemical damage.
Sex tonic for men and women. Stimulates the CNS. It reduces CNS degeneration from cerebellar ataxia, CVA's, Parkinsons disease and special sense organ disease. Adaptogenic --increases one's ability to resist stress.
It supports softening of the skin by increasing dermal secretion.

Preparations
With Carduus, Chelidonium, Taraxacum or Rosmarinus.

Dosage and mode of application
Dried fructus Sig 3g
Tincturae Sig 4ml
Liquidum extractum Sig 3ml

References
192 p496. 239 p170. 263, 1991, 57, [1], p11. 285, 1994, 8 [8] 445-51. 286, 2000, 28 [3] p351-60.

Scrophularia nodosa [Figwort]

Constituents
Flavonoids. Iridoids - bitter principles. Amino acids.

Primary pharmacological action:
Vasotonic alterative [blood cleanser].

Therapeutic classes
Allays inflammation. Depurative. Deobstruent. Relaxant and moderately
stimulant. Antifungal – Trichophyton.
Cardiac. Mild diuretic. Renal tonic.
Laxative.
Anodyne - mild. Dermatological agent. Vulnerary.
Antineoplastic.
Medicinal indications [Venus]
Appendicitis. Haemorrhoids.
Lymphadenopathy. Tuberculosis – lymph glands.
Oedema. Testicular problems. Syphilis.
Eczema. Psoriasis. Pruritus. Dermal ulcerations. Vesicular eruptions. Tinea.
Mastitis. Breast tumours.
Tissue conditions
Slow and persistent acting upon the lymphatics, mesentery and kidneys.
Glandular disorders associated with skin conditions. Works by cleansing the
system of impurities. Valuable in itchy skin and for skin eruptions, abscesses and
wounds. Clears uric acid conditions. Ulcerations of the skin with especial
influences for face, nose and eye ulcers. Traumatic ulcerations of the skin.
External use
Fol applied as a poultice.
Sprains, swelling, inflammation, wounds, abscess – fomentation.
Mammary and testicular inflammation – Ung.
Tinea.
Preparations
Skin disease/blood disorders with Stillingia and Rumex.
Skin conditions with Iris, Rumex and Trifolium.
Dosage and mode of application
Dried herba Sig 8g
Tincturae Sig 2ml
Liquidum extractum Sig 8ml
References
36. 43 p193. 111 686. 176 p372. 188 p184. 228 p120. 246 p405.

Scutellaria baicalensis [Baical skullcap]

Constituents
Flavone glycosides [flavones, flavonoids] - Baicalin. The three flavonoids wogonin, baicalein and baicalin significantly inhibited interleukin-1 production by monocytes exposed to E. coli. Baicalein inhibits cancer cells. Flavonoids inhibit prostaglandin release. Melatonin – 7.11ug/g.

Primary pharmacological action: Antiallergic.

Therapeutic classes
Antibacterial. Antimicrobial – E. Coil. Antiviral - Epstein barr, HIV, influenza.
Allays inflammation.
Antioxidant. Hypotensive. Antiplatelet activity.
Bitter. Periodontal infections. Cholagogue. Hepatic.
Diuretic. Anti rheumatic.
Sedative.
Antineoplastic.

Medicinal indications
Infection.
Hypertension. Scarlet fever. Hyperlipidaemia. Atherosclerosis.
Respiratory allergies. Asthma. Colds. Bronchitis. Influenza. Bronchial carcinoma.
Cholecystitis. Hepatitis. Bacillary dysentery. Gout. Inflammatory joint disease.
Dermatitis.
Cervical carcinoma. Sarcoma.

Tissue conditions
Following oral administration the aglycone baicalein peaks at 2, 4 and 12 hours.
Supports the repair of damaged DNA. Inhibits reverse transcriptase and is an HIV viral inhibitor. Inflammation and lipid peroxidation is blocked. Inhibits leucotrines which are in part responsible for inflammation. Enzyme precursors which stimulate neutophil activity are inhibited. Inhibits platelet aggregation. Enhances and stimulates the production of haematopoesis in carcinoma. Blocks mast cell histamine. Stimulates glomerular filtration.

Cautions
Coldness. Lethargy.

Dosage and mode of application
Dried rad Sig 2g
Tincturae Sig 5ml
Liquidum extractum Sig 4ml

References
48 p75. 219. 220 p40. 223. 230 p91. 263, 61, 1995, 150. 296, 1997, 350 1598.

Scutellaria lateriflora [Skullcap]

Constituents
Flavonoid glycoside – apigenin, scutellarin [bitter]. Iridoids catalpol and catalpolesters. Volatile oil – limonen, terpinol. Lignans. Resin. Tannin. Melatonin – 0.09 ug/g.

Primary pharmacological action:
CNS vasodilator. Tonic and antispasmodic.

Therapeutic classes
Allays inflammation. Anticonvulsant. Sedative. Anodyne. Antipyretic.
Medicinal indications
Coughs with headache. Nervous dyspepsia. Hiccups.
Nervous restlessness. Depression. Excitability. Headaches. Irritability. Sensitivity. Neuralgia. Panic. Hypochondria. Hydrophobia. Insomnia. Chorea. Delirium tremens. Epilepsy. Convulsions. Pain. Tetanus. Withdrawal from drugs. Intermittent fever. Rickets.
Tissue conditions
Nerve tonic for the complete CNS & ANS. Acting as a diffusive and peripheral nervine remedy. Weakness [hypotrophicity] of the nerves with sensitivity, anger, obsessional behaviour, rage, anxiety, tremors - treat over a long period of time. Sleeplessness due to exhaustion, aching eyes with a dull headache and poor attention. Irritability of the nerves. Panic and nervous tension. Poor concentration with amnesia. Convulsions - petit or grand mal epilepsy. Muscular twitching or jumpiness.
Preparations
Nerve disorders with: Humulus, Passiflora, Turnera, Valerian, Verbena or Viscum
Tension states and Chorea with Valeriana.
Cranial nerve disease with Cimicifuga.
Tetanus with Lobelia.
Heart weakness with Capsicum and Hydrastis.
Dosage and mode of application
Requires fairly full dosage.
Dried herba Sig 2g
Tincturae Sig 5ml
Liquidum extractum Sig 4ml
References
43 p193. 111 p687. 176 p123. 246 p367. 251 p141. 297, 1997, 350, p1598.

Selenicerus grandiflorus

[Echinocereus/Night blooming cactus].

Constituents
Isoquinoline alkaloids. Amines. Flavonoids - rutin.

Primary pharmacological action:
Cardiac tonic nervine and trophorestorative.

Therapeutic classes
Stimulates the ANS. Cardiac tonic. Diuretic.
Thyroactive. Tobacco addiction.

Medicinal indications
Anaemia. Atonic heart. Angina. Arrhythmia. Palpitations. Cardiac hypertrophy.
Hypotension. Valvular disease. Aneurysm. Arteritis. Endocarditis. Mitral
regurgitation. Myocarditis. Pericarditis. Cerebro vascular disease including
incipient CVA. Pulmonary haemorrhage from tuberculosis.
Indigestion.
Cystitis. Prostatic diseases. Congested kidneys from oedema of cardiac origin.
Rheumatism.
Thyrotoxicosis. Depression. Fatigue. Headache. Panic attacks.

Tissue conditions
Regulates functional activity of the heart, the pulse and increases the blood
pressure. Influence is through the vasomotor centre and vagus nerve. It slowly
increases contractile power of the myocardium.
When the circulation becomes congested and the patient sighs it is suggestive of
air hunger and the requirement is for Selenicerus. Dyspnoea, a sense of weight or
oppression of the chest. Endocarditis and pericarditis and in feeble heart action
following pneumonia. Calms a rapid and feeble pulse. Cardiac irregularities and
gastric irritability. Heart weakness of the tobacco addict. Cardiac disorders with
nervousness, panic or apprehension of danger or death.
Similar in action to Digitalis.

Cautions
Avoid in hypertension

Preparations
Enhanced activity with Leonurus or Avena.
Angina with Cimicifuga.
Used alone or with Hydrastis, Lycopus, Capsicum, Convallaria or Leonurus.

Dosage and mode of application
Tincturae flos. Sig 2ml
Liquidum extractum Sig 0.6ml

References. 126 p253. 176 p212. 189 p80. 192 p 381. 254 p90. 262 p91.

Sempervivum tectorum [Houseleek]

Constituents
Malic acid. Mucilage. Tannin.

Primary action: Astringent.

Therapeutic classes
Ophthalmic. Allays inflammation. Refrigerant. Antiviral - Herpes zoster.
Diuretic. Antipyretic.
Dermatological agent. Vulnerary.
Analgesic.
Medicinal indications [Jupiter]
Inflamed eyes. Earache.
Tongue scirrhous carcinoma. Aphthous ulceration. Haemorrhoids.
Burns. Corns. Erysipelas. Inflamed dermis. Nettle stings. Urticaria. Warts.
Migraine. Cervical carcinoma. Breast carcinoma.
Tissue conditions
Bartrum argues the fresh juice is more effective than alcoholic preparations. John
Lust advises fresh fol only.
External use
Acute opthalmia – fresh succus.
Inflamed dermis, Herpes zoster, warts, freckles etc – poultice of fresh fol succus.
Dosage and mode of application
Succus Sig 15ml
Infusium fol Sig 2g
Tincturae Sig 1ml
References
16 p79. 111 p689. 147 pp236. 188 p235. 189 p149.

Seneco aureus [Liferoot]

Constituents
Alkaloids – senecifoline, senecine. Volatile oil. Resin.

Primary pharmacological action: Uterine and prostate tonic.

Therapeutic classes
Astringent. Expectorant - mild.
Diuretic. Haematuria.
Uterine tonic. Atonic amenorrhoea. Emmenagogue.
Medicinal indications
Dyspepsia. Hyperchlorhydria.
Gonorrhoea. Urinary irritability. Haematuria.
Menopausal flushes, neurosis, vasomotor imbalance. Malpositions of the uterus - prolapse. Uterine atony causing amenorrhoea. Dysmenorrhoea. Menorrhagia. Metrorrhagia. Obstruction of the fallopian tubes. Slow parturition. Impotency.
Tissue conditions
Atony with impairment of uterine/prostate function and heaviness or dragging feeling within the pelvis. Tonic to the nerve and muscular structure of the uterus and prostate.
Dragging feeling within the testes and scrotum. Improves functional action of the uterus or ovaries. Allays nerve irritability of the uterus and prostate. Perineal sense of weight and fullness. Increases ovarian activity. Uterine and prostate ganglionic vasorelaxant.
Preparations
Uterine malpositions with Chamaelirium and Mitchella.
Amenorrhoea with Avena, Sanguinaria.
Dosage and mode of application
Dried herba Sig 4ml
Tincturae Sig 4ml
References
BHP 194. 111 p690. 126 p625. 176 p476. 188 p269. 224 p1810. 254 p106.

Seneco vulgaris [Groundsel]

Primary pharmacological action: Vermifuge.

Therapeutic classes
Ophthalmic. Antiseptic.
Antiflatulent. Emetic. Laxative.
Dermatological agent. Vulnerary.
Nervine.
Medicinal indications [Venus]
Conjunctivitis. Flatulence. Jaundice.
Gravel. Sciatica.
Memory loss.
Preparations
A useful remedy for localised dermatitis.
External use
Eye disorders - apply an eye pack.
Furunculosis, wounds, sore nipples - bruised fol.
Lymphadenopathy - poultice.
References
246 p478. 251 p91.

Seneco jacobaea [Ragwort]

Constituents
Volatile oil. Pyrrolizidine alkaloids.

Primary pharmacological action: Anticatarrhal.

Therapeutic classes
Allays inflammation. Mucous membrane detergent.
Diaphoretic.
Antineoplastic.
Medicinal indications [Venus]
Catarrh. Colds. Influenza. Mucous membrane inflammation.
Tonsillitis.
Gout. Rheumatism. Myalgia.
Tumours internal and external.
Cautions
Restrictions apply. Dosage is determined by the relief of symptoms.
External use
Rheumatic conditions with pain, gout, sciatica, synovitis – liniment.
Dosage and mode of application
Liquidum extractum Sig 3ml
Oleum infused for use as a liniment.
References
6. 43 p121. 192 p455. 246 p477.

Serenoa repens [Sabal/Saw palmetto]

Constituents
Flavonoids. Fatty acids – capric, caprylic, palmitic, oleic acid. Free and conjugated sterols - beta sitosterol. Fixed oils up to 26%. Volatile oil. Polysaccharides. Resin.

Primary pharmacological action:
Genito urinary and reproductive tonic for male and female.

Therapeutic classes
Vasotonic alterative. Allays inflammation. Antiexudative.
Expectorant.
Nourishing tonic.
Diuretic. Urinary antiseptic. Prostatic disorders.
Aphrodisiac.
Endocrine stimulant. Anabolic properties. Hirsutism. Sexual tonic.
Galactogogue. Inhibits prolactin.
Antineoplastic.
Sedative. Antispasmodic.

Medicinal indications
Catarrh. Laryngitis. Asthma. Bronchitis. Pertussus. Respiratory catarrh.
Dysentery. Malnutrition [underweight]. Muscle wasting.
Sterility of male and female. Decreased sperm. Testicular atrophy. Sex hormone disorders. Impotence/sexual dysfunction.
Enuresis. Incontinence. Cystitis. Orchitis. Epididymitis. Urethritis. Prostatic carcinoma/enlargement/hyperplasia. Prostatitis.
Pelvic cellulitis. Salpingitis. Ovaritis. Puerpural fever. Uterine enlargement.
Polycystic ovary disease. Underdeveloped mammary glands. Breast carcinoma.
Hirsutism – excessive hair growth.

Tissue conditions
Maximum serum strength occurs in 2 hours. Inhibits 5 alpha reductase and the conversion of testerone to its more active form of dihydrotestosterone [DHT] to androgen receptors in the prostate. High levels of DHT are associated with BPH and prostate carcinoma. Berries inhibit the activity of the enzyme lipoxygenase and are antioestrogenic.

Serenoa is a stimulating vasotonic alterative. Acts upon all the pelvic viscera to cleanse and tone the tissue of the genito urinary and reproductive systems of the male and female. It acts upon the mucous membranes of the genito urinary tract. Used in impotency, male infertility and reduced libido. Catarrh of the respiratory system. Retarded sexual development - atrophy of the testes, ovaries or mammary glands, excessive hair [female androgenisation], malabsorption, under developed muscle. Serenoa increases tissue nutrition.

Preparations

Prostate disease with Barosma, Agropyron or Piper.

Pelvic inflammatory disease with Calendula, Echinacea.

Dosage and mode of application

Dried fructus/bacc Sig 1g

Dry extract Sig 300mg

Tincturae Sig 4ml

Liquidum extractum Sig 2ml

References

43 p196. 192 p491. 179 p527. 192 p492. 239 p151. 285 1997, Vol. 11, 558-563 394 p335.

Silybum marianum [St Mary's thistle/Carduus marianus]

Constituents
Flavanone lignans – silymarin up to 3% – antioxidant and protein restorer.
Silymarin consists of three isomers [structurally similar compounds] called
silybin [50%], silidanin and silicristin. A flavolignan derivative silibinin is
considered as the most important as it stimulates ribosome RNA. Fixed oil up to
30% and of this 60% as linoleic acid. Protein up to 30%.

Primary pharmacological action:
Hepatic trophorestorative, cholagogue and choleretic.

Therapeutic classes
Allays inflammation. Demulcent. Antibacterial – Pseudomonas aeruginosa.
Antiviral – hepatitis A,B,C,D,E.
Antioxidant. Venous tonic. Anticholesterolaemic.
Silybum is a potent liver detoxifier – hepatoprotective. Antiemetic. Cholelithiasis.
Splenic tonic.
Emmenagogue. Galactagogue.
Vulnerary. Dermatological agent.
Antineoplastic. Antivenomous.
Antidepressant.

Medicinal indications
Improves low platelet count. Anaemia. Varicose veins.
Pleurisy.
Beneficial for liver health. Cholagogue. Choleretic. Reduces biliary cholesterol.
Cirrhosis – fatty liver. Cholelithiasis. Hepatitis – A, B, C, D, E. Fatty
degeneration of the liver. Cholangitis - bile duct inflammation. Jaundice. Spleen
enlargement. Meleana. Pruritus. Haemorrhoids.
Oedema. Urethral caruncle.
Passive uterine haemorrhage. Cholestasis of pregnancy.
Rabies. Epilepsy.
Burns. Eczema. Erythema. Psoriasis. Wounds. Alcohol abuse.

Tissue conditions
Poorly absorbed from the gastro intestinal tract. Pain in the spleen, liver or
kidneys with debility. Congestion with dull aching of the spleen. Infective,
inflammatory and degenerative liver disease. Silybum protects the liver from
damaging toxins [alcohol, carbon tetrachloride, Amanita phalloides toxin
[Martindale], galactosamine, organophosphates, thioactamide] and has been
shown to be an active cholagogue. Stimulates DNA ribosomal protein synthesis
increasing the production of hepatocytes. Stabilises the outer membrane of

hepatocytes [trophorestorative] and is a powerful antioxidant, a scavenger of free radicles. Increases glutathione [antioxidant] levels by 35%. Blocks histamine release. Increases liver enzymes.

Passive uterine haemorrhage from congested pelvic veins associated with liver disorders. Carcinoma of the skin, ovary and breast.

External use

Dermatitis, eczema, wounds, ulcers - apply fol [remove prickles] or crushed sem. poultice

Dosage and mode of application

Dried sem/flos/herba Sig 4g

Dry extract Sig 200mg

Decoctum Sig 3g

Tincturae Sig 10ml

Liquidum extractum Sig 2ml

References

188 p295. 192 p359. 224 p1810. 230 p70/79. 239 p135. 246 p485. 263 1992, 58, Suppl I A580. 285 9, 1995, 281-286. Phytotherapy LXVI, 1995, 1. 394 p260.

Smilax aristolochiae/
folia/febrifuga/ornata/regelii [Sarsaparilla]

Constituents
Steroidal saponins around 2% - sarsapogenin, smilagenin, sitosterol, stigmasterol.
Resin. Volatile oil.

Primary pharmacological action: Vasotonic alterative.

Therapeutic classes
Antiseptic. Tonic. Allays inflammation. Hepato protective.
Diuretic. Diaphoretic. Antirheumatic. Febrifuge.
Adrenal tonic. Hormonal enhancer. Oestrogenic. Pituitary stimulant.
Immune enhancer. Dermatological agent. Antipruritic. Antineoplastic.

Medicinal indications [Mars]
Catarrh of the respiratory tract. Expectorant.
Mercury poisoning. Hepatic atony. Bacillary dysentery. Anal itching.
Gout. Rheumatic disorders. Rheumatoid arthritis.
Syphilis. Impotence/sexual dysfunction. Infertility. PMS. Vaginal itching.
Supports the adrenal glands. Muscle builder.
Skin disease - psoriasis, eczema. Leprosy. Remittent fever - typhoid, malaria.

Tissue conditions
Used as a blood purifier [vasotonic alterative] for all conditions affecting the
blood. Builds up muscle – steroidal like activity. Menispermum is similar.

Preparations
Combines well with Arctium, Guaiacum, Rumex, Sassafras and Stillingia.
Dermal conditions with above.
Syphilis with Echinacea and Hydrastis.
Rheumatics with Cimicifuga, Guaiacum, Populus tremuloides and Salix alba.

Dosage and mode of application
Dried rad Sig 4g
Liquidum extractum Sig 4ml
>   **Decoctum Sarsae Compositum.** [Dec. Sars. Co].
>   Compound decoction of Sarsparilla.
>   Smilax 100g with Guaiacum 10g, Sassafras 10g, Daphne mezereon 10g
>   and Glycyrrhiza 10g. Decoct ingredients in a closed vessel with 500ml
>   aqua for 20 minutes. Cool and bottle. Dispense et aqua. Sig 30ml.

References
BPC 1949. 43. 111 p694. 176 p372. 192 p486. 233 p194. 239 p170. 224 p614.
246 p506.

Solanum dulcamara [Bittersweet]

Constituents
Saponin. Alkaloids and the glycoside dulcamarin.

Primary pharmacological action: Sedative.

Therapeutic classes
Vasotonic alterative. Expectorant.
Diuretic. Antirheumatic. Sexual sedative.
Uterine stimulant. Antigalactagogue.
Dermatological agent. Antipruritic.
Antineoplastic.
Antispasmodic.
Medicinal indications [Mercury]
Asthma. Tuberculosis. Acute bronchitis. Dyspnoea.
Jaundice. Hepatic disease. Haemorrhoids.
Cutaneous, including scaly skin diseases - eczema, pityriasis, scabies and
psoriasis. Pruritus. Warts. Leprosy. Scurvy.
Bruising and ecchymosis absorption. Oedema. Rheumatic disease - gout as a
painkiller. Chronic rheumatism. Myalgia.
Amenorrhoea. Breast tumours. Syphilis.
Anxiety. Mania. Panic. Epilepsy. Nymphomania.
Tissue conditions
Regulates the secretions. Indicated for acute disorders from cold or chills with
suppressed secretions. Deficient capillary circulation with cold skin and limbs.
Opens obstructions of the liver and spleen. Tumour inhibitor. Obstinate skin
eruptions.
Cautions
The full dose may cause giddiness in delicate types. Overdosage causes paralysis.
External use
Itching use a lotion or cream.
Preparations
Ulcers and cutaneous disease with Rumex and Stillingia.
Whitlows –ung.
Dosage and mode of application
Infusium 1:10 Sig 60ml
Tincturae rad/bacc Sig 2ml
Liquidum extractum Sig 4ml [390]
References
126 p346. 176 p371. 224 p1753. 236 p8-10. 246 p254/398. 262 p66. 390 p2012.

Solidago virgaurea [Goldenrod]

Constituents
Flavonoids up to 1.5% – hyperoside, quercetin, rutin - allays inflammation,
vulnerary. Triterpine saponins up to 6%. Essential oil 0.5% before and 1.9% after
flowering. Volatile oil - borneol. Catechin tannins up to 10%. Bioflavonoids.
Flavonoids released by infusion: 21% after 5mins, 28% after 10min.
Tannins released by infusion 22%after 5mins, 28% after 10mins.

Primary pharmacological action: Astringent [tonic] diuretic.

Therapeutic classes
Antiseptic. Allays inflammation. Antihaemorrhagic. Antioxidant. Antifungal.
Antiallergic. Anticatarrhal. Antitubercular. Carminative. Antidiarrhoeal.
Diuretic. Diaphoretic. Antilithic. Urinary tract inflammation.
Dermatological agent. Vulnerary.
Medicinal indications [Venus]
Nasopharyngeal catarrh. Hay fever. Influenza. Asthma. Bronchitis with purulent
mucus. Tuberculosis.
Oral candida. Tonsillitis. Hiccups. Heartburn. Nausea. Vomiting. Flatulent
dyspepsia. Diarrhoea. Enterocolitis. Ano genital soreness.
Backache. Lithuria. Cystitis. Haematuria. Scanty urination. Acute or chronic
nephritis. Prostatitis. Oedema. Genito urinary infections. Arthritis. Pyrexia.
Dermal ulcers. Wounds. Eczema. Exhaustion. Fatigue. Spasm.
Tissue conditions
Antiseptic and astringent to mucous membranes. Cleanser of internal viscera.
Stimulating and tonic antiseptic diuretic, increasing renal blood and glomurular
filtration rate. Nephritis with anuria or oliguria.
Preparations
Oropharyngeal infections with Capsicum, Gnaphalum, Hydrastis. Infusium with
apple cider vinegar.
Diuretic – Betula, Uva ursi.
External use
Oropharyngeal infections – garg.
Rheumatism – poultice. Wounds – compress to clear infections and aid healing.
Dosage and mode of application
Dried flos/herba Sig 4g
Tincturae Sig 10ml
Liquidum extractum Sig 4ml
References. 43. 111 p698. 192 p243. 236 p62. 246 p449. 263, 1993, 59 p281.
Biologia [Bratislava] 1994, 49 [3] p359-64. 394 p178.

Spigelia marilandica [Pinkroot]

Constituents
Alkaloid - Spigeline. Bitter principle. Volatile oil. Tannin. Resin. Mucilage.

Primary pharmacological action: Anthelmintic.

Therapeutic classes
Cardiotonic.
Purgative.
Nervine.
Medicinal indications
Optic neuralgia. Migraine.
Chronic catarrh.
Toothache.
Violent palpitations. Pericarditis. Weak and irregular pulse. Dyspnoea. Angina.
Rheumatic carditis. Febrile disease.
Threadworms.
Neuralgia [extending to the arm].
Tissue conditions
Has a marked affinity for the eye, heart and brain. Specific for neuralgia of the
fifth cranial nerve. Typically used as an anthelmintic.
Preparations
Purgative with Cassia.
Cautions
Restrictions apply. Dosage is determined by the relief of symptoms.
Antidote - stimulants. Once a laxative action has been achieved there is less
likelihood of toxic symptoms.
Dosage and mode of application
Powdered fol and rad. Children up to 4 years of age 500mg - 4g. Adults Sig 5g
Liquidum extractum Sig 5ml
References
111 p699. 126 p651. 176 p504. 188 p339. 189 p217.

Spilanthes achmella/oloracea [Spilanthes]

Constituents
Isobutylamine.

Primary pharmacological action:
Stimulating Vasotonic alterative [Blood cleanser]

Therapeutic classes
Antibacterial. Antifungal – candida, tinea, trichophyton. Antiviral - herpes simplex.
Immunostimulant. Antimalarial.
Medicinal indications
Ear infections. Colds. Influenza. Respiratory tract infections.
Lymes disease. Malaria.
Tissue conditions
Stimulates mucous membrane secretions.
External use
Fungal or viral infections – lotion, crem.
Urogenital candida – pessary or vaginal douche. Sig once or twice daily.
Preparations
Fungal or viral infections with Echinacea, Tabebuia, Usnea, Origanum, Melaleuca.
Dosage and mode of application
Tincturae herba/rad. Sig 4ml
References
King 434.

Spirulina [Blue green algae]

Constituents
Cell walls are composed of protein and sugars. Phycocyanin is antiviral, antineoplastic, stimulates RBC's & WBC's, cytokines and antibodies. Quercetin – inhibits PGE2. Beta carotine. Vitamin A, B1, B2, B3, B12. E. Nicotinic acid. Calcium. Copper. Iron. Manganese. Phosphorus. Selenium. Zinc. GLA at 29% of the total fatty acid. Protein up to 62%.

Primary pharmacological action: Nutritive.

Therapeutic classes
Antiviral – Aids, Candida, HIV1, HSV1, Herpes simplex, Human cytomegalovirus, Influenza.
Anaemia. Hyperlipidaemia. Supports haemopoesis.
Hepatic. Antiobesity.
Renal toxicity. Antirheumatic.
Antineoplastic. Immunostimulant. Infectious mononucleosis.
Radiation protective.
Medicinal indications
Stimulates white and red blood cell production [anaemia].
Oral carcinoma. Oral leucoplakia. Liver damage. Hypoglycaemia. Diabetes.
Pancreatitis. Peptic ulcers. Colitis. Malabsorption. Obesity.
Arthritis.
Inhibits cancer colony formation.
Radiation exposure.
Eczema. Psoriasis. Varicella.
Tissue conditions
Stimulates the immune system – Bone marrow stem cells, Macrophages, Natural killer cells, T lymphocytes. Supports the repair of damaged DNA.
Dosage and mode of application
Dried algae Sig 1.5g
References
192 p520. 230 p163. 327, 1993, p235-241.

Stachys betonica [Wood betony]

Constituents
Alkaloids – betonicine and stachydrine. Tannin.

Primary pharmacological action: Tonic.

Therapeutic classes
Ophthalmic. Vasotonic alterative. Aromatic. Astringent. Stimulant.
Stomachic. Hepatic. Splenic.
Antispasmodic. Sedative – mild. Dermatological agent.
Antivenomous. Vulnerary.
Medicinal indications [Jupiter]
Cataract. Conjunctivitis. Heart and arterial disease. Hypertension. Gangrene.
Nausea. Dyspepsia. Abdominal cramps. Diarrhoea. Colic. Haemorrhoids.
Gout. Enuresis. Scrotal hernia + external application.
Rheumatism. Sciatica. Chicken pox. Ulcers.
Chorea. Epilepsy. Nervous eye disorders. Amnesia. Headaches. Menopausal
depression. Cerebral atrophy. Myalgic encephalitis. Anxiety. Panic attacks.
Nightmares. Vertigo. Phrenitis. Rabies.
Tissue conditions
A gentle cerebral tonic improving cerebral blood circulation. Tonic to the
stomach and intestine. Neuralgic and ischaemic conditions affecting the head.
Antirheumatic alterative. Removes obstructions of the liver and spleen
Preparations
Heart disease with Crataegus, Convallaria.
Nervous headaches with Scutellaria or Valeriana.
Headache from a cold or chill with Sambucus.
Rheumatic conditions with Cimicifuga and Scutellaria.
Neuralgia or Ischaemia of the head with Rosmarinus and Scutellaria.
Nervine and stomach tonic with Acorus and Scutellaria.
Memory loss with Cardiuus.
Hydrocephalus with Parietaria.
External use
Wounds - apply the fresh succus.
Scrotal hernia - apply ung.
Dosage and mode of application
Dried herba. Sig 4g
Tincturae Sig 4ml
Liquidum extractum Sig 4ml
References. 228 p101/249. 246 p373. 251 p157.

Stellaria media [Chickweed]

Constituents
Saponins. Flavonoids. Triterpenoids. Coumarins. Vitamin C.

Primary pharmacological action: Demulcent.

Therapeutic classes
Ophthalmic. Refrigerant. Resolvent. Vasotonic alterative. Discutient.
Antihaemorrhagic.
Expectorant. Pectoral. Laxative – mild.
Antirheumatic. Antipyretic.
Dermatological agent. Antipruritic. Vulnerary. Emollient.
Medicinal indications [Moon]
Inflamed eyes. Blood cleanser.
Coughs. Colds. Bronchitis. Pleurisy.
Sore throats. Inflammation of the stomach or intestine. Stomach ulcers.
Appendicitis.
Encourages weight loss. Scrotal oedema. Gout. Rheumatism.
Skin disease – dry, eczema, itching, psoriasis, erysipelas, urticaria. Abscesses.
Burns. Dermal ulcers. Furunculosis. Insect stings and bites. Wounds.
Tissue conditions
Heals, soothes and allays icterus and inflammation of the skin. Soothes the
respiratory mucous membranes. Antihaemorrhagic to the pulmonary and gastro
intestinal tracts. Rheumatic pain of a shifting nature.
Eaten fresh - excellent in obesity. Appendicitis use the enema and fomentation.
Give also a decoction.
Preparations
Respiratory tract inflammation with Althea and Primula.
External use
Conjunctivitis – collyr.
Inflamed surfaces - abscess, burns, furunculosis, gout, mastitis, ulcers and skin
eruptions – poultice add Althea or Ulmus.
Cuts, ulcerated legs, penetrating wounds - Ung.
Dosage and mode of application
Tincturae herba Sig 10ml
Liquidum extractum herba Sig 4ml
References
192 p138. 246 p104. 251 p48. 262 p94.

Stephania tetrandra [Han Fang Ji]

Constituents
Isoquinoline alkaloids. Tetandrine inhibits interleukin I and tumour necrosis factor. Demethyltetrandrine. Fanchinine. Flavonoids.

Primary pharmacological action: Antirheumatic.

Therapeutic classes
Allays inflammation.
Antiallergic. Antifibrotic in chronic lung disease - pulmonary silicosis.
Diuretic.
Antineoplastic. Immunodepressant.
Analgesic. Muscle relaxant.
Medicinal indications
Arrhythmia. Hypotensive.
Abdominal oedema. Amoebic dysentery.
Leg oedema.
Arthritic conditions.
Tissue conditions
Calcium channel blocker in cardiovascular disease. It dilates the coronary arteries and eases arrhythmia including supra ventricular tachycardia. It is hypotensive and a striated muscle relaxant. Stimulating to tissue in chronic inflammatory conditions. Destroys malignant lymphatic and myeloid cells.
Dosage and mode of application
Dried rad Sig 3g
Tincturae Sig 5ml
Liquidum extractum Sig 2ml
References
48 p80. Journal of Rheumatology, 1997, 24 [3] p436.

Sterculia lychnophora [Purple mallow]

Constituents
Sterculin a bitter.

Primary pharmacological action: Vasoconstrictor.

Therapeutic classes
Relieves inflammatory conditions.
Medicinal indications
Diarrhoea. Haemorrhoids.
Genito urinary conditions - cystitis, lithiasis, urethritis, prostatitis, pyelitis.
Dysmenorrhoea.
Tissue conditions
The seed has a distinct action upon the vein walls as a vasoconstrictor. It removes
congestion and inflammation through improved drainage of the pelvis and
kidneys. Clearing utero - ovarian congestion.
Dosage and mode of application
Liquidum extractum Sig 1g

Sterculia urens – Karaya gum is used to form gum, gel and as a
base for toothpaste and in pharmacy and cosmetics.

Sticta pulmonaria [Lungwort]

Primary pharmacological action: Soothing pectoral tonic.

Therapeutic classes
Astringent. Demulcent.
Medicinal indications
Conjunctivitis.
Sinus disturbances. Hay fever. Laryngismus stridulus. Asthma. Bronchitis.
Haemoptysis. Pertussus. Influenza. Tubercular night sweats.
Rheumatic pain.
Tissue conditions
Sticta should not be confused with Pulmonaria. Sticta is a lichen which grows on
oak trees and suffers from atmospheric pollution.
A primary remedy for sinus congestion. It will soothe upper respiratory
conditions. Rheumatic reflex stiffness and pain of the neck and shoulders. Sharp
irritating, hacking or wheezing coughs, chest soreness or pain. Pyrexia with
cough and diaphragmatic irritation. Muscular and rheumatic pain.
Preparations
Blepharitis, Conjunctivitis use the Collyr.
Pulmonary haemorrhage with Lycopus.
Dosage and mode of application
Dried lichen Sig 2g
Liquidum extractum Sig 4ml
References
126 p655. 246 p572. 254 p96.

Stillingia sylvatica [Queens delight]

Constituents
Volatile oil. Terpenoids. Resin. Tannin.

Primary pharmacological action:
Stimulating vasotonic alterative.

Therapeutic classes
Astringent.
Circulatory stimulant.
Expectorant.
Sialagogue. Emetic. Hepatic. Cathartic.
Diuretic. Diaphoretic.
Dermatological agent.
Antineoplastic. Immunostimulant. Lymphatic.
Antispasmodic.
Medicinal indications
Laryngitis. Laryngismus stridulus. Bronchitis. Tuberculosis. Irritable coughs.
Hepatic congestion. Constipation. Haemorrhoids.
Sexually transmitted disease. Syphilis. Rheumatism. Hip arthritis.
Lymphadenopathy. Elephantiasis. Skin eruptions. Eczema. Scrophula.
Tissue conditions
An all-round cleansing and depurative agent for the lymphatics, skin and blood.
Irritable and inflamed conditions of the mucous membranes with deficient
secretions. Dry irritable, hypotrophic skin. Skin disease is relieved if persisted in.
Preparations
It is often combined with other alterative vasotonics for best effect in dermal,
blood or lymph disease – Iris, Smilax, Guaiacum, Phytolacca, Rumex, Trifolium.
Dosage and mode of application
Dried rad Sig 2g
Tincturae Sig 4ml
Liquidum extractum Sig 2ml
References
43 p199. 111 p702. 126 p655. 176 p375. 188 p364.

Strophanthus species [Strophanthus]

Constituents
Glycosides up to 10%, strophanthidin is cardioactive and poorly absorbed from the gastro intestinal tract.

Primary pharmacological action: Cardiotonic.

Therapeutic classes
Anti cholesterolaemic.
Diuretic.
Medicinal indications
Acute heart failure. Coronary insufficiency - Angina. Cardiac atony. Fatty degeneration of the heart. Arterial atheroma. Cardiac dyspnoea. Extrasystoles. Acute endocarditis. Mitral regurgitation. Mitral stenosis. Heart irritability of tobacco smokers. Hypotension. Tachycardia with hypotension. Pulmonary congestion with cardiac disturbances. Pertussus. Goitre.
Cholera.
Tissue conditions
Digitalis like action - slows and strengthens the heart. Half life after IM injection is 90 hours with half of the drug being excreted unchanged. Increases the contractility of the myocardial non striated muscle and arteries inducing arterial tension; it raises blood pressure.
Cautions
Restrictions apply. Dosage is determined by the relief of symptoms.
Will enhance ectopic beats. Myocardial infarction. Diabetes. Toxicity is common from overdose or acute intolerance. Induces respiratory paralysis.
Dosage and mode of application
Tincturae sem Sig 0.3ml administered carefully.
Tincturae 1:2 Sig 60mg. [390]
References
BP 1948. 126 p659. 142 p140. 176 p220. 188 p408. 189 p261. 224 p498. 390 p630.

Strychnos ignatii [Ignatius beans]

Constituents
Indole alkaloids - strychnine.

Primary pharmacological action: Stimulating nervine tonic.

Therapeutic classes
Ophthalmic. Stimulant.
Uterine atony. Sterility. Impotence/sexual dysfunction.
Nervine tonic.

Medicinal indications
Conjunctivitis. Asthenopia. Palpebral twitching. Facial twitching. Dullness of hearing.
Atonic dyspepsia. Gastrodynia. Intestinal spasm.
Cerebral anaemia. Panic. Depression. Hypochondria. Fullness of the head.
Backache. Dragging ache or spasm in the lumbar area. Neuralgia. Paralysis.
Epilepsy. Grief.
Amenorrhoea. Ovarian pain. Dysmenorrhoea. Uterine enlargement.

Tissue conditions
Atonic conditions. Nervous debility. Tendency to grieve. Panic or hypochondriacal disorders. Dragging aches in the loins or low back. Pelvic congestion. Frigidity or impotence/sexual dysfunction. Cold extremities.

Cautions
Restrictions apply. Dosage is determined by the relief of symptoms.
Similar in action to nux vomica. Avoid in excitable conditions of the nervous system.

Dosage and mode of application
Dried sem Sig 120mg [390]
Tincturae Sig 0.6ml
Safer dosage is Tincturae 10 gtt in 120 ml aqua. Sig 5ml

References
126 p425. 176 p162. 189 p152. 224 p255. 390 p327.

Styrax benzoin [Gum benzoin]

Constituents
Gum resin. Benzoic acid stimulates phagocytosis.

Primary pharmacological action: Antiseptic astringent.

Therapeutic classes
Stimulant. Antifungal - tinea.
Stimulates phagocytosis.
Expectorant.
Aromatic. Carminative.
Genito urinary antiseptic. Vulnerary.
Medicinal indications
Coughs. Colds. Hoarseness. Respiratory disease. Respiratory dyspnoea.
Oral candida. Aphthous ulcers. Gingivitis. Sore throats.
Wounds. Dermal ulcers. Skin infections. Scabies.
A chief ingredient in Friars balsam.
Tissue conditions
Protects oral mucous membranes and allays inflammation.
External use
Wounds, ulcers, skin infections – spray wounds.
Aphthous ulcers, gingivitis - topically dilute Tr.
Coughs, colds, bronchitis – inhalation.
Dosage and mode of application
Tinctura gum resin Sig 2.5ml
Ung Antifungal @ 10% strength.
Inhalation Benzoin Tincturae Inhalation of Benzoin tincture
Sig 5ml et aqua cal 500ml. Inhale vapour.
Tinctura Benzoini composita Compound Benzoin tincture [Friars Balsam]

Styrax coarse powder	60g
Storax	45g
Balsam of Tolu	15g
Aloes crushed	150g
Alcohol	550ml

Internal use Sig 3ml
Storax is a furified balsam obtained from the bark of Liquidambar orientalis.
Tincture Benzoin compound spray
Compound Benzoin tincture 15% et ethanol. Aerosol spray for reducing skin
sensitivity, irritation and infections.
References. 189 p29. 192 p49.

Strychnos nux vomica [Nux vomica]

Constituents
Yields several indole alkaloids of which strychnine constitutes about 50%.
Strychnine inhibits glycine at post synaptic sites. Bitters.

Primary pharmacological action: Potent CNS stimulant.

Therapeutic classes
Ophthalmic. Tonic. Digestive. Antidiarrhoeal. Hepatic. Splenic. Anthelmintic.
Bladder activity. Uterine tonic.
Anticonvulsant. Nervine tonic. Alcohol habit.

Medicinal indications [Mars]
Nervous eye tics. Asthenopia. Conjunctivitis. Keratitis. Choroiditis. Purulent
otitis media. Hypotension.
Asthma. Pneumonia with depressed breathing.
Appetite stimulant. Dyspepsia. Heartburn. Flatulent colic. Hepatic disorder with
jaundice. Atonic diarrhoea or atonic constipation. Dysentery. Cholera. Tanea.
Typhoid. Alcohol habit.
Vomiting of pregnancy or where there is panic. Post partum haemorrhage.
Frigidity - female. Amenorrhoea. Dysmenorrhoea [cramps].
Impotence/sexual dysfunction. Spermatorrhoea. Relaxed or paralysed sphincters
of the bladder inducing enuresis or retention of urine. Chorea. Neuralgia.
Paralysis - hemi and para. Spinal innervation. athletic constitution.

Tissue conditions
The hallmark is atony of the tissues. Stimulates the medulla and vasomotor
system. Heart and pulmonary stimulant. Stimulates the special sense neurones.
Stimulates the portal circulation in hepato-splenic congestion. Stimulates the
eliminative organs. Tongue - pale or yellow with flaccidity. Hepatic tenderness,
right hypochondrial or right sub scapula pain. Depressed spinal and circulatory
activity with consequent disorders of the liver, pancreas, intestine and gastro
intestinal tract. It has a tendency to stimulate to exhaustion.

Cautions
Restrictions apply. Dosage is determined by the relief of symptoms.
Care in acute inflammation. Spinal nerve stimulant which produces convulsions
at high dosage. Poisoning includes muscle stiffness, spasm and lock jaw,
respiratory arrest, convulsions.

Dosage and mode of application
Dry extract sem. [BPC 1963] Sig 60mg
Tincturae sem 1:10 Sig 1.5ml. Contains 0.125mg Strychnine; 2.5mg in 2ml.
Liquidum extractum Sig 0.2ml. Contains 3mg Strychnine in 0.2ml.

Pharmacopoeia

Strychnos Preparata [Powdered Nux vomica sem.] sem. Sig 250mg.
[390 p327]
Elixir Strychnos. Sig 5ml.
References
126 p205/485. 142 p42/299.176 p157. 188 p344. 189 p202. 224p255

Succisa pratensis [Devils bit scabious]

Constituents
Saponin glycosides - Scabioside.

Primary pharmacological action: Vasotonic alterative.

Therapeutic classes
Allays inflammation. Demulcent.
Ecchymosis.
Anthelmintic.
Diaphoretic. Antipyretic. Dermatological agent.
Menstrual disturbances.
Antivenomous. Vulnerary.
Nervine.
Medicinal indications [Mercury]
Coughs. Tonsillitis. Pyrexia.
Vaginitis. Venereal disease. Plague.
Epilepsy. Chorea. Panic. Irritability.
Tissue conditions
Purifies the blood.
External use
Pustules, freckles, wounds, ulcers, ecchymosis - infusium, lotion, succus.
Dosage and mode of application
Dried flos/rad/herba Sig 5g
References
189 p101.

Symphytum officinale [Comfrey]

Constituents
Allantoin up to 2.5% is a cell proliferant, it encourages cellular regeneration and tissue healing. Alkaloids act upon the CNS and are haemostatic and sedative. Mucilage is demulcent. Tannin is haemostatic. Sterols. Resin. Volatile oil. Gum. Triterpenes - sitosterol. Rosemarinic acid – allays inflammation and microvascular injury in the lungs. Pyrrolizidine alkaloid - echimidine has not been isolated in S. officinale.

Primary pharmacological action: Demulcent.

Therapeutic classes
Astringent. Cell proliferant. Stimulant. Antibacterial – Pseudomonas aeruginosa. Antihaemorrhagic.
Antitussive. Expectorant. Pectoral. Anti ulcer.
Vulnerary. Dermatological agent. Emollient.
Uterine tonic.
Analgesic.
Medicinal indications [Saturn]
Asthma. Bronchitis. Coughs. Haemoptysis. Tuberculosis. Pleurisy. Pneumonia. Gastro intestinal ulceration. Gastritis. Hiatus hernia. Peptic ulcers. Haematemesis. [Ulcerative] Colitis. Diarrhoea. Dysentery.
Furunculosis. Bruises. Sprains. Wounds. Fractures. Dermal ulcers. Gangrene.
Tissue conditions
Demulcent activity gives the plant a healing action in ulcers [internally and externally] and inflamed surfaces. Demulcent action make it of service in expectorant mixtures. Tones the bronchi and allays irritability of the mucosa. For irritating coughs and bronchitis. Ideal as a pulmonary tonic for the elderly or those of a weak constitution.
Haemostatic in haematemesis, meleana and in haemoptysis of pulmonary tuberculosis. Enhances callus formation in fractures. Stimulates fibroblast & osteoblast activity.
It is the writers opinion that pyrrolizidine alkaloids have stimulating effects upon hepatocytes, whereby the hepatocytes are stimulated to increased activity. Is it only when large doses of pyrrolizidine alkaloids are given that they become damaging influences? As an example alcohol initially stimulates hepatocytes and with excess use poisons hepatocytes.

Pharmacopoeia

External use
Bruises, ulcers, wounds, inflamed skin – fol poultice or with Arctium.
Damage to muscles, ligaments, bone [fractures] or joints apply fresh fol or liniment.
Preparations
Peptic ulcer with Althea, Geranium maculatum, Filipendula or Ulmus.
Tuberculosis with Allium. Inula.
Pleurisy/Pneumonia with Asclepias, Hyssopus, Marrubium.
Renal inflammation with Eupatorium purpureum.
Dosage and mode of application
Dried rad/rhiz Sig 4g
Liquidum extractum rad Sig 4ml
Dried fol Sig 8g
Liquidum extractum fol Sig 4ml
Ung Symphytum. [Comfrey ointment]
Pwd Symphytum 10g. Paraffin Molle to 60g. Mix together.
References
43 p201/2. 111 p708. 230 p25. 246 p351. 251 p57. 285, 9, 1995, p281-286.

Symplocarpus foetidus [Skunk cabbage]

Constituents
Alkaloids. Glycosides. Phenols. Volatile oils. Resin. Tannin.

Primary pharmacological action: Bronchial antispasmodic.

Therapeutic classes
Expectorant.
Sedative.
Medicinal indications
Asthma. Bronchitis. Pertussus.
Tissue conditions
Bronchial spasm and tightness affecting the trachea and bronchus.
Dosage and mode of application
Dried rad/rhizoma Sig 1g
Tincturae Sig 2ml
Liquidum extractum Sig 1ml
References
43 p203/4. 111 p709. 189 p251.

Syringia vulgaris [Liliac]

Therapeutic classes
Infusion of flowers as a digestive tonic.
Antiperiodic. Febrifuge.
Vermifuge.
Medicinal indications
Malaria.
External use
Infused oil of the flowers as a liniment in rheumatic aches and pains.

Syzygium aromaticum [Syzygium, Cloves]

Constituents
Up to 20% volatile oil primarily consisting of eugenol at 80%. Eugenol is anodyne and antiseptic. Gallotannic acid. Sterols.

Primary pharmacological action: Astringent and Antiseptic.

Therapeutic classes
Allays inflammation. Antifungal – Candida. Bacteriocide. Antiseptic.
Circulatory diffusive stimulant. Antioxidant.
Expectorant. Antihistamine.
Aromatic. Carminative. Antiemetic. Stomachic. Antidiarrhoeal. Hypoglycaemic.
Anthelmintic.
Diuretic. Glycosuria.
Analgesic. Antispasmodic – mild. Antipyretic.
Galactogogue. Oxytocic. Dermatological agent. Local anaesthetic. Vulnerary.

Medicinal indications
Cold extremities. Influenza. Colds. Bronchitis. Asthma. Pleurisy.
Aphthous ulcers. Oral infections. Toothache. Halitosis. Dyspepsia. Nausea.
Vomiting. Flatulence. Diabetes. Diarrhoea. Dysentery.
Candida. Wounds. Dermal ulcers. Neuralgia.

Tissue conditions
Stimulates vasomotor arteries to the pancreas and kidneys. Promotes the digestion. Dilates gastric blood vessels and stimulates hydrochloric acid.
Palpitations with flatulent dyspepsia. Disinfects the lungs, stomach, liver, kidneys and skin. Raises the temperature. Orbell recommends an infusion for influenza.

External use
The oil is spasmolytic, anodyne and has antihistamine effects.
Halitosis, aphthous ulcers – garg.
Toothache – 2gtt oleum applied on cotton wool - will ease the pain & is antiseptic
Insect bites – oleum.
Tinia pedis can be controlled with tincturae.
Liniment as a stimulant with relaxing agents produce a counter-irritant effect that is, blood is drawn to the surface to give relief from pain.

Dosage and mode of application
Powdered sem Sig 1g
Infusium siccatus Syzygium 1:40 Sig 30ml. Infusium - Influenza Sig 5 cloves.
Liquidum extractum Sig 4ml
Oleum Syzygium Sig 0.2ml
References. 176 p453. 189 p80. 192 p149/296/297. 262 p97.

Tabebuia impetiginosa & avelleneda

[Pau d'arco]

Constituents
Naphthaquinones [antiviral] - lapachol [antineoplastic], alpha and beta lapachone. Beta lapachone blocks viral enzymes – DNA and RNA polymerase and retrovirus reverse transcriptase. Vitamin K complexes. Tannin. Benzoic acid derivatives - coumarins, flavones – quercetin. Xyloidone – anti infective, virucidal. Vitamin K. Lapachol is not detected in bark samples.

Primary pharmacological action:
Anti infective. Antiparasitic. Immunostimulant.

Therapeutic classes
Antifungal - Candida, Cryptococcus, Dermatophytes, Trichophyton.
Antiviral – Herpes simplex 1 & 2. AIDS/HIV. Epstein barr virus, Polio virus, Stomatitis virus.
Antibacterial - gram positive organisms, Staphylococcus. Gram negative – Brucella. Antiparasitic – Plasmodium falciparum, Schistosomia mansoni, Trypanosoma cruzi. Antiprotozoal. Inhibits: Crithidia fasciculata. Astringent. Decongestant. Depurative. Tonic.
Allays inflammation. Antioxidant. Antiallergic.
Vasotonic alterative [Blood purifier].
Cardiotonic. Antihaemorrhagic. Hypotensive.
Hepatic. Diuretic.
Antineoplastic. Immunostimulant. Antimalarial.
Dermatological agent. Vulnerary. Antipyretic. Antivenomous.
Analgesic. Sedative.

Medicinal indications
Anaemia. Builds healthy blood. Hypertension. Syncope. Nervous palpitations.
Colds and fevers. Bronchitis.
Toothache. Oral candida. Stomatitis. Peptic ulceration. Gastritis. Diabetes.
Dysentery. Intestinal polyps. Fistula. Hepatic carcinoma.
Bladder polyps. Cystitis. Enuresis. Prostatitis. Prostate carcinoma. Gonorrhoea.
Syphilis. Hernia. Incontinence.
Uterine inflammation. Cervicitis. Vaginal candida. Breast carcinoma.
Rheumatic conditions. Backache. Pyrexia.
Headache. Improves vitality. Myalgic encephalitis.
Leukaemia. Carcinoma. Hodgkins disease. Skin carcinoma.
Rabies. Snakebite. Malaria.

Eczema. Furunculosis. Lupus erythematosus. Psoriasis. Skin ulcers. Scabies. Warts. Wounds.

Tissue conditions

Maintains a healthy immune system. Lapacho flowers are deadly to insects and inhibit solid tumours. They keep the host tree immune from virus, pests and fungi. Inhibits: Brucella organism that causes disease and abortion in animals.

Cautions

Pregnancy.

External use

Skin disease – eczema, psoriasis, fungal infections, skin cancers - poultice, wash, crem, ung of the decoction or diluted tincture.

Dosage and mode of application

Decoctum bacc Sig 30ml

Dried bacc/fol Sig 1.5g

Tincturae bacc Sig 2ml

References

192 p411. 267. 230 p83. 304, 1994, 2 [4] p27-43.

Austin. American Journal of Tropical Medicine. 3, 23, p412. 1974.

Tanacetum parthenium [Feverfew]

Constituents
Sesquiterpine lactones of which 85% is Parthenolide. Parthenolide affects smooth muscle in the walls of the blood vessels in the brain to block the action of vasoconstrictors like serotonin, prostaglandins and norephinephrine. Flavonoids. Volatile oil – camphor, terpenes.
Melatonin content –

T. parthenium [fresh green leaf]	2.45 ug/g
T. parthenium [fresh golden leaf]	1.92
T. parth. [freeze-dried green leaf]	2.19
T. parth. [freeze-dried golden leaf]	1.611
T. parth. [oven-dried green leaf]	1.69
T. parth. [oven-dried golden leaf]	1.37

Primary pharmacological action: Antispasmodic.

Therapeutic classes
Antibacterial – Escherichia coil, Salmonella, Staphylococcus aureus. Antifungal. Allays inflammation. Inhibits platelet aggregation. Antithrombotic. Vasodilator.
Bitter. Carminative. Anthelmintic.
Diuretic. Antipyretic.
Emmenagogue.
Insect repellent.
Sedative.
Medicinal indications
Toothache. Coughs - infusion. Asthma.
Flatulence. Atonic dyspepsia.
Arthritis. Rheumatic diseases. Rheumatoid arthritis.
[Panic associated with] amenorrhoea. Menorrhagia. Dysmenorrhoea.
Fever. Insect bites. Psoriasis.
Migraine. Tinnitus. Vertigo. Meniers disease.
Tissue conditions
Vasoconstrictors narrow blood vessels, subsequent vasoconstriction is one of the main causes of migraine. Tanacetum activity is vasodilatory. Soothes nervous conditions.
Only 5 randomised, double blind, placebo-controlled trials have been found. Three trials found a positive effect of the herb compared with placebo, whereas the other two did not. One explanation for the negative findings is that these trials used extracts standardised for the concentration of parthenolides, thought to be feverfew's active constituents. This could suggest that other compounds found

in whole leaf preparations may be important - a potential blow to those who are promoting standardisation as the way forward in herbal medicine [Lancet 1999].

Cautions

Sore mouth. Pleurisy. Uterine inflammation. Phrenitis. Pregnancy.

Preparations

Sciatica, sprains, rheumatic joints use a fomentation to ease pain.

Intestinal pain and swelling - fomentation.

Often used with nervines.

Keeps away flies.

Dosage and mode of application

Fresh fol Sig 2g

Dried fol Sig 200mg

Tincturae Sig 4ml

Liquidum extractum Sig 2ml

References

230 p37. 233. 241. 246 p466. 251 p78. 296, 1997, 350, p1598. 296, 1999, 353, [9154] p731.

Tanacetum vulgare [Tansy]

Constituents
Essential oil - beta thujone and camphor. Steroidal components as beta sitosterol. Mucilage. Terpenes. Tannins. Resin. Melatonin - 0.57ug/g.

Primary pharmacological action: Anthelmintic.

Therapeutic classes
Astringent. Allays inflammation. Tonic. Antibacterial – Pseudomonas aeruginosa. Circulatory stimulant.
Carminative. Abdominal viscera stimulant. Flatulence. Hepatic. Choleretic. Cholagogue.
Nephritic. Diaphoretic.
Antispasmodic. Emmenagogue. Intermittent fever.

Medicinal indications
Ocular inflammation. Hordeolum.
Hypertension. Varicose veins.
Colds and influenza. Sore throat. Diphtheria.
Tonsillitis. Anorexia. Nausea. Nematodes - Ascaris and Oxyuris [threadworm] infestation. Hepatitis. Jaundice. Diarrhoea.
Renal disease. Strangury. Gout. Oedema. Sciatica. Pyrexia. Muscle spasm. Amenorrhoea.
Headache. Panic attacks.
Fleas, lice, scabies.

External use
Bruises, earache, toothache, hordeolum, ocular inflammation – lotion.
Fleas, lice, scabies - infusium wash.
Pruritus ani - unguentum.
Nematodes expulsion – enema.
Varicose veins - lotion.
Rheumatism apply the Oleum.
Fol repels flies. The oil rubbed on the body will help repel insects.

Cautions
Avoid in pregnancy.

Dosage and mode of application
Dried herba Sig 2g
Liquidum extractum Sig 2ml

References
43 p205. 111 p710. 142 p121. 188 p415. 192 p536. 246 p465. 296, 1997, 350, p1598. 285, 9, 1995 p281-286.

Taraxacum officinale [Dandelion]

Constituents
Around 40% inulin is present in the root which is at its highest in the autumn. Fructose is produced on hydrolysis. Sesquiterpine lactones – [terpenoids]. Resin - bitter [taraxacin] content is choleretic. Sterols – sitosterol, stigmasterol, taraxasterol. Volatile oils. Acids – caffeic, linolenic, oleic. Potassium up to 297mg per 100g in the fol. Mucilage. Vitamin A, C.

Primary pharmacological action:
Relaxing cholagogue and choleretic.

Therapeutic classes
Ophthalmic. Cholelithiasis. Pancreatic. Hypoglycaemic. Splenic. Laxative. Diuretic. Antirheumatic.
Dermatological agent.
Antineoplastic. Antivenomous.

Medicinal indications
Anorexia. Cholelithiasis. Cholecystitis. Atonic dyspepsia. Portal congestion. Cirrhosis. Diabetes. Hepatomegaly. Jaundice. Hyperglycaemia. Constipation. Haemorrhoids.
Oedema. Oliguria. Urinary infections. Calculi. Rheumatism. Gout.
Abscess. Eczema. Snakebite. Used as a drink – dandelion coffee.

Tissue conditions
Taraxacum brings uric acid levels into solution from between the muscle fibres thereby aiding rheumatic and arthritic conditions. Specific for dyspepsia with cholecystitis from overcontracted conditions [biliary or intestinal spasm]. Obstructed conditions of the liver, gall bladder or spleen.
Dandelion coffee is made by grinding up the root and drying. 30g is added to 550 ml and used as ordinary coffee.

External use
Complexion aid – flos to remove freckles.

Preparations
The leaves are diuretic and contain potassium.
The root is cholagogue.
IV route has twice the action upon biliary secretion.
Gall bladder disease with Leptandra, Berberis or Chelone.
Anorexia and stomach complaints with Chamomilla.

Dosage and mode of application
Dried fol Sig 10g
Liquidium extractum fol Sig 10ml

Dried rad Sig 8g
Tincturae rad Sig10ml
Liquidium extractum rad Sig 8ml
Succus rad Sig 5ml
References
43 p206/7. 111 p711. 230 p27. 233 p73-77. 236 p53. 246 p495. 251 p66. 394 p78.

Taxus baccata/brevifolia [Yew]

Constituents
Diterpenes - Taxol. Alkaloids – taxine. Taxusines, taxagifin, and baccatins I, II, and III. Lignans – isotaxiresinol. Paclitaxel. Docetaxel.
Corylus avellana [Hazel tree] contains paclitaxel [282, No 49].

Primary pharmacological action: Antineoplastic

Therapeutic classes
Expectorant. Purgative.
Emmenagogue.
CNS depressant. Analgesic. Antispasmodic. Antimitotic.
Medicinal indications
Asthma. Coughs. Catarrh. Lung carcinoma.
Oesophageal carcinoma. Hepatic disturbances. Stomach carcinoma.
Bladder carcinoma. Rheumatism. Arthritis.
Dysmenorrhoea. Breast carcinoma. Uterine and ovarian carcinoma.
Carcinomas of the head and neck. Melanoma.
Epilepsy.
Tissue conditions
Paclitaxel and Docetaxel as found in the pacific variety inhibit the depolermerisation of tubulin, this leads to bundles of microtubules in the cell. The cell becomes blocked during the G2 and M phases of the cell cycle thus being unable to form a normal mitotic spindle. Cellular division is effectively stopped.
Cautions
Depresses motor neurons. Toxicity – nausea, gastric irritation. Leucopenia. Pallor. Collapse. Cardiac arrest.
Dosage and mode of application
Bacc/fol.
References. 189 p325. 192 p596. 246 p569. 268. 283, 1998, 28 [4] p569-75.

Tephrosea [Turkey pea]

Constituents
Bitter. Rutin.

Primary pharmacological action: Tonic.

Therapeutic classes
Deobstruent. Anti flatulent. Laxative.
Diuretic.
Medicinal indications
Bronchitis. Flatulence. Haemorrhoidal bleeding.
Syphilis. Typhoid.
Dosage and mode of application
Decoctum Sig 25ml

Terminalia arjuna [Arjun]

Constituents
Flavonoids – arjunone. Tannin. Triterpenoid saponins – arjungenin. Sterols.

Primary pharmacological action: Cardioprotective.

Therapeutic classes
Antibacterial. Anticholesterolaemic.
Hepatoprotective.
Diuretic. Antineoplastic.
Medicinal indications
Angina. Arrhythmia. Congestive heart failure.
Hepatic cirrhosis. Diarrhoea. Dysentery.
Tissue conditions
Improves left ventricular stroke volume.
Dosage and mode of application
The bark [cort] is mainly used.
Dried cort/fol Sig 1g
Liquidum extractum Sig 2ml
References
48 p131. 271, No 17. 281, Spring 2002.

Teucrium chamaedrys [Wall germander]

Constituents
Flavonoids. Bitters. Tannin. Volatile oil.

Primary pharmacological action: Stimulant tonic.

Therapeutic classes
Anti catarrhal. Allays inflammation. Antimicrobial. Antiseptic - mild.
Bitter.
Diuretic. Diaphoretic. Antirheumatic.
Emmenagogue.
Dermatological agent.
Vulnerary.
Antispasmodic.
Medicinal indications
Nasal catarrh. Bronchitis.
Pyorrhoea. Anorexia. Dyspepsia. IBS. Diarrhoea.
Oedema.
Rheumatoid arthritis. Gout.
External use
Dermal disorders.
Nasal polyps - use the snuff.
Preparations
Pectoral disorders e.g. bronchitis - Marrubium.
Rheumatoid arthritis with Apium, Guaiacum, Menyanthes.
Dosage and mode of application
Dried herba 4g
Liquidum extractum Sig 4ml
References
189 p126. 246 p366.

Teucrium scordonia [Wood sage]

Constituents
Diterpenes. Iridoids. Essential oil. Tannin.

Primary pharmacological action: Astringent tonic.

Therapeutic classes
Stimulant. Allays inflammation. Antiseptic. Vasotonic alterative. Anticatarrhal.
Carminative.
Diuretic. Diaphoretic. Febrifuge. Antirheumatic.
Emmenagogue.
Vulnerary.
Antineoplastic.
Medicinal indications
Nasal polyps. Upper respiratory infections. Bronchitis. Bronchiectasis. Pertussus.
Pneumonia.
Flatulent dyspepsia.
Pyrexia.
Amenorrhoea. Mastitis.
Wounds.
Tissue conditions
Inflammatory conditions with cold and pyrexia. Carcinoma external applications.
External use
Mastitis, carcinoma, abscess, hordeolum – decoction lotion.
Wounds – decoction wash.
Preparations
Colds with/out fever - combine with Achillea or Sambucus and Mentha piperita.
Dosage and mode of application
Dried herba/rad Sig 4g
Liquidum extractum herba Sig 4ml
References
188 456. 192 p210. 246 p365.

Thuja occidentalis [Arbor vitae]

Constituents
Volatile oil - thujone. Lignans - antineoplastic. Tannin. Bitter - pinipicrin.

Primary pharmacological action:
Lymphatic vasotonic alterative.

Therapeutic classes
Astringent. Stimulant. Antiseptic. Antibacterial. Antifungal. Antiviral – HIV.
Expectorant. Diuretic. Emmenagogue. Uterine tonic.
Anthelmintic. Antineoplastic. Antipyretic. Nerve tonic.
Remittent and intermittent fevers. Dermatological agent. Vaccination antidote.

Medicinal indications
Conjunctivitis. Pterygeum. Trachoma. Gangrene.
Tonsillar enlargement. Polyps. Laryngeal papilloma. Bronchitis. Pneumonia.
Tuberculosis. Anal and rectal prolapse.
Cystitis. Enuresis - all ages. Spermatorrhoea. Impotence/sexual dysfunction.
Prostate hypertrophy. Bladder irritability/infections. Syphilis. Fistula. Pyrexia.
Amenorrhoea. Cervical carcinoma & ulceration. Endometriosis. Fibroids.
Rheumatism. Skin ulcers. Warts – dermal and genital. Verrucae. Tinea.
Epithelioma. Psoriasis. Smallpox.

Tissue conditions
Stimulates mucous and serous membranes. Glandular vasotonic alterative e.g.
prostate, uterus. Stimulates the myocardium and removes oedema.
Malignant backgrounds – dermal carcinoma - internal and *external use.*
Vaccinations - supports the elimination of the vaccine and its unwanted effects.

Preparations
Pulmonary disease with Grindelia, Polygala or lobelia.
Open wounds - diluted lotion.

Cautions
Lactation. Pregnancy.

External
Warts, fungal growths - use an LE or floral water.
Skin carcinoma use the fresh plant tincture or floral water.
Eczema with Aqua Hamamelis or floral water.
Anal fissure, pruritus ani.

Dosage and mode of application
Tincturae Sig 1ml
Liquidum extractum Sig 1ml
References. 1 p103-4. 43 p210. 126 p677. 188 p421. 192 p540.

Thymus serphyllum/vulgaris [Thyme]

Constituents
Volatiel oil [spasmolytic] up to 3.4%. Essential oil in which thymol and carvacrol are present at around 70%. Thymol is bactericidal and antifungal. Flavonoids – thymonin [bronchial antispasmodic]. Phenolic monoterpenoids – rosmarinic acid. Saponins.

Primary pharmacological action: Antiseptic.

Therapeutic classes
Allays inflammation. Astringent. Tonic.
Anti bacterial – gram positive and gram negative bacteria; Corynebacterium parvum, Helicobacter pylori, Porphyromonas gingivalis, Salmonella typhimurium, Sarcina sp, Selenomonas artemidis, Streptococcus sombrinus.
Anti fungal – Aspergillus flavus and parasiticus, Colletotrichum lindemuthianum, Cryptococcus neoformans, Fusarium solani, Penicillium sp, Pytheum ultimum, Antiviral – Candida, Trichomonas – oleum, Rhizoctonia solani.
Antioxidant.
Expectorant. Mucous membrane disinfectant. Antitussive.
Oropharyngeal conditions. Carminative. Hepatic. Splenic tonic. Anthelmintic.
Antirheumatic.
Local anaesthetic. Antipyretic.
Dermal disinfectant. Counterirritant/Rubefacient.
Vaginal discharge/leucorrhoea. Mastitis.
Antispasmodic. Analgesic. Alcohol habit.

Medicinal indications
Hypolipidaemic.
Inflammatory conditions of the oral cavity and upper respiratory tract.
Otitis media. Sinus infection. Laryngitis. Bronchitis. Asthma. Pertussus. Influenza
Dental hygiene. Aphthous ulcers. Halitosis. Dyspepsia. Flatulence. Heartburn.
Gastritis. Hepatitis. Colic. IBS. Diarrhoea. Nematode infestation - Ascaria, Hookworm.
Enuresis. Gout. Sciatica. Pyrexia.
Menorrhagia. Parturient. Salpingitis. Uteritis. Mastitis.
Leprosy.
Panic. Giddiness. Nightmares. Headaches.

Tissue conditions
Catarrh, sore throats and bronchial irritation. Thymus arrests gastric fermentation, eases spasm associated with flatulent colic. Antioxidant compounds have been isolated in the fol these are known as a biphenyl compound and a flavonoid –

eriodicytol, they inhibit microsomal and mitochondrial peroxidation. Infective conditions of the respiratory, gastro intestinal and genito urinary tracts.

Cautions
Pregnancy.

External use
An antimicrobial in collyr, toothpaste, cream, unguentum and lotions.
Visual disturbances - infection, inflammation - use collyr.
Otitis media – oral and ear guttae.
Tonsillitis, aphthous ulcers, gingivitis - oral antiseptic and anaesthetic.
Testicular swelling from inflammation – ung.
Warts - use the ung.
Respiratory difficulties and infections - use the inhalation.
Wounds/ulcers.
Essential oil repels aphids.

Preparations
Infections with Commiphora.

Dosage and mode of application
Dried herba Sig 4g
Dry extract Sig 2g
Tincturae Sig 5ml
Liquidum extractum Sig 5ml
        Elixir Thymus Sig 8ml
        Gargarisma – infusium 10%.

References
43 p211/12. 179 p564. 239. 246 p382/383. 251 p154. 263, 41, 1981 p219. 263, 63, 1996 p217. 270, 1996, p279. 271 No 23. Nutr. Pract.. 1999, 1 [3] 24.6. 394 p376.

Tilia cordata/platyphylos/europaea

[Linden/Lime flower tree]

Constituents

Flavonoids up to 1% [known as flavone glycosides] are diaphoretic - quercitrin, hesperidin. Infusion extraction of flavonoids – 17% after 2.5 minutes, 17% after 10 minutes. Steroidal saponin - oestrogen molecule. Triterpenoid saponin. Mucilage polysaccharides up to 10%. Condensed tannins up to 2%. Sterol - tocopherol. Amino acids. Caffeic acid. Volatile oil. Phenolic acids [diaphoretic].

Primary pharmacological action: Antispasmodic and sedative.

Therapeutic classes

Aromatic. Mild astringent. Stimulant. Demulcent. Antifungal. Antibacterial.
Anti coagulant. Antisclerotic. Hypocholesterolaemic. Hypotensive. Vasodilator.
Stomachic.
Diuretic. Diaphoretic.
Antipyretic. Emollient.
Nervine relaxant. Sedative.

Medicinal indications

Arteriosclerosis. Hypertension. Inadequate peripheral circulation. Palpitations.
Catarrh. Infective colds with pyrexia. Irritable coughs. Bronchitis.
Vomiting. IBS. Diarrhoea.
Pyrexia.
Migraine/Headache. Panic. Anxiety. Restlessness. Hyperactivity. Insomnia.

Tissue conditions

Relaxes the myocardium – requires full dosage.
Upper respiratory infective conditions. Diaphoretic in acute and chronic conditions to relieve capillary pressure and tension. A gently acting medicine.

External use

Sedative – foot balneum

Preparations

Influenza tea – Chamomilla, Fillipendula, Salix alba & Auranti.
Hypertension with Viscum and/or diuretics.
Inadequate peripheral circulation - Achillea, Crataegus, Viscum or Zanthoxylum.

Dosage and mode of application

Dried flos/fol Sig 4g. Use as a tea for acute conditions.
Tincturae Sig 10ml
Liquidum extractum Sig 4ml

References

BPC 1934. 43 p214. 142 p227. 189 p171. 246 p237. 394 p240. 394 p240.

Trifolium pratense [Red clover]

Constituents
Isoflavonoids - daidzein, formononetin. Coumarin. Saponins. Volatile oil. Resin.

Primary pharmacological action: Vasotonic alterative.

Therapeutic classes
Ophthalmic. Deobstruent.
Anticoagulant.
Expectorant.
Hormonal balancer. Oestrogenic.
Dermatological agent. Lymphatic deobstruent. Vulnerary.
Antineoplastic. Antivenomous.
Antispasmodic. Sedative.
Medicinal indications
Throat carcinoma. Respiratory catarrh. Pharyngitis. Laryngitis. Laryngismus stridulus. Bronchitis. Irritable coughs. Pertussus. Tuberculosis. Aphthous ulcers. Chronic skin disease. Eczema. Psoriasis. Scrophula. Measles. Tibial ulcers. Dermal carcinoma.
Menopausal and hormonal imbalance. Menorrhagia. Ovary carcinoma. Breast carcinoma.
Tissue conditions
A general stimulating and relaxing blood vasotonic alterative with emphasis upon the larynx, salivary glands and bronchial mucous membrane. Heals and soothes the mucous membrane in those weakened by chronic coughing in cases of spasmodic [pertussus] and bronchial affections.
Supports the oestrogen and progesterone balance within the bone and uterus.
Used in dermal and mucus membrane carcinomas of the throat. Promotes granulation tissue.
External use
Carcinoma locally as a plaster and internal prescription
Psoriasis, eczema.
Preparations
Suitable for children with respiratory disturbances.
Pertussus with lobelia.
Skin disease with Rumex.
Combines well with Arctium, Larrea, Panax, Stillingia and Zanthoxylum.
Dosage and mode of application
Dried flos Sig 4g
Tincturae Sig 10ml

Liquidum extractum Sig 4ml

Ung Trifolium @ 15%

Compound Trifolium

Arctium 4ml Berberis vulgaris 4ml Phytolacca 4ml Rhamnus purshiana 4ml Stillingia 4ml Trifolium 8ml Zanthoxylum 1ml

Sig LE 2ml. Blood cleansing vasotonic alterative for dermal and septicaemic blood disease.

References

43 p216. 111 p716. 126 p681. 188 p367. 192 p463. 228 p110. 233 p183/4. 236 p40. 239 p149. 242 p161. 251 p136.

Trigonella foenum graecum [Fenugreek]

Constituents
Pyridine type alkaloids - trigonelline. Protein around 25%. Flavonoids. Steroidal saponins - Diosgenin. Mucilage up to 30%. Vitamins A, B1, C. Calcium. Minerals.

Primary pharmacological action: Astringent.

Therapeutic classes
Demulcent. Nutritive. Allays inflammation. Antibacterial.
Expectorant.
Diuretic. Hypoglycaemic. Laxative.
Uterine tonic. Galactagogue. Orexigenic. Oxytocic. Male aphrodisiac.
Dermatological agent. Antipyretic. Emollient. Vulnerary. Lymphatic.
Analgesic – mild.

Medicinal indications
Hypolipidaemic. Reduces total cholesterol and triglycerides. Reduces platelet aggravation. Thrombosis. Embolus. Weakness and oedema of the legs.
Coughs. Bronchitis. Tuberculosis.
Anorexia. Aphthous ulcers. Gingivitis. Anorexia. Dyspepsia. Gastritis. Hiatus hernia. Diabetes. Peptic ulcers. Diverticulitis. Diarrhoea. Colitis. IBS. Crohn's disease. Dysentery. Fistula. Intestinal carcinoma – anodyne. Constipation.
Gout. Impotence/sexual dysfunction.
Menopausal hormonal imbalances - flushes. Breast developer. Mastitis.
Fever. Eczema. Dermal ulcers and wounds. Myalgia. Lymphadenitis.

Tissue conditions
Mucilage has demulcent effects upon mucous membranes and skin. Gastro intestinal disorders with irritation or inflammation. Increases body weight.
Suitable in pregnancy.

External use
Oropharyngeal disorders – aphthous ulcers: collutoria - emollient and vulnerary.
Throat pack poultice - ground sem.
Abscesses, furunculosis, ulcers, wounds – antiseptic and emollient wound dressing [ground sem].
Myalgia. Lymphadenitis.

Dosage and mode of application
Sem Sig 10g daily. Tincturae Sig 30ml
Liquidum extractum Sig 6ml
References. 43 p217. 188 p182. 192 p207. 247 p82. 270 1996, [4], p372. 272, 1995, 7 [4] 67. 394 p130.

Trillium erectum [Bethroot]

Constituents
5% saponins, trillarin - steroidal glycoside. Tannin.

Primary pharmacological action:
Stimulating tonic to the prostate, uterus and pelvic organs.

Therapeutic classes
Vasotonic alterative. Antiseptic. Antifungal. Astringent. Tonic.
Antihaemorrhagic.
Pectoral. Expectorant.
Uterine stimulant. Parturient.
Dermatological agent. Antivenomous.
Medicinal indications
Gangrene.
Asthma. Bronchitis. Haemoptysis.
Diarrhoea. Dysentery.
Haematuria. Menorrhagia. Metrorrhagia. Candida. Vaginal discharge/vaginal
discharge/leucorrhoea. Uterine fibroids with haemorrhage.
Parturient and oxytocic - increases contractions at birth.
Tissue conditions
Astringent and tonic acting upon the mucous membranes to astringe back a
profuse catarrhal discharge or internal haemorrhage. Relaxed tissues with chronic
mucus discharge. Antihaemorrhagic to the uterus, lungs, nose, gastro intestinal
and genito urinary tract. Menopausal menorrhagia.
Preparations
Assists cardiac medicines when given for functional conditions.
External use
Epistaxis – snuff.
Vaginal haemorrhage - douche with Geranium Maculatum.
Vaginal discharge/leucorrhoea – douche 1:40.
Gangrene/ulcers – poultice with Ulmus.
Tumours - fol poultice.
Dosage and mode of application
Pwd rad Sig 2g
Tincturae Sig 4ml
Liquidum extractum Sig 2ml
References
43 p218. 111 p716. 176 p273. 192 p53. 235 p204. 254 p106. 262 p61.

Tropaeolum majus [Nasturtium]

Constituents
Glucoside - glucotropaeoline hydrolyses to sulphur, an antimicrobial compound.
Iodine. Iron. Phosphate.

Primary pharmacological action: Anti infective.

Therapeutic classes
Relaxing vasotonic alterative. Antimicrobial. Antifungal – Candida.
Antitussive. Expectorant.
Diuretic.
Antidepressant.
Medicinal indications
Influenza. Acute respiratory catarrh. Pharyngitis. Bronchitis. Pneumonia.
Emphysema.
Tonsillitis. Anorexia.
Cystitis. Pyuria in children. Candida infection of the genito urinary tract.
Tissue conditions
Fol and flos can be used as a salad vegetable it has a peppery taste.
External
Alopecia - massage tincture/succus into the scalp.
Dosage and mode of application
Fol/flos Sig 5g.
Succus Sig 5ml
References
147 p289. 188 p306.

Tsuga canadensis [Hemlock spruce]

Constituents
Oligomeric procyanidins. Volatile oil – pinine. Resin. Tannin - up to 14%.

Primary pharmacological action: Astringent.

Therapeutic classes
Tonic. Antimicrobial. Antifungal – Candida. Antiseptic.
Antioxidant. Circulatory stimulant.
Anticatarrhal.
Diuretic. Diaphoretic.
Uterine tonic.
Mild rubefacient.

Medicinal indications
Oropharyngeal inflammation. Catarrh. Pharyngitis.
Aphthous ulcerations. Gingivitis. Stomatitis. Vomiting. Colitis. Diarrhoea.
Diverticulitis. Haemorrhoids.
Cystitis. Arthritis. Rheumatism.
Vaginal discharge/leucorrhoea.

Tissue conditions
Asthenia. Atonic digestion with pale mucous membranes. Broncho pulmonary irritation.

External use
Vaginal discharge/leucorrhoea, gonorrhoea, prolapsus ani, prolapsus uteri, cervical ulcers - injection dect.

Preparations
The bark is an ingredient of Composition essence.
Haemorrhoids with Hamamelis.
Diarrhoea - use the enema.

External use
Arthritis with painful joints - poultice.
Aphthous ulcers, gingivitis, stomatitis with Commiphora.

Dosage and mode of application
Dried cort Sig 2g
Tincturae Sig 2ml
Liquidum extractum Sig 2ml
Injection dect.

References
43 p218. 127 p638. 176 p350. 189 p217.

Turnera diffusa [Damiana]

Constituents
Cyanogenic glycoside - Tetraphyllin B. Phenolic glycoside - Arbutin. Volatile oil up to 1%. Bitter acid - Damianin up to 7%. Tannin up to 3.5%. Gum. Resin.

Primary pharmacological action:
Central nervous system and Pelvic tonic.

Therapeutic action
Stomachic. Laxative. Diuretic.
Thymoleptic. Antidepressant. Aphrodisiac. Nervine trophorestorative.
Medicinal indications
Mucous membrane astringent. Nervous dyspepsia. Atonic constipation.
Enuresis. Prostatic enlargement. Irritable bladder. Impotence/sexual dysfunction.
Premature ejaculation. Spermatorrhoea.
Amenorrhoea. Dysmenorrhoea. Frigidity. Acne at menarche or with uterine dysfunction.
Neurohormonal disorders. Anxiety. Depression. Paralysis. Debility. Exhaustion.
Pituitary disorders.
Tissue conditions
Nervine trophorestorative. Stimulating tonic to all nerves - CNS & ANS.
Weakness of the nervous system with debility and lack of general nerve power.
Sensitivity of feelings - fears, weepiness etc.
Impotence/sexual dysfunction associated with sexual inadequacy from fear or panic. Lack of libido in males [impotence/sexual dysfunction] and females [frigidity]. Improves the trophic state of the desire to action responses through the CNS to spinal level and then through the sacral nerve pathways. Tonic to the kidneys and urinary mucous membrane
Preparations
Nerve disorders, anxiety, depression, sensitivity etc. with Panax, Scutellaria.
Impotence/sexual dysfunction - with Pulsatilla and or Scutellaria or Strychnos nux vomica.
Impotence/sexual dysfunction with Cola and Serenoa.
Senility with Avena and Scutellaria.
Dosage and mode of application
Dried herba Sig 4g
Tincturae Sig 4ml
Liquidium extractum Sig 4ml
References
43 p219. 176 p459. 189 p100. 254 p80.

Tussilago farfara [Coltsfoot]

Constituents
Alkaloids. Flavonoids. Tannins around 17%. Mucilage. Inulin. Phytosterols.
Volatile oil. Bitters. Glycosides. Zinc - up to 3%.

Primary pharmacological action: Tonic expectorant.

Therapeutic classes
Allays inflammation. Antiseptic. Demulcent. Astringent. Stimulant.
Diffusive. Anticatarrhal. Antitussive.
Haemostatic.
Dermatological agent. Emollient. Vulnerary.
Antispasmodic.
Medicinal indications
Allergies. Sinusitis. Asthma. Bronchitis. Coughs. Dyspnoea. Pertussus.
Trachieitis. Pneumonia. Pleurisy. Tuberculosis.
Dried leaves are used as a tobacco substitute.
Cystitis.
Bites. Wounds. Ulcers.
Tissue conditions
Stimulates the respiratory mucous membrane as a soothing demulcent. Loosens
phlegm in coughs, asthma, bronchitis, pertussus. A favourite remedy in cough
prescriptions.
External use
Wounds and cutaneous eruptions - fol.
Sinusitis - use the spray.
Lung conditions - poultice.
Preparations
Chest conditions with Asclepias, Inula, Lobelia or Marrubium.
Cough mist. Glycyrrhiza, Tussilago and Marrubium.
Dosage and mode of application
Dried flos/herba Sig 2g
Tincturae Sig 8ml
Liquidum extractum Sig 2ml
Syrupus Tussilago. Tussilago syrup. Extract Tussilago fol et flos 25g aqua
400ml and syrup 100ml. Sig 5ml
References
BPC 1949. 43 p220. 111 p719. 192 p157. 246 p473. 251 p54. 254 p94.

Tylophora indica [Indian ipecac.]

Constituents
Alkaloids around 0.3%.

Primary pharmacological action: Antiasmatic.

Therapeutic classes
Allays inflammation. Antiallergic.
Immunorelaxant.
Medicinal indications
Allergic asthma. Rhinitis. Hay fever. Bronchitis. Nocturnal dyspnoea.
Amoebic dysentery.
Rheumatism.
Autoimmmune disease. Chronic fatigue if auto intoxication is suspected.
Eczema. Urticaria.
Dosage and mode of application
Dried herba Sig 0.3g
Tincturae Sig 1ml
References
48 p134. 191 p156. 271 Nos. 47 & 48, 1995.

Ulmus fulva/glabra [Slippery elm/Wych elm]

Constituents
Mucilage polysaccharides – hexose and pentose. Hydrolysis yealds glucose.
Tannin up to 6.5%. Sterols. Sesquiterpenes. Minerals.

Primary pharmacological action: Demulcent.

Therapeutic classes
Ophthalmic. Antimicrobial. Allays inflammation.
Pectoral. Antitussive. Expectorant.
Nutritive. Antacid.
Diuretic.
Dermatological agent. Emollient. Vulnerary.
Antivenomous. Antidote.

Medicinal indications
Ocular inflammation. Sore throats. Pharyngitis. Pneumonia. Pleurisy.
Gastro intestinal inflammation or ulceration. Nutritive food for infants and the
elderly, suitable as a food during convalescence.
Gastric or duodenal acidity. Gastritis. Travel sickness. Heartburn. Oesophagitis.
Reflux. Enteritis. Inflammatory bowel disease. Intestinal irritability. IBS. Colitis.
Diarrhoea. Dysentery. Crohn's disease. Diverticulosis/itis. Anal fissures.
Typhoid.
Skin inflammation. Externally – Abscesses, Burns, Furunculosis, Gangrene,
Haemorrhoids, Scalds, Ulcers, Vaginitis, Varicose ulcers, Wounds.

Tissue conditions
Suitable for all age groups. Nutritive food taken as a gruel.
Finely powdered it makes an excellent food [sold as slippery elm food but only
contains around 10% slippery elm].
Soothing to all mucous membranes of the respiratory, gastrointestinal and urinary
systems as it disperses irritation and inflammation. Coats over ulcers and
inflamed tissue. Ulmus gathers toxins from the mucous membranes and
eliminates these via the intestine. Taken at night it will induce sleep. An antidote
to many poisons use internally to support expulsion of toxins.

External use
Stimulates new cellular growth. Encourages the healing process. Used both
internally and externally as an antiseptic poultice. Antisepsis is enhanced with
Commiphora – use a small amount as it becomes too drawing and will cause pain
on denuded surfaces.
Purulent opthalmia - poultice.
Toothache - apply some powder into a cavity to stop a toothache and delay decay.

Poultice - mix with a little water [and glycerine to prevent it drying out] use in abscesses, furunculosis, thorns - to draw and bring to a head.

Abrasions, abscess, burns, ulcers, whitlows [to soothe and heal] - poultice.

Apply on sterile lint and renew as required usually 2-4 hourly depending upon the severity of the case.

Nappy rash - use direct upon the area or mix with egg white and leave until it dries before covering area.

The unpowdered bark inserted into the vagina is used to soothe the vaginal walls.

The pessary will expel the contents of the uterus.

Rectal and vaginal troubles with inflammation or infection – suppository, pessary.

Preparations

Pleurisy with Althea and Glycyrrhiza.

Reflux oesophagitis with Chamomilla and Zingiber.

Thorns - with Althea.

Dosage and mode of application

Decoctum 1:8 Sig 16ml

Capsules powder Sig 4g.

Powdered inner cort Forms a thick jelly on contact with liquid.

Make by:

[1] the cold method - steep in appropriate vehicle overnight

[2] or use heat - and whisk while simmering

Flavour with Cinnamon or Nutmeg.

Sig 4g in aqua or other vehicle, oat, goats, rice, soya milk.

Enemata Sig 10g mixed with vehicle and administer.

References

43 p222. 111 p719. 127. 224 p929. 230 p93. 246. 254 p88.

Uncaria tomentosa [Cats claw]

Constituents
Pentacylic oxindole alkaloids are immunostimulant, antineoplastic, activate T lymphocytes and macrophages and are vasodilatory. Rhynophylline – vasodilatory. Dimeric and trimeric proanthocyanidins are antineoplastic. Quinovic acid glycosides allay inflammation and are antiviral. Catechins combat the toxic effects of alcohol. Beta sitosterol – allay inflammation. Hyperin - protects the liver. Tannin.

Primary pharmacological action:
Immunostimulant and vasotonic alterative.

Therapeutic classes
Antiallergic. Allays inflammation. Depurative.
Antiviral – Candida, Epstein barr, Feline crown virus, Herpes zoster, Herpes simplex, genital herpes, HIV/AIDS - impedes the virus, Lamb Maed visna virus and Vesicular stomatitis virus.
Antioxidant. Vasodilator. Hypotensive. Hypocholesterolaemic. Antioxidant. Inhibits platelet aggregation. Enhances phagocytosis. Increases lymphocytes.
Antiulcerogenic. Hepatoprotective. Vermifuge.
Diuretic. Sexually transmitted diseases. Antirheumatic. Febrifuge.
Antineoplastic. Antimutagenic. Cytostatic. Radiation disorder.
Contraceptive.

Medicinal indications
Vesicular stomatitis virus. Vasotonic alterative [blood cleanser]. Increases T4 lymphocytes. Stimulates phagocytosis. Environmental toxin poisoning. Systemic Candidiasis. Hypertension. Tachycardia. Allergies. Asthma.
Gastritis. Gastric ulcer. Cirrhosis. Dysentery. Diabetes. Chronic infections and congested conditions of the gastro intestinal tract. Chrohn's disease. Leaky intestine. Diverticulitis. Dysentery. Fistulas. Haemorrhoids. Systemic Candidiasis.
Urinary tract carcinoma. Urinary inflammation. Gonorrhoea. Arthritis. Rheumatism.
Depression. Neuralgia. Chronic fatigue. Debility. Myalgic Encephalomyelitis. Lupus erythematosus.
Radiation burns. Acne. Abscesses. Cysts. Wounds.
Fungal infections - Genital and oral herpes.
Menstrual irregularities. Birth control.

Tissue conditions
A cleanser of the intestinal tract. Detoxifying effects upon the liver and reduces alcohol poisoning. Protects against tobacco smoke.

Alkaloids are responsible for immune activity. Normalises the immunoglobulins by activating T-Lymphocytes and macrophages. Lowers blood cholesterol, inhibits platelet aggregation, relaxes blood vessels - vasodilatory and lowers the heart rate. Immune function is improved by up to 50%.

Cats claw has been shown to enhance immunity in cancer patients by increasing immunoglobulin counts. Protects against radiation damage.

Herpes zoster, genital herpes, aids and carcinoma are beneficially affected. Enhances DNA repair, improves mitogenic response and leukocyte recovery.

Birth control – Decoct 6 kilos of bark in water and reduce to 500ml. Taken for three months during each menstrual cycle. Should give protection for three to four years.

Cautions

Avoid in pregnancy.

External use

Wounds, fungal infections, fistulas, haemorrhoids - use the wash.

Preparations

Immune supportive with Echinacea or Tabebuia.

Dosage and mode of application

Dried rad/bacc Sig 7g

Liquidum extractum Sig 4ml

References

30/31. 192 p120. 195. 230 p15. 270 2001, 8, [4], p275-82. 271 No 73. 274, 1993, 38, 63-7. 299, Aug/Sept. 1995. 273, Special Supplement.

Urgenia maritima [Squills]

Constituents
Cardiac glycosides - scillaren A, scillaren and other minor glycosides. The aglycones are similar to Digitalis in action. Aglycones are poorly absorbed from the GI tract. Flavonoids. Stigmasterol. Tannin. Volatile oils.

Primary pharmacological action: Stimulating expectorant.

Therapeutic classes
Cardioactive. Diuretic.
Emetic. Cathartic. Rubefacient - fresh juice.

Medicinal indications
Hoarseness. Unproductive coughs. Bronchial catarrh. Asthma. Bronchitis. Pertussus.
Cardiac insufficiency with oedema. Hypotension. Effusion. Emetic.
Impaired renal function. Oedema. Nephritis. Uric acid. Ascites.
Amenorrhoea. Dysmenorrhoea.

Tissue conditions
Atony of the tissues. Effusion of the pleura, pericardium or peritoneum – promotes absorption of oedema. Glycosides are poorly absorbed from the intestine. Increases the stroke volume of myocardial contractions [a positive inotropic effect]. Increases systolic blood pressure. Diuretic action results from increased cardioactivity. An gastric irritant causing expectorant activity for dry and irritating coughs with scanty bronchial secretions.
Emetic action is centrally induced through gastric irritation. Given to induce stomach lavage in cases of poisoning.

Cautions
Cardiac toxicity is rare. Pregnancy. Acute inflammation. Nausea and vomiting. Check renal health. Antidote emesis.

External use
Dandruff and seborrhoeic dermatitis - lotion.

Dosage and mode of application
Dried bulb Sig 200mg
Tincturae Sig 1ml
Liquidum extractum Sig 0.5ml
> **Urgenia Oxymel**. Oxymel of Squill. 5% Urgenia, in apple cider vinegar and sucrose to 100ml. Sig 5ml.
> **Syrupus Urgenia**. Urgenia syrup. Apple cider vinegar 45ml, sucrose 80g, aqua to 100ml. Sig 5ml.

References. 43 p223. 142 p144. 189 p256. 224 p604/5. 233 p205.

Urtica dioica/urens [Nettle]

Constituents

Indole alkaloids - histamine this increases gastric acid. 5 hydroxytryptamine.
Sterols. Amines in the stem hairs. Acids - Citric acid. Silica around 5mg in 1g.
Vitamin C. Tannin. Formic acid. Lectins are glycoproteins and composed of
isolectins, they bind to sugars. Potassium. Coumarin. Phenolic acids – caffeic and
malic, inhibit cyclo-oxygenase and 5-lipoxygenase derived reactions.
Polysaccharides stimulate T-lymphocytes. Research has been published since
1950 on BPH activity. Calcium. Potassium. Silicon.

Primary pharmacological action: Astringent diuretic.

Therapeutic classes

Vasotonic alterative - Blood purifier. Antiseptic. Allays inflammation.
Depurative. Antiallergic. Antiscorbutic. Mucous membrane astringent.
Antibacterial – Staphylococci, Sporozoa,
Circulatory stimulant. Hypotensive. Vasodilator. Haemostatic. Venous
insufficiency.
Anti allergic. Antihistamine. Antiasthmatic.
Oral inflammation. Nutritive. Hypoglycaemic. Splenic
Diuretic-uric acid eliminative. Prostatic disease. Urinary tract inflammation.
Uterine relaxant. Galactagogue.
Dermatological agent. Vulnerary. Rubefacient. Antirheumatic.
Antineoplastic.
CNS depressant.

Medicinal indications

Arteriosclerosis. Thrombosis. Anaemia. Cardiac insufficiency – fresh succus.
Hypertension.
Epistaxis - snuff. Coughs. Allergic rhinitis. Respiratory allergies. Asthma.
Tuberculosis.
Aphthous ulcers. Hypoglycaemic - mild. Diabetes. Diarrhoea. Dysentery.
Enteritis. Colic. Haemorrhoidal bleeds. Cholera.
Oedema. Cystitis. Prostatic enlargement. BPH. Calculi. Menorrhagia.
Lymphadenopathy.
Cutaneous eruptions – acne, eczema, urticaria, pruritus. Wounds – old. Warts.
Promotes hair growth. Varicella.
Mild attacks of rheumatism and associated backache. Gout. Sciatica. Muscle
spasm.
Paralysis [weak muscles].

Pharmacopoeia

Tissue conditions
Modulates inflammatory responses in allergies. Inhibits prostatic growth factor interactions by inhibiting membrane potassium and sodium adenosine triphosphatase in the prostate – this results in rebalancing of prostate cellular metabolism and modulation of sex hormone binding globulin [SHBG] to its receptor sites upon prostate cell membranes. Lignans selectively bind with sex hormone binding globulin [SHBG] on the prostate, this action controls hormones and BPH. Isolectins influence T-lymphocytes, compliment system and trigger tumour necrosis factor also inhibit cell proliferation and block binding of epidermal growth factor to tumour cell line receptor. The enzyme aromatase is a steroid hormone and mediates the conversion of androgens to oestrogens, enzyme inhibition has been detected by GLC. Ulcerations and inflammations of mucous membranes. Supports the elimination of chlorides and urea. Used for all types of haemorrhage. Builds up the blood in anaemic states. Venous insufficiency – succus. Paralysis and rheumatic conditions - an old fashioned treatment is to rub the area allowing the nettle sting to encourage warming of the area - rubefacient.
External use
Dry nettles cut into small pieces, cover with surgical spirit in a wide necked bottle, seal. Shake every day. Strain off the spirit after the seventh day.
Uses -Liniment for backache, rheumatic pain.
Epistaxis, wounds, eczema, dermatitis - succus upon cotton wool and apply.
Dandruff - use an infusium.
Urinary irrigation – cystitis.
Burns, gout, neuralgia, sciatica, sprains, tendonitis – infusium.
Stings - fresh fol.
Wounds, old, limb pain from injuries – poultice fresh succus. Rheumatic pain – poultice. Rheumatic pain – apply nettle to produce a wheal [see Lancet 2000].
Preparations
Prostatic hypertrophy – Urtica rad and Serenoa.
Mild attacks of rheumatism take an infusion wineglassful TDS.
Stings – Rumex.
Dosage and mode of application
Full dosage in acute urticaria.
Dried rad/fol Sig 5g
Dry extract fol Sig 2.1g
Dry extract rad Sig 1.3g
Tincturae rad/fol Sig 7.5ml
Liquidum extractum rad/fol Sig 5ml
Succus Sig 10ml. Poultice.
References. 43. 192 p379. 179 p491. 228 p373. 239 p139. 246 p 83. 251 p119. 263, 61, 1995, p31 &138. 263, 1997, 63 p529. 270, 1, 1994, p213. 270, 1977, 5, p387-402. 296, 2000, 355 [9219] 1975. 394 p372.

Usnea barbata [Old mans beard]

Constituents
Lichenic acid [usnic acid] – antimicrobial. Vitamin C. Sterols.

Primary pharmacological action: Antimicrobial.

Therapeutic classes
Antifungal – Candida, Tinea, Trichomonas, Trichophyton.
Antibacterial – gram positive organisms; Mycobacterium, Pneumococcus,
Staphylococcus and Streptococcus.
Expectorant.
Oropharyngeal agent. Gastro intestinal anti infective.
Urinary anti infective. Vaginal anti infective.
Dermatological agent.
Antineoplastic.
Medicinal indications
Sore throats. Sinusitis. Respiratory infections. Bronchitis. Pleurisy. Pneumonia.
Tuberculosis – lung & skin.
Intestinal infections. Dysentery. Cholera.
Urinary tract infections. Renal infections.
Cervical dysplasia. Mastitis.
Furunculosis. Impetigo. Wounds.
Sarcoma 180. Ehrlich tumour cells.
Tissue conditions
All round anti infective medicine for the respiratory, gastro intestinal and urinary
tracts.
External use
Nasal infections – use the spray.
Infected throats – garg.
Dermatological conditions – apply undiluted tincturae as a lotion.
Cervical dysplasia with Echinacea and/or Hydrastis.
Dosage and mode of application
Tincturae 5ml
Liquidum extractum lichen. Sig 3ml
References
246 p572. 394 p386.

Vaccinum macrocarpon [Cranberry]

Constituents
Berry with a pH of less than 2.5. The polyphenols are responsible for the astringency of the berry. It contains vitamin C.

Primary pharmacological action: Urinary antiseptic.

Therapeutic classes
Antiscorbutic.
Urinary infections. Genito urinary inflammation.
Renal calculi with an alkaline urine.
Tissue conditions
A disinfectant berry for the urinary tract when infection is present. It reduces the ability of bacteria to adhere to the mucosal lining of the tract. Breaks down calcium carbonate and struvite calculi. Calculi and infective processes are often found with an alkaline urine. Bone quotes a study 'whereby Cranberry increased the excretion of hippuric acid and nephron activity which indicates that it is inadvisable in patients with renal insufficiency or those with a tendency to develop uric acid or calcium oxalate stones due to high oxalate content'.
Constitutionally blue and mixed iris clients have a tendency to uric acid diathesis – most caucasians.
Preparations
Barosma, Crataeva, Uva ursi.
Dosage and mode of application
Tincturae Bacc Sig 4ml
References
142 p101, 276. 188 p133. 271. No. 72, Nov 1999.

Vaccinium myrtillus [Bilberry]

Constituents
Bioflavonoids - Anthocyanins [proanthocyanidins] are antioxidants and prevent free radicle damage, protect capillaries and strengthen collagen matrix.
Flavone glycosides – astragalin, hyperoside, quercitrin.
Catechin tannin up to 10% – thickens the surface protein layer of mucous membranes.
Phenolic acids – caffeic acid. Triterpenes – ursolic acid up to 25%. Pectin.
Fructose up to 30%. Vitamin A, C.

Primary pharmacological action: Optic vasoprotective.

Therapeutic classes
Ophthalmic. Allays inflammation. Astringent. Antibacterial – Escherichia coli.
Antioxidant. Vasoprotective. Hypercholesterolaemia. Venous tonic. Antiplatelet.
Antiemetic. Antidiarrhoeal. Hyperglycaemia [fol].
Antilithic. Diuretic. Urinary antiseptic.
Antihaemorrhagic – general.
Dermatological agent. Vulnerary.
Antineoplastic. Antigalactagogue.

Medicinal indications
Myopia. Retinal damage – strengthens retinal capillaries. Retinitis. Macular degeneration. Night blindness. Glaucoma. Cataract. Diabetic retinopathy.
Cerebral ischaemia. Atherosclerosis. CVA. Vascular tonic. Raynauds disease.
Inhibits platelet aggregation. Venous insufficiency. Varicose veins.
Leucoplakia. Oropharyngeal inflammation. Anti ulcer. IBS. Diverticulosis.
Gastro enteritis. Diarrhoea. Colitis. Crohn's disease. Dysentery. Haemorrhoids.
Urinary tract infections. Oedema.
Dermal ulcers. Vaginal discharge/leucorrhoea.

Tissue conditions
Short duration of action and remedy utilisation within two hours. Free radicle scavenger. Anthocyanosides encourage the production of rhodopsin [visual purple] which improves night vision and visual adaptation to glare. A vision enhancer which reduces visual fatigue. Glaucoma preventer. Vascular eye health is improved by improving capillary strength, reducing capillary fragility [strengthens capillary walls] and is antihaemorrhagic to the retinal vessels.
Increases the amount of blood to the eye [vasodilatory].
Inhibits platelet aggregation and prevents spider naevi from forming. The anthocyanosides are powerful antioxidants which protect against free radicle

Pharmacopoeia

damage. Collagen cross linkage is also protected from free radicles. Anti ulcer activity as it stimulates gastric mucus production.
Clinical trials date back to 1964.

Preparations
Intestinal disorders with Filipendula.

Dosage and mode of application
Dried bacc/fruct Sig 20g
Dry extract Sig 160mg
Liquidum extractum Sig 4ml
Garg. @ 10%.
Succus Sig 200ml
Lotion dect. @ 10%

References
34/35, p138-141. 179 p299. 192 p57. 230 p7. 246 p311. 266. 271, No 59, 1977. 394 p18.

Valeriana officinalis [Valerian]

Constituents
Iridoid alkaloids up to 2% known as Valpotriates are sedative and depress the CNS. Some 80% are known as valtrates - valerianine. Flavonoids. Tannin. Essential oil around 1%. Sesquiterpenes up to 1.4%. Gum. Resin.

Primary pharmacological action: Antispasmodic nervine.

Therapeutic classes
Bactericidal. Carminative.
Hypotensive.
Emmenagogue.
Antipyretic.
Anodyne. Anxiolytic. Hypnotic. Muscle relaxant. Sedative.

Medicinal indications
Palpitations. Scarlatina. Measles.
Flatulence. Intestinal colic. Intestinal spasm [cramp].
Urinary tract infections. Rheumatic pain.
Dysmenorrhoea. Pyrexia.
Migraine. Headache. Anxiety. Excitability. Nervous tension. Neuralgia.
Depression from excess anxiety. Stress. Panic. Insomnia. Muscular cramp/spasm.
Convulsions. Chorea. Epilepsy.

Tissue conditions
At times in certain individuals an abreaction has been observed with the use of Valerian. The abreaction is due to the sudden release of pent up vital nerve energy within the patient [due to the obstruction of nerve current]. Lower the dose or withdraw until the patient settles down. Valpotriates considered toxic are rendered neutral by gastric acid but still have sedative activity.
Volatile oils and Iridoids relax coronary smooth muscle, are inotropic with a negative chronotropic effect; allaying arrhythmias.
Calming and relaxing nerve remedy when irritable or excitable with an active mind that refuses to switch off and causes restlessness or insomnia. Tendency to worry with associated mental depression due to depleted nerve innervation. Smooth muscle relaxant.

Preparations
Neuralgia, nervous tension states, hypnotic action with Scutellaria or Viscum. With essence of anise to control the taste.

Pharmacopoeia

Dosage and mode of application

As the valpotriates break down the root gives off more odour.
Low dosage relax, while higher dosage have a sedative action.
Dried rad/rhizome Sig 3g
Infusium Conc. Concentrated infusion 1:5. Sig 4ml
Soft extract Sig 300mg.
Tincturae Sig 10ml
Liquidum extractum Sig 2ml
Balneum Sig 100g in muslin

References

43 p225. 111 p723. 179 p582. 224 p1828. 246 p431. 251 p149.
270, LXVI 1995, 2, 99-112. 394 p395.

Veratrum album/viride [Hellebore]

Constituents
Alkaloids – protoveratrine. Sterols. Chelidonic acids.

Primary pharmacological action: Hypotensive.

Therapeutic classes
Allays inflammation. Pectoral.
Cardiac depressant.
Hepatic. Nephritic.
Dermatological agent & anaesthetic. Analgesic. Anticonvulsant.

Medicinal indications
Bronchitis. Pleurisy. Pneumonia. Pulmonary oedema. Tuberculosis.
Aneurysm. Palpitation. Hypertension. Tachycardia. Venous obstruction.
Septicaemic convulsions. Rheumatic fever.
Tonsillitis. Gastritis. Emetic. Hepatitis. Peritonitis. Typhoid fever.
Nephritis. Gonorrhoea.
Meningitis - active cerebral hyperaemia. Chorea. Myasthenia gravis. Panic.
Tetanus. Neuralgia. Erysipelas. Thyrotoxicosis.
Puerperal convulsions. Eclampsia. Toxaemia of pregnancy. Epilepsy.

Tissue conditions
Vasomotor inhibitor. Acting through the reticular formation and the motor area
within the medulla, this causes a reduction in sympathetic outflow and is an
arterial sedative. Reduces the pulse rate. Active hyperaemia [acute inflammation],
serous inflammation. Convulsions from meningitis. Irritability of nerve centres,
full bounding pulse, tachycardia, hypertension. Acute inflammatory disorders.

Cautions
Poisoning is uncommon. Vomiting. Bradycardia. Syncope.

External use
Dermal inflammation.
Neuralgia especially facial – ung.

Dosage and mode of application
Acutes - use hourly.
Tincturae 1:10 Sig 2ml. [Ref 390 p816].
Injection [Acute hypertensive crisis] Sig 100mcg – 400 mcg. Increasing doses by
10-20mcg every hour until the desired response is obtained. Maximum response is
obtained in 1 to 2 hours.
Unguentum 2%.

References
126 p687. 142 p161/304. 176 p84. 92 p266/268. 224 p680. 245. 246 p505.

Verbascum thapsus [Mullein]

Constituents

Flavonoids up to 4% – hesperidin, verbascoside. Iridoid monoterpenes. Triterpene saponins. Mucilage polysaccharides up to 3%. Volatile oil. Gum. Resin. Bitter glycosides – aucubin.

Primary pharmacological action:
Vasotonic alterative. Respiratory demulcent.

Therapeutic classes

Absorbent. Antiseptic. Astringent. Antiviral – herpes simplex type 1, influenza.
Antihaemorrhagic. Anticatarrhal.
Soothing expectorant. Pectoral.
Oropharyngeal agent. Laxative – mild.
Diuretic. Lymphatic.
Emollient. Vulnerary.
Antineoplastic.
Anodyne. Sedative – mild.

Medicinal indications

Deafness. Earache. Otitis media. Ear ulceration. Ear eczema.
Respiratory tract haemorrhage. Hoarseness. Hay fever. Sinus disturbances.
Influenza. Asthma. Bronchitis. Trachieitis. Pleurisy. Pulmonary fibrosis.
Tuberculosis. Haemoptysis.
Sore throat. Tonsillitis. Aphthous ulcers. Dysentery. Peritonitis. Diarrhoea. Gastro intestinal haemorrhage.
Cystitis. Testicular swelling. Rheumatism.
Mastitis.
Infectious mononucleosis. Lymphadenopathy.

Tissue conditions

Gentle soothing and demulcent remedy for the mucous membranes of the respiratory, gastro intestinal, urinary tracts and serous structures. Promotes absorption of cellular effusions in pleuritic and other lung conditions. Allays nervous irritability and bronchial coughs. Palliates harsh and dry coughs. Allays inflammation in acidity of the urine. Removes hardened secretions from the meatus – Oleum. Flos are sedative in insomnia.

External use

Tonsillitis - fomentation.
Otitis media, Ear wax – Oleum 2 guttae BD/TDS.
Haemorrhoids, chilblains use boiled fresh leaves and apply as a poultice.
Lymphadenopathy - fomentation.

Abscess, tendon and synovial swelling – fomentation.
Rheumatic pain – oleum.
Preparations
Use with a diffusive.
Allergic conditions, hay fever with Sambucus.
Bronchitis with Grindelia, Lobelia, Marrubium or Tussilago.
Lymphadenopathy – fomentation with an internal prescription of Sambucus, Sanicula europaea, Smilax and Trifolium.
Dosage and mode of application
Dried fol/flos Sig 8g
Tincturae Sig 10ml
Liquidum extractum Sig 5ml
Oleum Verbascum 1:5
References
111 p726. 192 p371. 224 p934. 233 p403. 246 p403. 251 p116. 394 p270.

Verbena officinalis [Vervain]

Constituents
Iridoid glycosides - Verbenalin and Verbenin. Volatile oil. Bitters. Saponin.
Tannin. Vitamin K.

Primary pharmacological action:
Renal and Autonomic nerve relaxant.

Therapeutic classes
Ophthalmic. Astringent.
Expectorant.
Bitter. Cholagogue. Emetic. Vermifuge.
Antilithic. Diuretic. Diaphoretic. Antirheumatic.
Dermatological agent.
Emmenagogue. Galactogogue. Uterine tonic stimulating.
Antiparasitic. Antineoplastic.
Antidepressant. Anodyne. Antispasmodic. Nerve tonic. Hypnotic.
Medicinal indications
Ocular inflammation. Anaemia. Hypertension.
Sinus disturbance. Hay fever. Colds. Asthma. Bronchitis. Pneumonia. Pertussus.
Dyspnoea. Tuberculosis.
Aphthous ulceration. Cholelithiasis. Cholecystalgia. Jaundice. Splenic disorders.
Ascarides. Haemorrhoids.
Gravel and urinary obstruction. Dysuria. Oedema. Renal calculi. Aphrodisiac.
Partum pain.
Paralysis. Paranoid states. Muscle spasm. Neuritis. ME.
Pyrexia. Smallpox. Intermittent fever. Icterus. Plague to reduce contagion.
Anxiety, panic. Depression. Epilepsy. Insomnia. Nervous exhaustion. Delirium.
Tissue conditions
Action is upon the parasympathetic.
Stimulates the liver and spleen. Helps to relieve miscarriage. Tones and cleanses
the lining of the uterus.
Verbena is a mild nervine it works best when combined with other nervines e.g.
Scutellaria, Valeriana or Viscum.
Preparations
Infected gums and teeth, sore throat and halitosis – Collut.
Hay fever and sinus troubles with Achillea, Marrubium and Salvia.
Nervous exhaustion and weakness with Avena, Chamomilla and Scutellaria.
External use
Ear neuralgia - use the poultice.

Opthalmia, sore gums, oral ulcers use the infusion.

Wounds, sunburn – apply infusium lotion.

Dosage and mode of application

Infusium herba Sig 30ml

Tincturae Sig 4ml

Liquidum extractum Sig 4ml

References

43 p228. 142 p318. 127 p813. 192 p557. 246 p359. 254 p82. 265, 1995, Vol 7, issue 4, 105. 314, 2000, 15 [2] p139-43.

Viburnum opulus [Guelder rose]

Constituents
Bitter principle vibernine is a gastro intestinal tonic. Resin - viburnin. Valeric acid. Tannin.

Primary pharmacological action: Antispasmodic.

Therapeutic classes
Astringent - mild. A general muscular relaxant.
Nervine - sedative.
Medicinal indications
Palpitations. Angina. Intermittent claudication. Arteritis.
Asthma.
Enuresis. Stricture of the bladder. Epididymitis.
Polymyalgia. Rheumatoid arthritis.
Ovarian or uterine pain. False labour pain. Menopausal metrorrhagia. Partus preparator. Spasmodic dysmenorrhoea.
Nervous and muscular tension. Panic. Cramp.
Tissue conditions
A neuromuscular relaxant for voluntary and involuntary muscular cramp.
Balances both sides of the autonomic nervous system.
Spasm in hollow viscera - stomach, intestines, bladder, prostate and uterus.
Preparations
Circulatory disturbances – Achillea, Crataegus, Lavandula, Leonurus, Zanthoxylum, Zingiber.
Cramp with Dioscorea and Zanthoxylum.
Pregnancy with Caulophyllum.
Dosage and mode of application
Tincturae bacc Sig 5ml
Liquidum extractum Sig 4ml
References
43 p230. 111 p730. 1126 p694. 88p133. 246 p427. 254 p82.

Viburnum prunifolium [Black haw bark]

Constituents
Salicin – anodyne. Coumarins - scopoletin [antispasmodic]. Volatile oil. Bitter glycoside - Viburnin [acts upon the uterus]. Isovaleric acid. Tannin. Resin.

Primary pharmacological action:
Gastro intestinal trophorestorative. Antispasmodic.

Therapeutic classes
Astringent - mild. Haemostatic.
Anti asthmatic.
Diuretic. Prostate irritability.
Uterine antispasmodic. Parturient. Sedative. Analgesic.

Medicinal indications
Asthma. Hypertension. Cramp.
Spasm of the hollow viscera. Diarrhoea. Enuresis.
Morning sickness. Partus preparator. Post partum haemorrhage. Uterine haemorrhage. Dysmenorrhoea. Menorrhagia. Metrorrhagia. Sterility. Prevents miscarriage.
Panic. Anxiety. Insomnia. Chorea. Muscle cramp.

Tissue conditions
Allays irritability associated with pelvic disturbances. Used to remove spasm of the heart, intestine, uterus and bladder. Relaxes the motor nerves. Tonic influence upon the uterus and prostate. Uterine irritability, during pregnancy, as it regulates sympathetic activity and is regulatory at the menopause. Calf cramp. Checks haemorrhage from the uterus during and post partum. Providing the membranes have not ruptured abortion can be prevented [threatened miscarriage]. Promotes normal contractions. Post partum promotes normal uterine tone by preventing sub involution, prolapse or malposition.

Preparations
Uterine activity – Chamaelirium luteum, Hydrastis.

Dosage and mode of application
Requires to be given in large dosage for antispasmodic action.
Tincturae bacc Sig 10ml
Liquidum extractum Sig 8ml

References
BPC 1949. 43 p231. 111 p731. 126 p694. 176 p474. 192 p67. 246 p427. 254 p146.

Vinca major/rosea [Periwinkle/Catharanthus roseus]

Constituents
Indole alkaloids have been isolated. Vinblastine and vincristine are two of the major compounds. The alkaloid reserpine. Volatile oil in the leaf. Tannin.

Primary pharmacological action: Lymphatic vasotonic alterative.

Therapeutic classes
Ophthalmic. Astringent.
Hypoglycaemic.
Antigalactagogue.
Dermatological agent.
Antineoplastic.
Medicinal indications
Eye disease. Sore throat. Laryngitis. Haemorrhoids.
Menorrhagia. Metrorrhagia. Vaginal discharge/leucorrhoea. Galactorrhoea.
Enuresis.
Choriocarcinoma - uterus, ovary and testes. Hodgkin's disease. Lymphoblastic leukaemia. Breast carcinoma.
Dermal inflammation.
Cramp.
Tissue conditions
Inhibits cellular division in the metaphase. Detoxifying remedy for the blood, lymphatics and immune system.
External use
Inflammatory eye disease - collyr.
Haemorrhoids - ung.
Wounds.
Cramp – poultice.
Dosage and mode of application
Dried herba Sig 4g
Liquidum extractum Sig 5ml
References
43 p232. 189 p214. 246 p332. 265 2001, 13 [1] p24.

Vinca minor [Lesser periwinkle]

Constituents
Indole alkaloid - Vincamine.

Primary pharmacological action: Cerebral tonic.

Therapeutic classes
Ophthalmic. Astringent.
Cerebrovascular stimulant. Circulatory stimulant. Vasodilator.
Bitter stomachic tonic. Hypoglycaemic.
Styptic. Febrifuge.
Medicinal indications
Optic atrophy. Hearing deficit.
Hypotensive rad. Arteriosclerosis. Cerebral atherosclerosis.
Epistaxis. Pulmonary haemorrhage.
Gingivitis. Gastric haemorrhage. Dyspepsia. Flatulence. Diarrhoea.
Headaches. Vertigo. Poor memory. Behaviour disorders. Irritability. Restlessness.
Tinnitus. Meniers disease.
Mastitis. Galactorrhoea. Vaginal discharge/leucorrhoea.
Menorrhagia/Metrorrhagia. PMS.
Bruises. Lacerations. Wounds.
Tissue conditions
Improves cerebral arterial activity and oxygen consumption. Increases EEG
activity. Cerebral disturbances - lack of attention and restlessness. Post CVA.
Cautions
Brain tumour. Raised intracranial pressure. Cerebral bleeding.
External use
Vaginal discharge/leucorrhoea – douche.
Preparations
Menorrhagia/metrorrhagia with Alchemilla vulgaris.
Dosage and mode of application
Dried herba Sig 4g
Liquidum extractum fol/rad Sig 4ml
References
142 p180. 188 p334. 246 p331.

Viola odorata [Sweet violet]

Constituents
Saponins. Salicylic glycosides. Flavonoids. Mucilage. Volatile oil. Vitamin C.
Carotenoids.

Primary pharmacological action: Demulcent expectorant.

Therapeutic classes
Ophthalmic. Antiseptic. Antibacterial – trichomonas. Antiviral – Aids/HIV.
Cardiac.
Emetic. Hepatic. Laxative.
Nephritic. Diuretic. Febrifuge. Antirheumatic.
Antineoplastic.
Anodyne. Nerve relaxant. Hypnotic.

Medicinal indications
Conjunctivitis. Oropharyngeal inflammation. Throat/tonsil epithelioma.
Chronic catarrh/coughs. Peritonsillar abscess. Bronchitis. Pleurisy. Tuberculosis.
Bronchial carcinoma.
Aphthous ulcers. Cholelithiasis. Jaundice. Haemorrhoids. Intestinal carcinoma.
Inflamed and painful conditions of the urinary tract – cystitis, vaginal
trichomonas, urethritis. Fibroids. Rheumatism of the wrists.
Abscesses. Furunculosis. Papules.
Lymphadenopathy. Breast carcinoma.
Improves the memory. Headache. Epilepsy – purple fol.

Tissue conditions
Used as a blood cleanser [vasotonic alterative] in malignant conditions of the
breast and intestine. It is slightly laxative as it cools and moistens. It eases
headache from lack of sleep. Moderates anger.

External use
Ophthalmic disease – inflammation – collyr.
Inflammation, pain, swelling, haemorrhoids   plaster, poultice of Green fol.
Fibroids – douche.

Preparations
With Galium for the above conditions.

Dosage and mode of application
Dried herba Sig 4g
Tincturae Sig 4ml
Liquidum extractum Sig 4ml

References
BPC 1923. 43 p233. 142 p202. 246 p252. 251 p152. 274 14, p45, 1985.

Viola tricolor [Heartsease, Pansy]

Constituents
Bitter. Flavonic glycoside. Saponins. Salicylates. Rutin. Mucilage. Resin.

Primary pharmacological action:
Depurative to the skin and genito urinary tract.

Therapeutic classes
Allays inflammation. Demulcent. Vasotonic alterative. Antibacterial –
Mycobacterium tuberculosis. Antifungal – Trichophyton.
Anti allergic. expectorant.
Circulatory stimulant to the eliminative organs.
Laxative.
Diuretic. Febrifuge. Antirheumatic.
Antineoplastic. Dermatological agent.
Mild sedative.
Medicinal indications
Capillary fragility. Asthma. Bronchitis. Pertussus. Tuberculosis.
Diarrhoea.
Urinary infections. Cystitis. Rheumatism.
Skin eruptions – acne, cradle cap, eczema, with Scrophularia, Urticaria. Dermal
tuberculosis.
Pyrexia. Epilepsy.
Tissue conditions
Cleansing vasotonic alterative medicine for the mucous membranes and skin.
Effecting detoxification of the skin and mucous membranes to allay infections and
skin eruptions. Stated to relieve capillary haemorrhage from steroids.
Preparations
Pertussus with Pilosella.
Cystitis with Agropyron.
Eczema with Galium, Rumex, Stellaria, Trifolium or Urtica.
Dosage and mode of application
Dried herba Sig 4g
Tincturae Sig 5ml
Liquidum extractum Sig 4ml
References
43 p234. 142 p331. 188 p221. 192 p397. 228 p146. 246 p255.

Viscum album [Mistletoe]

Constituents
Viscotoxin is a polypeptide and is cardioselective, it reduces the ventricular rate. Lectins - a polysaccharide extract of Viscum has a stimulating effect on neutrophils and use in the treatment of neutropenia. Some sugar and protein fractions showed marked carcinostatic activity. The protein fractions act on nucleic cellular control mechanisms. Flavonoids - [Flavones] are antineoplastic. Oleic acid 80%, palmitic acid. Amines. Lectins. Terpenoids. Sterols. Mucilage. Tannin.

Primary pharmacological action: Antispasmodic to the ANS.

Therapeutic classes
Antisclerotic. Cardioselective. Haemostatic. Hypotensive.
Antiasthmatic.
Anaphrodisiac. Oxytocic.
Antineoplastic. Immunostimulant. Cytotoxic.
Stimulating and relaxing nervine. Sedative. Tonic.

Medicinal indications
Atherosclerosis. Arrhythmia. Hypertension. Hypertensive headache. Tachycardia. Oedema. Menorrhagia. Sterility. Post partum haemorrhage.
Anxiety. Chorea. Depression. Epilepsy. Headache. Insomnia. Nervousness. Panic attacks. Vertigo.
Carcinoma of the breast, stomach, colon, rectum or cervix.

Tissue conditions
Influences the solar plexus - to relax abdominal nerve tension [vasoconstriction] which is a frequent precursor of general arterial troubles. For this reason Viscum is a tonic to the abdomen. Relaxes blood vessels and relieves hypertension.
Cardiac tonic as it lessens reflex irritability of the heart and acts as a cardiac tonic to strengthen the beat whilst raising the frequency of a slow pulse.
Allays inflammation exerting an action upon capillary permeability and oedema. It stimulates granulation and the new formation of connective tissue.
Viscum contracts the longitudinal muscles of the uterus and is helpful in uterine haemorrhage and to induce labour. It will help to expel the placenta when difficulties arise from non expulsion following labour. In menorrhagia and post partum haemorrhage it is of value.
Enhances cytotoxic and immunostimulant properties of NK [natural killer] cells. One study supports the immunological action of Viscum where post Chernobyl nuclear respiratory disease in children who showed decreases in fatigue, headache, pyrexia, emotional instability and musculoskeletal pain.

Cautions
Pregnancy.
Preparations
Two remedy prescription - Viscum and Humulus in hypertension.
Hypertension, tachycardia with Tilia, Crataegus.
Rheumatism, inflamed haemorrhoids –lotion.
Nervous complaints with Valeriana and Verbena.
Dosage and mode of application
Freshly squeezed extracts contain free amino acids.
Dried fol Sig 6g
Infusium Sig 30ml
Tincturae Sig 2ml
Liquidum extractum Sig 3ml
References
43 p236.192 p363/365. 239 p137. 246 p87. 301,1998, 3 [1]. 328, 1997, 5, 141-6.
329, 2001, 7;57-78.

Vitex agnus castus [Chaste tree]

Constituents
Up to 35 constituents; the main ones in the fruits are alpha-pinene, limonene 1,8-cineole and sabinene. Iridoid glycosides - acubin and agnuside. Ketosteroid hormones. Flavonoids - casticin. Volatile oil up to 0.5%. Triterpenoids and an alkaloid – viticin. Essential oil – alpha and beta pinine. Vitex binds to dopamine receptors in the pituitary. It is a dopamine receptor blocker in the pituitary gland which diminishes prolactin secretion and thereby reduces FSH. Linoleic acid.

Primary pharmacological action: Hormonal adaptogenic.

Therapeutic classes
Allays inflammation.
Endocrine gland disorders - pituitary, ovary, adrenal and thyroid.
Hyperprolactinaemia. Galactogenic.
Dermatological agent.
Antivenomous.
Medicinal indications
Diarrhoea.
Acne – male and female.
Prostatic hyperplasia.
Amenorrhoea. Dysmenorrhoea. Infertility. Sterility. Mastalgia. Mastitis. PMS – breast swelling. Uterine fibroids. Corpus luteum insufficiency. Menopause.
Depression.
Pituitary imbalance. Hypotrophic breast tissue.
Thyroid dysfunction.
Tissue conditions
Acts upon the pituitary. Increases lutenising hormone and reduces the follicular phase [reduces FSH]. Reduces prolactin levels. Significant increase in the levels of progesterone and oestrogen. Vitex has an adaptogenic action on the hormones. In hypo-oestrogenicity – flushes, night sweats and palpitations Vitex may benefit. Hyper-oestrogenicity – PMS and fertility cycle mastalgia – Vitex balances. Progesterone deficiency may complicate infertility. Endometriosis, fluid retention, hyperprolactinaemia, or polycystic ovary disease. Male impotence/sexual dysfunction with high prolactin levels – high doses. Vaginal bleeding if outside of the normal cycle must be investigated.
Vitex does not affect testosterone.

V

Cautions
Avoid with HRT and oral contraceptives.
Dosage and mode of application
Small doses should be administered so as not to unbalance the other hormonal levels. Low doses may stimulate, high doses reduce prolactin.
PMS - Tincturae Sig 5ml Aq cal daily for 10 days prior to menses.
Anovulatory Tr up to 10 ml per week.

Dry extract Sig 40mg [0.04g]
Tincturae fruct Sig 2ml
Liquidum extractum Sig 0.5ml
References
142 p317/318. 143. 239 p93. 243. 246 p358. 262 p93. 293, 6, 1994, 341-344. 271 No 15. 295, 322 [7279] 134-137. 394 p62.

Withania somnifera [Ashwagandha - winter cherry]

Constituents
Steroidal lactones known as withanolides. Tropane alkaloids - withanine.
Saponins. Iron.

Primary pharmacological action: Tonic nervine. Adaptogen.

Therapeutic classes
Vasotonic alterative. Allays inflammation. Astringent. Antibacterial –
tuberculosis. Deobstruent. Antianaemic. Hypotensive. Increases leucocytosis.
Diuretic.
Anxiolytic. Aphrodisiac. Sedative - mild. Hypnotic. Spasmolytic.
Emmenagogue.
Antineoplastic. Immunemodulator.
Medicinal indications
Hypertension. Leucocytosis.
Asthma. Bronchial disease.
Cholecystitis. Anthelmintic.
Diuretic. Impotence/sexual dysfunction. Improves sperm count and motility.
Arthritis. Joint pain from autoimmune disease. Rheumatoid arthritis with pain
and swelling. Lumbago.
Fever and chills. Infantile pyrexia. Smallpox.
Anxiety states. Senile dementia. Exhaustion. Debility. Headache.
Tissue conditions
Influences the endocrine, cardiopulmonary and central nervous systems. Cardiac
muscle tonic. Depleted leukocytes resulting from toxic conditions. Increases
neutrophil count.
An adaptogenic tonic controlling anxiety with it's myriad symptoms -
palpitations, sweating, tension. Improves memory, poor concentration and
fatigue. It augments cerebral function. Impotence/sexual dysfunction from stress
or exhaustion.
Smooth muscle antispasmodic. Uterine muscle tonic.
External use
Wounds, ulcers, inflammation - rad powder as antiseptic dressing.
Dosage and mode of application
Dried rad Sig 2g
Liquidum extractum Sig 4ml
References
48 p137. 191p161. 265, 1996, 8 [3], 78. 281, 1996, 8 [3].

Yucca bacata/glauca [Yucca, Yucca schidigera]

Constituents
Terpenoids as saponins [outer bark] - titogenin, chlorogenin. Stimulates prostaglandins. Phospholipase PA2 is restricted.

Primary pharmacological action: Antirheumatic.

Therapeutic classes
Vasotonic alterative.
Anticholesterolaemic. Anticoagulant. Cardiotonic. Hypotensive.
Cholagogue.
Diuretic.
Hormonal balancer.
Medicinal indications
Headaches
Aphthous ulcers. Improves stomach disorders and gastro intestinal function.
Hypertension. Improves circulation. Corrects cholesterol and triglyceride levels.
Articular pain, stiffness and swelling.
Tissue conditions
Rebalances progesterone.
External use
Shampoo use fresh or dry.
Preparations
Larrea and Yucca - fibroids.
Dosage and mode of application
Inner pith used internally as the outer bark is too strong.
References
188 p460. 231 p703. 409. 410.

Zanthoxylum americanum/clava herculis [Prickly ash]

Constituents
Alkaloids - isoquinolines – chelerythrine [antimicrobial], laurifoline, nitidine and magnoflorine. Tannin. Volatile oils. Resin. Lignans.

Primary pharmacological action: Arterial vasostimulant.

Therapeutic classes
Vasotonic alterative. Antimicrobial. Tonic. Circulatory stimulant.
Sialagogue. Carminative. Antidiarrhoeal.
Diaphoretic. Antipyretic. Antirheumatic.
Emmenagogue.
Dermatological agent. Immunostimulant.
Antispasmodic.

Medicinal indications
Cramp. Raynauds syndrome. Peripheral circulatory insufficiency e.g. cold hands and feet. Cold skin. Raynauds disease. Intermittent claudication.
Pharyngitis.
Toothache. Flatulence. Dyspepsia. Gastritis. Hypochlorhydria. Constipation from deficient mucus secretion. Abdominal pain - costiveness. Intestinal spasm.
Typhoid. Typhus. Dysentery. Cholera [40].
Syphilis. Impotence/sexual dysfunction.
Arthritis. Lumbago. Rheumatism. Pyrexia.
Skin - eruptive disease with recession of blood from the skin. Dermal ulcers.
Psoriasis.
Epilepsy. Paralysis - general, vocal cord. Hemiplegia. Locomotor ataxia. Nervous headaches.

Tissue conditions
A good general arterial stimulant. Stimulating vasotonic alterative for atonic conditions. It encourages diaphoresis. Used for general stimulation of the tissues and whenever a stimulant is required. Dry mucus membrane of the oropharynx. Stimulates saliva flow, appetite and hydrochloric acid. It is a tonic for a debilitated stomach, with fermentation of food and gastro intestinal tract e.g. cramp, colic and cholera. Calms the stomach and intestine, removing flatus and dyspepsia. Hypersecretion from relaxed mucus tissues. Hypotonic nervous system.

Often applied with other medicines to stimulate circulatory effect to the tissues and organ areas, enhancing the primary pharmacological action of other medicines.

Preparations

Nervous exhaustion with LE Avena.

External use

Ulcers or wounds to stimulate the tissue – Powdered bacc.

Rheumatic pain – fomentation.

Dosage and mode of application

Baccae are more active than the rad.

Dried bacc Sig 2g

Tincturae bacc Sig 4ml

Liquidum extractum bacc Sig 2ml

Dried cort Sig 3g

Tincturae cort Sig 5ml

Liquidum extractum cort Sig 3ml

References

6 p66. 40. 43 p238. 69 p166. 111 p751. 126 p697. 254 p66.

Zea mays [Corn silk]

Constituents
Saponins up to 3%, in the female flowers. Stigmas contain tannin up to 13%. Allantoin. Phytosterols. Flavonoids. Resin. Volatile oil – carvacrol, a-terpinol, thymol. Fixed oil. Bitters. Potassium. Vitamin C, K.

Primary pharmacological action:
Antiseptic. Demulcent diuretic.

Therapeutic classes
Tonic diuretic. Antilithic.
Uterine tonic.
Anodyne.
Medicinal indications
Urinary infections and inflammation. Prostatitis. Urethritis. Cystitis. Nephritis. Pyelitis. Lithuria. Nocturnal enuresis. Oedema. Gonorrhoea.
Tissue conditions
Soothing and tonic for all urinary conditions.
Purulent urine - which appears cloudy and is often due to mucus or infection. Frees the circulation of urea and uric acid. Administered in cystitis [with urinary phosphates]. Mucus inflammation of the genito urinary tract. Zea strengthens uterine muscle tone.
Preparations
Urinary infections with Althea.
Bladder disorders - Barosma, Capsella, Eupatorium purpureum, Hydrangea, Parietaria.
Gonorrhoea with Arctium, Rumex and Stillingia.
Nephritis with Solidago.
Enuresis with Agrimonia.
Uterine pain and inflammation with Aletris.
Vaginal discharge/leucorrhoea with Eupatorium, Pipsissewa.
Dosage and mode of application
Dried stigma Sig 8g
Tincturae Sig 10ml
Liquidum extractum Sig 8ml
References
43 p239. 126 p698. 188p128. 233 p69. 246 p545. 254 p84.

Zingiber officinale [Ginger]

Constituents
Free fatty acids - caprylic acid, linoleic acid, linolenic acid. Oleoresin up to 7.5% - phenols gingerol.
Volatile oils up to 3% - sesquiterpine lactones up to 70% – bisabolene, zingiberine.
Amino acids. Carbohydrates as starch up to 60%. Protein up to 10%.

Primary pharmacological action:
Arterial vasostimulant especially to the capillary function.

Therapeutic classes
Allays inflammation. Antiseptic. Aromatic.
Antifungal. Antiviral – rhinovirus IB.
Antimicrobial to gram positive and gram negative bacteria – Escherichia coli, Proteus vulgaris, salmonella, Staphylococcus aureus, Streptococcus viridans.
Cardio vascular stimulant. Circulatory diffusive stimulant. Peripheral vasodilator.
Antioxidant. Anticholesterolaemic. Antiplatelet.
Antitussive. Expectorant.
Sialagogue. Carminative. Anti nausea. Antiemetic. Cholagogue. Antiparasitic.
Diaphoretic. Antirheumatic.
Uterine tonic.
Rubefacient - topical. Antineoplastic.
Antispasmodic.
Medicinal indications
Atherosclerosis. Atony of the circulatory and digestive organs. Faint pulse.
Colds. Sore throat. Bronchitis. Pneumonia. Influenza.
Aromatic. Anorexia. Alcoholic gastritis. Atonic, flatulent dyspepsia. Gastric atony. Peptic ulcers. Nausea [from food poisoning]. Hepatic disease. Relaxed bowel [diarrhoea]. Intestinal colic [contraction spasm]. Intestinal fermentation and putrefaction. Diarrhoea. Dysentery. Cholera. Schistosomes.
Vomiting of pregnancy. Amenorrhoea from cold or chills. Dysmenorrhoea.
Rheumatic complaints. Arthritis. Musculoskeletal pain.
Headache. Migraine. Vertigo - Motion sickness. Paralysis.
Tissue conditions
Around 40% of the active remedy is eliminated within 12 hours. For atony of the gastro intestinal tract with associated flatulence. Zingiber stimulates saliva and hydrochloric acid secretion. Tonic and antispasmodic action upon intestinal smooth muscle, it increases peristalsis.

Pharmacopoeia

A strong tasting diffusive to the circulation and is diaphoretic. It inhibits blood platelets from sticking together and lowers cholesterol levels.

Preparations

Lung conditions with appropriate combination.

Laxative prescriptions to prevent griping of laxatives.

Motion sickness – Sig 2g PRN –2/3 hourly.

External use

Rubefacient action in rheumatic conditions – arthritic pain, sprains.

Dosage and mode of application

Dried rad/rhizome Sig 9g

Fresh rad/rhiz Sig 9g

Infusium Sig 2g

Tincturae Sig 10ml

Tincturae forte [1:2] 0.5ml

Liquidum extractum Sig 2ml

Succus Sig 7.5ml.

References

40 p157. 111 p755. 192 p228. 230 p43. 278 1994, 57 [5] p658. 271 no 52 & 53. 330, 2001, 50, 8, 720. 304 p153.

Zizyphus jujube [Chinese sour date]

Constituents
Saponins – jujubosides A and B. Betulin. Betulinic acid. Alkaloids. Volatile oil.
Vitamins A, B2, C. Iron. Mucilage.

Primary pharmacological action: Tonic nervine.

Therapeutic classes
Astringent.
Hypotensive.
Antiallergic. Antitussive.
Hepatoprotective.
Immunemodulator. Antineoplastic.
Anticonvulsant. Antidepressant. Analgesic. Anxiolytic. Hypnotic. Sedative.
Medicinal indications
Hypertension. Palpitations. Night sweats.
Coughs.
Cirrhosis. Hepatitis. Diarrhoea.
Melanoma.
Insomnia. Nervous exhaustion. Anxiety. Impotence/sexual dysfunction. Elevates
the mood and improves psychomotor tasks. Chronic fatigue syndrome.
Tissue conditions
Sympathetic nervous system irritability, tension states together with the usual
anxiety state. GMP enhances sexual performance. Cyclic GMP is a chemical that
declines with age. Nitric oxide leads to an increase in cyclic GMP this increases
sexual function in the male. Zizyphus enhances the level of nitric oxide which in
turn increases GMP. Panax also has the same effects. Leaves and roots are
anodyne.
Cautions
Colic, flatus.
Dosage and mode of application
Dried sem/fruct Sig 3g
Tincturae sem/fruct Sig 3ml
Liquidum extractum Sig 3ml
References
48 p87. 187p291. 282 No. 38. 331, 33 [suppl] 5-16. 332, 1995,
1, 10, p1046-1050.

Medical Astrology

- Jupiter – Agrimonia eupatoria, Agropyron repens, Borago officinalis, Castanea sativa, Cichorium intybus, Datura stramonium, Geum urbanum, Hyssopus officinalis, Melilotus officinalis, Melissa officinalis, Panax species, Phyllitis scolopendrium, Pulmonaria officinalis, Quercus robur, Rumex crispus, Salvia miltiorrhiza, Salvia officinalis, Salvia triloba, Sempervivum tectorum, Stachys betonica, Taraxacum officinale, Tilia cordata/platyphylos/europaea, Vaccinum myrtillus.
- Mars – Allium sativa, Armoracia rusticana, Artemesia absinthum, Berberis aquifoleum, Berberis vulgaris, Bryonia alba, Capsicum species, Cinchona species, Cnicus benedictus, Crataegus, Cytissus scoparius, Galium odoratum, Gentiana lutea, Geranium maculatum, Humulus lupulus, Linaria vulgaris, Ocimum basilicum/sanctum, Ononis spinosa, Pinus sylvestris, Pulsatilla vulgaris, Ranunculus ficaria, Rheum palmatum, Ruscus aculeatus, Sanicula europaea, Strychnos nux vomica, Teucrium chamaedrys, Urgenia maritima, Urtica dioica/urens, Zingiber officinale.
- Mercury – Anethum graveolens, Apium graveolens, Artemesia abrotanum, Avena sativa, Ballota nigra, Carum carvi, Cassia acutifolia, Convallaria majalis, Daucus carota, Foeniculum vulgare, Galega officinalis, Glycerrhiza glabra, Inula helenium, Lavandula angustifolia, Linum usitatissimum, Marrubium vulgare, Menyanthes trifoliata, Origanum vulgare, Parietaria diffusa, Petroselinum crispum, Podophyllum peltatum, Solanum dulcamara, Succisa pratensis, Teucrium scordonia, Valeriana officinalis.
- Moon - Eschscholzia californica, Galium aparine, Iris versicolor, Lactuca virosa, Ligustrum lucidum, Lilium tigrinum, Nymphaea odorata, Papaver somniferum, Pimpinella saxifrage, Salix alba, Salvia sclarea, Stellaria media, Vitex agnus castus.
- Saturn – Aconitum napellus, Adonis vernalis, Atropa belladonna, Cannabis sativa, Capsella bursa pastoris, Colchicum autumnale, Conium maculatum, Dryopteris felix mas, Epilobium parvifoleum, Equisetum arvense, Fumaria officinalis, Gaultheria procumbens, Hedera helix, Helleborus niger, Hieracium pilosella, Hyoscyamnus niger, Pilosella officinarum, Polygonum bistorta, Populus tremuloides, Rhamnus frangula, Symphytum officinale, Taxus baccata, Ulmus campestris, Veratrum album/viride, Verbascum thapsus, Viola tricolor.
- Sun – Angelica archangelica, Arnica montana, Calendula officinalis, Centaurium erythraea, Chamomilla recutita, Chamaemelum nobile,

Chelidonium majus, Commiphora molmol, Drosera rotundifolia, Echium vulgare, Euphrasia officinalis, Fraxinus excelsior, Hypericum perforatum, Juniperus communis, Levisticum officinale, Paeonia lactiflora, Petasites hybridus, Potentilla reptans, Rosmarinus officinalis, Ruta graveolens, Sanguisorba officinalis, Viscum album.

- Venus – Achillea millefoleum, Ajuga reptans, Alchemilla vulgaris, Alnus glutinosa, Althea officinalis, Aralia, Arctium, Aristolochia serpentaria, Artemesia vulgaris, Bellis perennis, Betula alba, Cynara scolymus, Digitalis species, Dipsacus fullorum/sylvestris, Erigeron canadense, Filipendula ulmaria, Lamium album, Leonurus cardiaca, Mentha piperita, Mentha pulegium, Morus alba, Nepeta cataria, Nepeta hederacea, Plantago species, Potentilla erecta, Primula veris, Prunella vulgaris, Rumex acetosella, Sambucus nigra, Saponaria officinalis, Scrophularia, Seneco jacobaea, Seneco vulgaris, Solidago virgaurea, Tanacetum parthenium, Tanacetum vulgare, Thymus serphyllum/vulgaris, Tussilago farfara, Verbena officinalis, Vinca minor/major/rosea, Viola odorata.

Summary
Those of a scientific mind may ask where is the scientific proof?
Proof comes from already existing evidence about the herbal medicines given in the above profiles and also:
1] practitioner use and case history notes of herbalists from around the world
2] over many years of traditional use throughout the world
3] writings from books in particular British Pharmacopoeia [BPC], British Herbal Compendium, British Herbal Pharmacopoeia, Martindale 7th and 27th Ed., Culpeper, Potters Cyclopaedia, King, Felter & Lloyd, Herbal Medicine – Blumenthal, Goldberg & Brinckmann, German Commission Monographs also see bibliography.
4] research material reviews e.g. British library, Greenfiles.
5] audit of cases.
6] Culpeper and Heinrich Daath works provide Astrological data, this has been included for those wishing to avail themselves of medical astrology.

Perhaps the question that should be asked requires a change of thought process for the scientific mind to ponder, as the usual question asked is why and how does it work?
It is far more scientific to prove that the remedy will not do what it is stated to do. Conduct your own research by trying to disprove the facts stated in a remedy monograph.

Human perception is biased not evidence based i.e. it is not objective. One selects certain things according to our perception and bias. Evidence in books is selected.

It will also be noticed that the monographs have few indications on herb and drug interactions. Intentionally avoided, herb drug interactions are out of place in this work. It is not intended that the medicines described here are to be relegated to a second place in medicine, that is behind synthetic drugs. Rather that this pharmacopoeia be the mainstream medical treatment in primary care.
Adverse reactions can be found in Ernst et al [239] also German E Commission Monographs.

36
EMERGENCY HERBAL MEDICINE

Treatments of acute medical emergencies.
Specific medication is found under the name of the condition and dosage of an individual remedy will be found in the pharmacopoeia [Chapter 35] and the quick reference guide [Chapter 39].

Assess and observe the patient
1] Conscious or unconscious.
2] Breathing normal?
3] Heart rate normal?
4] Haemorrhage?
5] What are they complaining of and what are the symptoms?

The above accounts of primary symptoms within each condition bring attention to the causes and to the treatment of the syndrome. Study of the above gives the correct indications for immediate treatment.
The more severe the symptoms the more life-threatening the condition. With a large number of casualties each would be assessed upon life threatening symptoms and treated accordingly.
Triage system in practice concentrates upon the most life threatening symptoms and the patient is triaged as red - this means immediate treatment. Some emergencies are medical while others are surgical. For the benefit of clarity the main causes of emergencies are listed here. In some cases herbal medicine is adequate for those emergencies *where the practitioner has the skill* to treat and manage the condition.
A low Sa O2 means low oxygen saturation and requires for the patient to be on oxygen.
Many emergencies are life threatening.

917

Emergency Medicine Chest

Medications
Anaesthetic - Piper methysticum, Solanum dulcamara. Oleum Lavandula.
Analgesic – Phenobarbitone Herbal [PB]. A compound for the relief of pain:
Passiflora, Pulsatilla, Salix nigra, Valeriana equal parts of each.
Antiseptic for gargle/wash – Commiphora, Salvia. Oleum Lavandula.
Antiseptic cream - use Thymus and Oregano oleum.
Catarrh pastilles
Cream – antiseptic/healing/anti itch – Plantago. Ol. Ti tree.
Diarrhoea mist. – Quercus.
Dyspepsia mist. – Filipendula. Expectorant mist. – Glycyrrhiza.
Injections [needles suitable for sc, im, iv, 23g x 30mm and syringes 2, 5, 10ml].
Pasco injections 5 ampoules of each:
      1] Sedativa – sedative
      2] Allya – Inflammations of musculoskeletal system
      3] Rheuma pasc – acute rheumatic pain
      4] Dolo – neuritis, neuralgia.
Liniment for massage – Oleum Cajuput, Camphor and Gaulthera. Ol. Hypericum.
Medications:
      Capsicum drops provide intense stimulation.
      Commiphora drops provide intense antisepsis.
      Lobelia drops provide intense relaxation/antispasmodic activity.
      Salvia herba or Tr.
      Zingiber – anti nauseant, anti emetic.
      Rescue remedy.

Medical equipment
Adhesive strapping
Antiseptic disinfectant – use Thyme and Oregano oil.
Bandages 5-7.5cm
Bandages crepe 7.5cm
Cotton wool
Dressing pack: with forceps, cotton wool swabs, tray, sterile field, yellow disposable bag.
Dropper bottle
Elastoplast adhesive strip
Eye bath. Gauze – plain
Gloves Lint
Medicine measure
Melolin - non stick. Paraffin gauze, Plasters .
Safety pins medium and large, Scissors – blunt ended, Spatula .
Sterilised eye pad with bandage
Thermometer , Torch, Triangular bandage .

Emergency conditions

Abdominal pain/Trunk injury
Check the following:
Airway, breathing, haemorrhage, shock. Is this a surgical or medical case?
Poultice
Arnica, Calendula, Symphytum, Trigonella.

Abscess – as inflammation with hot fomentations.
Medicine
Blood vasotonic alterative. Althea, Arctium, Calendula, Dioscorea, Echinacea, Galium, Iris, Rumex, Trifolium.

Acidity, heartburn
Medicine
Px Vegetable charcoal with Ol. Caraway/Anise, Elettaria, Cinnamomum, Filipendula and Rheum.
Centaurium, Filipendula, Mentha piperita.

Allergic rhinitis
Medicine
Echinacea, Ephedra, Pulsatilla, Sambucus, Verbascum.

Allergies to food
Fast on water.
Test suspected food substances with a pulse test and antibody blood test.
Support detoxification via the intestine with a cathartic.

Anaemia
Avoid tea.
Medicine
Agrimonia. Gentiana. Medicago. Urtica. Spinach. Watercress. Vitamin C.

Angina [See chest pain]

Anorexia
Medicine
Centaurium. Gentiana. Marsdenia. Flower remedy - Holly.

Anthrax
Medicine
Blood, hepatic and splenic medicines. Pulmonary anthrax is fatal.

Herbal Medicine - Keys

Achillea, Allium, Baptisia, Capsicum, Commiphora, Echinacea, Euphorbia, Hamamelis, Hydrastis, Hydrangea, Humulus, Juglans cinera, Lonicera caprifoleum, Mitchella, Nymphaea, Sticta pulmonaria. [176, 1 p91-93]

Appendicitis
Management - Avoid all food.
Medicine
Aconitum napellus. Atropa, Baptisia, Bryonia, Chamomilla, Capsicum, Commiphora, Dioscorea, Echinacea, Gelsemium, Hamamelis, Hydrastis, Iris, Lobelia, Nepeta, Olea, Papaver, Stellaria, Trigonella.
Enema
Dioscorea and Nepeta.
Poultice
Oleum Ricinus, Chamomilla or Linum usit.

Arthritis - pain
Medicine
Achillea, Arctium, Dioscorea, Guaiacum, Harpagophytum, Menyanthes, Phytolacca, Populus tremuloides, Salix alba, Sambucus, Urtica, Zanthoxylum, Zingiber plus nervines.

Anxiety
Medicine
Avena, Humulus, Panax, Piper methysticum, Scutellaria, Valeriana, Verbena, Viscum, Zizyphus.

Asphyxia
Medicine
Thomsons No 6. Commiphora and Capsicum. Sig 2ml. Administer as drops onto the tongue and base of the neck.

Asthma
Medicine
Tincturae Antispasmodic Sig 20gtt aqua frig. PRN. Apply Tr Antispasmodic to the neck and spinal nerves.
Antispasmodics – Aspidosperma, Datura, Ephedra, Euphorbia, Galeopsis. Lobelia with Capsicum.

Acute infections of the upper respiratory system
Medicine
Allium, Althea, Baptisia, Echinacea, Phytolacca, Thymus, Composition essence.
Inhalation Friars balsam.

Emergency conditions

Inhalation with dilute Essential Ol - Caryophylum, Eucalyptus, Thymus, Rosmarinus, Melaleuca.

Backache/pain
Check the following: Airway, absence of leg pulses, shock, pain, pyrexia. Check renal function, urinary infection, prostate/uterine function, vertebral structure/disc prolapse/rheumatic/arthritic disorders, circulatory/venous return.
Treatment
Soreness of the lumbar spine and general weakness of the latissimus dorsi and associated musculature are benefited by:
External
Arnica, Fucus, Gaultheria, Hypericum, Seneco jacobea, Symphytum.
Medicine
Antispasmodic Tr., Apium, Cimicifuga, Lobelia, Gaultheria, Gelsemium, Harpagophytum, Hypericum, Juniperus, Populus tremuloides, Salix alba.

Bites see insect below

Botulism
Infection caused by Clostridium botulinum occurs from infected food.
Medicine
Baptisia, Berberis sp., Capsicum, Cinnamomum Zeylandicum, Commiphora molmol, Echinacea, Hydrastis.

Bronchitis - acute.
Steaming with volatile oils of Eucalyptus, Melaleuca, Mentha piperita, Origanum and/or Thymus.
Pectoral diffusives and demulcents
Althea, Glycyrrhiza, Hyssops, Lobelia, Marrubium, Thymus, Tussilago.
Antiseptics and expectorants
Allium, Baptisia, Bryonia, Echinacea, Eucalyptus, Pilosella, Thymus.
Bronchodilators
Datura, Ephedra, Euphorbia, Grindelia, Lobelia, Thymus,
Antispasmodic Tr.

Bruises
Rest the area. Limb bruises - elevate the limb.
Apply a cold compress or fomentation for bruises, sprains, aching in the muscles and tendons. Apply cold and renew frequently.
External
Arnica is specific to bruised, sore, lacerated and contused muscular tissue - [See injury]. Aqua Hamamelis. Symphytum fol - fomentation or oleum.

Herbal Medicine - Keys

Cellulitis
Encourage lymph and venous drainage.
Use antimicrobials, diuretics, and circulatory tonics.
Medicines
Antimicrobials – Baptisia, Commiphora, Echinacea, Tabebuia.
Diuretics - Daucus, Eupatorium purpureum.
Venous tonics – Aesculus, Capsicum, Crataegus, Centella, Zingiber.

Cerebro vascular accident [Stroke]
CVA due to haemorrhage
Arnica will support the reabsorption of haemorrhage. Indicated for threatened CVA.
Tincturae 1:10 Sig 1-10 gtt
Or as a safer dosage: Tincturae 40 gtt
120ml aqua. Sig 5ml every one/two hours

Medicines
Aesculus, Arnica, Capsicum, Centella, Crataegus, Equisetum, Helleborus niger, Hydrastis, Centella, Piper methysticum.
CVA from an embolus.
Cases require stimulation to circulation .
Medicines
Capsicum. Ginkgo. Centella. Panax. Rosmarinus. Zanthoxylum. Zingiber.
Vitamin C, E.
Chronic cases, bedridden etc. Local treatment for the skin and mobilisation of the joints.

Chest pain
Check the following: Airway, shock, life threatening arrhythmia, history/? ECG suggestive of MI, altered consciousness. Low Sa O2, severe cardiac or pleuritic pain, acute dyspnoea, hypotension, dizzyness, persistent vomiting.
Treat the cause e.g. Arrhythmia, MI, Chest infection, Pleurisy, Pneumonia, Pulmonary embolus.
Anginal pain
Ease vasospasm as it causes anginal pain. Hydrotherapy – elbow bath.
Medicines
Antispasmodics and Vasodilators: Antispasmodic Tincture, Avena, Ballota, Chamomilla, Cannabis – sedative, Capsicum, Crataegus, Leonurus, Phytolacca, Scutellaria, Vitamin E.

Myocardial infarction
Treat the causative factors atherosclerosis, stress, hypertension.

Emergency conditions

Treatment
Vigorous and repeated coughing with a deep breath between coughs encourages more O2 into the lungs and the coughing movements squeeze the heart and support a return to a more normal rhythm. [BNA News update 008, Health cares, Rochester Hospital, Kent].
Vital stimulation to circulation in order to keep the blood flowing.
Anticoagulants to reduce the risk of further myocardial damage.
Ease the pain - antispasmodics.
Medicines
Antispasmodic tincturae, Allium, Avena, Ballota, Capsicum, Cannabis, Colchicum, Crataegus, Gelsemium, Lobelia, Phytolacca, Selenicerus, Tilia, Viscum, Zanthoxylum. Co enzyme Q10 up to 100mg daily. Vitamin E.

Chilblains
Warm the area by wrapping it up.
Medicines
Angelica archangelica, Capsicum, Zanthoxylum, Zingiber, Vitamin E.

Colds
Hot face and a dry throat. Thick yellow discharge from the nares. Pyrexia.
Frequent colds/catarrh indicate a lowered immune response.
Treatment
Fluids, rest and a short fast.
Diaphoretic [see below, sore throat]
Medicines
Antiseptic; Allium/Baptisia/Echinacea/Thymus.
Profuse watery secretion use Euphrasia or Ephedra.
Inhalation for catarrh and colds:
[1] menthol crystals [2] Ol thymus [3] Ol Eucalyptus or [4] Ol Melaleuca.

Cold sores [herpes]
Keep the area dry. Locally Baptisia/Commiphora /Hydrastis/Hypericum/Melissa.

Colic and flatulence [See physiomedical pain treatments].

Colitis
Medicines
Althea, Atropa, Dioscorea, Glycyrrhiza, Geranium maculatum, Hyoscyamnus, Lobelia, Potentilla, Ulmus, Zingiber.

Herbal Medicine - Keys

Collapse
Check the following: Airway. Are there fits. Shock, ECG arrhythmia's, low Sa O2, Severe pain, dyspnoea, hypoglycaemic, hyperglycaemic with ketosis, altered consciousness, rash, pyrexia, hypothermia, urine infection.
Medicines
Capsicum [Thomsons No 6], Composition Essence.

Constipation
Medicine
Aloe, Syrup of Cassia or Syrup of figs. Sig full dosage.

Confusion
Check the following: Airway, hypoglycaemia, shock. Low Sa O2, altered consciousness, overdose or poisoning? Pyrexia. hypothermia. Check the psychiatric history.
Check the blood sugar and urine for evidence of infection. Neurological test and Co ordination test.

Cough
Is the patient choking? Clear the airway.
A cough is always a symptom of a deeper syndrome. However cough relief will allow rest for the patient.
Medicine
Glycyrrhiza, Lobelia, Prunus serotina, Tussilago.
Steam inhalation with one of the following:
Ol Eucalyptus 5gtt/Ol Thymus 5gtt/Ol Camphor 5gtt.

Cystitis - acute
Micturition with dysuria, pyuria or haematuria.
Treatment
Advise plenty of fluids. Warm pack to the bladder alternating with cold packs.
Medicine
Demulcents and antiseptics - Agropyron, Althea, Allium, Barosma, Echinacea, Hydrangea, Piper methysticum, Uva ursi, Zea.

Deep vein thrombosis/DVT
Check the following: Airway, shock, low Sa O2, pain, dyspnoea.
Treatment
Fluids. Stimulation to circulation. Movement.
Medicine
Aesculus, Allium, Capsicum, Colchicum, Galium odoratum, Lobelia, Trigonella, Zanthoxylum. Vitamin E.

924

Emergency conditions

Depression
Observe the patient. Are there suicidal tendencies.
Medicine
Avena, Hypericum, Panax, Piper methysticum, Rosmarinus, Scutellaria, Turnera, Flower Medicines. Avoid Humulus.

Dermatology - Burns. Cuts. Scalds. Ulcers. Wounds.
Burns and scalds cool the area first with copious amounts of clean cold water or cold Aloe succus. Aloe can be frozen as ice cubes for immediate use.
Sunburn - avoid the sun and cover up.
Cuts, ulcers and wounds
Aseptically clean the area. Sterile dressing or poultice.
Crem for burns
LE Urtica 5% Arnica 1% Oleum Lavandula 1% Base to 60g

Dermal anaesthetic, antiseptic vulnerary:
1. Acanthus mollis [Bears breech] – fresh fol or dect. rad is astringent: dermal inflammation, burns and scalds. [Ref. 246 p415].
2. Ajuja reptans - ulcers, wounds including stab wounds, haematomas
3. Aloe vera gel is one of the most suitable lotions to use apply neat.
4. Althea with Ol Linum. Renew every 2/3 hours.
5. Calendula lotion/crem.
6. Carica papaya - wound healer - infected or purulent wounds, following surgery with incomplete healing, necrotic damage. It arrests local inflammation and is a topical debriding agent. Dry scaly skin conditions.
7. Chamomilla - allays dermal irritation and swelling from any cause.
8. Carica papaya - wound healer - infected or purulent wounds, following surgery with incomplete healing, necrotic damage. It arrests local inflammation and is a topical debriding agent. Dry scaly skin conditions.
9. Choerospondias axillaris [water extract from the bark] was compared with saline gauze treatment of second degree burns, and resulted in faster healing and fewer infections. The commentary criticizes the size and potential bias of the trial, but suggests further investigation as the bark is cheap and convenient to use. Ref. 301, 1997, 2 [2]. 334 1996, 30, p139-144.
10. Hydrocarpus laurifolia - a dressing for wounds and ulcers.
11. Hypericum – eases oedema
12. Linum usitatissimum oleum or crushed sem as a wound dressing.
Poultice of crushed seed alone or combined with mustard for bronchitis, ulceration, superficial or deep inflammation.

Herbal Medicine - Keys

13. Plantago's effects on cuts and open wounds rank it as a haemostatic comparable to Calendula and Achillea.
14. Honey is antiseptic apply to any wound - cover with a sterile dressing. Honey should not be diluted as its loses its efficacy.
    Manuca honey - effective against Staphylococcus aureus.
15. Passiflora tetrandra is a climbing vine found in New Zealand, the oil from the seeds are used by the Maori to treat chronic sores and obstinate wounds. Antibacterial - Escherichia coli, Bacillus subtilis, and Pseudomonas aeruginosa. 263, 1991 57 [2] 129-31.

16 Polygonum bistorta has a powerful faculty to resist poisons used as a wash.

17 Sanguisorba officinalis – burns, eczema, wounds.

18 Sempervivum tectorum/Houseleek - analgesic, astringent, dermal ulcers.

19 Trigonella - Wound dressing/poultice [ground sem] is antiseptic - abscesses, furunculosis, ulcers, wounds.

20 Verbesina encelioides - Goldweed [Anil de muestro]
    Finely ground leaves mixed with olive oil are placed on open wounds or sores.

21 **Astringent lotion** made from powdered Quercus and powdered Polygonum rad - invaluable for open wounds it has enormous cleansing power.

22 **Oleum** Lavandula diluted to 1% and spray onto a burn wound or ulcer.

23 **Poultice** - ulcers/wounds
    Rad Symphytum 20g. Rad Althea 20g. Flos Calendula 10g.
    Mix the powders with water. Spread onto sterile gauze apply to the wound. Cover and leave. Replace daily or less often as improvement occurs.

24 **Crem Stellaria** [Chickweed cream].
    Handful of chickweed and mix with warmed lard, leave, the herb will become crisp. Strain and use. Apply to cuts, bruises, dermal ulcers.

25 **Tincture Benzoin co spray.** Compound Benzoin Tincture 15% with alcohol.
    Aerosol spray is vulnerary for reducing skin sensitivity, irritation, infections, chilblains, dermal ulcers, eczema, fissure, gingivitis, herpes, nipple fissure, wounds [Benzoin formula see Styrax benzoin].

26 **Unguentum Eucalyptus**
    Px Ol Eucalyptus   1ml
    Paraffin molle   90g
    Melt the paraffin and stir in the oil. Pour into jars and stir until cool.
    Used as an antiseptic dressing.

27 **Unguentum Lavandula**
    Px Ol Lavandula   1ml
    Paraffin molle   90g
    Melt the paraffin and stir in the oil. Pour into jars and stir until cool.
    Used as an antiseptic dressing.

Emergency conditions

28 **Oleum Oenothera** – use neat.

Gangrenous wounds
Strong stimulation to the vital force and circulation is required in gangrene.
<u>Medicine</u>
Capsicum, Commiphora, Echinacea, Hydrastis, Juglans, Pineapple. Stachys, betonica/palustris, Zanthoxylum, Zingiber.
<u>Inflammatory wounds</u> need soothing demulcents - Allium, Carica papaya, Commiphora molmol, Echinacea, Hydrastis, Juglans, Symphytum, Ulmus.
Px Althea with Ulmus as a poultice. Use both as powdered roots and renew before it dries.

Dermal ulcers
Check the cause of ulcers which are mainly from deficient circulation of the area - varicose, rheumatoid, hyperlipidaemia, diabetes, raynauds disease.
<u>Treatment</u>
Encourage movement and elevation of the limb.
Dietary changes should be made - use baked apples, stewed prunes, figs and dates.
Various preparations may be used to heal ulcers. It is not advisable to use strong drawing preparations which can cause an increase in ulcer pain.
<u>External antiseptics</u>. These can be applied upon sterile gauze.
Allium succus, Aloe, Baptisia, Calendula, Chamomilla, Carica papaya, Commiphora, Cynoglossum officinale, Echinacea, Honey, Hydrastis, Onion juice, Papaya, Pineapple, Plantago, Populus tremuloides, Symphytum, Thuja.
Poultice - Centella asiatica in syphilitic ulcers
Fomentation - Calendula.

Green surgical dressing for wounds
Poultice the area with the appropriate remedy or cover wound with sterile gauze and a dressing.

Sterile dressing – Should be aseptically dressed. An aerosol spray can be used to spray the wound.
When a sterile dressing is unobtainable a freshly laundered sheet is considered sterile and will be suitable for cutting up to required sized dressings.

Dermal poultices - A poultice allays irritation and pain and promotes suppuration.
Allium - fresh paste – antiseptic, Althea & Ulmus – drawing poultice [abscesses], Bran – sciatica, Berberis vulgaris – antiseptic, Calendula – wounds, Capsicum – stimulation, Humulus – pain, Linum – poultice of crushed seed alone or combined

with mustard for bronchitis, ulceration, superficial or deep inflammation. chest infections, burns/scalds, Hydrastis – antiseptic, Lobelia – pain, Mango and Potato - wounds, Symphytum – fractures and ulcers, Ulmus – drawing and soothing to ulcers, Zingiber - stimulation.
Usually muslin is used to contain the herb used for the poultice.

Vulnerary - wound medicines are also styptics and antiseptics - used as lotions, washes, poultices, creams or ointments.
Achillea, Aloe, Agrimonia, Allium, Althea, Baptisia, Bellis, Calendula, Chamomilla, Capsella, Centella, Commiphora, Echinacea, Geranium maculatum, Hamamelis, Hypericum, Oleum Lavandula, Linum usittitassimum, Oleum Melaleuca, Nymphaea, Plantago, Prunella vulgaris, Oleum Ricinus, Sanguisorba officinalis, Stachys palustris, Stellaria, Styrax, Symphytum, Trigonella, Ulmus, Urtica, Viola.
Vitamin E – antioxidant. Zinc – vulnerary.

Diarrhoea
Check the following: Airway, shock.
Diarrhoea may follow over eating, sudden change of diet, food poisoning etc.
Treatment
Fast for 48 hours with water only. Then introduce fruit juices. Look for the cause. Use astringents to ease the ferocity of the diarrhoea. Do not suppress it. Any infection may otherwise stay around for longer when the intestine is really trying to clear itself of accumulations.
Astringe the intestine – Filipendula, Geranium maculatum, Hamamelis, Plantago, Polygonum, Potentilla, Quercus, Rubus.
[See Chapter on tropical disease re dysentery].

Dizzyness see EENT p165

Diverticulitis
Medicine
Demulcent/antispasmodics.
Althea, Antispasmodic Tr., Chamomilla, Glycyrrhiza, Hamamelis, Linum, Lobelia, Ulmus.

Diuretic
Acute retention. Immerse the pelvis in warm water for acute retention of urine. Catheterisation may be necessary.
Stimulating diuretics:
Alchemilla arvensis, Barosma, Capsicum, Juniperus, Uva ursi, Zingiber.

Emergency conditions

Drowning
Immediate treatment: CPR
<u>Medicine</u>
Thomsons No 6. Commiphora and Capsicum. Sig 2ml. Administer as drops onto the tongue and base of neck.

Dysmenorrhoea
Warm pack to the lower abdomen.
<u>Medicine</u>
Antispasmodic Tr, Capsicum, Caulophyllum, Cimicifuga, Lobelia, Pulsatilla, Viburnum species.

Dyspnoea
Check the following: Airway, altered conscious level, shock, life threatening arrhythmia's, ECG abnormal, MI, cardiac pain, pyrexia, exhaustion, low peak expiratory flow rate. Treat the cause.

Ear disturbances
Pain due to cold, draughts, dampness, exposure give - Pulsatilla.
Perforations and deafness: Pilocarpus jaborandi, Plantago, Verbascum.
Otitis media - use and. Support elimination via the intestine.
<u>Medicine</u> - antiseptics
Allium/Baptisia/Echinacea/Hydrastis/ Plantago/ Pulsatilla/Solidago.

Eczema
<u>Medicine</u>
Calendula, Echinacea, Fumaria, Hypericum, Rumex, Stellaria, Urtica, Viola tricolor.

Electrocution
Immediate treatment CPR.
<u>Medicine</u>
Thomsons No 6. Commiphora and Capsicum. Sig 2ml. Administer as drops onto the tongue and base of neck.

Emetic
Ipecac. induces vomiting within 20 minutes.
Px LE Ipecac 7ml vegetable glycerine to 100ml
Sig: child 6 – 18 months - give 10ml
          child over 2 - give 20ml
          adults - give 30ml. Follow with 200 ml of water, flavoured if required.
May be repeated after 20 minutes if vomiting has not occurred.

Herbal Medicine - Keys

Epilepsy [See fits]

Epistaxis
First aid - sit the patient up.
    Apply nasal pressure for 5-10 minutes.
    Cold pack to the nose and back of the head.
    Pack nares with ribbon gauze soaked in a styptic. Capsicum is a styptic
for severe cases. Keep the patient on bedrest. Repack for up to 48 hours.
Give a mouthwash afterwards.
Astringent and styptics
Calendula, Geranium maculatum, Hamamelis, Plantago,
Give a diaphoretic – Achillea, Nepeta, Sambucus. Treat the cause.

Eyes
Injuries - lacerations use styptics - dilute Collyr Capsicum et Hamamelis.
Conjunctivitis - Collyr Calendula/Euphrasia. Collyr guttae Ol Allium
Iritis - Collyr guttae Allium, Baptisia, Calendula or Echinacea.

Falls
Check the following: Arrhythmia's, airway, fitting, shock, hypoglycaemia.

Fits
Check the following: Life threatening ECG arrhythmia's, airway, purpura, fitting,
shock, hypoglycaemia. Altered consciousness level, overdose, meningism, rash,
low Sa O2, pyrexia. Prevent injury
Medicine
Capsicum, Lobelia, Hyssopus, Scutellaria, Viscum, Antispasmodic Tr.

Fear – see below [grief]

Fever [pyrexia]
[Various types of fever are explained in Chapter 14 & Naturopathy].
Fever is a response to tissue injury. Local and general inflammations may result
in fever. Infections often bring about a fever. Fever must be kept adequate for the
ejection of toxins through the skin and to resolve the pyrexia adequately. No
fever should be reduced until the perspiration phase has been completed. A level
of 38c [102 F] is adequate for resolution of the febrile phase.

Two responses to fever are worth noting:
Athletic habitus and sanguine temperament give rise to high fever with local
inflammations. Cerebral symptoms may occur.
Treatment: Diffusive relaxants [diaphoretics] **relax the skin.**

Emergency conditions

Medicine
Angelica archangelica, Asclepias, Chamomilla, Nepeta, Pulsatilla, Sambucus.
Asthenic habitus often have a feeble febrile reaction. Cerebral symptoms include restlessness.
Treatment: **diffusive stimulation** [Achillea, Zingiber] diffusives are to be preferred as Asthenics tend to react inadequately to the febrile response and often need nervine tonics and trophorestoratives rather than stimulants.

Flatulence [See colic]

Food poisoning
Fast for a minimum of 24 hours on water.
Medicines
To allay vomiting use Althea, Ballota, Cetraria, Glycyrrhiza.
To ease diarrhoea use appropriate astringents e.g. Hamamelis, Plantago sp., Polygonum bistorta.
Anti salmonella – grape seed extract, Allium, Arctium, Armoracea, Centaurium, Gentiana, Hydrastis, Larrea, Ocimum, Origanum, Salvia.

Fractures
Observe for haemorrhage. Immobilise. Avoid food. Treat shock if present.
Medicine
Artemesia absinthium, Cinnamomum, Equisetum, Hypericum, Medicago, Pilosella, Symphytum, Trigonella, Verbascum. Flower remedies.
Poultice
Hypericum, Symphytum, Arnica [diluted] for bruising. See also injury.

Frostbite
Medicine
Capsicum, Equisetum, Zingiber.

Gangrene [See inflamed wounds].

Gastritis
Fluids and fasting.
Medicine
Althea, Cetraria, Chondrus, Glycyrrhiza, Ulmus.

Gout
For pain and to allay inflammation - cold water applications.
Medicine
Apium, Arctium, Dioscorea, Menyanthes, Urtica.

Herbal Medicine - Keys

Grief/fear
Medicine
Tincturae antispasmodic Sig 20gtt Aq frig 2 hourly, Ignata.
Bach flowers:
Grief - Sweet chestnut, Fear - Aspen, Cherry plum, Mimulus, Rock rose.

Haematemesis & Melena
Check the following: Airway, shock, pain. Passage of blood by vomiting or rectum.
Styptic medicine
Agrimonia, Capsella, Capsicum, Composition essence, Geranium maculatum, Hydrastis, Lycopus, Myrica, Polygonum, Potentilla, Quercus.

Haemorrhoids
Acute pain - reduce the haemorrhoids using warm water. To prevent recurrence use cold water or an ice pack wrapped in a towel and applied to the anus – one minute at a time.
Medicine
Aesculus. Collinsonia. Geranium maculatum. Hamamelis. Potentilla.
Apply ung Ranunculus.

Hay fever
Vasoconstrictor medicine
Euphrasia, Ephedra, Plantago, Sambucus, Urtica.

Headache/Head pain
Check the following: Airway, fitting, purpura, shock. Severe pain, abrupt onset, altered conscious level, sudden loss of vision, meningism, rash, pyrexia.
Ascertain the cause.
Treatment
Head pain or Migraine - Full dose of Gelsemium, Piper methysticum, Piscidia, Scutellaria, Stachys, Tanacetum parthenium or Valeriana.

Head injury [concussion]
Check the following: Airway, haemorrhage, fitting, shock. Pupils.
Treatment depends upon the causes and effects of the injury.
Medicine
Arnica, Avena, Capsicum, Cola, Hypericum, Scutellaria, Stachys.

Heartburn
Fluids. Restricted food intake. Treat the stomach, gall bladder, liver or nervous system.

Emergency conditions

Heartburn medicine
Althea, Cetraria, Chondrus, Filipendula, Glycyrrhiza, Mentha piperita/ spicata/viridis, Ulmus.

Heat, high humidity, sunstroke
Management
Fluids. Cool the patient. Keep in the shade. Sponging with cold water.
Medicine
Cold infusium - Mentha piperita/spicata, Paullinia, Portulaca oleracea, Zizyphus.
Bartrum recommends stimulation to circulation in **heat exhaustion** with Capsicum or Zanthoxylum. Heat exhaustion can kill – keep casualty cool.

Heart
Arrhythmia
Digestive disturbances e.g. flatulence. Fear, terror, panic.
Medicine
Capsicum, Crataegus, Convallaria, Cytissus, Gelsemium, Leonurus, Lobelia, Melissa, Passiflora, Pulsatilla, Scutellaria, Strophanthus, Valeriana, Viscum, Zingiber.
Heart block
Medicines - Capsicum, Convallaria, Selenicerus, Zanthoxylum, Zingiber. Oleum camphor 2gtt on a sugar lump.
RVF – Right ventricular failure
Crataegus, Hydrastis, Diuretics.
LVF – Left ventricular failure
Avena, Capsicum, Crataegus, Convallaria, Cytissus, Digitalis, Astringents – Myrica. Diuretics.

Hernia – strangulated
Reduce if possible using Lobelia internally and externally [254].

Hyperactivity
Sedate the nervous system. [See Chapter on nervous system for treatments].

Hypertension
Treatment
Rest.
Nervine sedatives – Humulus, Passiflora.
Circulatory diffusives – Achillea, Nepeta, Sambucus, Viscum.
Arterial sedatives – Crataegus, Rauwolfia, Tilia, Veratrum, Viscum.
Diuretics – Juniperus, Parietaria, Taraxacum fol.

Herbal Medicine - Keys

Hyperglycaemia

Check the following: Airway, Breathing, Shock, Dehydration, Dry tongue, Glycosuria, Ketonuria, Hyperglycaemia with ketosis > 11m/mol, Vomiting, altered conscious level, pyrexia, Infection, Hypokalaemia.

Treatment - Hyperglycaemia

Reduce the blood sugar level. Once controlled advise upon the correct diet etc.

Medicine

Capsicum sp, Chionanthus, Galega officinalis, Gymnema sylvestre, Hydrastis, Pterocarpus marsupium, Syzygium cumini, Syzygium aromaticum, Urtica, Vinca, Mineral – Chromium.

Hyperventilation

Increased respiratory rate. Check the blood sugar level.

Treat for anxiety, shock or panic.

Medicine

Antispasmodic tincture, Cannabis, Lobelia.

Hypoglycaemia

Re-establish the blood sugar levels. Check the blood sugar level.

Honey is absorbed very quickly to rebalance the blood sugar levels. Increase fluids. Treat any shock. Take regular meals.

Medicine

Chamomilla, Capsicum, Chelone, Composition essence, Glycyrrhiza, Myrica, Taraxacum rad, Pterocarpus marsupium. Mineral – Chromium.

Indigestion

Treat as heartburn.

Infection

Medicines

Allium, Baptisia, Echinacea, Hydrastis.

Grapefruit seed extract is effective against - campylobacter jejuni, candida, E. coli, giardia, helicobacter pylori legionella, lysteria, pseudomonas, salmonella, staphylococci, streptococci, and tinea. [273].

Influenza

Fast. Oral fluids. Diaphoresis with antiviral and bacteriostatic medicines PRN.

Px 1. Influenza infusion – Syzygium flowerbuds x 5. Aqua 100ml. Pour boiling water upon the buds, cover and leave 10 minutes, strain and add honey to cover the taste.

Sig 100ml QDS.

Emergency conditions

Insect bites [See also Chapter 29]
Check the following: Airway, haemorrhage, stridor, shock. Severe pain, history of allergy, acute dyspnoea, wheeze, facial oedema, tongue oedema - any degree, a blistering or discharging eruption > 10% of body surface.
Insect bites can prove very annoying and itchy. Scratching causes damage to the skin which could allow infection to be introduced. Treatment see itch below.

Shock resulting from a bite or sting
Aconite, Capsicum with Lobelia, Star of Bethlehem flower remedy.

Herbal insect repellent against biting anthropods
Allium, Basilicum, Cedarwood, Citrus limon, Cymbopogon nardus [Citronella], Commiphora, Eucalyptus, Juniperus, Lavandula, Mentha pulegium, Palmarosa, Pinus, Rose geranium, Rosmarinus and Syzygium. Mix 20gtt aa essential oil and base oil to 50ml into a spray bottle. Use as required.

Candle burning impregnate with an herbal oil is effective to drive away insects – use Cymbopogon nardus [Citronella], Szygium.

Cockroaches
Cedarwood, Laurus nobilis - fresh or dried bay leaves in cupboards, Machura pomifera [Osage orange], Mentha canadensis [Japanese peppermint] and M. gracilis [Scotch spearmint].
Dog/rabies/hydrophobia [See under rabies]
Fleas
Flea pillows or spray - dried leaves of Erigeron canadense, Mentha pulegium and California laurel, with Citrus limoneum and Pinus oils.
Chrysanthemum leucanthemum [White ox eye daisy] destroys fleas.
Horsefly
Hypericum, Rumex, Urtica.
Housefly
Spray –
Acorus, Citronella, Chamomilla, Cymbopogon citratus, Eucalyptus globulus, Juniperus Palmarosa, Rose geranium, Santalum and Vetivera zizanoides-Vetiver.
Midges
Myrica gale oleum [Bog myrtle] protects against midges.
Ticks [See Chapter 29]

Insomnia
See Chapter on the nervous system for treatments.

Herbal Medicine - Keys

Ischaemia [Anoxaemia/hypoxia]
An accumulation of metabolites build up in the tissues from insufficient O2 and reduced blood supply to the tissues. From spasm or lack of local blood supply occurs angina, intermittent claudication or cramp.
Relax the blood vessels by:
Manipulation. Compresses. Spray – alternating hot and cold.
Antispasmodic and cerebral vasostimulants prescribed as appropriate to the presenting condition.
Medicine
Crataegus, Dioscorea, Ginkgo, Panax, Scutellaria, Viburnum species, Zanthoxylum. Vitamin E.

Itching
Is there any jaundice?
Medicines – use internally and externally.
Anti itch medication
Asperula, Calendula, Echinacea, Hedera, Hypericum, Hydrastis, Mentha piperita, Rumex, Stellaria, Symphytum, Urtica. Tr or LE can be used in an emergency – the infusion or decoction is considered more effective.
External
Aloe, Arnica, Plantago, Rumex, Stellaria, Urtica.
Apply one of the following.
A] Cream or lotion made from an infusion or decoction of the above
C] Fresh Rumex fol can be rubbed upon a sting as an anti itch.
D] Dist Hamamelis.
E] Acid tincture of Lobelia
F] Spray of oils. See above.
G] Cold compress.

Kidney infection
Check the following: Airway, signs of shock.
Treatment
Fluids. Rest the digestive tract
Stimulate the renal dermatomes with a cold water spray.
Medicine
Agropyron, Barosma, Equisetum, Eupatorium purpureum, Galium, Zea.

Labyrinthritis
Can cause severe vertigo.
Medicine – Baptisia, Cochleria, Echinacea, Phytolacca, Pulsatilla, Scutellaria.

Emergency conditions

Laryngitis
Medicine
Demulcents – Althea, Glycyrrhiza, Ulmus.
Antiseptics – Phytolacca, Populus candicans, Salvia, Thymus, Tussilago.

Listeria
A gram positive bacterial infection.
Causes - Anti partum and intra partum infection e.g. abortion. Sometimes contracted infection can be caused by ingestion of infected dairy products, meat or raw vegetables. It can survive refrigerator temperatures. Infection can cause meningitis, bacteraemia, dermatitis.
Medicine
Allium, Baptisia, Echinacea, Grape seed extract.

Liver failure
Isolate the cause and treat as appropriate
Medicine
Berberis sp., Capsicum, Silybum, Zingiber.

Lumbago see backache

Lymphoedema
Medicines
Arctium, Baptisia, Calendula, Dipteryx odorata [Tonka bean 192 p544], Echinacea, Galium, Hydrastis, Iris, Phytolacca, Scrophularia, Smilax, Stillingia, Thuja, Trifolium.

Mastitis
Is the patient pregnant?
Poultice with Althea, Chamomilla, Phytolacca. Dist Hamamelis. Cold pack.

Measles
Check for signs of otitis or pneumonia.
Antiseptics
Baptisia, Calendula, Commiphora, Echinacea, Thymus and diaphoretics – Achillea, Capsicum, Chamomilla, Eupatorium perfoliatum, Hyssopus, Nepeta, Pulsatilla, Sambucus, Tilia with the emphasis upon elimination. Vitamin C.

Meleana [See haematemesis]

Herbal Medicine - Keys

Meningitis
Medicine
Helleborus niger, Papaver somniferum, Passiflora, Phytostigma venenosum, Pilocarpus jaborandi.

Migraine [See headache]

Myocardial infarction
See angina

Nausea
Check the diet, blood sugar, gall bladder, liver or stomach.
Medicine - antinausea
Atis [inhalation], Ballota, Chamomilla, Chondrus, Cinnamomum, Mentha Species, Zingiber.

Neck pain
Check the following: Airway, purpura, meningism, shock, pain, rash, pyrexia.
Causes - Neck spasm, Neuritis, Arthritis. Treat the cause.

Nervous restlessness and tension
Full dose of one of the following:
Asafoetida, Bacopa, Humulus, Lactuca, Lobelia, Passiflora, Piper me, Scutellaria.
General antispasmodic nervine
Valeriana 2ml Humulus 0.5ml Scutellaria 2ml Ferrula 0.5ml Gentian 0.5ml.
Sig 5ml TDS Aq cal PRN.

Neuritis/Neuralgia
Occurring from muscular spasm e.g. trapezium spasm.
Antispasmodics – Antispasmodic tincture, Ferrula, Filipendula, Piper methysticum, Piscidia, Scutellaria, Valeriana, Viburnum opulus.

Oesophageal varices
The veins are prone to burst with severe haemorrhage and instant death.
Medicine
Capsicum, Lycopus.

Otitis [See ear]

Parasites
Medicine
Allium, Juglans, Ol Melaleuca. Grape seed extract.

Emergency conditions

Peritonitis
Fast.
Medicine
Althea, Dioscorea, Echinacea, Lobelia, Ulmus, Veratrum album/viride, Zingiber.
External – Oleum Ricinus pack.

Physiomedical Pain treatments
- Pain is not a disease and a search must always be made for the cause.
- Pain is often severe and can cause shock.
- Painful conditions must be allayed to relieve suffering.
- Pain can also be a cause of depression as pain depletes the vitality.
- Secretory organs. Pain may be felt as a result of secretory organ tension – treat using relaxants e.g. Lobelia, Dioscorea, Levisticum, Sambucus.
- Inflammatory disease can create pain - see appropriate section.

Psychogenic aetiology
Pain which is unremitting or remains constant with no remission is most likely to have a psychological cause.
Nervine medicine
appropriate to the area concerned - Cannabis, Humulus, Hyoscyamnus, Lactuca, Passiflora, Piscidia.

Analgesic
Cimicifuga 50, Guaiacum 7.5, Gaultheria 25, Humulus 50, Hypericum 25, Passiflora 7.5, Valerian 25, alcohol 25
Sig 2.5-5ml PRN Aq cal. Any of the above can be used singly to full dosage.
Antispasmodic tincturae to relieve spasmodic pain.
Analgesic – Phenobarbitone Herbal [PB]. A compound for the relief of pain - Passiflora, Pulsatilla, Salix nigra, Valeriana of each equal parts.

Colic - intestinal
Empty the bowel and stomach with: fast and enema if severe.
Carminatives:
Acorus, Alpinia, Anethum, Carum, Centarium, Cardomomum, Cinnamomum, Dioscorea, Foeniculum, Lobelia, Melissa, Mentha species, Pimpinella, Zingiber.
Antispasmodics: Hyoscyamnus. [See also paediatrics/specific conditions]

Colic - renal
Medicine
Relaxing diuretics - Agropyron, Aphanes arvensis, Eryngo, Eupatorium purpureum, Hydrangea, Lobelia, Verbena.

Herbal Medicine - Keys

Colic - biliary

Medicine

Hepatic, gall bladder and duct relaxants.

Chionanthus, Leptandra, Podophyllum, Taraxacum.

In all colics a warm enema of – Dioscorea, Lobelia or Nepeta, [Cypripedium].

Inflammation [See also Chapter 6].

Treatment

Careful dietary adjustment and adequate fluids.

Fomentations/plasters. Stimulate elimination. Remove infection. Relieve tension and congestion by – relaxants and diffusives.

Injury

Treatment

Packs hot and/or cold. Soft tissue manipulation/movement/massage.

Injury con't

Hamamelis, Symphytum, Arnica, Stachys palustris [woundwort] - bruises.

Hypericum – injured nerves, spinal injuries, crushed fingers or toes.

Aloe or Urtica – burn or scald pain.

Arnica is specific to bruised, sore, lacerated and contused muscular tissue.

Internal use with care. Tr 1:20 Use 30 gtt in 120ml aqua. Sig 5ml every hour will relieve the muscular soreness and extreme feebleness from severe protracted muscular strain.

External use

Arnica one part to five of warm water can be applied on a compress over the affected parts. Renew every two to three hours.

Caution

> Should a patient become nervously excited, experience tingling of the tongue, mouth or skin followed by numbness, a weak slow pulse, clammy skin, dizzyness, vertigo or dyspnoea, then discontinue its use immediately.

Arnica must never be prescribed in large doses.

Phlebitis

Inflammation of a vein with tenderness, burning and erythema.

Medicine

Aesculus, Centella, Polygonum bistorta, Vitamin E.

Pleural effusion

Medicine

Urgenia maritima.

Emergency conditions

Pneumonia, pneumothorax and pleurisy
To relieve congestion and equalise the circulation - Asclepias, Zingiber.
Inhalation – Friars balsam. Adequate fluids. [See also SARS]
Medicine
Achillea, Aconite, Allium, Asclepias, Atropa, Baptisia, Barosma, Chondrus, Convallaria, Echinacea, Eupatorium perfoliatum, Gelsemium, Linum usitatissimum, Mentha piperita, Nepeta, Sambucus, Taraxacum, Thymus, Veratrum viride, Verbascum, Zingiber. Vitamin C, E.
External
Poultice with Angelica arch., Linum usit., Oleum Camphor diluted.

Poisoning
Acids
Treatment – Milk, Chondrus crispus, Cetraria, Ulmus decoctions.

Poisoning
Carbon monoxide – Confusion, Dizzyness, Extreme tiredness, Persistent headache, Vomiting.
Treatment – Capsicum.
Drugs
Treatment – Stop the drug, Arctium, Capsicum, Plantago plus eliminative medicines e.g. diaphoretics, diuretics etc.
Foods, toadstools
Treatment – Emetic, Silybum.

Pulmonary embolism
Medicine
Allium, Capsicum, Colchicum, Zanthoxylum, Zingiber.

Radiation sickness [See also burns]
Medicine
Agaricus, Aloe, Chamomilla, Eleutherococcus, Fagopyrum, Fucus, Medicago, Oenothera, Panax, Rhodiola, Smilax, Spirulina, Uncaria. Vitamin C.

Rabies/hydrophobia
Infected dog bite transmits the virus.
Treatment
Suck out the poison. Clean the wound with Allium, Calendula, Commiphora, Hypericum. And then poultice with Commiphora and Ulmus.
Anti infective Medicine
Antispasmodic - Antispasmodic Tr., Lobelia.

Herbal Medicine - Keys

Alisma plantago [188 p450], Baptisia, Capsicum, Commiphora molmol, Cynoglossum officinale [Houndstongue – mercury], Echinacea, Rhodea japonica [188 p365].

Rashes
Check the following: Airway, purpura, meningism, shock, stridor. Severe pain or itching, allergy, facial oedema, tongue oedema, dyspnoea, purpura, pyrexia, wide spread discharging or blistering skin. Treat the cause.

Retention of urine
Potentially a serious condition in the acute stage. Acute renal failure must be ruled out. Aetiology – bladder or spinal injury, infections, poliomyelitis, prostate disorders, fibroids, post operatively, uterine prolapse.
Treatment of the cause.
Catheterisation PRN, Warm hip bath.
Medicine
Gelsemium, Lobelia, Verbena, Zea.

Rheumatic pain [See arthritic pain].

SARS
An infection by a corona virus. It is infective in the early stages. Initally the virus attacks the lungs causing pneumonia which can be fatal.
Medicine
Glycerrhiza [HFB August, 2003 quoting German scientific paper in the Lancet].
Lonicera confusa/dasystyla/hypoglauca/japonica – flos.
Constituents - chlorogenic acid.
Anticholesterolaemic, antiviral – herpes, influenza, allays inflammation, anti infective, antitoxin, antioedema. Endotoxin, furunculosis, diarrhoea, dysentery– bacillary, pneumonia, pyrexia, sore throat. Stimulates white blood cells.

Sciatica
Treatment – Rest and relaxation to the back, spinal nerves and legs.
Medicine
Full dose of Harpagophytum, Hypericum and/or Lobelia with a few drops of capsicum. Antispasmodic Tr, Cimicifuga, Gelsemium, Hypericum, Juniperus, Piscidia, Valeriana, Viburnum opulus.
External
Warm fomentation to the painful area – Seneco Jacobaea.
Liniment – Oleum - Camphor, Cajuput, Capsicum, Hypericum or Lobelia.

Emergency conditions

Septicaemia
Bacterial infection of the blood with fever and often a very ill patient.
<u>Medicine</u> septicaemia
Arctium, Baptisia, Capsicum, Commiphora, Echinacea, Iris, Phytolacca.

Shingles
<u>Medicine</u>
Piscidia, Scutellaria.
<u>External</u>
Commiphora, Hypericum.

Shock
Px 1 Antispasmodic tincture Sig 1ml PRN.
Px 2 Star of Bethlehem flower remedy or Rescue Remedy. Sig 4gtt every 15 minutes.
Px 3 Infusium: Arnica, Chamomilla, Melissa, Scutellaria or Stachys.

Sinusitis
Aetiology - Catarrh, fumes e.g. petrol, paint, infection, polyps, stress.
<u>Medicine</u>
Sambucus 4ml with Pulsatilla 0.5ml for immediate pain relief.
Glechoma, Plantago, Solidago.
<u>Crem</u> made of paraffin molle with Ol Menthol, Ol Eucalyptus, Ol Pinus, Ol Mentha pip. Sig 1gtt aa and mix into base.
<u>Steam inhalation</u> boiling water into a bowl add Ol Szygium/Ol Eucalyptus/Ol Mentha piperita/Ol Thymus 2gtt aa. then cover head and bowel with a towel and inhale. Keep the eyes closed.

Snake bites
They defend and attack only when provoked and the snake becomes frightened. Cobra snakes can spit venom up to 3.5 metres distance. Venom is spat into the victim's eyes.
<u>Treatment</u>
Venom should be washed off immediately with copious amounts of water or sucked out of any wound. Snake bites should be treated using a pressure bandage and giving anti venom immediately.
<u>Medicine</u>
Abrus precatorius, Allium, Arctium, Echinacea, Polygala senega, Rauwolfia, Rumex.

Sore throat
Often caused by an infection, tonsillitis, colds, influenza, urinary disease.

Herbal Medicine - Keys

<u>Treatment</u> sore throat
Plenty of fluids, possible short fast. Cold pack to the throat.
Px antiseptic gargle – Salvia, apple cider vinegar.
<u>Medicine</u> to clear the cause – tonsillitis:
Baptisia/Commiphora/Echinacea/Phytolacca.
When pyrexia is present use diaphoretics: Eupatorium perfoliatum or Sambucus [both relaxing]
Achillea/Zingiber [stimulating]
Pulsatilla [nervine for pain].

Splinters/thorns
Remove the splinter if possible. Apply a poultice of Plantago.

Stings [Also see bites]
<u>Shock</u> resulting from a bite or sting.
Aconite, Capsicum with Lobelia, Star of Bethlehem flower remedy.

Bee sting
A bee sting is acid so apply an alkaline - Bicarbonate of soda solution or onion.

Poisonous stings [scorpions, jelly fish, snake, rat]
1] Remove the poison if possible - tourniquet and suck out the poison.
2] Keep the patient calm – give Ferula [asafoetida], Chamomilla or Scutellaria.
3] Antivenomous mixture:
Px1 Allium, Asclepias, Berberis aquifolium, Menispermum canadense, Smilax, Stephania, Zingiber or
Px2 Artemesia vulgaris, Ruta and Salvia - as a warm poultice.

Stonefish, stingray stings
<u>Medicine</u>
Dodonea viscosa.
Cover with apple cider vinegar bandage.

Wasp sting
is alkaline apply lemon juice or apple cider vinegar.

Strain/sprain/fractures
Immobilise the fractured limb to aid rest.
Arnica, Calendula, Hypericum, Symphytum.
<u>External</u>
Hot fomentation to a strained/sprained muscle. Poultice of Symphytum.
Infusion of Calendula 30g to 550ml of water. Sig 15ml TDS.

Emergency conditions

Sunburn [See under burns].

Tetanus
An acute infectious disease caused by Clostridium tetani. It causes tetanic spasm of the involuntary muscles commonly the masseter [jaw] muscle. Infection most commonly supervenes from a wound.
Medicine
Capsicum, Larrea tridentata, Lobelia, Papaver somniferum, Phytostigma venenosum, Scutellaria, Veratrum album/viride.

Tendonitis
Treatment
Rest the limb and apply a cold pack.
Poultice
Arnica - dilute, Gaultheria, Harpagophytum, Ruta, Seneco jacobea, Symphytum.

Toothache
Apply on cotton wool a few drops of Ol. Szygium.

Teething pain
Very suitable for children. Chamomilla - make an infusion and apply to the gums.

Pain after root extraction
Used as a surgical dressing Aloe vera can be put into extraction sockets to encourage healing. Its sedative effects help ease pain. Szygium 2gtt applied upon cotton wool to the tooth/socket.

Painful erupting wisdom teeth
Treatment
Aloe sprayed onto the tooth and gum help ease pain.
Ol Szygium applied upon cotton wool and placed upon the crown of the tooth for a few minutes. Chamomilla tincture applied to the gum eases pain.

Tonsillitis [See sore throat]

Trench foot
As a result of prolonged wet. White wrinkly skin which breaks down rapidly and becomes infected.
Treatment
Clean and dry the feet. Expose to the air to allow healing. When sores or ulcers are present cover with a dry dressing. Px Powder the feet with powdered Symphytum/Ulmus. Commiphora in infected states.

Herbal Medicine - Keys

Ulcers see burns/cuts/scalds/wounds/inflamed wounds.

Ulcers stomach and duodenal - perforated
Fast patient because peritonitis can ensue.
Medicine
Ulmus, Astringents.

Urinary tract infections [See kidney infections above].

Vomiting
Check the following: Airway, fitting, shock.
Commonly caused by infected food, over eating/drinking.
Treatment
Fast with sips of water only, until all the vomiting clears, then introduce food in very small amounts only.
Medicine
antiemetics and demulcents
Ballota, Cinnamomum, Cetraria, Glycyrrhiza.

Wounds
See dermatology in this chapter

.

37
Vitamins, Minerals & Trace Elements

A quick reference guide to dosing with minerals and vitamins

Caffeine, nicotine and alcohol interfere with nutrient absorption.
Alpha –Linolenic acid
An unsaturated fatty acid. It is converted into a omega series 3 fatty acid. Immunoregulator. Reduces cholesterol and is hypotensive. Psoriasis, Eczema, MS, lupus erythematosus, cancer. It is found in flaxseed oil, linseed oil, soya oil, pumpkin and walnuts.
Amino acids
22 amino acids are needed by the body. Amino acids are proteins and all but 8 are made in the body. Current knowledge suggests all but tryptophan are present in Aloe vera.
Antioxidants
A family of chemicals which have specific properties. They neutralise dangerous activity of free radicles.
Sources - Allium, Anethum, Origanum, Petroselinum, Salvia, Thymus [392].
Vit A, C, E, Beta carotine, Selenium and Zinc.
Red wine, green tea are anti oxidant.
Alpha Lipoic acid is a co-enzyme essential in mitochondrial electron transport [energy] reactions. Also a powerful anti oxidant [33]. Supports liver detoxification. Chelates toxic metals and anaesthetics from the blood [230 p111]. Sources – broccoli, spinach, kidney, beef.
DHEA – natures steroid. Supports heart function and allays aging.
Melatonin – a pineal gland secretion that balances the bodies circadian rhythm - sleep and wakefulness. Used in lung cancer, depression, fatigue, insomnia, MS epilepsy. Dark stimulates it's release. Sources – Soya. Sig 3mg nocte. Cancer Sig 50mg daily [230 p149]
Phenyllalanine - natural pain killer, allows endorphines to rise, lowers perception of pain
green lipped muscle - builds up bone and cartilage, contains glycos amino glycans act to allay inflammation.
L. methionine is a component of glycos amino glycans. A potent allayer of inflammation in excess of ibuprofen.
Dairy produce
Lactobacillus is a bacteria that forms upon sour milk and other CHO foods. It produces lactic acid. Lactic acid helps to rebalance the intestinal flora.
Enzymes
Aid digestion to break down sugars and starches. Some enzymes act as catalysts, lipase acts on fats. Aloe vera has lipase, amylase, peroxidase and others.

Herbal Medicine - Keys

Co enzyme Q10 [Ubiquinone].
A fat soluble substance made by the body. Q10 releases energy from food. Adenosine triphosphate [ATP] cannot be produced without Q10. Deficiency causes: cardiomyopathy [35].
The primary treatment is for the heart and blood vessels, hypertension, atherosclerosis, angina, mitral valve trouble, congestive heart failure and enlarged heart [39]. Periodontal gum disease, loose teeth, bleeding and tender gums. Increased cellular damage. Q10 is a free radicle scavenger. It helps to regulate mitochondrial function.
Dose: 15-30mg daily for maintenance
Up to 100mg daily for specific conditions.

Glucosamine
Glucosamine is found in tendon, ligament and cartilage. Glucosamine in clinical trials proved more effective than ibuprofen. Pain showed a significant decrease, along with joint swelling and tenderness. [135]

Vegetable and fish oils
Activity - Stimulate prostaglandins - allay inflammation. Cardiovascular protective. Anti allergic. Auto immune disease.
Suggested intake ratio omega 3 to omega 6 fatty acids is 1:1.

Essential fatty acid oils
The following contain omega 3 & 6 EFA's.
Sources - safflower, sunflower oils.
Blackcurrant seed oil. Borage oil. Evening primrose oil. Linum usititassimum oil. Olive oil. Fish oils – cod liver, mackerel, salmon, herring.
Pumpkin seeds.

Minerals – upper safe daily level. Maximums include USA [FNB and SCF].

Boron	mg	20
Calcium	mg	1500
Chromium	mcg	10
Copper	mg	10
Iodine	mcg	1100
Iron	mg	45
Magnesium	mg	400
Manganese	mg	15
Molybdenum	mcg	600
Phosphorus	mg	1500
Potassium	mg	3500
Selenium	mcg	450
Zinc	mg	40

Vitamins, Minerals & Trace elements

It needs to be remembered that some individuals require more than the typical amounts stated, of vitamins and minerals. Long term shortage of nutrients create hypotrophic cells.

Aluminium
Poisoning from aluminium induces the following effects.
Nausea, diarrhoea, skin rashes, bad tempered children. Long term effects include exhaustion, severe arthritis, loss of memory and [green hair in excessive poisoning in acute cases].

Boron may protect against atherosclerosis [24] Boron combines with calcium to help prevent osteoporosis.

Calcium - Calcium functions in bone and teeth structure. Helps in the transmission of nerve impulses. Enzyme regulation and blood clotting.
It needs phosphorus and magnesium for effective action. Vitamin D helps absorption.
Sources - dairy produce, soya, bread, shellfish, green vegetables, eggs.
Supplementation - calcium citrate.

Chlorine – extracellular anion which combines with sodium.
Source - salt.

Chromium – plays a vital role in sensitising the body's tissues to the hormone insulin. Weight gain tends to impair sensitivity to insulin and thus in turn makes it harder to lose weight. Chromium picolinate helps to preserve muscle and burn more fat. Found in brewers yeast, molasses, grapes, beer, wholegrains.

Cobalt
Sources - meat, fish, dairy foods, eggs.

Copper – deficiency causes higher LD Lipoproteins and lower HD therefore increase in bad cholesterol. Glucose clearance reduced. anaemia, reduced encephalines [pain killers produced by the body]. Where a high copper is found use zinc to rebalance.

Iodine – is essential for normal thyroid function. Thyroid action affects sexual function via neuroendocrine links.
Sources - kelp, salt, seafoods.

Iron – iron uptake may be inhibited by phytates in bread, tannin in tea, carbonates, phosphates, lack of protein.
Sources - pulses, liver, eggs, millet, molasses, dried fruit, green leafy vegetables, wheat. Supplementation - ferrous gluconate.

Magnesium - around 25 grams are distributed in bone and soft tissue. It is involved with ATP and other enzyme reactions. Protein dissemination and energy metabolism are enhanced.
Magnesium levels are frequently low in asthma. Low magnesium status caused a relative lack of the neurotransmitter, dopamine. [25]. A MAFF report in 1994 explains 79% of women do not receive an adequate Mg intake.

949

Herbal Medicine - Keys

Magnesium works on the heart muscle. Natures calcium channel blocker, it blocks the entry of calcium into the heart muscle cells. Resulting in reduced blood pressure. Strengthens heart muscle contraction. The Lancet in 1985 says Magnesium decreases the stickiness of the blood and helps in coronary disease.

Sources - walnuts, almonds, whole grains, wheat germ, green leafy vegetables, molasses. When flour is refined 82% Mg is lost in the process. Rice loses 83% by refining. Refined white sugar 99% is lost.

Supplementation - magnesium citrate.

Manganese – enhances enzymes. It is involved in steroid synthesis, CHO, lipid and protein synthesis. Required for cerebral functioning. Supports the pancreas – diabetes. Epilepsy – prevents seizures. Bone health [osteoporosis], prevents sclerosis, RA.

Sources –
unrefined cereals, whole grains, almonds and pecans, legumes, liver and kidney.

Phosphorus – functions in bone and teeth structure. Fractures, osteoporosis, osteomalacia, rickets. Involved with ATP and RNA/DNA in the utilisation of cellular energy [vital force]. An intracellular buffer. Impaired response to insulin. Renal relaxation or atony enables loss of phosphorus to occur.

Sources - meats - all types, whole grains.

Potassium – an intracellular electrolyte and osmotic balancer. Sodium and chloride outside of the cell results in cell membrane charge. Charges are transferred into nerve impulses creating activation of vital force. Potassium is a diuretic.

Sources - avocados, broccoli, prunes, halibut, bacon, almonds, kale, potatoes, celery, mushrooms, bananas, grapes, meat, milk.

Selenium - selenium and Vit E repair cartilage, inhibits action of lysosomal enzymes, inhibits inflammatory prostaglandins to allay inflammation. Selenium helps detoxification. Selenium is involved in the production of glutathamine oxidase - breaks down rancid fat and free radicles A low selenium intake is associated with higher cancer rates [prostate]. Used in coronary artery disease, liver disease, skin disease, myotonic dystrophy, prostate health, foetal development. Selenium is destroyed by food processing.

Sources - soya, coconut, sesame seeds, herring, tuna, cows and pigs kidney, wheatgerm, pistachios, garlic, seaweed.

Silicon – restores the elasticity of connective tissue of the skin and lungs. Strengthens the skin and hair, prevents greying.

Sources - cereals, beer.

Sodium – an extracellular electrolyte and osmotic cation. Regulates the body fluids: blood and tissue fluid. Sodium is a bone component.

Sources - salt, olive, tuna, beans, cheese, pretzels, bread, celery, oats.

Vitamins, Minerals & Trace elements

Sulphur – a constituent of amino acids. Sulphur is present in some enzyme reactions. Part of glycose – aminoglycans. It is present in the skin, hair, nails, cartilage and connective [collagen] tissue. Sulphur is required to make bile acids, influence fat absorption and is a component of insulin. Used in acne, body odour, itchy, dry skin. Diarrhoea, vomiting. Depression.
Sources - meat, poultry, organs, fish, beans, garlic, dairy produce, pulses and onions.
Vanadium – bone and teeth strength. Diabetes. Hypercholesterolaemia.
Sources - cereals, nuts, Anethum, buckwheat, carrots, green beans, oats, parsley, pepper, turnips. Olive oil.
Zinc around 200 enzymes are zinc dependent. Major groups are: RNA integrity, alkaline phosphatase, carbonic anhydrase. Zinc is vulnerary.
Deficiency of zinc can cause:
Macular degeneration. Night blindness.
Gastrointestinal – anorexia, improves sense of taste and smell, diarrhoea, intestinal dysfunction. Blood sugar control - Type 2 diabetes NIDDM have low plasma zinc.[18]
Enlarged prostate gland.
Dermatological – alopecia, blepharitis, dermatitis, psoriasis, acne.
Neuropsychiatric –depression, irritability, impaired concentration.
Impaired cell mediated immunity. Improves fertility.
Various actions of zinc combinations
Zinc, copper and manganese break down free radicles.
Zinc can deplete copper. Zinc competes with copper for absorption in the GI tract.
Lead excess creates zinc deficiency.
Sources - oysters, shrimps, crab, meat, whole grains, nuts, pulses.
Supplementation – zinc citrate and zinc picolinate.

Vitamins – upper safe daily level. Maximums include USA [FNB and SCF].

Vitamin A	ug	3000
Vitamin C	mg	5000
Vitamin D	ug	1000 [Reference BNJ Vol 15 no3]
Vitamin E	mg	1000
Vitamin B1	mg	100
Vitamin B2	mg	200
Vitamin B3	mg	450
		[synonyms - Nicotinamide, Nicotinic acid, Niacin]
Vitamin B6	mg	200
Folic acid	ug	1000
Vitamin B12	ug	2000

[High dose – 1000ug are indicated in pernicious anaemia, usually 2000ug for the first month].

Herbal Medicine - Keys

Biotin	ug	900
Pantothenic acid	mg	500
Vitamin K	mcg	1000

Vitamin individual effects

Vitamin A + D - help bind calcium.

Vitamin B

B2 reduces migraine attacks.

B3 Derived from vitamin B3 is an ingredient called NADH. NADH increases ATP to improve cellular energy. It is used in energy deficient states e.g. chronic fatigue, depression etc. Dosage of NADH is up to 15mg daily.

Sources - muscle tissue of poultry and cattle.

B6 and B12 help to prevent the risk of dementia.

B12 - comfrey, spinach

Biotin – essential for cellular growth and RNA and DNA production. Deficiencies include grey hair, splitting nails, hair loss, candidiasis.

Sources – organ meats, eggs, chocolate, whole grains, fish.

Vitamin C acts as an anti oxidant. Vit C , lowers total cholesterol and lowers triglycerides. It breaks down histamine.

Vitamin C – buffered form may work better in asthma such as sodium ascorbate or calcium ascorbate.

Vit C and E are destroyed by tobacco, nicotine and caffeine.

Ascorbic acid may appear to aggravate an arthritic condition in some cases, persist with the treatment and adjust the dose accordingly.

Vitamin E can help against Alzheimers disease Sig 2000 iu per day [23]

Excessive vitamin E can leach out calcium from the bones.

Bioflavonoid - [flavonoid] e.g. citrin, hesperidin, quercetin.

Bioflavonoids correct abnormal capillary permeability. They strengthen intercellular cement substances [astringent]. Bioflavonoids are needed with Vitamin C. Bioflavonoids are antioxidant. They restore capillaries to normal. Bioflavonoids counter the ill effects of free radicles. Bioflavonoids strengthen collagen as does vitamin C. Flavonoids are anti viral, anti fungal, antineoplastic, anti microbial, acaricidal. Lipoxygenase inhibitor, Immunemodulator, anti thrombotic.

Sources - apricots, blackcurrants, blackberries, broccoli, cabbage, cantaloupe, cherries, citrus fruit - large amounts in the white layers of the inner skin [pith], dandelion greens, grapes, lemons, melons, mustard greens, onions, peppers, plums, rose hip syrup, sprouts, tomatoes. Crataegus.

Rose hip – is astringent, cholagogue, diuretic & tonic. Contains Vit C, B2, P, K.

Sources from herbs for vitamins and minerals

Fucus and Medicago contain the required elements for building blood as they contain Vitamin C, Chlorophyll, Iron and Iodine.

38
Running a Practice

What this Chapter is about
Herbal practice consists of two businesses. The medical herbalist has to split time
into two parts. The practice of seeing patients/clients will take most of the time. It
must be remembered to be successful one must have a good business plan.
Business will only be rewarding if enough ground work is put in to find the
suitable premises in the best location possible.
Starting a practice will require [1] a business plan [2] finance.

Patient or client?
It could be argued use of the word patient is seen as disempowering to that
individual. A patient may believe them self to be a patient who has an incurable
illness. Whereas the use of the word client suggests a sort of autonomy on behalf
of the client where they take responsibility for their health rather than the medical
herbalist taking all responsibility for their health. The term client can be more self
empowering to the individual.

Where will you practice?
Setting up a practice in the best location is the first point to consider.
Can clients get to you if they use public transport? How far from the bus or rail
station are you likely to be? If a patient has to travel even a short distance it takes
time and older patients want you in a fairly handy place. Can they park easily? Is
access available for wheelchairs?

Are you a lone worker or do you want to work with others in a group practice?
Sometimes a patient will say something to your assistant they may have not
mentioned to you. Remarks can be good for you, even if negative. They help us
grow as people. And to develop a better practice.
A group practice provides support and can encourage you to feel more at home in
an environment which if a lone worker can be a little lonely. Loneliness can rob a
practitioner of self confidence.

Will you work while developing your herbal practice?
A regular income from employment helps keep a roof over your head while
developing your herbal practice. When you work for an employer it takes time
and energy, these qualities are needed for your developing herbal practice. You
only have a finite amount of energy available if you give to an employer then it
means you will have less for your practice.

Herbal Medicine - Keys

What do you wear?
Maybe you are surprised by this question. White coats are out of fashion as they encourage 'white coat syndrome' whereby the patient feels at a distance from the practitioner or may even feel anxious. Patients may perceive incorrectly that you might find the worst. The writer has known of cases where patients blood pressure has risen as a result of 'white coat syndrome'.

Receptionist or do it all yourself?
Having a receptionist eases the transition from the outside to the practitioner. A receptionist can bridge that gap between the two of you. It can provide support and a nice cup of herbal tea for us all.

Male herbalist?
For a male practitioner you must cover yourself and have a female assistant around the place, for your own protection. It will avoid comebacks and litigation. It is best to have others around as it helps to give you support and it is good for patients to see others.

How successful do you want to be?
You may be happy just seeing a few clients a week to start with. As your confidence grows you will take on more difficult cases. Your practice is an extension of yourself. So when you feel happy it reflects upon the business. Likewise when you get low or depressed it will also affect the patient and your relationship with them. Everyone understands that we all have differing moods but you must keep control over your mood at all times. There are some people to whom nothing will be right whatever you try to do for them. It may be necessary to say sorry, I cant help you and refer them to a colleague. You cant treat everyone.

Will you do home visits?
Personally the writer discourages home visits because it takes time and all too often people will not pay for the extra travel time. It's better to get them to see you at the practice. You have all your equipment and medicine available for dispensing straight away.

How much will you charge?
There are no fixed rules on charges. What will the market stand. Is there competition? Find out about competitors and their charges. Check your own outgoings. Consultation time must be charged on an hourly or half hourly basis. No professional herbalist should charge less then £30 per consultation hour.

Running a Practice

Costs of medicines etc: As a guide many health food shops make 25-35% profit on a single product. Some herbs taken as teas are very cheap to buy. People wanting your service will find the money if they really want to see you. Never make your prices too cheap as this devalues the product and the service that you offer.

The herbal business is judged on its ability to provide a reasonable lifestyle for the practitioner from the amount of surplus profit left after business expenditure. Everything that is done within the business must increase sales, enhance margins and reduce overheads so that the business will produce better results.

S is sales, C is cost of sales, GPM is gross profit margin, O is overheads, NP is net profit.

The formula for that result is:

$$S - c = GPM - o = NP$$

[capitals emphasise the most important aspects] [152].

Do you offer reductions?

Reductions can be offered to low wage earners, single parent families or unemployed. Those retired may also qualify for a reduction in fees. You may want to charge only for medicine for some patients. If you offer reductions make sure the patient is worthy of the reduction. Poor people don't as a rule ask. The better off clients, often fuss about the cost. There are no rules for reductions.

Can the patient access you easily?

There is nothing more confusing for people than not knowing who to speak to or being unable to get hold of you. Its bad for business. If you are busy use an answer phone with a clear message and check it regularly. Get back to the client as soon as possible.

Marketing the business.

Marketing any business requires that you sit down and do some homework. We mentioned earlier about setting charges 'How much will you charge'. It will depend upon whether you work from home or a multi practice. Have a shop or private rooms. Your overheads will determine some of your costs. You must charge accordingly.

Marketing the business image may not be as useful to your practice as you imagined it to be. Rather stimulate the prospective buyer of your service and your product [the treatment] to want what you have to offer.

The patient is not interested in your business they want something else. This is an improvement in their well being; for which they will pay you, for the time spent with them and the treatment that you prescribe.

Herbal Medicine - Keys

Telephone
An essential part of a business. A land line is preferable to a mobile number. Patients may not call for information if they have to pay for a costly call to get information on the service you offer. The telephone manner should always be caring and clear, never rushed. Many patients are elderly and may not take in all that you say. Why not send a brochure?

Talks
Giving talks can be productive and bring in new cases for treatment. Some referrals call you up years later and say I heard your talk at such and such! When you give a talk the person may not need your services at that moment in time. Always take brochures along to talks or some home-made preparations for them to see and try. Personally I charge for talks now. When starting off you may wish to talk for free.

Literature
A good image is important for your practice. Create an image and stay with it. Business cards and headed note paper are examples. Your practice information should say what you offer and what will happen when they get to your place. Don't make your leaflet/brochure look like a high street takeaway.

Radio
Short talks on the radio can be helpful to get your name around. Dont expect a lot of business from it. Be careful giving advice over the air because it could come back to haunt you.

Television
If you have a good story line television could well be interested.. Unfortunately there is often too little time to put your point across. It may help further publicity.

Newspapers
Advertising is often a waste of money. First, you should be in the telephone directory yellow pages, Thomson etc. Most people would look first at one of these publications. Newspapers and magazines are full of adverts. The chances are you will waste a lot of money in that sort of media. Internet advertising and web sites are becoming more widely used by the public accessing a practitioner.

Internet
Developing the practice through the internet may be helpful by using a web page. Various courses teach design principles. Email is a necessary these days, don't forget to read them.

Running a Practice

Accountant
Always keep receipts and enter them in an expenses book.
Get a good accountant. Large firms are often only interested in businesses with large turnovers. It is better to go for a smaller firm. Small firms are usually more available to see you when you need help and can answer questions because it is easier to get hold of your accountant. Check the costs and make a note of it. Look around a number of firms to see what they offer. You could do your own accounts to start with, at least until business is sufficient to warrant the cost of an accountant. Get advice in order to make an informed decision.

Summary
To be a good medical herbalist takes time.
A qualification does not make one caring - it has to come from the heart. It is not just about making money - one needs money to live. Charging must reflect your level of competence in the work that you do and the service that you give. Remain accountable to your clients/patients at all times. Treat them with care and they will return to you whenever they have a health problem.

Three points must always be taken into account in any business - the three point prosperity plan. Sales, gross profit margin and overheads govern the business - use the plan as outlined above to improve your level of awareness for successful business and patient care.

****

'It is not clever to pay too much but it is even worse to pay too little. If you pay too much you lose some of your money: that is all.

But if you pay too little, you may occasionally lose everything, since the object you bought cannot serve its intended service.
The law of economics prohibits receiving considerable quality for little money.

If you accept goods at the lowest price you must take the risk of having to add something to it.
And if you do that, then you also have enough money to pay for something better'.

John Ruskin, English philosopher and social reformer, 1819-1900.

39
Herbal Medicines Preparation Formulary with Doses

A quick reference guide to dosing

A
Abies alba
Linamentum Abies resin.
Abrus precatoreus
Restrictions apply. Dosage is determined by the relief of symptoms.
Collyr 1:12
Contraceptive - a single dose 200mg of the powdered seeds give up to 13 months protection.
Acacia catechu
Powdered cort Sig 5g. Tincturae Sig 5ml. Acacia mucilage
Pwd Acacia et aq 1:16 can be used as an internal drink to allay inflammation.
Acacia syrup. Acacia 10g, sucrose 80g, aqua to 100ml
Acacia senegal
Cough linctus Sig 15ml.
Syrup Acacia Acacia syrup Acacia 10g, sucrose 80g, aqua to 100ml.
Employed as a demulcent in linctus for mucous membrane inflammation.
Sig 15ml. Cholesterolaemia Sig up to 50g daily
Achillea millefoleum
Dried herba/flos. Sig 4g
Infusium Sig 2g
Tincturae Sig 10ml
Liquidum extractum Sig 4ml
Succus Sig 5ml
Balneum Sig 100g in muslin.
Acorus calamus
Dried rad Sig 3g. Decoctum 30ml. Tincturae Sig 4ml.
Liquidum extractum Sig 3ml
Aconitum napellus
Restrictions apply. Dosage is determined by the relief of symptoms.
Tincturae rad/fol. 5gtt aqua 120ml Sig 5ml
Tincturae 1:10 Sig 0.3ml [BPC 1949]
Linamentum Aconitum. Tincturae 2% qs Dist. Hamamelis to 100ml.
Ung 3%
Adhatoda
Dried herba Sig 10g. Tincturae Sig 4ml. Liquidum extractum Sig 3ml
Adiantum
Dried herba Sig 2g. Infusium 10ml. Liquidum extractum Sig 2ml

Formulary

Adonis vernalis
Restrictions apply. Dosage is determined by the relief of symptoms.
Dried herba Sig 1g
Infusium herba 1:40 Sig 15ml
Tincturae 1:5 Sig 0.9ml. Liquidium extractum Sig O.12ml
Aesculus
Powdered sem. stripped of bark. Sig 2g. Dect. sem. Sig 15ml.
Dry extract Sig 200mg. Tincturae sem Sig 10ml.
Liquidum extractum sem Sig 2ml. Liquidum extractum cort Sig 4ml.
Agaricus blazei
Decoction Sig 30g. Succus Sig 25ml
Agrimonia
Infusium herba Sig 4g. Tincturae Sig 4ml. Liquidum extractum Sig 3ml
Agropyron repens
Dried rhizome Sig 8g. Tincturae Sig 15ml. Liquidum extractum Sig 4ml
Ajuga reptans
Infusium herba Sig 30ml. Liquidum extractum Sig 4ml
Albizia lebbeck
Powdered cort Sig 2g. Liquidum extractum Sig 3ml
Alchemilla mollis/vulgaris
Dried herba Sig 2g. Tincturae Sig 15ml. Liquidum extractum Sig 4ml
Aletris farinosa - Dried rhizome Sig 0.6g. Liquidum extractum Sig 1ml
       Elixir Sig 4.25ml
Allium Sativa
Dried/fresh bulb Sig 1.5g. Tincturae Sig 10ml
Liquidum extractum Sig 4ml. Succus Allium Sig 8ml. Ol. Allium Sig 0.12ml.
Alnus glutinosa
Infusium fol/bacc Sig 30ml. Liquidum extractum Sig 4ml.
Aloe vera
Succus gel Sig 10-15ml
Laxative - Tincturae 1:10 with LE Glycyrrhiza Sig 0.5-2ml
Laxative & tonic - Tinctura aloes 1:30 with Gentiana, Rhei and Zingiber
Sig 4-8ml
Powder 200mg. Tincturae 1:10 Sig 2ml. Liquidum extractum resin Sig 1ml
Alyosa citriodora
Infusium herba Sig 30ml
Alpinia officinarum
Dried rhizome/rad Sig 2g. Decoctum/decoctum Sig 15ml. Tincturae Sig 4ml.
Alstonia constricta/scholaris
Infusium powdered bacc Sig 30ml. Tincturae Sig 4ml. Liquidum ext. Sig 3ml.
Althea officinalis/Althea Rosea
Dried rad/fol Sig 5g. Dried extract Sig 1g. Decoctum rad Sig 60ml.

Herbal Medicine - Keys

Tincturae Althea fol/rad Sig 25ml. Liquidum extractum fol/rad Sig 5ml.
Syrupus Althaea Althea syrup. Sig 10ml.
Ung extractum 10%
Amenopsis californica
Decoctum rhiz Sig 4g. Tincturae Sig 3ml
Amni visnaga
Powdered sem/herba Sig 30ml. Tincturae Sig 5ml. Liquidum ext. Sig 0.5ml.
Anamirta cocculus
Restrictions apply. Dosage is determined by the relief of symptoms.
Liquidum extractum Sig 0.06ml. Lotion @ 1%. Crem @ 1%.
Andrographis
Dried herba Sig 2g. Liquidum extractum Sig 3ml
Anethum graveolens
Dried sem Sig 4g. Aqua Anetha distillata Sig 4ml. Oleum Anethi Sig 0.2ml.
Angelica archangelica
Dried herba Sig 5g or infuse.
Dried rad/rhiz Sig 2g or as a decoction. Tincturae herba. Sig 5ml. Tr rad. Sig 2ml
Liquidum extractum herba Sig 5ml. Liquidum extractum rad Sig 3ml.
Angelica sinensis
Powder Sig 1g. Tincturae Sig 5ml. Liquidum extractum Sig 2ml
Aphanes [Alchemilla] arvensis
Dried herba 4g. Infusium 4g. Tincturae Sig 10ml. Liquidum extractum Sig 4ml.
Apium graveolens
Action is potentiated by Taraxacum.
Dried fruct/sem Sig 3g. Decoctum Sig 2g. Tincturae Sig 5ml.
Liquidum extractum Sig 2ml. Apium vinegar Sig 15ml.
Apocynum cannabinum/androsaemifoleum
Restrictions apply. Dosage is determined by the relief of symptoms. Dried rad
and rhizome Sig 0.3g. Tincturae Sig 0.5ml. Liquidum extractum Sig 0.25ml.
Aralia racemosus
Liquidum extractum rad/rhiz Sig 4ml
Arctium lappa
Dried fol/ sem/radix Sig 4g. Decoction Sig 15ml. Solid extract Sig 1g
Tincturae Sig 6ml. Liquidium extractum Sig 4ml.
Arctostaphylos uva ursi
Dried fol Sig 4g. Dry extract Sig 210mg. Infusium Uva ursi conc. Sig 4ml.
Tincturae Sig 2ml. Liquidum extractum Sig 4ml. [1ml = 70mg arbutin].
Areca catechu
Restrictions apply. Dosage is determined by the relief of symptoms.
Powder sem [nuts] Sig 4g. Decortum 1:20.
Liquid extractum sem/fruct/rind Sig 4ml. Enema decoction Sig 1:20

Formulary

Aristolochia serpentaria
Restrictions apply. Dosage is determined by the relief of symptoms.
Powdered rad,rhiz Sig 100mg. Concentrated infusion 2:5 Sig 4ml.
Tincturae Sig 4ml. Liquidum extractum Sig 2ml.
Armoracia rusticana
Fresh rad Sig 6g. Powder Sig 250mg. Decoctum 1:20 Sig 120 ml BD.
Tincture Sig 10ml. Liquidum extractum Sig 2ml.
Oleum @ 2% strength.
　　　Poultice - Grated fresh rad 15g and wrap in muslin then apply.
　　　Acetum Armoracea Armoracea vinegar. Sig 5-10ml.
　　　Spiritus Armoraciae composit. Compound spirit of Armoracia. Sig 4ml
　　　Tincturae Armoraciae com. Compound tincture of Armoracia. Sig 30ml
Arnica montana
Restrictions apply. Dosage is determined by the relief of symptoms.
Advisable to start with a very small dose and observe the patient.
Potency of 3x or 6x. Oropharyngeal treatment – 10% strength.
Dried rad Sig 2g.
Tincturae 1:10 Sig 0.25ml [5gtt]. Safer dosage is 5ml aqua ad 100 Sig 5ml TDS
Liquidum extractum flos Mix LE 30gtt with Aqua 120ml. Sig 5ml TDS
Oleum 1:5 Dilute with five times the volume.
Ung. up to 25% Tr. Oleum @ 15%
Artemesia abrotanum
Dried herba Sig 4g. Liquidium extractum Sig 4ml.
Artemesia absinthium
Dried herba Sig 2g. Infusium Sig 30ml.
Tinctura Sig 1ml. Liquidum extractum Sig 2ml
Artemesia annua
Dried herba Sig 3g. Liquidum extractum Sig 5ml.
Larger doses to effect in malaria up to 13ml TDS.
Artemesia tridentata
Liquidum extractum fol/flos Sig 4ml.
Artemesia vulgaris
Dried herba Sig 2g. Infusium herba Sig 15ml.
Liquidum extractum Sig 2ml.
Asarum canadense
Restrictions apply. Dosage is determined by the relief of symptoms. Taken hot it
is a strong diaphoretic.
Infusium rad/rhiz Sig 30ml
Parturition -
Sig Tincturae 5gtt aqua 100ml - Sig 5ml every 10 minutes for pain or weakness.
Asclepias tuberosa
Dried rad Sig 4g. Infusium Sig 4g. Tincturae Sig 2.5ml. Liquidum ext. Sig 2ml.

Herbal Medicine - Keys

Asparagus racemosus
Liquidum extractum Sig 4ml.
Aspidosperma quebracho blanco
Restrictions apply. Dosage is determined by the relief of symptoms.
Dried bacc/rad/fol Sig 50mg. Tincturae Sig 4ml. Liquidum extractum Sig 2ml.
Asphaltum -
Astragalus membranaceus
Dried rad Sig 2g. Liquidum extractum rad Sig 3ml.
Interferon effect Sig up to 8g daily. Oncology patients - Sig up to 20g daily.
Atropa belladonna
Restrictions apply. Dosage is determined by the relief of symptoms.
Dried herba Sig 50mg. Dried rad Sig 30mg. Dry extract Sig 60mg.
Tincturae Atropa radix. 1:10 Sig 0.5ml.
Liquidum extractum Atropae Rad. Sig 0.2ml. Ung Atropa @ 2%.
Mist Atropa paediatric [prepare fresh]
Tr Atropa rad 0.15ml, Tr Auranti 0.01ml, Glycerol 0.5ml, Syrup 1ml aq add 100.
Sig up to one year 5ml. 1-5 years 10ml. 5ml contains 45 micrograms of alkaloids
    Ung Atropa 2%.
    Oculentum Atropa 1%.
    Guttae pro oculus Atropa 1g Aqua sterile to 100ml. Sig 5gtt.
    Linimentum Atropinae – Atropa 1ml, Ol Olive 15ml, Ol Ricinus
    15ml Ol Lavandula 1ml Alcohol to 100. Apply with gentle friction.
Avena sativa
Tincturae Avenae herba or sem 10ml. Liquidum extractum Sig 4ml.
Azadirachta
Infusium fol/fruct/sem/bacc/rad 1:20 Sig 30ml. Tincturae bacc,fol. Sig 4ml

B
Backhousia myrtifolia
Tincturae Sig 4ml
Bacopa monniera
Dried herba 2g. Liquidum extractum Sig 4ml
Ballota nigra
Dried herba Sig 4g. Tincturae Sig 2ml. Liquidum Extractum Sig 3ml
Baptisia tinctoria
Small doses are stimulant. Large doses are emetic.
Powder rad Sig 1g. Decoctum Sig 1g. Tincturae 5ml.
Liquidum extractum Sig 1.3ml. Ung 1 Part LE to 8 parts base.
Barosma betulina
Dried fol Sig 2g. Tincturae Sig 4ml. Liquidum extractum Sig 4ml

Formulary

Bellis perennis
Dried flos/herba/rad Sig 5g
Berberis aquifolium
Dried rad/rhiz Sig 2g. Decoctum Sig 2g.
Tincturae Sig 4ml. Liquidum extractum Sig 2ml.
Berberis vulgaris
Dried cort/bacc Sig 2g. Decoctum 2g. Tincturae Sig 4ml.
Liquidum extractum Sig 2ml
Betula alba/pendula
Fol and sap - diuretic. Cort - antiseptic. Inner cort - astringent. Buds - laxative.
Dried fol Sig 2g. Tincturae fol Sig 5ml. Succus Sig 10ml.
Borago officinalis
Oleum Sem Sig 500mg. Infusium herba Sig 5g. Tincturae Sig 10ml
Borrea verticillata
Boscia senegalensis
Boswellia serrata
Use small dose initially. Liquidum extractum Oleo gum resin Sig 4ml
Bryonia alba
Restrictions apply. Dosage is determined by the relief of symptoms. The physiological dose is small. Given alone or alternate with other medicines. Preferable in a syrup form to aid the taste.
Liquidum extractum Sig 10gtt in 120ml aqua. Sig 5ml hourly in acutes.
Maximum dosage
Dried rad Sig 0.6g. Tincturae 1:10 Sig 0.6ml. Liquidum extractum Sig 0.7ml
Bupleurum falcatum
Dried rad Sig 2g. Liquidum extractum Sig 4ml
Butyrospermum paradoxum
External.

C
Caesalpinia bonducella
Powdered kernals Sig 1.5g
Cajunus cajun
Calendula officinalis
Dried florets Sig 2g. Infusium Sig 2g.
Tincturae Sig 10ml. Liquidum extractum Sig 4ml. Ung Calendula @ 10%.
Calluna vulgaris
Dried herba/flor Sig 2g. Tincturae Calluna Sig 4ml. Liquidum extractum Sig 2ml
Cannabis indica
Restrictions apply. Dosage is determined by the relief of symptoms.
Dried herba Sig 1g. Sem Sig 10g. Resin Sig 1g. Tincturae Sig 1ml

Capsella
Dried herba Sig 4g. Tincturae Sig 10ml. Liquidum extractum Sig 4ml.
   Conc. Inf. Capsella. Concentrated Infusion of Capsella Sig 10ml
Capsicum
Fructus Sig 120mg. Tincturae 1:5 Sig 1ml. Tincturae 1:20 Sig 2ml.
External oleoresin up to 5%
   Compound Tincture of Capsicum et Lobelia.
   Antispasmodic. Relaxant. Advised in spasm and tetanus. Sig 20gtt PRN.
   Stimulating Linimentum 1
   Capsicum 4 Camphor 3 Guaiacum 4
   Stimulating Linimentum 2
   Capsicum 40 Cypressus 1 Mentha piperita 1 Origanum 1 Pinus 1

   Diptheria & Scarlatina gargle It can be used in an atomiser.
   Sig Gargle and paint on the tonsils every two hours.
   Sprains, bruises & neuralgia lotion
   Capsicum 3 parts. Lobelia 16 parts. Artemesia absinthium 1 part.
   Rosmarinus 1 part Mentha viridus 1 part.
   Linimentum Capsicum
   Painted on the skin or applied on lint in rheumatic conditions, sciatica, or
   chest affections.
   Unguentum Capsicum
   Capsicum 10% in a base of yellow paraffin molle 60%.
Carica papaya
Fresh fruit may be consumed as a desert.
Wounds - apply strips over the wound and dress.
Carum carvi
Powdered fructus Sig 2g. Infusium Sig 2g. Tincturae Sig 4ml.
Liquidum extractum Sig 2ml.
   Oleum Cari Sig 0.2ml
   Aqua Cari distillata 1:10 Sig 30ml. **Aqua Cari concentrate** Sig 1ml
Cassia acutifolia/angustifolia
Use with aromatics or carminatives.
Give at night a full dose for relief of constipation. Fol is stronger than the pods.
Dry extract 0.5g. Dried fol Sig 2g. Dried sem pods Sig 2g.
Liquidum extractum fol Sig 2ml.
   Composita carminative, laxative and tonic.
   Cassia. Rheum. Mentha piperita
   Antibilious physic
   Cassia. Ipomaea. Zingiber
   Confection Cassia Sig 10-15ml
   Syrupus Cassia Sig 8ml

Formulary

Infusium Cassia concentratum Sig 2-8ml
Tincturae Cassia composita Sig 2-4ml
For stat dose Sig 8-16ml.
Mistura Cassia composita Sig 60ml.
Castanea sativa
Infusium bacc/fol Sig 4g. Liquidum extractum fol Sig 4ml
Castanospermine australe
Catha edulis
Restrictions apply. Dosage is determined by the relief of symptoms.
Fresh/dried fol chewed or infused. Sig 200g
Catharanthus roseus [see Vinca]
Caulophyllum
As an antispasmodic it requires to be given in large doses.
Dried rad/rhiz Sig 5g. Decoctum Sig 30ml. Tincturae Sig 2ml.
Liquidum extractum Sig 2ml
    Liquor Caulophyllum et Pulsatilla For antispasmodic effect. Sig 4ml
    Liquor Caulophyllum et Pulsatilla compositus
Prescribed as Antispasmodic and Uterotonic. Sig 4ml
Centaurium erythraea
Taste may be improved with Angelica or Mentha piperita AC.
Infusium Sig 60ml. Dried herba Sig 4g. Liquidum extractum Sig 4ml
Centella asiatica
Dried fol Sig 0.6g. Liquidum extractum Sig 4ml
Cephalis
Full dosage will produce a free emesis Sig 2g
Dried rad Sig 120mg. Tincturae Sig 1ml.
Liquidum extractum Sig 0.12ml. Alkaloidal content 0.1%
    Elixir Cephalis Sig 2ml. **Mist Pertussus** Sig 5ml
    Syrupus Cephalis Sig 30ml.
Paediatric under 1 year of age Syrupus Cephalis Sig 10ml
Cetraria islandica
Decoctum thalus 1:20 Sig 120ml. Jelly is often employed. Infusium Sig 6g
Tincturae Sig 30ml. Liquidum extractum Sig 6ml
Chamaelirium luteum
Small doses often produce remarkable results.
Dried rad/rhizome Sig 2g. Tincturae Sig 4ml. Liquidium extractum Sig 2ml
Chamomilla recutita
Dried flos Sig 8g. Tincturae Sig 15ml. Liquidum extractum Sig 4ml.
Garg infusium. Sig 3g. Inhalation Sig Inhale steam from an aqueous infusion.
Balneum 100g in muslin. Ung Chamomilla 10%

Chamaemelum nobile
A bitter remedy.
Dried flos Sig 4g. Tincturae Sig 4ml. Liquidum extractum Sig 4ml
Chasmanthera dependens -
Chelidonium majus
Restrictions apply. Dosage is determined by the relief of symptoms.
Collyr Infusium Chelidonium in an eyebath aqua frig.
Dried herba 2g. Tincturae herba Sig 2ml. Liquidum extractum Sig 2ml
Chelone
Liquidum extractum Sig 4ml
Chenopodium olidum
Restrictions apply. Dosage is determined by the relief of symptoms. Powdered
sem Sig 4g. Infusium herba Sig 30ml. Liquidum extractum Sig 4ml
Chenopodium ambrosioides
Restrictions apply. Dosage is determined by relief of Symptoms.
Oleum et sucrose/emulsion mane - adult dose Sig 16gtt. 6-8 years 6gtt [Bartrum].
Dose for two days follow with cathartic each dose - Oleum Ricinus 15-30ml.
Weiss recommends only robust children be treated at 1 gtt for each year and
followed by a second dose two hours later. After the second dose Oleum Ricinus
15-30ml.
Powdered sem boiled in milk Sig 4g. Liquidum extractum Sig 4ml
Chimaphilla umbellata
Dried fol Sig 3g. Liquidum extractum Sig 5ml
Chionanthus virginicus
Liquidum extractum rad/bacc Sig 2ml
Chlorophora excelsa
Decoctum cort Sig 2ml
Chondrodendron tomentosum
Solid extract Sig 1.5g.
Liquidum extractum rad/stip. Sig 10ml.
Chondrus crispus
Dried thalus Sig 10g. Infusium thalus Sig 10g. Decoctum Sig 120ml.
    Jelly - Sig drink freely.
Cichorium
Decoctum rad Sig 30ml. Succus Sig 15ml.
Cimicifuga racemosus
Dried rad/rhizome Sig 2g. Standardised extract Sig 8mg.
Tincturae Sig 2ml. Liquidum extractum Sig 4ml
Cinchona species
Restrictions apply. Dosage is determined by the relief of symptoms.
Powdered cort Sig 1g. Tincturae Sig 4ml. Liquidum extractum Sig 1ml

Formulary

Cinnamomum zeylandicum
Dried bark Sig 1.5g. Tincturae Sig 6ml. Liquidum extractum Sig 1.3ml.
    Aqua Cinnamomum Sig 30ml. **Ol Cassia** Sig 0.2ml
Citrus aurantium/limon
Oleum Auranti/citrus Sig 0.2ml. Infusium Auranti Sig 4ml. Tincturae Sig 4ml.
Liquidum extractum Sig 2ml. **Elixir simplex** Simple elixir Sig 8ml
Clutia abyssinica
Rad Sig 2g
Cnicus benedictus [Carbena benedicta - holy thistle]
Dried herba Sig 3g. Infusium Sig 3g. Tincturae Sig 10ml. Liquidium Ext. Sig 4ml
Codonopsis pilusula
Dried rad Sig 5g. Tincturae Sig 5ml
Cola acuminata/nitida
Dried sem Sig 3g. Dry extract Sig 0.75g
Tincturae Sig 10ml. Liquidum extractum Sig 2ml
Colchicum autumnale
Restrictions apply. Dosage is determined by the relief of symptoms.
Dried corm Sig 200 mg. Dry extract Sig 30mg. Tincturae corm Sig 2ml
Coleus forskohlii
Collyr - 4 gtt and dilute with aqua in an eyebath QDS.
Dried rad Sig 4g. Liquidum extractum Sig 4ml
Collinsonia canadensis
Dried rad Sig 4g. Tincturae Sig 4ml. Liquidum extractum Sig 4ml
Mist Collinsonia and Hamamelis
LE Sig 30gtt aa every 2 hours. Indications: Haemorrhoids and haemorrhages.
Combretum micranthum
Commiphora molmol
Give in small doses, you will often find that drop doses are sufficient.
Tincturae resin Sig 2.5ml. Liquidum extractum Sig 2ml.
Gargle Sig 60gtt aq frig. Dental powder @ 10% strength
Thompsons no 6 [Capsicum 1 part and Myrrh 4 parts] Highly stimulating
compound for asphyxia, drowning, electrocution, where a vital positive stimulant
is required. Sig 2ml. Tincturae resin Sig 2.5ml
Commiphora mukul
Tincturae Sig 2ml
Conium maculatum
Restrictions apply. Dosage is determined by the relief of symptoms.
Pwd. fol/fruct Sig 0.5g. Liquidum extractum Sig 0.4ml. Ung Conium fol/fruct 7%
Convallaria majalis
Restrictions apply. Dosage is determined by the relief of symptoms.
Acute conditions full dose.

Herbal Medicine - Keys

Convallaria continued
Infusium flos/herba Sig 15ml. Tincturae 1:8 Sig 1ml. Liquidum extractum Sig 2ml. IV injection in dilution over 4 minutes.
Coptis trifolia/chinensis/teeta
Powdered Rhiz Sig 1.2g. Tincturae Sig 3.5ml. Liquidum extractum Sig 4ml
Corallorhiza odontorhiza
Infusium Sig 30ml. Liquidum extractum Sig 2ml
Corydalis ambigua/yanhunuo
Dried rad 3g. Liquidum extractum Sig 3.5ml
Crataeva nurvala
Decoctum dried rad/cort Sig 10ml. Liquidum extractum Sig 3ml
Crataegus species
Dried fol Sig 3g. Infusium flos Sig 30ml. Tincturae flos/bacc/fol Sig 10ml. Liquidum extractum Sig 2ml.
Croton eleuteria
Restrictions apply. Dosage is determined by the relief of symptoms.
Dried bacc/fruct/sem Sig 2g. Infusium Sig 30ml.
Tincturae fruct/sem. Sig 4ml. Liquidum extractum Sig 3ml
Curcuma longa
Dried rhiz Sig 4g. Liquidum extractum Sig 4ml.
Cyamopsis tetragonolobus [Guar gum].
Fibre from sem Sig 10g
Cymbopogon citratus
Herba 5g. Rad Sig 2g.
Cynara scolymus
Dried fol Sig 3g. Dry extract 1:12 0.5g. Rad Sig 4g.
Tincturae Sig 6ml. Liquidum extractum Sig 2ml
Cypripedium
Dried rad Sig 4g. Tincturae Sig 4ml. Liquidum extractum Sig 4ml
Cytisus scoparius
Dried herba/fol Sig 2g. Infusium 1:10 Sig 60ml
Decoctum 1:20 Sig 120ml. Tincturae Sig 2ml. Liquidum extractum Sig 4ml

D
Datura stramonium
Restrictions apply. Dosage is determined by the relief of symptoms.
Dry extract Sig 60mg. Up to 500mg in Parkinsons.
Cigarettes each contains 1g Stramonium.
Infusium fol/fleur Sig 200mg. Tincturae 1:10 Sig 2ml.
Liquidum extractum Sig 0.2ml
Daucus carota
Dried herba Sig 4g. Liquidum extractum Sig 4ml

Formulary

Delphinium
Powder decoction sem Sig 150mg. Tincturae 1:10 Sig 0.25ml.
Tr Delphinium 4ml aqua to 120ml. Sig 5ml TDS.
Ung Staphysagria @ 20%.
Lotion Staphysagria. Stavesacre lotion.
Desmodium ascendans
Tincturae herba Sig 5ml
Dicentra canadensis
Infusium rad Sig 30ml. Liquidum extractum Sig 4ml
Digitalis lanata/purpura
Treatment is determined by the glycoside requirement and level of tolerance.
In heart failure a small to very small dose is required. Duration of use- short term.
Standardised powder
Infusium fol Sig 7ml [Ellingwood. p215]. Infusium fol Sig 15ml [174 p226].
Tincturae D. purpura 1:10 fol Sig 1 ml [174 p226].
Tincturae D. purpura 1:10 fol Sig 1.75ml [184 p49].
Tincturae D. purpura 1:10 fol Sig 1ml [188 p189].
Tincturae D. purpura Sig 1ml [BPC 1959].
Dioscorea villosa
Full dose expected to work quickly, within 2 hours – otherwise change medicine.
Dried rad/rhizome Sig 4g. Tincturae Sig 5ml. Liquidum extractum Sig 4ml
Dipsacus fullorum/sylvestris
Infusium flos/rad Sig 5g.
Dodonea viscosa
Infusium Sig 30ml. Tincturae fol/rad Sig 4ml.
Drima altissima [see Urgenia].
Drosera rotundifolia
Dried herba Sig 2g. Tincturae Sig 1ml. Liquidium Extractum Sig 2ml
Dryopteris felix mas
Restrictions apply. Dosage is determined by the relief of symptoms.
Powdered rhiz/fronds Sig 10g. Liquidum extractum Sig 6ml.
Follow with Oleum Castor or saline to promote rapid expulsion of the remedy.

E
Echinacea species
Dried rad/rhiz Sig 1.5g. Tincturae Sig 5ml. Liquidum Extractum Sig 2ml.
Succus Echinacea Sig 3ml
Echium vulgare
Infusium herba Sig 30ml
Eclipta alba
Tincturae herba. Sig 4ml
Elaeis guineensis

Herbal Medicine - Keys

Elettaria cardamomum
Dried sem Sig 2g. Tincturae Sig 4ml. Liquidum extractum Sig 4ml
    Tinctura Composita Cardamomum [Compound Tr Cardamom] Sig 4ml
Eleutherococcus senticosus
Dried rad/bacc. Sig 1.3g. Inf. Sig 3g. Tincturae Sig 15ml. Liquidum ext. Sig 3ml.
Embelia schimperi
Restrictions apply. Dosage is determined by the relief of symptoms.
Powdered fruct. Sig 4g. Embelia ribes/robusta fruct. Sig 16g.
Liquidum extractum Sig 4ml.
Ephedra sinica
Restrictions apply. Dosage is determined by the relief of symptoms.
Dried cut herba 23g provides 300mg of ephedrine.
Children Sig 40mg herba per kg of body weight. Dried rad Sig 2.5g. Inf. Sig 2g.
Tincturae Sig 10ml. Liquidum extractum Sig 3ml.
Epilobium angustifoleum
Decoctum Sig 15ml. Tincturae rhizome Sig 5ml. Ung fol @ 10%.
Equisetum arvense
Dried herba Sig 4g. Tincturae Sig 10ml. Liquidum extractum Sig 4ml. Lotion and
poultice – steep 20g herba in 250ml aqua covered for 10 minutes. Balneum 60g
Erigeron canadense
Oleum as a haemostatic is more effectual. Tincturae herba/sem Sig 10ml.
Liquidum extractum herba/sem Sig 4ml
Eryngium maritimum
Dried rad Sig 4g. Tincturae Sig 5ml. Liquidum extractum Sig 4ml
Erythrina Senegalensis
Decoctum bacc Sig 1g.
Erythroxylum catuaba
Infusium Sig 30ml. Tincturae Sig 1ml
Erythroxylum coca
Restrictions apply. Dosage is determined by the relief of symptoms.
Liquidum extractum Sig 2ml
Eschscholzia californica
Dried herba Sig 3g. Infusium Sig 3g. Tincturae Sig 4ml. Liquidum ext. Sig 4ml
Eucalyptus globulus
Infusium fol Sig 2g. Tincturae Sig 10ml. Liquidum Extractum Sig 4ml.
Ol Eucalyptus Sig 0.2ml. Inhalation Ol 5gtt diluted in water.
Euonymous atropurpureus
Dried rad/cort Sig 1g. Tincturae Sig 2.5ml. Liquidum extractum Sig 1ml.
Eupatorium perfoliatum
Dried herba Sig 2g. Tincturae Sig 4ml. Liquidum extractum Sig 2ml.
Eupatorium purpureum
Dried rad Sig 4g. Tincturae Sig 2ml. Liquidum Extractum Sig 4ml.

Formulary

Euphorbia capitata/hirta/pilulifera
Herba Sig 300mg. Tincturae Sig 2ml. Liquidum extractum Sig 0.5ml
Euphrasia officinalis
Dried herba Sig 4g. Tincturae Sig 4ml. Liquidum extractum Sig 4ml

F
Ferrula asafoetida
Powdered resin Sig 1g. Tincturae resin Sig 4ml
      Emulsion Asafoetidae Sig 15ml. **Enema Asafoetida** Sig 120ml.
      Mistura Asafoetida composita Sig 10ml. **Tablet** containing 1g. Sig 2.
Filipendula ulmaria
Infusium herba/flos Sig 5g. Decoctum rad Sig 5g. Tincturae herba Sig 10ml.
Liquidum extractum Sig 6ml
Foeniculum vulgare
Infusium crushed dried fruct Sig 3g. Liquidum extractum Sig 3ml.
      Conc. Aqua Foenic. Concentrated Fennel water Sig1ml
Fraxinus elselsior
Liquidum extractum fruct/fol/bacc. Sig 2ml
Fucus vesiculosis
Gradually increase dosage. Check the thyroid function.
Dried thallus Sig 10g. Tincturae Sig 10 ml. Liquidum extractum Sig 8ml.
Fumaria officinalis
Dried herba Sig 4g. Tincturae Sig 4ml. Liquidum extractum Sig 4ml

G
Galanthus nivalis See Narcissus
Galega officinalis
Dried fol. Sig 2g. Tincturae Sig 5ml. Liquidum extractum Sig 2ml.
Galeopsis ochroleuca
Liquidum extractum Sig 4ml
Galium aparine
Dried herba Sig 4g. Tincturae Sig 10ml.
Liquidum extractum herba Sig 4ml. Succus Sig 10ml.
Galium odoratum
Dried herba Sig 5g. Infusium Sig 30ml
Ganoderma lucidem
Dried mushroom Sig 10g. Powder 0.5g.
Garcinia cambogia
Dried rind Sig 5g
Gaultheria procumbens
Dried fol Sig 1g. Tincturae Sig 2ml. Liquidum extractum Sig 1ml
Geijera parvifolia Tincturae 3ml

Herbal Medicine - Keys

Gelsemium sempervirens
Restrictions apply. Dosage is determined by the relief of symptoms.
Dried rad and rhizome Sig 60mg. Tincturae 1:10 Sig 1ml. 1ml contains 0.03 –
0.034 alkaloids. **Compound** Gelsemium & Hyoscyamnus. Sig 1ml.
Gentiana lutea
Combine with an aromatic or demulcent to make it more palatable.
Dried rad/rhiz Sig 2g. Tincturae Sig 10ml. Liquidum extractum Sig 4ml
 Concentrated Compound Gentiana Infusium
 Con. Co. Infusion Gentian. Sig 2ml.
 Compound Gentiana Tincturae Compound Gentian tincture. Sig 5ml.
Geranium maculatum
Dried rhiz Sig 2g. Tincturae Sig 4ml. Liquidum extractum Sig 4ml
Geum urbanum
Infusium herba Sig 4g. Liquidum extractum Sig 4ml
Ginkgo biloba
Dried fol/sem Sig 3g. Dry extract Sig 50mg. Tincturae Sig 10ml.
Liquidum extractum Sig 4ml
Glechoma hederacea
Dried herba Sig 4g. Tincturae Sig 10ml. Liquidum extractum Sig 4ml
Glycyrrhiza glabra
Dried rad/rhiz Sig 4g. Dry extract Sig 600mg
Tincturae Sig 5ml. Liquidum extractum Sig 5ml
Glycyrrhiza uralensis
Dried rad Sig 2g. Tincturae Sig 3ml
Gnaphalum ulignosum
Infusium Sig 4g. Tincturae Sig 4ml. Liquidum extractum Sig 4ml
Gossypium hirsutum
Solid extract Sig 1.25g. Tincturae bacc. Sig 4ml
Liquidum extractum Sig 4ml
Grifolia frondosa
Dried mushroom Sig 10g
Grindelia camporum/robusta
Dried herba Sig 3g. Tincturae Sig 1ml. Liquidum extractum Sig 1ml
Guaiacum officinale
Dried bark/heartwood/resin Sig 2g. Tincturae Sig 4ml.
Liquidium extractum Sig 2ml
Gymnema sylvestre
Dried fol Sig 5g. Infusium Sig 30ml. Liquidum extractum Sig 3ml

H
Hagenia abyssinica
Liquidum extractum flos Sig 4ml

Formulary

Hamamelis virginiana
Dried fol/bacc Sig 2g. Decoctum Sig 3g. Tincturae Sig 5ml.
Liquidum extractum Sig 4ml
Garg. Sig 3g.
    Dist Hamamelis. Apply to affected area PRN.
    Ung Hamamelis @ 10%
    Suppository – 1g decoctum extract.
    Compress @ 10 % decoctum.
    Poultice @ 30%
    Spray hydrosol dist hamamelis

Harpagophytum procumbens
Dried rhiz/tub Sig 2g. Tincturae tub Sig 10ml. Liquidum extractum Sig 2ml

Hedera helix
Infusium fol Sig 2g. Tincturae Sig 5ml. Liquidum extractum Sig 1ml.

Helleborus niger
Restrictions apply. Dosage is determined by the relief of symptoms.
Liquidum extractum rhiz Sig 0.6ml

Hemidismus indica
Dried herba. Sig 3.5g. Tincturae Sig 5ml

Heracleum mantegazzianum
Herba/fruct/rad.

Hieracium pilosella
Dried herba. Sig 4g. Liquidum extractum Sig 4ml. Syrup Sig 20ml

Humulus lupulus
Small doses are advised in nervous anxiety while larger doses in insomnia and where sedation are required. Dried strobile Sig 1g. Dry extract Sig 80mg [0.08g]. Soft extract 1g. Tincturae Sig 10ml. Liquidum extractum Sig 2ml

Hydrangea arborescens
Dried rhizome Sig 4g. Tincturae Sig 10ml. Liquidum extractum Sig 4ml

Hydrastis canadensis
Dried rad/rhizome Sig 1g. Dry extract Sig 120mg. Tincturae Sig 2ml.
Liquidum extractum Sig 1ml.
Collyr Sig 2-3gtt in an eyebath with tepid aqua.

Hyoscyamnus niger
Restrictions apply. Dosage is determined by the relief of symptoms. Small doses stimulate and large doses sedate.
Dried fol/flos Sig 1g. Tincturae Sig 1ml. Liquidum extractum Sig 0.25ml

Hypericum perforatum
Dried herba/flos Sig 2g. Dry extract Sig 300mg. Tincturae Sig 4ml. Liquidum extractum Sig 4ml

Hyssopus officinalis
Dried herba Sig 4g. Tincturae Sig 4ml. Liquidum extractum Sig 4ml

Herbal Medicine - Keys

I

Ilex paraguariensis
Dried herba/fol Sig 4g. Infusium Sig 30ml. Tr. Sig 10ml. Liquidum ext. Sig 4ml.
Inula helenium
Dried rad Sig 4g. Tincturae Sig 5ml. Liquidium Extractum Sig 4ml
Iris versicolor
Cathartic - full dose. Dried rad/rhiz Sig 2g. Tincturae Sig 10ml.
Liquidum extractum Sig 2ml

J

Jateorhiza calumba
Powdered rad Sig 2g. Tincturae Sig 2ml. Liquidum extractum Sig 2ml
Juglans cinera
Dried fol Sig 3g. Liquidum extractum cort Sig 6ml
Juniperus communis
Always use a small dose and administer with a demulcent. Dried bacc Sig 3g.
Oleum Juniperus Sig 0.2ml. Tincturae Sig 10ml. Liquidum extractum Sig 3ml.

K

Krameria triandra
Gargarisma - Tincturae diluted with 10 parts aqua. Sig gargle QDS
Gargarisma - Infusium 2g aqua 150ml Sig gargle QDS
Dried rad Sig 2g. Decoctum 30ml. Tincturae Sig 4ml

L

Lactuca virosa
Dried fol Sig 3g. Tincturae Sig 4ml. Liquidum extractum Sig 4ml
Lamium album
Infusium Sig 10ml. Tincturae Sig 5ml
Larrea tridentata
Infusium fol Sig 5g
Lavandula angustifolia
Dried flos/fol Sig 2g. Tincturae Sig 10ml. Liquidum extractum Sig 4ml. Oleum
Sig 4gtt on sugar cube. Spray Aqua Lavandula.
Ledum latifoleum
Dried fol Sig 5g. Infusium Sig 60ml
Leonurus cardiaca
Dried herba Sig 4g. Tincturae Sig 10ml. Liquidum extractum Sig 4ml
Leptandra virginica
Tincturae rad Sig 4ml. Liquidum extractum Sig 4ml
Leptospermum petersoni
Tincturae Sig 1ml

Formulary

Levisticum officinale
Dried fruct/rad/rhiz Sig 4g. Liquidum extractum Sig 2ml
Ligustrum lucidum
Decoctum fol/bacc Sig 15ml. Tincturae fol/bacc Sig 4ml
Ligustrum porteri
Tincturae rad Sig 3ml
Lilium tigrinum
Tincturae herba Sig 0.5ml
Linaria vulgaris
Infusium Sig 30ml.
Linum usitatissimum
Unstable and destroyed by heat, light and air. Take with water.
Infusium sem Sig 30ml
Sem whole or crushed Sig 10g. Granulated gruel used for mucilaginous action.
Oleum Sig 30ml
Tincturae Sig 10ml
Liquidum extracum Sig 2ml
     Fomentation Sig 60g Linum flour.
Liriosma ovata
Powder rad/stem Sig 2g. Liquidum extractum Sig 5ml
Lobelia inflata
Restrictions apply. Dosage is determined by the relief of symptoms. Always
combine with Capsicum or Mentha sp. to diffuse the Lobelia around the tissues.
Powdered herba Sig 2g [Ref 390]. Solid extract Sig 4g.
Simple Lobelia tincturae [1:8] Sig 2ml. Tincturae herba 1:8 Sig 2ml
Liquidum extractum herba Sig 0.6ml
     Syrupus Lobelia 1:4 Sig 2ml
     Emulsion expectorant et Linum usitatissimum.
     Acidum Tincturae Lobelia Acid tincture of Lobelia. 1:10 Sig 4ml
     Topically as per above dosage.
Lotus corniculus
Infusium Sig 10g. Liquidum extractum Sig 1ml
Lyceum chinense
Dried rad Sig 5g. Tincturae Sig 5ml
Lycopus europaeus
Dried herba Sig 3g. Infusium Sig 30ml. Tincturae Sig 5ml.
Liquidum extractum Sig 2ml

M
Malva sylvestris
Infusium Sig 30ml. Liquidum extractum Sig 8ml

Herbal Medicine - Keys

Marrubium vulgare
Dried herba Sig 5g. Liquidium extractum Sig 4ml. Syrupus Sig 4ml
Marsdenia condurango
Use small doses in irritable stomach conditions.
Powdered bark Sig 4g. Liquidum extractum Sig 4ml
Maytenus buchanani
Dried cort 1g
Medicago sativa
Infusium Sig 10g. Liquidum extractum Sig 10ml
Melaleuca alternifolia
Oleum Sig 5gtt. Inhalation. Crem et Ung Sig 20gtt et 60ml base.
Melia azederach
Berries and seeds are very strong and used as an anthelmintic, they can cause gastro intestinal haemorrhage.
Powdered fol/flos/rad/bacc Sig 0.5g. Tincturae fol/flos/rad Sig 1ml
Melilotus officinalis
Infusium herba Sig 30ml. Tincturae Sig 5ml
Melissa officinalis
Dried herba Sig 5g. Dry extract Sig 1g.
Tincturae Sig 10ml. Liquidum extractum herba Sig 4ml
Menispermum canadense
Powdered rad Sig 2g. Liquidum extractum Sig 4 ml
Mentha piperita
Dried herba Sig 4g. Dry extract Sig 1g..Infusium herba Sig 30ml.
Tincturae Sig 10ml. Liquidum extractum Sig 4ml
> **Conc Aqua** Mentha piperita Concentrated peppermint water Sig 0.25ml.
> **Oleum** Mentha Sig 0.2ml
> **Essence** Mentha piperita Sig 2ml

Mentha pulegrum
Dried herba Sig 4g. Liquidum extractum Sig 4ml
Menyanthes trifoliata
Dried fol Sig 2g. Tincturae Sig 5ml. Liquidum extractum Sig 2ml
Mitchella repens
Dried herba Sig 4g. Liquidum extractum Sig 4ml
Morus alba
Succus 5ml. Tincturae bacc/cort/fol/fruct Sig 4ml
Myrica cerifera
Diaphoretic effect Infusium Sig 15ml every 15 minutes until diaphoresis occurs.
Powdered bark Sig 4g. Liquidum extractum Sig 2ml

Formulary

Myristica fragrans
Fructus Sig 2g
Oleum Sig 0.2ml
Myroxylum balsamum
Tincturae balsam [oleo resin]. Sig 2ml
Tolu Syrupus @ 10%. Sig 8ml
Myrrhis odorata
Decoction herba/rad/sem Sig 30ml

N
Nardostachys jatamansi
Decoctum rad/rhiz Sig 3g. Tincturae Sig 2ml
Narcissi
Emetic dose of pwd flos. Sig 8g. Tincturae bulb Sig 0.5ml
Nepeta cataria
Frequent dosing in acute cases.
Infusion herba Sig 30ml. Liquidum extractum Sig 4ml
Nepeta hederacea
Dried herba Sig 4g. Tincturae Sig 10ml. Liquidum Extractum Sig 4ml.
Nymphaea odorata
Dried rad/rhiz Sig 5g. Liquidum extractum Sig 4ml

O
Ocimum basilicum
Dried herba Sig 3g. Infusium herba Sig 30ml. Tincturae Sig 4ml
Ocimum tenuiflorum
Dried herba Sig 3g
Oenothera biennis
Ol Oenothera Sig 1-8g daily. Approximately 100mg GLA per 1g Oleum.
Olea europaea
Dried fol Sig 500mg. Liquidum extractum fol Sig 2ml. Oleum can be freely used.
Ononis spinosa
Infusium is to be preferred Sig 30ml
Opuntia vulgaris
Dried flos Sig 1g. Liquidum extractum Sig 1ml
Origanum vulgare
Dried herba Sig 3g. Infusium Sig 30ml

P
Paeonia lactiflora
Dried rad Sig 2g. Liquidum extractum Sig 4ml

Herbal Medicine - Keys

Panax ginseng
Large doses are required in neoplasm.
Dried fol/rad Sig 1g. Decocturm Sig 2g. Tincturae Sig 10ml.
Liquidum extractum Sig 2ml.
Papaver somniferum
Restrictions apply. Dosage is determined by the relief of symptoms.
Long duration of activity - up to three days.
Powder Sig 200mg. Maximum 500mg in 24 hours.
Dry extract Sig 60mg
Tincturae 1:10 unripe capsules Sig 1ml [equivalent to 10mg morphine per ml].
Liquidum extractum Sig 2ml
Papaver syrupus Syrup of Papaver [BPC 1949] Sig 4ml
  Enema Papaver 6% in starch mucilage.
  Lin. Papaver. Papaver liniment.
  Ung @ 7.5%
Parietaria diffusa
Dried herba Sig 5g. Tincturae Sig 5ml. Liquidum extractum Sig 4ml
Passiflora incarnata
Dried herba Sig 2g. Dry extract Sig 0.4g. Tincturae Sig 10ml.
Liquidum extractum Sig 2ml
  Nerve sedative prescription
  LE Passiflora 1ml. LE Pulsatilla 0.5ml. LE Salix nigra 3.5ml.
  Sig Full dose to effect.
Paullinia cupana
Slow absorption. Powdered sem Sig 4g. Tincturae Sig 6ml. Liquidum ext. Sig 4ml
Pausinystalia yohimbe
Restrictions apply. Dosage is determined by the relief of symptoms.
Liquidum extractum bacc. Sig 4ml.
Petasites
Decoctum flos/rad/rhiz Sig 9g. Tincturae Sig 3ml
Petroselinum crispum
Full dose to allay skin irritations. Dried herba/rad/sem Sig 4g. Tincturae Sig 10ml.
Liquidum extractum herba/rad/sem Sig 4ml.
Peumus boldus
Start with a small dose as large dose can be too stimulating in sensitive individuals.
Dried fol Sig 1g. Infusium Sig 3g. Tincturae Sig 5ml. Liquidum ext. Sig 1.5ml.
Pfaffia paniculata
Dried rad Sig 2g
Phyllanthus amarus/niruri
Dried herba infusium Sig 30ml. Dried powder Sig 200mg
Liquidum extractum fol Sig 2ml

Formulary

Phyllanthus emblica
Tincturae herba/flos/rad/fruct. Sig 4ml
Phyllitis scolopendrium
Dried fol/fronds. Sig 4g. Tincturae Sig 6ml. Liquidum extractum Sig 4ml
Phytolacca americana
Emetic dose Sig 1g. Dried rad Sig 0.3g. Tincturae 1:5 Sig 0.3ml.
Liquidum extractum Sig 1ml
Phytostigma venenosum
Tincturae Sig 0.6ml
Picrasma excelsa
Dried lignum Sig 0.6g. Concentrated Quassia infusium 1:2 Sig 4ml
Tincturae Sig 4ml.
Enemata 1:20 Sig 150ml PR each day for three days with suitable anthelmintic
per oram E.g. Tanacetum.
Picrorrhiza kurroa
Dried rhiz Sig 4g. Liquidum extractum dried rad Sig 1.5ml
Pilocarpus jaborandi
Restrictions apply. Dosage is determined by the relief of symptoms.
Minute doses relieve excessive perspiration.
Dried fol Sig 500mg. Tincturae 1:5 Sig 2ml. Lotion 5%.
Pilosella officinarum
Syrupus Sig 10ml. Infusium herba Sig 30ml. Liquidum extractum Sig 4ml
Pimento dioica
Powdered fructus Sig 2g. Liquidum extractum Sig 4ml. Oleum Pimento Sig 0.2ml
Pimpinella saxifrage
Infusium rad Sig 30ml. Tincturae Sig 1ml
Pimpinella anisum
Infusium dried fructus Sig 1g. Tincturae Sig 5ml.
Syrupus Anisi Sig 4ml. Aqua Anisi Conc BPC Sig 1ml.
Pinellia ternata
Tincturae rhiz/rad Sig 4ml
Pinus sylvestris
Powdered needles/tur Sig 400mg. Tincturae 1:20 Sig 0.5ml.
    Inhalation composita. Essential oleum Sig 20gtt aqua frig.
    Balneum Pinus. Pine oil bath. Add Oleum Pinus 5gtt to a warm bath.
Piper cubeba
Powdered fruct Sig 4g. Tincturae Sig 2ml. Liquidum extractum Sig 4ml
Piper methysticum
Restrictions apply. Dosage is determined by the relief of symptoms.
Dried rad/rhiz. Sig 1g. Dry extract Sig 400mg [0.4g]. Tincturae Sig 10ml.
Liquidum extractum Sig 4ml.

Herbal Medicine - Keys

Piscidia erythrina
Dried rad/cort Sig 4g. Tincturae Sig 5ml. Liquidum extractum Sig 8ml
Plantago lanceolata/major
Dried herba Sig 30ml. Tincturae rad/fol Sig 7ml. Liquidum extractum. Sig 4ml.
  Garg infusium Sig 1.5g. **Poultice. Ung** @ 10%
Plantago ovata/psyllium
Semen Sig 10g. Soak the seeds in boiling water for two plus hours before ingestion. Take with plenty of fluid. Liquidum extractum Sig 5ml.
Podophyllum peltatum
Restrictions apply. Dosage is determined by the relief of symptoms.
Always give in small doses.
Resin Sig 0.06g
Tincturae rad/rhiz Sig 0.25ml. Liquidum extractum Sig 0.3ml.
Polygala senega
Dried rad Sig 3g. Infusium 1:2 Sig 5ml. Tincturae Sig 4ml.
Liquidum extractum Sig 4ml. Syrupus Sig 5ml.
Polygonum bistorta
Powdered rad Sig 2g. Tincturae Sig 5ml. Liquidum extractum Sig 2ml.
Polygonum multiflorum
Dried rad Sig 5g. Tincturae Sig 5ml. Liquidum extractum Sig 4ml
Polymnia uvedalia
Liquidum extractum Sig 3ml
Populus candicans/giliadensis
Preferable to mix with a demulcent [Gum Arabic] or a syrup to cover the disagreeable taste.
Dried gem Sig 4g. Infusium gem Sig 4g. Tincturae Sig 8ml.
Liquidum extractum Sig 8ml. Syrupus Sig 5ml. Ung @ 30%.
Populus tremuloides
Dried bacc Sig 4g. Tincturae Sig 4ml. Liquidum extractum Sig 4ml
Poria cocos
Decoctum fungus Sig 5g. Tincturae Sig 4ml
Potentilla erecta
Tincturae rad/rhiz. Sig 4ml. Liquidum extractum Sig 4ml
Potentilla reptans
Infusium Sig 30ml. Liquidum extractum herba/rad. Sig 4ml
Primula veris
Dried flos/rad/rhiz. Sig 3g. Tincturae Sig 6ml. Liquidium extractum Sig 2ml
Propolis
5g per day in capsule form. Asthma and bronchitis - alcoholic Tr Sig 20gtt TDS.
Garg. Sig 5gtt PRN. Emulsion 1:4 with sunflower oleum.
Prunella vulgaris
Infusium herba Sig 30ml.

Formulary

Prunus serotina
Powdered cort Sig 2g . Tincturae Sig 4ml. Liquidum extractum Sig 4ml.
Syrupus Prunus Sig 10ml
Pueraria lobata
Tincturae rad Sig 4ml
Pulmonaria officinalis
Dried herba Sig 4g. Tincturae Sig 4ml. Liquidum extractum Sig 4ml
Pulsatilla
Infusium herba Sig 0.3g. Tincturae Pulsatilla herba Sig 1.5ml.
Liquidum extractum Sig 1ml
Pygeum africana
Tincturae stem/bacc. Sig 5ml

Q
Quercus robur
Infusium Sig 3g. Liquidum extractum cort Sig 5ml

R
Ranunculus ficaria
Dried herba Sig 5g. Liquidum extractum Sig 5ml. Ung @ 5%
Rauwolfia serpentina
Restrictions apply. Dosage is determined by the relief of symptoms.
Reduction of hypertension may take six weeks.
Dried extract Sig 60mg. Rad has been used in doses up to 2g.
Dry extract Sig 60mg.
Tincturae 1:10 alcohol 60%. Sig 0.5ml
Rehmannia glutinosa
Dried rad Sig 3g. Decoctum Sig 10g. Tincturae Sig 5ml.
Liquidum extractum Sig 4ml
Rhamnus frangula/cathartica
Dried cort Sig 3g. Dry extract Sig 30mg. Decoctum Sig 2.5g.
Liquidium extractum Sig 5ml.
Rhamnus purshiana
For a prompt cathartic action give a full dose at night. Dried cort Sig 1g.
Dry extract 300mg. Dry extract 300mg. Infusium Sig 2g.
Tincturae cort Sig 5ml. Liquidum extractum Sig 4ml. Elixir Sig 2ml in syrup.
Rheum palmatum/officinale
Suitable for children. Dried rad/rhizome Sig 4g as a laxative.
Dried rad/rhizome Sig 1g astringent/antidiarrhoeal. Dry extract Sig 500mg.
Tincturae Sig 5ml. Liquidum extractum Sig 4ml
Rhodiola rosea
Liquidum extractum rad Sig 2ml

Rhus aromatica/glabra
Pulv bacc Sig 2g. Liquidum extractum rad/rhiz/bacc Sig 4ml.
Ribes nigrum/rubrum
Succus fructus. Sig 20ml
Ricinus communis
Ol Ricinus expressed from the sem Sig 20 ml. With fruit juice to cover the taste.
Rosa damascena
Tincturae flos Sig 4ml
Rosmarinus officinale
Dried fol/herba Sig 4g. Dry extract Sig 0.5g. Tincturae Sig 10ml.
Liquidum extractum Sig 4ml
Balneum. Oleum Sig 4gtt. Ung @10%. Liniment with 10% oleum
Rubus idaeus
Dried fol Sig 8g. Liquidum extractum Sig 8ml
Rubus parvifolius
Tincturae Sig 5ml
Rumex acetosella
Infusium Sig 30ml
Rumex crispus/aquaticus
Dried rad Sig 4g. Tincturae Sig 2ml. Liquidum extractum Sig 4ml
Ruscus aculeatus
Decoction fol/rhiz/rad Sig 7.5ml.Liquidum extractum Sig 1ml.
Ruta graveolens
Powdered herba Sig 1g. Liquidum extractum Sig 2ml. Ung @ 15%.

S
Salix alba
Dried cort Sig 3g. Tincturae Sig 8ml. Liquidum extractum Sig 3ml
Salix nigra
Liquidum extractum Sig 4ml
Salvia miltiorrhiza
Dried rad Sig 2g. Liquidum extractum Sig 4ml
Salvia officinalis
Dried/fresh fol Sig 4g. Dry extract Sig 0.36g. Essential oil Sig 0.3ml.
Tincturae Sig 10ml. Liquidum extractum Sig 4ml.
      Acetum Salvia Sage vinegar Sig 5ml Aqua cal PRN.
Salvia sclarea [Clary sage]
Liquidum extractum herba. Sig 4ml
Salvia triloba
Liquidum extractum Sig 4ml
Sambucus nigra
Dried flos Sig 5g. Infusium Sig 4g. Tincturae flos/fol Sig 10ml. Liq. ext. Sig 4ml

Formulary

Sanguinaria canadensis
Give in very small dosage and well diluted.
Dried rad Sig 0.5g. Tincturae Sig 1ml [Sig 2-5ml as an emetic].
Liquidum extractum Sig 0.3ml [1ml as an emetic]
Sanguisorba officinalis
Dried herba 5g. Tincturae Sig 8ml. Liquidum extractum Sig 6ml
Sanicula europaea
Liquidum extractum fol/rhiz Sig 4ml
Santalum album
Oleum Sig 5gtt in a maple syrup vehicle.
Liquidum extractum heartwood Sig 4ml
Saponaria officinalis
Dried rad Sig 5g. Decoctum Sig 30ml. Liquidum extractum Sig 4ml
Saracena purpura
Powdered rad Sig 2g. Liquidum extractum Sig 4ml
Sassafras officinale
Dried cort/bacc Sig 4g. Tincturae Sig 2ml. Liquidum extractum Sig 2ml
      Essence Oleum Sassafras 1% alcohol to 1000ml.
      Lotion – max 2% strength. Used as a flavouring agent.
Schizandra chinensis
Dried fructus Sig 3g. Tincturae Sig 4ml. Liquidum extractum Sig 3ml.
Scrophularia nodosa
Dried herba Sig 8g. Tincturae Sig 2ml. Liquidum extractum Sig 8ml
Scutellaria baicalensis
Dried rad Sig 2g. Tincturae Sig 5ml. Liquidum extractum Sig 4ml
Scutellaria lateriflora
Dried herba Sig 2g. Tincturae Sig 5ml. Liquidum extractum Sig 4ml
Selenicerus grandiflorus
Tincturae flos Sig 2ml. Liquidum extractum Sig 0.6ml
Sempervivum tectorum
Infusium fol Sig 2g. Tincturae Sig 1ml. Succus Sig 15ml.
Seneco aureus
Dried herba Sig 4ml. Tincturae Sig 4ml
Seneco vulgaris
Eye disorders - apply an eye pack. Furunculosis, wounds, sore nipples - bruised fol. Lymphadenopathy - poultice.
Seneco jacobaea
Restrictions apply. Dosage is determined by the relief of symptoms. Liquidum extractum Sig 3ml. Oleum.
Serenoa repens
Dried fructus/bacc Sig 1g. Dry extract Sig 300mg
Tincturae Sig 4ml. Liquidum extractum Sig 2ml

Herbal Medicine - Keys

Silybum marianus
Dried sem/flos/herba Sig 1g. Dry extract Sig 200mg. Decoctum Sig 3g.
Tincturae Sig 10ml. Liquidum extractum Sig 2ml.
Smilax aristolochiaefolia/febrifuga/ornata/regelii
Dried rad Sig 4g. Liquidum extractum Sig 4ml.
   Decoctum Sarsae Compositum Compound dec. of Sarsparilla Sig 30ml
Solanum dulcamara
Restrictions apply. Dosage is determined by the relief of symptoms.
Infusium 1:10 Sig 60ml
Tincturae rad/bacc Sig 2ml. Liquidum extractum Sig 4ml.
Solidago virgaurea
Dried flos/herba Sig 4g. Tincturae Sig 10ml. Liquidum extractum Sig 4ml.
Spigelia marilandica
Restrictions apply. Dosage is determined by the relief of symptoms.
Powdered fol and rad. Children up to 4 years of age 500mg – 4g. Adults Sig 5g.
Liquidum extractum Sig 5ml.
Spilanthes achmella/oleracea [Spilanthes].
Tincturae herba/rad. Sig 4ml
Spirulina
Dried algae Sig 1.5g
Stachys betonica
Dried herba Sig 4g. Tincturae Sig 4ml. Liquidum extractum Sig 4ml
Stellaria media
Tincturae herba Sig 10ml. Liquidum extractum Sig 4ml
Stephania tetrandra
Dried rad Sig 3g. Tincturae Sig 5ml. Liquidum extractum Sig 2ml
Sterculia lychnophora
Liquidum extractum Sig 1g
Sticta pulmonaria
Dried lichen Sig 2g. Liquidum extractum Sig 4ml
Stillingia sylvatica
Dried rad Sig 2g. Tincturae Sig 4ml. Liquidum extractum Sig 2ml
Strophanthus species
Restrictions apply. Dosage is determined by the relief of symptoms.
Tincturae sem Sig 0.3ml administered carefully.
Tincturae 1:2 Sig 60mg.
Strychnos ignatii
Restrictions apply. Dosage is determined by the relief of symptoms.
Dried sem Sig 120mg.
Tincturae Sig 0.6ml. Safer dosage is Tincturae 10 gtt in 120 ml aqua. Sig 5ml.

Formulary

Stryax benzoin
Tinctura gum resin Sig 2.5ml.
    Ung antifungal @ 10% strength.
    Tinctura Benzoini composita Compound Benzoin tincture [Friars Balsam]. Sig 3ml.
    Inhalation Benzoin Tincturae Inhalation of Benzoin tincture.
5ml et aqua cal 500ml. Inhale vapour.
    Tinctura Benzoini composita Compound Benzoin tincture.
Internal use Sig 3ml
    Tincture Benzoin compound spray 15% et ethanol.
Strychnos nux vomica
Dry extract sem. Sig 60mg.
Tincturae sem 1:10 Sig 1.5ml. Contains 0.125mg Strychnine; 2.5mg in 2ml.
Liquidum extractum Sig 0.2ml. Contains 3mg Strychnine in 0.2ml.
    Strychnos Preparata [Powdered Nux vomica sem.] sem. Sig 250mg.
    Elixir Strychnos. Sig 5ml.
Succisa pratensis
Dried flos/rad/herba Sig 5g
Symphytum officinale
Dried fol Sig 8g. Liquidum extractum fol Sig 4ml.
Dried rad/rhiz Sig 4g. Liquidum extractum rad Sig 4ml Ung @ 10%.
Symplocarpus foetidus
Dried rad/rhizoma Sig 1g. Tincturae Sig 2ml.
Liquidum extractum Sig 1ml
Syringia vulgaris
Linimentum Syringia.
Szygium aromaticum
Powdered sem Sig 1g. Infusium siccatus Szygium 1:40 Sig 30ml.
Liquidum extractum Sig 4ml. Oleum Szygium Sig 0.2ml

T
Tabebuia
Decoctum bacc Sig 30ml. Dried bacc/fol Sig 1.5g. Tincturae Sig 2ml
Tanacetum parthenium
Fresh fol Sig 2g. Dried fol Sig 200mg.
Tincturae Sig 4ml. Liquidum extractum Sig 2ml
Tanacetum vulgare
Dried herba Sig 2g. Liquidum extractum Sig 2ml
Taraxacum officinale
Dried fol Sig 10g. Liquidium extractum fol Sig 10ml.
Dried rad Sig 8g. Tincturae rad Sig10ml. Liquidium extractum rad Sig 8ml.
Succus rad Sig 5ml

Taxus bacata
Bacc/fol.
Tephrosea
Decoctum Sig 25ml
Terminalia arjuna
Dried cort/fol Sig 1g. Liquidum extractum Sig 2ml
Teucrium chamaedrys
Dried herba 4g. Liquidum extractum Sig 4ml
Teucrium scordonia
Dried herba/rad Sig 4g. Liquidum extractum herba Sig 4ml
Thuja occidentalis
Tincturae Sig 1ml. Liquidum extractum Sig 1ml
Thymus serphyllum/vulgaris
Dried herba Sig 4g. Dry extract Sig 2g. Tincturae Sig 5ml. Liquid ext. Sig 5ml.
      Elixir Thymus Sig 8ml.
      Gargarisma infusium Sig 10%.
Tilia cordata/platyphylos/europaea
Dried flos/fol Sig 4g. Tincturae Sig 10ml. Liquidum extractum Sig 4ml
Trifolium pratense
Dried flos Sig 4g. Tincturae Sig 10ml. Liquidum extractum Sig 4ml
     Compound Trifolium Sig 2ml.
     Ung Trifolium @ 15%.
Trigonella foenum graecum
Sem Sig 10g daily. Tincturae sem Sig 30ml. Liquidum extractum Sig 6ml.
Trillium erectum
Pwd rad Sig 2g. Tincturae Sig 4ml. Liquidum extractum Sig 2ml
Tropaeolum majus
Fol/flos Sig 5g. Succus Sig 5ml.
Tsuga canadensis
Dried cort Sig 2g. Tincturae Sig 2ml. Liquidum extractum Sig 2ml. Enema dect.
Turnera diffusa
Dried herba Sig 4g. Tincturae Sig 4ml. Liquidium extractum Sig 4ml
Tussilago farfara
Dried flos/herba Sig 2g. Tincturae Sig 8ml. Liquidum extractum Sig 2ml
     Syrupus Tussilago. Sig 5ml.
Tylophora indica
Dried herba Sig 0.3g. Tincturae Sig 1ml

<u>U</u>
Ulmus
Decoctum 1:8 Sig 16ml. Enemata Sig 10g mixed with vehicle and administer.
Powdered inner cort Sig 4g in aqua [or other vehicle, oat, goats, soya milk].

Formulary

Uncaria tomentosa
Dried bacc/rad Sig 7g. Liquidum extractum Sig 4ml
Urgenia maritima
Dried bulb Sig 200mg. Tincturae Sig 1ml. Liquidum extractum Sig 0.5ml.
Urgenia oxymel Sig 5ml. Syrupus 5ml.
Urtica dioica
Full dose in acute urticaria.
Dried fol/rad Sig 5g. Dry extract fol Sig 2.1g. Dry extract rad Sig 1.3g.
Tincturae rad/fol Sig 7.5ml. Liquidum extractum rad/fol Sig 5ml.
            Succus Sig 10ml. Poultice.
Usnea barbata
Tincturae Sig 5ml. Liquidum extractum lichen. Sig 4ml.

V
Vaccinum macrocarpon
Tincturae bacc Sig 4ml
Vaccinium myrtillus
Dried bacc/fruct Sig 20g. Dry extract Sig 160mg. Liquidum extractum Sig 4ml.
Garg. @ 10%. Succus Sig 200ml. Lotion dect. @ 10%.
Valeriana officinalis
As the valpotriates break down the root gives off more odour.
Low doses relax, while higher doses have a more sedative action.
Dried rad/rhizome Sig 3g. Infusium Conc 1:5. Sig 4ml. Soft extract Sig 300mg.
Tincturae Sig 10ml. Liquidum extractum Sig 2ml. Balneum 100g in muslin.
Veratrum album/viride
Acutes - use hourly.
Tincturae 1:10 Sig 2ml.
Injection [Acute hypertensive crisis] Sig 100mcg – 400 mcg. Increasing doses by
10-20mcg every hour until the desired response is obtained.
            Unguentum 2%.
Verbascum thapsus
Dried fol/flos Sig 8g. Tincturae Sig 10ml. Liquidum extractum Sig 5ml.
Oleum Verbascum 1:5.
Verbena officinalis
Infusium herba Sig 30ml. Tincturae Sig 4ml. Liquidum extractum Sig 4ml
Viburnum opulus
Tincturae bacc Sig 5ml. Liquidum extractum Sig 4ml
Viburnum prunifolium
Requires to be given in large dosage for antispasmodic action.
Tincturae bacc Sig 10ml. Liquidum extractum Sig 8ml
Vinca major/rosea
Dried herba Sig 4g. Liquidum extractum Sig 5ml

Herbal Medicine - Keys

Vinca minor
Dried herba Sig 4g. Liquidum extractum fol/rad Sig 4ml
Viola odorata
Dried herba Sig 4g. Tincturae Sig 5ml. Liquidum extractum Sig 4ml
Viola tricolor
Dried herba Sig 4g. Tincturae Sig 5ml. Liquidum extractum Sig 4ml
Viscum album
Freshly squeezed extracts contain free amino acids.
Dried fol Sig 6g. Infusium Sig 30ml. Tincturae Sig 2ml.
Liquidum extractum Sig 3ml
Vitex agnus castus
Dry extract Sig 40mg [0.04g]. Tincturae fruct Sig 2ml.
Liquidum extractum Sig 0.5ml
      PMS - Tincturae Sig 5ml aq cal once daily for 10 days prior to menses.
      Anovulatory Tr up to 10 ml per week.

W
Withania somnifera
Dried rad Sig 2g. Liquidum extractum Sig 4ml

Y
Yucca
Inner pith used internally as the outer bark is too strong.

Z
Zanthoxylum americanum/clava herculis
Baccae are more active than the rad.
Dried bacc Sig 2g. Tincturae bacc Sig 4ml. Liquidum extractum bacc Sig 2ml
Dried cort Sig 3g. Tincturae cort Sig 5ml. Liquidum extractum cort Sig 3ml
Zea mays
Dried stigma Sig 8g. Tincturae Sig 10ml. Liquidum extractum Sig 8ml
Zingiber
Dried rad/rhizome Sig 9g. Fresh rad/rhiz Sig 9g. Infusium Sig 2g.
Tincturae Sig 10ml. Tincturae forte [1:2] 0.5ml.
Liquidum extractum Sig 2ml.
      Succus Sig 7.5ml.
Zizyphus jujube
Dried sem Sig 3g. Tincturae sem.fruct Sig 3ml. Liquidum extractum Sig 3ml

Formulary

Therapeutic classification of medicines

The lists of medicines are a quick reference guide as an aid to memory.
Refer to the Pharmacopoeia for detailed information on any particular medicine.

1] Medicines acting as <u>Sialogogues</u> - producing saliva
2] Medicines acting as <u>Stimulants</u> - stimulating the vital force to action
3] Medicines acting as <u>Astringents</u> – contract tissues
4] Medicines acting upon the <u>vasomotor system</u> –
Deobstruent – remove obstructions
5] Medicinal <u>Tonics</u> – restores normal tone to tissues
6] Medicines acting upon <u>Cardio vascular system</u>
7] Medicines acting upon the <u>capillaries-Antihaemorrhagic/Styptics/haemostatics</u>
8] Medicines acting upon the <u>blood and immune system including</u>
<u>Vasotonic alterative and immunostimulants</u>
9] Medicines acting upon tissues - <u>Discutient</u> – disperse swellings
10] Medicines acting upon the <u>respiratory system</u> including Respiratory sedatives
11] <u>Expectorants</u>
12] Medicines acting upon the <u>stomach</u> - <u>Emetics</u>
13] Medicines acting upon the <u>stomach</u> - <u>Stomachic</u>
14] Medicines acting upon the <u>liver and gall bladder – choleretic/cholagogue</u>
15] Medicines acting as <u>Hydragogue cathartics</u>
16] Medicines acting upon the <u>intestinal tract including Anthelmintics</u>
17] Medicines acting upon the <u>Gastro intestinal tract including</u>
<u>Carminatives, Choleretics, Cholagogues and hepatics</u>
18] Medicines acting upon <u>gastro intestinal tract - Aperient/cathartic/laxatives</u>
19] Medicines acting upon <u>gastro intestinal tract - Aromatics</u>
20] Medicines acting upon <u>mucous membranes and skin - Demulcents</u>
21] Medicines acting upon <u>skin Diaphoretic/Sudorific/Febrifuge/Antihydrotic/</u>
<u>Antipyretic</u>
22] Medicines acting upon the <u>skin – Emollient/Vulnerary –</u>
<u>wound healing and soothing.</u>
23] Medicines acting upon the <u>skin - Rubefacient - warming the skin.</u>
24] Medicines acting upon <u>genito urinary system - Diuretics</u>
25] Medicines acting on the <u>sexual organs includes Aphrodisiac/Anaphrodisiac</u>
26] Medicines acting upon head - <u>Cephalgic - ease head pain</u>
27] Medicines acting upon the <u>nervous system –</u>
<u>Anodyne, Nervine relaxant and Sedative.</u>
28] Medicines acting upon the <u>nervous system - Antispasmodics</u>
29] Medicines acting upon the <u>nervous system as Nervine Tonics</u>
30] Medicines acting upon the <u>uterus and prostate including Emmenagogues</u>
31] Medicines acting upon the <u>uterus & prostate - uterine & prostate tonics</u>

Herbal Medicine - Keys

1] Medicines acting as Sialogogues -producing saliva

Capsicum species - chillies
Pilocarpus jaborandi - jaborandi
Piper cubeba - cubeb
Sanguinaria canadensis – bloodroot
Zanthoxylum americanum – prickly ash

2] Medicines acting as Stimulants - stimulating the vital force to action

Alpinia officinalis – galangal
Angelica archangelica – angelica
Artemisia absinthium - wormwood
Arum maculatum – cuckoopint
Barosma betulina – buchu
Brassica sp. – mustard [Mars]
Capsella bursa pastoris – shepherds purse
Capsicum minimum – chillies
Cinnamomum zeylandicum – cinnamon
Commiphora molmol - myrrh
Coriandrum sativa – coriander
Cuminum cyminum - cumin
Daphne mezerium - mezerium
Daucus carota – wild carrot
Elettaria cardamomum – cardamom seed
Eucalyptus globulus – eucalyptus
Eupatorium purpureum – gravel root
Fabiana imbreicata - pichi
Ferula sumbul – musk root
Foeniculum offic. – fennel
Iris versicolor – blue flag
Juniperus communis - juniper
Marrubium vulgare – horehound
Mentha sp – mint
Mentha species – peppermint/spearmint
Myrica cerifera – bayberry bark
Origanum majorana - marjoram
Petasites vulgaris – butterbur
Pilocarpus jaborandi – jaborandi
Piper angustifolia – matico leaves
Polygonum hydropiper – smartweed
Polymnia uvedalia – bearsfoot
Populus candicans – balm of gilead
Rhus toxicodendron – poison ivy

Therapeutic classification of medicines

Ruta graveolens – rue
Salvia offic. – sage
Sassafras offic. – sassafras
Styrax benzoin – benzoin
Taraxacum offic. – dandelion
Zanthoxylum americanum/bungeanum – prickly ash
Zingiber offic. – ginger

3] Medicines acting as Astringents – contract tissues
Achillea millefoleum - yarrow
Agrimonia eupatorium - agrimonia
Alnus glutinosa - english alder
Arctostaphylos uva ursi - bearberry
Areca catechu – areca nut
Artemisia absinthium - wormwood
Calaminta ascendens – calamint [Mercury]
Cinchona sp. - peruvian bark
Conium maculatum - hemlock
Coptis trifolia - gold thread
Eriodictyon glutinosum – yerba santa
Euphrasia offic. - eyebright
Filipendula ulmaria - meadowsweet
Geranium maculatum - cranesbill
Geum urbanum - avens
Glechoma hederacea - ground ivy
Gnaphalum ulignosum - cudweed
Hamamelis virginia - witchhazel
Herniaria glabra - rupturewort
Hypericum perforatum - st johns wort
Inula helenium - elecampane
Limoneum carolinian
Linaria vulgaris – toadflax
Lycopus virginicus - bugleweed
Lysimachia vulgaris – loosestrife [Moon]
Myrica cerifera - bayberry
Myristiga fragrans - nutmeg
Peltigera canina – english liverwort [Jupiter]
Piper angustifolia – matico
Polygonum aviculare – knotgrass
Polygonum bistorta - bistort
Polygonum multiflorum - solomons seal
Potentilla reptans – cinquefoil

Potentilla tormentilla - tormentil
Prunella vulgaris - self heal
Prunus serotina - wild cherry
Quercus robur - oak
Ranunculus ficaria - pilewort
Rheum palmatum - rhubarb
Rhus glabra - sweet sumach
Rosmarinus offic. - rosemary
Rubus idaeus - raspberry
Rubus villosus - american blackberry
Salix alba - white willow
Salvia offic. - sage
Sanicula europaea - sanicle
Seneco aureus - liferoot
Stachys betonica - wood betony
Sticta pulmonaria - lungwort lichen
Trillium erectum - white pond lily
Urtica dioica - nettle

4] Medicines acting upon the vaso motor system –

Deobstruents – remove obstructions

Capsicum sp. – chillies
Myrica cerifera – bayberry
Phytolacca decandra – pokeroot
Quillaja saponaria – soap bark
Smilax offic. – sarsparilla
Teucrium scordonia – wood sage

5] Medicinal Tonics – restores normal tone to tissues
Achillea millefoleum – yarrow
Agrimonia eupatoria – agrimony
Alnus glutinosa – alder
Arctium lappa – burdock
Arctostaphylos uva ursi – bearberry
Aristolochia serpentaria – snake root
Artemisia absinthium – wormwood
Carum carvi – caraway
Cetraria islandica – iceland moss
Chelone glabra – balmony
Cinchona sp. – peruvian bark
Cnicus benedictus – holy thistle
Cola species – kola

Therapeutic classification of medicines

Commiphora molmol – myrrh
Coptis trifolia – golden thread
Crateagus sp. – hawthorn
Dicentra cucullaria – turkey corn
Eriodictyon californicum – yerba santa
Eupatorium purpureum – gravel root
Euphrasia offic. – eyebright
Fabiana imbricata – pichi
Ferrula sumbul – sumbul
Gentiana lutea – gentian
Glechoma hederacea – ground ivy
Grindelia camporum – grindelia
Hepatica nobilis – liverwort
Hieracium pilosella – mouse ear
Hydrastis canadensis – golden seal
Hyssopus offic. – hyssop
Jateorrhiza calumba – calumba
Juglans cinera – butternut
Leonurus cardiaca – motherwort
Marrubium vulgare – horehound
Menispermum canadensis – yellow parilla
Menyanthes trifoliata – bogbean
Nepeta cataria - catmint
Origanum majorana – marjoram
Picrasma excelsa – quassia
Polygonum bistorta – bistort
Polygonum multiflorum – solomans seal
Polypodium vulgare-polypody root - expectorant, cholagogue, alterative Sig 4ml.
Polytrichum juniperum – hair cap moss
Populus tremuloides – aspen
Potentilla reptans – cinquefoil
Potentilla tormentilla – tormentil
Prunus avium – cherry stalks
Quercus robur – oak bark
Rosmarinus offic. – rosemary
Rubus idaeus – raspberry
Rumex crispus – yellow dock
Ruta graveolens – rue
Salix alba – white willow
Salvia offic. – sage
Sassafras offic. – sassafras
Selenicerus grandiflorus – night blooming cereus

Serenoa serrulata – saw palmetto
Stillingia sylvatica – queens delight
Strophanthus kombi – strophanthus
Swertia chirata – chiretta
Thymus vulgaris – thyme
Trillium pendulum – beth root
Urtica dioica – nettle
Verbena offic. – vervain

6] Medicines acting upon Cardio vascular system
Apocynum androsaemifoleum - milkweed
Bellis perennis - daisy
Calendula offic. - marigold
Cinnamomum camphora – camphor
Convallaria majalis - lily of the valley
Crateagus - hawthorn
Leonurus cardiaca - motherwort
Scolopendrium vulgare - hearts tongue fern
Selenicerus grandiflorus - night blooming cereus
Tanacetum vulgare - tansy
Taraxacum - dandelion
Viola tricolor - heartsease

7] Medicines acting upon the capillaries
Antihaemorrhagic/Styptic/haemostatic.
Achillea millefoleum – yarrow
Angelica archangelica – angelica
Calendula officinalis - marigold
Capsicum minimum – chillies
Cinnamomum - cinnamon
Commiphora molmol – myrrh
Curcuma longa - turmeric
Ephedra sinica – ma huang
Equisetum arvense - horsetail
Geranium maculatum – cranesbill
Guaiacum offic. – lignum vitae
Hamamelis virginiana – witch hazel
Hydrastis canadensis – golden seal
Hypericum perforatum – St Johns wort
Krameria triandra – rhatany
Lycopus virginicus - bugleweed
Lycoperdon sp. – puff ball

Therapeutic classification of medicines

Myrica cerifera – barberry
Plantago major – plantain
Potentilla reptans - cinquefoil
Potentilla tormentilla – tormentil
Quercus robur – oak bark
Rumex crispus – yellow dock
Sanguinaria canadensis – blood root
Styrax benzoin – benzoin
Symphytum offic. – comfrey
Trillium pendulum – beth root
Uva ursi - bearberry
Verbascum thapsus – mullein

8] Medicines acting upon the blood and immune system including -
Vasotonic alterative and immunostimulant

Agrimonia eupatoria - agrimony
Allium sativa - garlic
Alnus glutinosa - alder
Anemone pulsatilla - pasque flower
Apocynum androsaemifoleum - milkweed
Arctium lappa - burdock
Artemesia abrotanum – southernwood
Astragalus membranaceus – membranous milk vetch
Baptisia tinctoria - wild indigo
Berberis aquifolium - mountain grape
Berberis vulgaris - barberry
Calendula officinalis - marigold
Catharanthus rosea - periwinkle
Chelidonium majus - celandine
Chimaphilla umbellata - pipsissiwa
Chionanthus virginicus - fringetree
Commiphora molmol - myrrh
Daphne mezerium - mezereon
Dicentra canadensis – turkey corn
Echinacea species - cone flower
Eucalyptus globlus - eucalyptus
Euonymous atropurpureus - wahoo
Guaiacum officinale - lignum vitae
Hamamelis virginiana - witch hazel
Iris versicolor - blue flag
Ligustrum porteri - osha
Menispermum canadensis – yellow parilla

Panax ginseng - ginseng
Phytolacca decandra - pokeroot
Picrorrhiza kurroa -
Plantago major - plantain
Polygonum multiflorum – flowery knotweed
Polypodium vulgare - polypody
Porea cocos – Hoelen/Chinese mushroom
Rehmannia glutinosa - chinese foxglove
Rhus glabra – sumach
Ribes nigrum - blackcurrant
Rumex crispus - yellow dock
Salvia miltiorrhiza - Mediterranean sage
Sanguinaria canadensis - bloodroot
Sanicula europaea - sanicle
Sassafras officinalis - sassafras
Scrophularia nodosa - figwort
Smilax officinalis - sarsparilla
Solanum dulcamera - woody nightshade
Stachys betonica - wood betony
Stillingia sylvatica - queens delight
Sutherlandia microphylla [392]
Tabebuia impetiginosa – pau D arco
Tanacetum parthenium - feverfew
Thymus sp. - thyme
Trifolium pratense - red clover
Trillium erectum - bethroot
Uncaria tomentosa - cats claw
Veronica beccabunga – brook lime
Veronica officinalis – speedwell
Viola odorata - sweet violet
Viscum album - mistletoe

9] Medicines acting upon tissues - Discutient – disperse swellings
Conium maculatum – hemlock
Digitalis purpura – foxglove
Fucus vesiculosis – bladder wrack
Hyoscyamnus niger – henbane
Populus nigra – black poplar
Smilax ornata - sarsparilla
Solanum dulcamera – bittersweet root

Therapeutic classification of medicines

10] Medicines acting upon the respiratory system including
Respiratory sedatives

Althea offic. – marshmallow fol and rad
Cetraria islandica – iceland moss
Chondrus crispus – irish moss
Drosera rotundifolia – sundew
Glycyrrhiza glabra – liquorice root
Grindelia camporum – grindelia
Hieracium pilosella – mouse ear
Lobelia inflata – lobelia
Myroxylon balsamum - tolu balsam
Prunus serotina – wild cherry
Tussilago farfara – coltsfoot
Ulmus fulva – slippery elm
Verbascum thapsus – mullein

11] Expectorants

Achillea millefoleum - yarrow
Adiantum vernalis – maidenhair
Aletris farinosa – true unicorn root
Allium sativa – garlic
Arum maculatum – cuckoopint
Asclepias tuberosa – pleurisy root
Calaminta ascendans – calamint
Cochleria armoracea – horseradish
Hypericum perforatum – st johns wort
Hyssopus offic. – hyssop
Inula helenium – elecampane
Lysimachia vulgaris – loosestrife
Malva sylvestris – mallow
Marrubium vulgare – horehound
Mentha piperita – peppermint
Origanum majorana – marjoram
Pimpinella anisum – aniseed
Plantago major – plantain
Polygala senega – senega
Polypodium vulgaris – polypody
Potentilla tormentilla – tormentil root
Pulmonaria offic. – lungwort
Rubus idaeus – raspberry leaves
Salvia officinalis – red sage
Sambucus nigra – elder flowers

Sanguinaria canadensis – blood root
Scolopendrum vulgare – hearts tongue
Seneco aureus – liferoot
Sticta pulmonaria – lungwort
Styrax benzoin – benzoin
Symphytum offic. – comfrey rad/fol
Symplocarpus foetidus – skunk cabbage
Thuja occidentalis – thuja
Thymus vulgaris – thyme
Trifolium pratense – red clover
Urgent maritima – squills
Veronica offic. – speedwell
Viola odorata – sweet violet

12] Medicines acting upon the stomach - Emetics
Apocynum androsaemifoleum – bitter root
Brassica nigra – mustard seed
Cephalis ipecacuanha - ipecacuanha
Eupatorium perfoliatum – boneset
Lobelia inflata – lobelia
Mentha piperita – peppermint
Nepeta cataria – catnep
Polygala senega – senega
Sambucus nigra – elder flowers
Sanguinaria canadensis – blood root
Urgent maritima – squill

13] Medicines acting upon the stomach - Stomachic
Acorus calamus – calamus root
Adiantum vernalis – maidenhair
Aletris farinosa – true unicorn root
Chamaemelum nobile – roman camomile
Citrus aurantium – orange peel
Collinsonia canadensis – stone root
Coptis trifoliata – golden thread
Drimys winteri – winters bark
Erythrea centaurium – centaury
Foeniculum vulgare – fennel
Gentiana lutea – gentian
Inula helenium – elecampane
Mentha piperita – peppermint
Mentha pulegium – pennyroyal

Therapeutic classification of medicines

Mentha spicata – spearmint
Myristica fragrans – nutmeg
Myrrhis odorata – sweet cicely
Pimpinella saxifraga – burnet saxifrage
Populus tremuloides – aspen
Saracena purpura – pitcher plant
Tanacetum vulgare – tansy

14] Medicines acting upon the liver and gall bladder – choleretic/cholagogue
Berberis aquifolium – mountain ash
Berberis vulgaris – barberry
Chionanthus virginica - fringetree
Corallorhiza odontorhiza – crawley root
Fabiana imbricata - pichi
Kickxia elatine – fluellen
Leptandra offic. – black root
Podophyllum peltatum - mandrake
Saracena purpura – pitcher plant
Taraxacum offic. – dandelion

15] Medicines acting as Hydragogue cathartics
Conium maculatum – hemlock
Tamus communis – black bryony

16] Medicines acting upon the intestinal tract including Anthelmintics
Prescribing of these Medicines often requires some vehicle to cover the taste.
Aloe vera - aloes
Areca catechu - areca nut
Artemisia absinthium - wormwood
Brayera anthelmintica - [Hagenia abyssinica] kousso
Chenopodium ambrosioides – wormseed
Delphinium staphysagria – stavesacre
Dryopteris felix- mas - promote fast elimination of this toxic product.
Juglans cinera - butternut
Mallotus philippines - kamala
Ruta graveolens - rue
Spigelia marilandica – indian pink
Tanacetum vulgare - tansy
Thuja occidentalis - tree of life

17] Medicines acting upon the Gastro intestinal tract including
Carminatives, Choleretics, Cholagogues and hepatics

Adiantum vernalis - maidenhair
Alpinia officinalis - galangal or chinese ginger
Anethum graveolens - dill
Angelica archangelica - angelica
Artemisia vulgaris - mugwort
Carum carvi - caraway
Chelone glabra - balmony
Chionanthus virginiana - fringetree
Cinnamomum zeylandicum – cinnamon
Coriandrum sativa - coriander
Dioscorea villosa - wild yam
Foeniculum - fennel
Hydrastis canadensis - golden seal
Juniperus communis – juniper
Levisticum officinalis - lovage
Mentha piperita - peppermint
Mentha pulegrum - spearmint
Nepeta cataria - catmint
Pimpinella anisum - aniseed
Pimpinella saxifrage - burnet saxifrage
Piper cubebs – cubebs
Polygonum erectum - knotgrass
Polypodium peltatum - mandrake
Rheum officinalis - rhubarb
Solidago virgaurea - golden rod
Szygium aromaticum - cloves
Taraxacum officinalis - dandelion
Thymus vulgaris - thyme
Zingiber species - ginger

18] Medicines acting upon gastro intestinal tract-Aperient/cathartic/laxative

Aloe vera - aloe
Apocynum androsaemifoleum – bitter root
Baptisia tinctoria - wild indigo
Berberis vulgaris - barberry
Brayera anthelmintica [Hagenia abyssinica] - kousso
Cassia angustifolia - senna
Chelidonium majus – celandine
Cytissus scoparius – broom
Eupatorium perfoliatum – boneset

Therapeutic classification of medicines

Garcinia hanburyi - gamboge
Hydrangea arborescens - hydrangea
Ipomoea orizabensis - scammony
Ipomoea purga - jalap
Iris versicolor - blue flag
Juglans cinera - butternut
Leptandra virginicus - blackroot
Linum catharticum - mountain flax
Menispermum canadense - yellow parilla
Phytolacca decandra – pokeroot
Phyllitis scolopendrium - heartstongue
Podophylum peltatum - mandrake
Polymnia uvedalia - bearsfoot
Rhamnus purshiana - cascara
Rhamnus frangula - buckthorn
Rheum officinalis - rhubarb
Ricinus communis - castor oil
Spigelia marilandica – pink root
Styrax benzoin - benzoin
Taraxacum officinalis - dandelion

19] Medicines acting upon gastro intestinal tract - Aromatics
Acorus calamus - calamus
Angelica archangelica - angelica
Carum carvi - caraway
Cinnamomum camphora - camphor
Cinnamomum zeylandicum - cinnamon
Drimys winteri – winters bark
Elettaria Cardomomum - cardamom
Foeniculum vulgare - fennel
Filipendula ulmaria - meadowsweet
Myrica gale – sweet gale
Myristica fragrans - nutmeg
Pimpinella saxifrage - burnet saxifrage
Piper cubeba - cubebs
Salvia officinalis – sage
Szygium aromaticum - cloves

20] Medicines acting upon mucous membranes and skin - Demulcents
Acacia catechu - acacia
Agropyron repens – couch grass
Alchemilla arvensis – parsley piert

Althea offic. – marshmallow fol and rad.
Astragalus gummifer – tragacanth gum
Calendula officinalis - marigold
Cetraria islandica – iceland moss
Chondrus crispus – irish moss
Glycyrrhiza glabra – liquorice root
Linum usitatissimum – linseed [flaxseed]
Malva sylvestris – mallow
Maranta arundinacea – arrowroot
Nymphaea odorata – white pond lily
Plantago psyllium - psyllium
Polygonum multiflorum – solomons seal root
Sticta pulmonaria – lungwort
Symphytum offic. – comfrey fol and rad
Tussilago farfara – coltsfoot
Ulmus fulva – slippery elm
Zea mays - corn silk

21] Medicines acting upon skin-Diaphoretic/Sudorfic/Febrifuge/antihydrotic
Achillea millefoleum – yarrow
Anagallis arvensis – scarlet pimpernel
Apocynum androsaemifoleum – bitter root
Aristolochia serpentaria – snake root
Asclepias tuberosa – pleurisy root
Barosma betulina – Buchu
Calaminthus – thymus
Capsicum sp. - cayenne
Chamomelum nobile – roman camomile
Corallorhiza odontorhiza – crawley
Dioscorea villosa – wild yam
Dorstenia contrayerva - contrayerva
Eupatorium perfoliatum – boneset
Fumaria offic.   fumitory
Gallium aparine - clivers
Gelsemium sempervirens – gelsemium
Leptandra virginicus – blackroot
Lobelia inflata – lobelia
Menispermum canadense – yellow parilla
Mentha piperita – peppermint
Nepeta cataria - catmint
Pilocarpus microphyllus – jaborandi
Polygala senega – senega

Therapeutic classification of medicines

Potentilla repens – cinquefoil
Sambucus ebulus – dwarf elder
Sambucus nigra – elder flowers
Sanguisorba officinalis – greater burnet
Sassafras albidum – sassafras
Scutellaria lateriflora - skullcap
Seneco jacobaea – ragwort
Solanum dulcamara – bitter sweet
Stillingia sylvatica - queens delight
Tanacetum parthenium - feverfew
Teucrium scordonia - wood sage
Zanthoxylum species – prickly ash
Zingiber officinale - ginger

22] Medicines acting upon the skin - Emollient/Vulnerary –
wound healing and soothing to the skin.
Althea officinalis - marshmallow
Ficus carica – fig
Nymphaea odorata – white pond lily
Trigonella foenum-graecum – fenugreek
Ulmus fulva – slippery elm

23] Medicines acting upon the skin - Rubefacient - warming the skin.
Brassica species - mustard
Capsicum minimum – capsicum
Tamus communis – black bryony
Zingiber officinalis – ginger

24] Medicines acting upon genito urinary system - Diuretics
Acorus calamus – sweet flag
Agrimonia eupatoria – agrimony
Agropyron repens – couch grass
Ajuga chamaedrys – ground pine
Alchemilla arvensis – parsley piert
Anagallis arvensis – scarlet pimpernel
Angelica archangelica – angelica
Apocynum androsaemifoleum – bitter root
Arctium lappa – burdock
Arctostaphylos uva ursi – bearberry
Barosma betulina – buchu
Brassica alba – white mustard
Capsella bursa pastoris – shepherds purse

Chelidonium majus – celandine
Chimaphilla umbellata – pipsissiwa
Chionanthus virginica – fringe tree
Chondrodendron tomentosum – pariera
Cimicifuga racemosus –black cohosh
Cola vera – cola
Collinsonia canadensis –stoneroot
Convallaria majalis – lily of the valley
Curcuma longa – turmeric
Cytisus scoparium – broom
Daucus carota – wild carrot
Dicentra canadensis – turkey corn
Eupatorium purpureum – gravel root
Fabina imbricata – pichi
Filipendula ulmaria – meadowsweet
Gallium aparine – Clivers
Glechoma hederacea – ground ivy
Guaiacum offic. – lignum vitae
Hamamelis virginiana - witch hazel
Hordeum distichon – barley
Humulus lupulus
Iris versicolor – blue flag
Juniperus communis – juniper
Levisticum offic. – lovage
Linum catharticum – mountain flax
Melissa offic. – balm
Menyanthes trifoliata – bogbean
Nepeta cataria – catmint
Parietaria offic. – parietaria
Peumus boldo – boldo
Piper angustifoleum – matico
Piper cubeba – cubebs
Piper methysticum   kava kava
Plantago major – plantain
Polygonum hydropiper – smartweed
Polytrichum juniperum – hair cap moss
Populus candicans – balm of gilead
Populus tremuloides – white poplar
Potentilla repens – cinquefoil
Rhus glabra – sumach
Ribes nigrum – blackcurrant
Sambucus ebula – dwarf elder

Therapeutic classification of medicines

Sassafras varifoleum – sassafras
Scolopendrum vulgare – harts tongue
Scrophularia nodosa – figwort
Seneco aureus – liferoot
Serenoa serrulata – serenoa
Tamus communis – black bryony
Tanacetum vulgare – tansy
Taraxacum offic. – dandelion
Turnera diffusa – damiana
Ulmus fulva – slippery elm
Urgent maritima – squill
Urtica dioica – nettles
Verbena offic. – vervain
Veronica offic. – speedwell

25] Medicines acting upon the sexual organs - Aphrodisiacs
Acorus calamus - calamus
Anemone pulsatilla - pasque flower
Apium graveolens – celery
Aristolochia serpentaria – virginia snakeroot
Avena sativa - oats
Byrsocarpus coccineus
Chamaelirium luteum – false unicorn root
Cola vera - kola
Eleutherococcus - ginseng
Foeniculum vulgare – fennel
Funtumia elastica - stem and twig latex
Jasminum officinale – jasmine
Liriosma ovata - muira puima
Microdesmis puberula
Microglossa pyrifolia
Neubouldia laevis
Panax ginseng - ginseng
Pausinystalia yohimbe - yohimbe
Ptychopetalum olacoides - muira puama
Pulsatilla – pasque flower
Salvia officinalis - sage
Schizandra chinensis
Scutellaria lateriflora - skullcap
Serenoa serrulata - saw palmetto
Smilax officinalis - sarsparilla

Tinospora cordifolia – [Guduchi] allays inflammation, uric acid diathesis, cleansing vasotonic alterative, tonic, autotoxaemia.
Trigonella foenum-graecum – fenugreek
Turnera diffusa – damiana
Vitex agnus castus – chaste tree
Withania somnifera - ashwaganda
Zizzyphus jujube – sour date

Anaphrodisiac
Anemone pulsatilla - pasque flower
Curcuma longa - turmeric
Chondrodendron tomentosum – pareria brava
Humulus lupulus – hops
Nelumbo nucifera – lotus [188]
Polygonum bistorta - bistort
Salix nigra - black willow
Viscum album - mistletoe

26] Medicines acting upon head - Cephalgic – ease head pain
Anemone pulsatilla – pasque flower
Avena sativa – oats
Coriandrum sativa – coriander
Elettaria officinalis – cardamoms
Gelsemium sempervirens - gelsemium
Hypericum perforatum – st Johns wort
Origanum majoranum - origanum
Rosmarinus offic. – rosemary
Ruta graveolens – rue
Salvia sclarea – clary sage
Sambucus nigra – elderflowers
Scutellaria lateriflora - skullcap
Stachys betonica – wood betony
Tilia europaea – lime flowers
Valeriana offic. – valerian

27] Medicines acting upon the nervous system –
Anodynes, Nervine relaxants and Sedatives
Aconitum napellus – aconite
Atropa belladonna - belladonna
Cannabis sativa - cannabis
Cypripedium pubescens - ladies slipper [endangered species]
Datura stramonium- thorn apple
Eschscholzia californica - californian poppy

Therapeutic classification of medicines

Gelsemium sempervirens - yellow jasmine
Humulus lupulus - hops
Hyoscyamnus niger - henbane
Hypericum perforatum - st johns wort
Lactuca virosa - wild lettuce
Lobelia inflata - lobelia
Mentha species - peppermint, spearmint
Papaver somniferum - poppy
Passiflora incarnata - passionflower
Piper methysticum - cava cava
Piscidia erythrina - jamaica dogwood
Scutellaria lateriflora - skullcap
Trillium erectum - bethroot

28] Medicines acting upon the nervous system – Antispasmodics

Anemone pulsatilla - pasque flower
Artemesia abrotanum - southernwood
Asclepias tuberosa - pleurisy root
Atropa belladonna - belladonna
Baptisia tinctoria - wild indigo
Chamomilla recutita - german camomile
Capsella bursa pastoris - shepherds purse
Chamomelum nobile - roman camomile
Cimicifuga racemosa - black cohosh
Cypripedium pubescens - ladies slipper
Datura stramonium- thorn apple
Dioscorea villosa - wild yam
Drosera rotundifolia - sundew
Echinacea sp. - ephedra
Eucalyptus globlus - eucalyptus
Ferula foetida - asafoetida
Gelsemium sempervirens - gelsemium
Hyoscyamnus niger - henbane
Lavandula officinalis - lavender
Leonurus cardiaca - motherwort
Lobelia inflata - lobelia
Mentha piperita - peppermint
Sanicula europaea - sanicle
Scutellaria lateriflora - skullcap
Symplocarpus foetidus - skunk cabbage
Thymus sp. - thyme
Valeriana offic. - valerian

Verbena officinalis
Viburnum opulus - cramp bark
Viscum album - mistletoe

29] Medicines acting upon the nervous system as Nervine Tonics
Anemone pulsatilla – pulsatilla
Artemisia vulgaris – mugwort
Avena sativa – oats
Cinchona sp. – peruvian bark
Cola vera – kola
Ferrula sumbul – musk
Gentiana lutea – gentian
Humulus lupulus – hops
Lactuca virosa – wild lettuce
Melissa offic. – balm
Passiflora incarnata – passionflower
Piper methysticum – kava kava
Piscidia erythrina – jamaica dogwood
Rosmarinus offic. – rosemary
Salvia officinalis – sage
Scutellaria lateriflora – skullcap
Symplocarpus foetidus – skunk cabbage
Tanacetum parthenium – feverfew
Turnera diffusa – damiana

30] Medicines acting upon the uterus and prostate including Emmenagogues
Ajuja chamaepitys – ground pine
Aloe vera – aloe
Artemisia abrotanum – southernwood
Artemisia vulgaris – mugwort
Baptisia tinctoria – wild indigo
Chenopodium olidum – arrach
Juglans cinera –butternut
Juniperus sabina – savin
Mentha pulegrum – pennyroyal
Origanum majoranum – marjoram
Salvia officinalis – sage
Sanguinaria canadensis – bloodroot
Seneco aureus – life root
Serenoa serrulata – saw palmetto
Tanacetum parthenium – feverfew
Thuja occidentalis – thuja

Therapeutic classification of medicines

31] Medicines acting upon the uterus and prostate - uterine & prostate tonics
Alchemilla vulgaris – ladies mantle
Aralia racemosa – spike yard
Chamaelirium luteum – false unicorn root
Mitchella repens - squaw vine
Myrica cerifera – bayberry bark
Polygonum bistorta - bistort
Rubus idaeus - raspberry
Seneco aureus - liferoot
Trillium erectum – beth root
Tsuga canadensis - hemlock spruce
Viburnum prunifoleum – black haw

Glossary definitions

Words sometimes have several meanings. The definition only gives the meaning, that the word has, as used, in this text.

Adaptogenic – balancing and adjusting medicine.

Aberration - disorder.

Vasotonic alterative – blood cleansing medicine, known as an alterative.

Angiogenesis – the growth of new blood vessels towards and within tissues.

Anodyne – analgesic – synonymous terms. Pain relieving.

Antibacterial – destroys bacteria. Bacteria e.g. - Escherichia, Proteus mirabilis, Pseudomonas aeruginosa, Staphylococcus aureus.

Antifungal – destroys fungus. Fungi e.g. - Candida, Cryptococcus, Dermatophytes, Trichophyton.

Antihydrotic – checks excessive perspiration.

Antimycotic = antibacterial.

Antiparasitic – Parasites e.g. Plasmodium falciparum, Schistosomia mansoni, Trypanosoma cruzi.

Antiperiodic – easing recurrent fevers e.g. malaria.

Antiphlogistic – relieving pain and allaying inflammation, fever and swelling.

Antipyretic - febrifuge, diaphoretic.

Antiscorbutic – cure scurvy.

Ant scrofulous – curing tubercular lymphadenopathy.

Antiviral – destroys fungi. Coxsackie [188p132]. Epstein barr virus Herpes 1 & 2. Influenza. Herpes. Listeria. Polio virus. Stomatitis virus. Trichomonas. Candida. Vesicular pox virus.

Apoptosis – a natural phenomena whereby the cell is programmed at birth to decay at a certain time. Immune cells ingest apoptotic cells and deliver the contents into the extravascular spaces. Apoptosis allows the rapid healing of wounds.

Bioplasm - the nuclear mass of the cell.

Chylification - Chyle, is a milk - white emulsion of fat globules in the lymph, formed in the small intestine during digestion.

Counter irritant – external application of Medicines which induce local inflammation or hyperaemia and act as a derivative to relieve irritation, inflammation & pain in some part adjacent or remote from the area of application.

Cytostatic – arrests the growth of cells.

Detergent – cleansing.

Deobstruent – removes obstructions in the tissues and eliminative organs.

Depurative/depurant – purifying the blood and tissues.

Detergent – cleansing to wounds.

Diaphoretic – enhances perspiration the same as sudorific.

Diathesis – a tendency to a certain condition.

Diffusive or Diffuse - stimulates the capillary circulation.
Discutient – allay inflammation. Dissolves tumours.
Emollient – soothes and softens the skin.
Empirical - basic, elementary, practical.
Eruptive fever - chickenpox, measles, scarlet.
Extrinsic - factors from outside of the cell.
Febrifuge – diaphoretic, antipyretic.
Flavonoid = flavone.
Fungus – candida, crytococcus, dermatophytes, trichophyton.
Galactogogue – produces milk.
Gram positive bacteria – e.g. staphylococcus.
Gram negative bacteria – e.g. brucella.
Haemostatic – antihaemorrhagic/styptic -
Hydragogue – purging which produces watery evacuations
Hydrophobia - rabies
Inimical - destructive and harmful. Adversely affecting cell function.
Intrinsic - occurring inside of the cell.
Insecticide – kills insects.
Kinetic - capable of producing motion within matter, where energy is seen as movement distinct from a resting energy.
La grippe – epidemic influenza
Maladies - conditions.
Mydriatic - dilates the pupil.
Myotic – contracts the pupil.
Neurasthenia – nervous exhaustion/depletion.
Orexigenic – stimulates the appetite.
Oxytocic – stimulates the contraction of the uterus.
Parasiticide – kills parasites.
Parturient - a remedy that hastens parturition the process of giving birth.
Partus preparator – brings on labour. Allays thirst.
Pathologic physiology –
Pathophysiology; the study of disordered functions modified by disease.
Prolactin depressor – reduces prolactin levels to reduce milk production.
Refrigerant – cooling and allaying inflammation or irritation. Dispels excess heat within the body. Relieving thirst.
REM - rapid eye movements
Remittent fever - typhoid, cholera, typhus, malaria.
Resolvent – promote resolution or dissipation or tumours. Disperses inflammatory products.
Scrophula – Tuberculosis of the lymph nodes.
Secernants - the eliminative organs:
liver & gall-bladder, bowel, skin, kidneys & lungs.

Herbal Medicine - Keys

Sensibility - sensitivity / responsiveness.
The ability of a nerve to send and receive impulses.
Sialagogue – stimulates saliva.
Sternutatory – medicines which cause sneezing.
Styptic - Antihaemorrhagic/ /haemostatic
Sudorific - produces perspiration same as diaphoretic.
Thermotaxis - heat production, the balance of heat and cold.
Tonic – an agent that increases tissue tone and energy. Tonics give tone to connective tissues of all organs. Some tonics are specific to organ areas. A blood tonic – Vasotonic alterative.
Trichophyton – ringworm fungus
Vasomotor - relates to the activity of the circulatory and nervous system as it produces physiological balance.
Vasotonic - an vasotonic alterative.
Blood cleansing remedy known as a vasotonic alterative - they can be relaxing or stimulating in their influences. A blood tonic and detoxifier.
Vasoconstrictor – contracts tissue and blood vessels.
Vasorelaxant – relaxes blood vessels and tissue.
Vulnerary - wound healer.

References

1 N.I.M.H. course in herbalism. 1975.
2 Griggs. B. Green Pharmacy. 1981.
3 The Herbal Practitioner. Vol 15. No 6. March 1964.
4 Paracelsus selected writings, Bolingen series xxviii, Pantheon books.
5 Fox. W. Family Botanic Guide. 1924.
6 Priest. A. Studies in Physiomedicalism. 1959
7 Beach. W. American Practice. 1842.
8 John Skelton. Science and practice of Medicine. 1870
9 Bynum. W & R. Porter. Medical Fringe & Medical Orthodoxy. 1750 - 1850.
10 Miley. U. & J.V. Pickstone. Medical Botany around 1850.
11 Cook. W.H. Science and Practice of Medicine. 1879.
12. Priest. A. Study notes on physiomedicalism. 1965
13 Thurston. J.M. The Philosophy of Physiomedicalism. 1900.
   Being a plea for a more exalted idea of the Vital integrity of the human organism.
14 Greer. J. Physician in the house. 1897.
15 Skelton. J. Science and Practice of Medicine. 1870.
16 Lyle. T. J. Physiomedical Therapeutics and Materia Medica. 1932.
17 Fleet & Mayer. Dietary selenium. Nutrition reviews 55 [7] 277-286. 1997.
18 Blostein. Journal of clinical nutrition. 66. 1997.
19 Paubert-Braquet. Prostaglandins, leucotrines and essential fatty acids. 57 [229] 1997.
20 Hill. European respiratory journal. 10 [2225]
21 Pool-Zobel. Carcinogensis. 18 [9] 1847.
22 Horn- Ross. American Journal of Epidemiology. 146 [2] 1997.
23 Sano. New England Journal of Medicine 336 [17] 1997.
24 Naghii. Biological trace element research 56 [3] 1997.
25 Christie. Female hormone imbalance systems. 1993.
26 Swain J. Witchcraft in 17th C England. 1994
27 Doyle W. Dietary survey during pregnancy in a low socio economic group. Journal of human nutrition, 36a 1982.
28 Crawford & Doyle. A comparison of food intakes during pregnancy and birthweight in high and low socio economic groups. Progress in lipid research, 25, 1986.
29 Endocrinology 1993, 132.
30 Senatore. Phytochemical and biological research of Uncaria.. Bol Soc Italy Sp 65, 1989
31 Rizza. Mutagenic & Antimutagenic activities of Uncaria Ethno pharmacology 38. 1993.
32 Bunello. Pharmaceutical Res. Comm. 17, 1985
33 Passwater. Whole foods. 1995

Herbal Medicine - Keys

34 J. Clin Microbiol 1990, 28
35 Journal Molecular aspects of medicine. 1994.
36 Lea & Febinger. Autonomic nervous system. Kuntz. Philadelphia USA 1945
37 Williams and Hemmings. Intestinal uptake & transport of proteins. Proc R Soc London Br. 203, 1979.
38 Gastroenterology 66. Uptake & transport of macromolecules by the intestine. 1974.
39 J Lab clin med 26, 1940
40 Newall and Anderson. Herbal Medicines. 1996.
41 J.R. Buchanan MD. Periodicity. Kosmos publishing co. Pre 1917
42 Lindlahr. Nature Cure.
43 British Herbal Pharmacopoeia. British Herbal Medicines Association. 1990
44 Taylor L. Herbal secrets of the rainforest. 1998.
45 BPC 1934
46 Wood. Book of Herbal Wisdom. 1997
47 Ayensu. E. Medicinal plants of West Africa. 1978.
48 Bone K. Clinical applications of Ayurvedic and Chinese herbs. 1996.
49 Duke. J. & E. Ayensu. Medicinal plants of China. 1985.
50 A Barefoot doctors manual. Cloudburst press. Seattle. 1977
51 Beech. BL. Midwifery today. Autumn 1999.
52 Ekeke. Planta Medica. 1985. Planta Medica. Iwu. 1986 and 1990.
53 Breyer-Brandwijk. JM. Medicinal and poisonous plants of Southern and Eastern Africa. Watt 1962. E. & S. Livingstone, Ltd., Edinburgh & London.
54 Pharmaceutical formulas - Vol 1. 1944.
55 Mutation research 1984
56 Gabrielle Hatfield. Memory, Wisdom and healing. 1999.
57 Opthalmology & visual science [38] 9 1997.
58 Mayo. J. Remarkable health benefits of soy protein. 1998
59 The Medical Herbalist. May 1933
60 Packer & Brand. Ophthalmology's botanical heritage. t Survey of opthalmology Vol 36 1992
61 Knight & Eden. Phyto oestrogens confer cancer protective effects. Review of phytoestrogens. Obstetrics & Gynaecology 1996: p87.
62 Beech. B. Birthing your baby. Aims. 2001.
63 Gosling. N. MNIMH. Herbs for bronchial troubles. Thorsons. MNIMH.
64 Gosling. N. Herbs for the heart and circulation. Thorsons.
65 Gosling. N. Herbs for constipation. Thorsons.
66 Gosling. N. Herbs for headaches. Thorsons.
67 Gosling. N. Herbs for colds and flu. Thorsons.
68 Smith. W. MNIMH. Herbs for constipation. Thorsons. 1976.
69 Ellingwood & Lloyd. Materia medica, therapeutics and pharmacognacy. 1919

70 McTaggart. L. The Vaccination Bible. 1998.
71 Calver A. Nitric oxide and the control of vascular tone in health and disease. Eur. J. Med. 1993
72 Petty. RG. Endothelium the axins of vascular health and disease. Journal Royal college of physicians, London. 1989
73 Moncada S. Nitric oxide discovery and impact on clinical medicine. Journal of the Royal society of medicine. 1999
74 Hawarth press. Journal of chronic fatigue syndrome. NY. Vol 8. 2001
75 Linford Rees. Short textbook of Psychiatry. English university press 1967
76 Kretschmer E. Physique & Character, Routledge, London. 1921
77 Tredgold & Wolff. UCH handbook of Psychiatry. Duckworth 1975
78 Sheldon. W.H. Typology 1966
79 Gauquelin. Michael. Cosmic influences on human behaviour. 1974
80 Krieger/Priest. Fundamental basis of Iridology 1980/1985
81 Jensen. Iridology volume 2. 1982
82 Hall. D. Iridology. 1986
83 Hay. Louise. You can heal your life. 1984
84 Edwards. N. Delivering your placenta. Aims. 1999.
85 Koch. Natural immunity. 1936
86 Douglas Hulme. E. Pasteur exposed. 1989
87 Bechamp. A. The blood and its third anatomical element. 1912 Veritas press, Australia
88 Mc Donagh. Nature of disease. 1948.
89 Allen. Roy. The microscopy of micro organisms associated with neoplasms. 1948 issue of The New York Microscopical Bulletin.
90 Livingston. Virginia. Cancer-a new breakthrough 1972 and The conquest of cancer 1984.
91 Wuerthele-Caspe, Alexander-Jackson and Anderson. Cultural properties & pathogenicity of certain micro-organisms obtained from various proliferative & neoplastic diseases. Am J. Med Sci 1950.
92 Mellon & Fisher. New studies on the filterability of pure cultures of the tubercle group of micro organisms. Journal of Infect Dis 1932.
93 Beinhauer & Mellon. 1937. Pathogenesis of noncaseating epithelioid TB of hypoderm and lymph glands
94 Alexander-Jackson. Eleanor. The cultivation and morphological study of a pleomorphic organism from the blood of leprosy patients. International journal of leprosy. 1951.
95 Mattman. L. Cell wall deficient forms. 1974.
96 Reich. Wilheim. The Bion Experiments. 1938.
97 Rosenow. Journal of infectious diseases 14. 1914.
98 Lutard. Etudes sur la Rage.
99 Coulter. Vaccination, social violence and Criminality. 1990.

Herbal Medicine - Keys

100 WDDTY. Major seizure link to jabs. 1994; 5:8.

101 Kretchsmer. Physique and Character. 1906.

102 Horrobin. EFA's, immunity & viral infections. Journal of Nutritional Medicine -1990

103 Romain. P. St. Lessons in loving. 1989.

104 Rowe. D. Depression. 1983.

105 Dhammandara. K. Why worry? No date advised.

106 Gottman J. Psychologist. University of Washington. Seattle.

107 BBC 1. CJD - documentary. 24.3.2001

108 Wren. R.C. Potter's new cyclopaedia of botanical drugs and *Preparations*. [1907 1st edition]. 1988.

109 Wallis Budge. E. The Divine Origin of the Craft of the Herbalist. Dover. 1996.

110 Thomson. New Guide to Health. 1831.

111 Cook. W. H. Physiomedical Dispensatory: Therapeutics, Materia Medica and Pharmacy. 1869.

112 Stein I. Royal jelly. Thorsons 1986.

113 Holmes. P. The Energetics of Western Herbs. Vol 1+2. NatTrop publishers. 1989/93.

114 Gruner, OC. Study of blood in cancer. Renouf, Montreal. 1942

115 Cantwell, A. AIDS: the mystery and the solution. Aries rising press. LA. USA. 1983

116 Bird, C. What has become of the Rife microscope? New age journal. Boston. 1976.

117 The Lee foundation for Nutritional research.. Rife microscope or facts and their fate. Reprint # 47. Milwaukee. Wi.

118 Livingstone -Wheeler, V. The conquest of cancer. Franklin Watts. 1984

119 Sonea, Sorin & Panisset, Maurice. A new bacteriology. Jones & Bartlett. Boston. 1983

120 Reich. Wilheim. The Bion experiments. 1938.

121 Mackenzie. Dr S. The nature and treatment of cancer. 1906.

122 Darbinyan V. Rhiodiola rosea in stress induced fatigue. Department of Neurology. Armenian medical university, 9 Astratyan St, Kanaker Yerevan, Armenia. 375000.

123 Fulder S. The drug that builds scientists. New scientist 21, s76. 1980.

124 Das. D. Contraceptive effects. 1976 India.

125 Indian Journal of Pharmacology. 1967. Pages 235-237.

126 Felter Lloyd. Kings American Dispensatory. 1898. Reprint. Eclectic medical publications. Sandy, Oregon. 1983.

127 Grieve. M. A Modern Herbal. 1931. Reprint 1978 .

128 Heitner. Paediatric medicine. 1987.

129 Medical science research 1996.

130 Red Cross magazine - issue 3. 1998.
131 Prescription from "Notes on Tropical diseases" Liverpool school of tropical medicine. Annals of Tropical Medicine and Parasitology Vol VI No3 B. Oct 1912.
132 Commission E. Monograph. 1988. Cynara folium. Artishockenblatter. BGA. Aufbereitungsmorografie, Bundeanzeiger.
133 Walker. Middleton. Petrowicz.. Artichoke leaf extract reduces IBS symptoms. Phytotherapy research.15[1] 2001
134 Tobler et al. Schweizerische Zeitschrift fur Ganzheitmedizen. Journal suisse de medicine holistique. Vol 5/94 & 6/94.
135 Vaz Al. Double blind clinical eval. Curr Med Res Opin 8 [3] 145.
136 Loehnis & Smith. Journal of agricultural research. July 1916.
137 Paediatric Infect Dis J. 1996.
138 Monboisse J. Oxygen free radicles as mediators of collagen breakage. 1984.
139 Magistrate M. Anti ulcer activity of Vaccinium myrtillus. 1988.
140 [1] ALA. D. Effect of anthocyanosides on visual performance. 1979
140 [2] Boniface R. Vaccinium treatment of diabetic microangiopathy. 1985.
141 Bottecchia D. Inhibitory effect of Vaccinium myrtillus on platelet aggregation and clot reaction. 1987
142 Weiss. R F. Herbal Medicine. Beaconsfield. 1988.
143 Sliutz 1993. Merz 1996.
144 Treben. Maria. Health from Gods garden. Thorsons. 1987.
145 De Biaracli Levi. Juliette. Herbal Handbook for everyone. Faber & Faber. 1966.
146 Cowper. A. Medicinal plants in Australia. Rose print. 1987.
147 Lust. J. B. The Herb Book. Bantam. 1979.
148 Leyel. C. Elixirs of Life. Faber. 1947
148 Leyel. C. Compassionate Herbs. Faber. 1946.
149 Schauenberg & Paris. Guide to medicinal plants. Lutterworth press. 1977.
150 Pharmacology dept. University of Wisconsin at Madison.
151 Erichsen-Brown. Charlotte. Medicinal & other uses of North American plants.
Dover. 1979.
152 Health Food Business. Jan 2002.
153 Observation chart. North Staffs Hospital. England. Dec 2001.
154 Triage assessment. MAU. North Staffs hospital. England. Dec 2001.
155 Conway. D. The Magic of herbs. Panther. 1985.
156 Stuart. Malcolm. The Encyclopaedia of Herbs and Herbalism. Caxton. 1989.
157 Bremness. L. The Complete book of Herbs and Spices. Dorling Kindersley. 1990.
158 Gerards herbal. Bracken books. 1985.
159 Barker. A. Herbal pocket prescriber. 1948.

160 Wordsworth. Culpepers herbal. 1995.
161 Densmore. F. How Indians use plants for food, medicine and crafts. Dover. 1974.
162 McIntyre. A. Herbs for Pregnancy and Childbirth. Sheldon press. 1988.
163 Messegue. M. Health Secrets of Plants and Herbs. Pan books 1983.
164 Yance D. Herbal Medicine, Healing and Cancer. Keats pub. 1999.
165 Budd. M. ND. DO. Why Am I So Tired? Thorsons. 2000
166 Chancellor. P. Handbook of Bach Flower Medicines. C. W. Daniel. 1977.
167 EJHM. Pub NIMH. Dec. 2001
168 BBC Panorama 3.2.2002.
169 Christopher. J.R. School of Natural Healing. By World publishing. 1976.
170 Boik. John. Natural Compounds in Cancer Therapy. Oregon medical press. 2001
171 Pharmaceutical Society. GB. The Pharmaceutical Pocket Book. 1933
172 Pharmaceutical Society. GB. The British Pharmaceutical Codex. 1934
173 The Chemist & Druggist. Pharmaceutical Formulas. Vol 1. 1944
174 Whitla. Pharmacy, Materia Medica & Therapeutics. 11th Edition. 1923
175 Gill. JM. Digitalis – Deadly poison or gentle healer. EJHM. Dec 2001.
176 Ellingwood. F. Ellingwoods Therapeutics. [358] pub Ellingwoods Therapeutist. 1919
177 Chamberlain. M. Old Wives Tales. Virago. 1981.
178 Channel 4 documentary. Secrets of the dead. 24.2.2002.
179 Mills S. & Bone K. Principles and Practice of Phytotherapy. Churchill/Living 2000.
180 BBC 1 news. 8/3/2002
181 Lust. John. B. 1961. Thorsons.
182 Reckeweg. Dr. Fresh Plant Extracts. Berliner Ring 32, D64625, Bensheim, Germany. Date unadvised.
183 Laurence. DR. Clinical Pharmacology. 4th edition. 1973. Churchill, Livingstone.
184 Conolly. J. MD. The Prescribers Pharmacopoeia. Churchill. 5th edition. 1864.
185 Mayo. J.L. Clinical Nutrition Insights. Vol 6. No 13. 1998.
186 Grady. D. Officials see no grounds for a mass smallpox effort. NY Times 29.3.2002
187 Conway. P. Tree Medicine. Piatkus. 2001.
188 Bartrum. T. Encyclopaedia of Herbal Medicine. Robinson. 1995.
189 Wren. RC. Potters New Cyclopaedia of Botanical Drugs and *Preparations*. Daniel. 1988.
   The 1973 edition contains some facts not available in later editions.
190 British Journal of Naturopathy. Spring 2002.
191 Jain. S. K. Medicinal Plants. National Book Trust. India. 1968.

192 Fetrow. C & Avila. J. The Complete Guide to Herbal Medicines. Pocketbooks. 2000.

193 Hobbs. C. Handbook for Herbal Healing. Botanica press. 1990.

194 Smith. Ed. Therapeutic herb manual. Published by author 1999.

195 Cabooses. Dr Freehand. The Saga of the Cats Claw. Via Lector editors. Lima. 1994.

196 Hanson. L. Breastfeeding Stimulates the Infant Immune system. Science & Medicine. Vol 4. No 6. Dec. 1997.

197 Mctaggart. L. The Cancer Handbook. 1999.

198 Leach. J. The evidence for a Nutritional approach to Cancer [Lecture]. BNA conference. April 2002

199 Webb. M. Ageing bone, osteoporosis & its diagnosis & treatment without conventional HRT. Lecture BNA conference. 2002.

200 Shamsuddin. A. M. Inositol hexaphosphate inhibits growth and induces differentiation of PC-3 human prostate cancer cells. Carcinogenesis. 16, 1975-1979.

201 Dobson. R. Article: Research identifies lifestyle cancers. The Times. 21/4/2002.

202 Schellenberg. R. Treatment for PMS with Vitex fruct extract, prospective, randomised placebo controlled study. BMJ. 2001. 20. 134-7.

203 Whorwood C.B. Shepard MC. Steward PM. Liquorice inhibits 11B-hydroxysteroid dehydrogenase ribonucleic acid levels and potentiates glucocorticoid hormone action. Endocrinology 1993. 132: 2287-92

204 Anderson JW. Allgood LD. Turner. Effects of Psyllium on glucose and serum lipid concentrations in men with type 2 diabetes and hypercholesterolaemia. American journal of Clinical Nutrition. 1999. 70. 466-73

205 Strandhagen. E. Hansson PO. Boseaus I. High fruit intake may reduce mortality among middle aged and elderly men. European Journal Clinical Nutrition. 2000; 54.

206 Koscielny J. Klubendorf D. Latza R. The antiathersclerotic effect os Allium sativa. Atherosclerosis. 1999; 144.

207 Koch HP. Lawson LD. Garlic: The Science and Therapeutic Application of Allium Sativa. 2nd edition. Williams and Wilkins. Baltimore. 1996. 62-64.

208 Legnani C. Frascaro M. Guazzaloca. Effects of dried garlic preparation on fibrinolysis/platelet aggregation in healthy subjects. Arzneimittelforschung. 1993:43. 119-22.

209 Melchior J. Palm S. Wilkman G. Controlled clinical study of standardised Andrographis paniculata extract in common cold. Phytomedicine 1996: 3, p314.

210 Bone K. The story of Andrographis paniculata. Nutrition and healing 1998; Sept 3.

Herbal Medicine - Keys

211 Zakay. Rones Z. Varsano N. Inhibition of several strains of influenza virus in vitro and reduction of symptoms with elderberry extract during an outbreak of influenza. Journal of alternative and complimentary medicine. 1995. 361.

212 Leuttig B. Steinmuller C. Gifford GE. Macrophage activation by the polysaccharide arabinogen isolated from plant cultures of Echinacea purpura. Journal of the National Cancer Institute. 1989; 81 669-75.

213 Braunig B. Dorn M. Kneik E. Echinacea purpura root for strengthening the immune response to flu like infections. Zeitschrift Phytotherapy. 1992; 13. 7-13.

214 Brinkeborn RM. Shah D. Echinaforce and other fresh plant *Preparations* in the treatment of the common cold. A randomised placebo controlled double blind clinical trial. Phytomedicine. 1999; 6. 1-6.

215 Melchart D. Walther E. Linde K. Echinacea root extracts for the prevention of upper respiratory tract infections. A double blind placebo controlled randomised trial. Arch. Family Medicine. 1998; 7. 541-5.

216 Nathan A. Health clinic fears dirty tricks after burglary. The Times. 28/4/2002.

217 Carson CF, Cookson BD, Farrelly et al. Susceptibility of methicillin-resistant Staphylococcus aureus to the essential oil of Melaleuca alternifolia. Antimicrobial Chemotherapy. 1995. Mar: 35 [3] 421.

218 Cox SD. Mann CM. Markham JL. The Mode of antimicrobial action of the essential oil of Melaleuca alternifolia. Journal of Applied Microbiology 2000. Jan; 88 [1] p170

219 Proline Botanicals newsletter. 2002. Vol 1 and Vol 2 Issue 1. Bourne Road, Stamford, Lincs.

220 Nishioka Y. Kyotani S. Influence of time on administration of a Shosaiko-To extract granule on blood concentration of its active constituents. Chem Pharm Bull. 1992. 40.

221 Alcarez MJ. Ferrandiz ML. Modification of arachidonic metabolism by flavonoids. Journal of Ethnopharmacology. 1987; 21 209-229.

222 Higashitanai A. Tabata S. Plant saponins can affect DNA recombination in cultured mammalian cells. Cell Structure Functions. 1989; 14:617-24.

223 Gildberg VE. Dry extract of Scutellaria Baicalensis as a haemostimulant in antineoplastic chemotherapy in patients with lung cancer. Eskp Klin Farmakol 1997.

224 Martindale The Extra Pharmacopoeia. 27th edition. The Pharmaceutical Press. 1979.

225 Barker A. Hall A. The National Botanic Pharmacopoeia. National Association of Medical Herbalists. 1932.

226 Duke. J. Handbook of biologically active phytochemicals & their activities. Boca Raton. FL. CRC press.

227 Ernst E. A Primer of Complimentary and Alternative medicine commonly used by cancer patients. Medical Journal of Australia. January 2001.

228 Pollington S. Leechcraft. Early English Charms, Plantlore and Healing. Anglo Saxon Books. 2000.

229 Czene K. Lichtenstein P & Henninki K. Environmental & Heritable Aetiology of Cancer among 9.6 million individuals in the Swedish family – cancer database. International Journal of Cancer. 99, 260-266 [2002]. Wiley - Liss Inc.

230 Forger L. Herbal companion to AHSDI. Washington society of health system pharmacists. 2001.

231 Murray M Pizzorno J. Encyclopaedia of Natural Medicine. Little, Brown & company. 1998.

232 Viola H. Apigenin a component of Matricaria recutita flos, a central benzodiazepine receptor lignans with anxiolytic effects. Planta medica. 1995; 61.

233 Bradley P. British Herbal Compendium. British Herbal Medicines Association. 1992.

234 Pole S. Pukka herbs newsletter. 2002.

235 Kloss J. Back to Eden. Longview publishing house. 1955.

236 Silverman M. A City Herbal. Ash Tree Publishing, Woodstock, New York. 1977.

237 Mauthner H & Schimmer O. Polymethoxylated xanthones from Centaurium erythraea with strong antimutagenic properties in Salmonella typhi. Planta medica. 1996. 62; 561-64.

238 Berkan. T. et al. Anti inflammatory, analgesic and antipyretic effects of an aqueous extract of Erythraea centaurium. Planta medica 57; 34-37. 1991.

239 Ernst, Pittler, Stevinson and White. The desktop guide to alternative and complimentary medicine. Mosby/Harcourt. 2001

240 Egawa H. Antifungal substances found in Eucalyptus species. Specialia. 1977 15;889

241 Murphy JJ. Randomised, double blind, placebo controlled trial of Feverfew in migraine prevention. Lancet. Lancet 2: 189, 1998.

242 Coffin A I. Botanic guide to health. Publisher author. Around 1860.

243 Amman VW. Acne vulgaris and agnus castus. Z allgemeinmed. 1975 51 [35] 1645.

244 Raman A. Weir U. Bloomfield SF. Antimicrobial effects of Tee tree oil and its major components on Staphylococcus aureus, Staphylococcus epidermis and Propionibacterium acnes. Lett Appl Microbiol 1995; 21 [4]: 242.

245 Turner P. Richens A. Clinical pharmacology. Livingstone medical text. 1973.

246 Barker. J. The Medicinal Flora of Britain and Northwestern Europe. Winter press 2001.

247 Fluck H. Medicinal Plants. Foulsham. 1973.

248 Christie S. Vitex agnus castus. EJHM. [3] 29. 1997.
249 Duker E. Effects of extracts from Cimicifuga racemosa on gonadotrophin release in menopausal women. Plant Medica. [5] 420. 1991.
250 Bethel M. The healing power of herbs. Wilshire book co. 1968.
251 Smith W. Wonders in weeds. C. W. Daniel .1983.
252 Webb. WH. Standard Guide to Non Poisonous Herbal Medicine. Visiter printers. 1916.
253 Harper-Shove. Prescriber and clinical repertory of medicinal herbs. CW Daniel. 1952
254 Priest A. Herbal Medication. Fowler. 1985
255 Ratsch. C. Marijuana Medicine. Healing arts press. 2001.
256 Manniche. L. An Ancient Egyptian Herbal. British Museum. 1989.
257 Felter. HW. The Eclectic Materia Medica, Pharmacology & Therapeutics. Eclectic medical publications. 1922
258 Lad. Vasant. The Complete book of Ayurvedic home remedies. Piatkus. 1998.
259 Samel G. Tibetan Medicine. Little Brown & Co. 2001.
260 Mc taggart L. What doctors don't tell you. Vol 12 no 12. March 2002.
261 British Naturopathic Journal. P40. Volume 19 No2.
262 Talalaj S & Czechowicz A. Herbal Remedies harmful and beneficial effects. Hill of Content. Melbourne. 1989.
263 Planta Medica 1991.
264 Greenfiles
265 Australian Journal of Medical Herbalism 1994, Vol 6 (2)
266 J. Urology 1984, 131, 1013-6 New England Jour. Medicine. 1991, 324, 1559
267 British Journal of Phytotherapy. 3, 3, 112-7
268 Gelmon K. The Lancet 1994, 344, [8932] 1267.
269 Canadian Journal of Herbalism
270 Phytomedicine [Fitotherapea].
271 Mediherb newsletter. Phytotherapy press PO box 276, Warwick, Queensland.
272 American Botanical Council - Herb Companion.
273 Beyond Nutrition
274 Journal of Ethno pharmacology
275 Aromatherapy
276 Hamdard Medicus
277 Journal of clinical Endocrinology & Metabolism. Vol. 77, No 5, p1215.
278 Journal of natural products.
279 Journal of Orthomolecular Medicine, Vol 5, No 3, 1990.
280 Recent Advances in Drug Research, Vol. 46, 1996.
281 American Herb Association Newsletter.
282 Herbalgram No 49.
283 Royal College of Physicians Edinburgh.

284 Positive health No 63, April 2001

285 Phytotherapy Research

286 American Journal of Chinese Medicine.

287 Herbs for health.

288 New Herbal Practitioner

289 Phytotherapy [Fitotherapy].

290 Wounds

291 Health Consciousness

292 Inhibition of human T-cell lipotrophic virus [HIV] in vitro by Acemannan [Aloe mucopolysaccharides]. Beyond Nutrition Press. Dept. Pathology, Texas, USA.

292 British journal of G. P's 1999, 49 [447] p823-8.

293 Journal of Essential oil Research.

294 Bio factors

295 British Medical Journal

296 The Lancet

297 New Scientist magazine.

298 Modern Phytotherapist journal

299 Townsend letter for doctors.

300 Hansard Medicus

301 FACT

302 European Neurology

303 Chem. Brit.

304 Journal of herbs, spices and medicinal plants.

305 International Journal of Immunopharmacology.

306 Nutritional Practice.

307 The Avant Gardener 1997, Courtesy American Herb Asso. News. 1998, XIV

308 Journal of Alternative & Complimentary medicine

309 Journal of Pharmaceutical Pharmacology

310 British Journal of Phytotherapy

311 Medical Herbalism

312 Journal of Clinical Psychiatry

313 British Journal of Dermatology.

314 Annali Italiana Di Medicina Interna.

315 Journal of Naturopathic Medicine.

316 Journal of antimicrobial Chemotherapy

317 Biotechnology & Applied Biochemistry

318 Journal of Applied Bacteriology

319 Antimicrobial Agents & Chemotherapy

320 Nutritional Research

321 International Journal of Clinical Pharmacology & Therapeutics

322 European Journal of Herbal medicine

Herbal Medicine - Keys

323 Journal of the Royal Society for the Promotion of Health
324 Biochemical & Biophysical Research Communications
325 Clinical drug investment
326 International Journal of Alternative and Complimentary Medicine
327 Journal of Applied Psychology
328 Complimentary therapies in medicine
329 Alternative Therapies Health Medicine
330 Family Practitioner
331 International Journal of Pharmacognosy. 332 Nature Medicine
333 Biohealth newsletter No 4 April 2001.
334 Journal of Plastic Reconstructive Surgery.
335 Indian Co. of Med. Res. New Delhi. Medicinal Plants of India, Vol 1. 1976.
336 Jain, SK. Med. Plants of India. Reference Publications, Algonac MI. 1991
337 Kapoor, L. CRC Handbook of Medicinal Plants, CRC Press, Inc., 2000 Corporate Blvd, N.W. Boca Raton, USA.
338 Bensky, D. & Barolet, R. Chinese Herbal Medicine. Formulas & Strategies. Eastland Press, Inc., Seattle, WA.
339 Foster, S. & Yue. Herbal Emissaries - Bringing Chinese Herbs to the West. 1992. Healing Arts Press, Rochester.
340 Leung, A. Chinese Herbal Remedies. Universe Books, New York, 1984.
341 Reichet, R. Yam and DHEA. Quarterly Review of Natural Medicine Winter: p257. 1996.
342 Time-Life. The Complete Guide to Alternative & Conventional Treatments. Time Life, Inc., Alexandria Va. 1996. 1152 pp.
343 Tyler, V.E. Herbs of Choice - The Therapeutic Use of Phytomedicinals. Pharmaceutical Products Press, New York. 1994.
346 CRC Press, Boca Raton, FL. 1992
347 Economic Plants. CRC Press, Boca Raton, FL.
348 Member of the Institute Oswaldo Cruz. [Suppl.I] p203. 1986
349 Tham. Benefits of phytoestrogens. Journal of Clinical Endocrinology. 1998.
350 Amyes Sebastian. Magic Bullets, Lost Horizons. Taylor and Francis. 2001.
384 Priest A. Studies in Irisdiagnosis. Paper 1. Physiomedical Values. No date.
386 Campbell – Atkinson F. Kos – A Journey Through Time. EJHM Vol 6 No 1
387 Crawford V. A Homelie Herbe: Medicinal Cannabis in Early England. EJHM Vol 6. No1
388 British Naturopathic Journal. Vol 19 No 4. Winter 2002/3.
389 Greenfiles. Winter 2002. 138 Oak Tree Lane, Mansfield, NG 18 3HR.
390 Martindale The Extra Pharmacopoeia. Twenty-sixth edition. 1972
391 Mercks Manual 1889
392 Greenfiles. Spring 2003
393 Veever – Carter. A Garden of flowers. Oxford uni press. 1990

394 Blumenthal, Goldberg, Brinckmann. Herbal Medicine Expanded Commission E Monographs. American Botanical Council. 2000.

395 Mycology News. Article by Dr Kenyon. Observational non controlled study of the use of Coriolus Versicolor supplementation in 30 cancer patients. Vol 1 Edition 7. March 2003.

396 Dr Tang. Article on Kava toxicity. University of Hawaii. CAM journal. May 2003. Honolulu Advertiser email: honoluluadvertiser.com/article/2003.

397 Heinrich Daath. Medical Astrology. LN. Fowler. No date - pre 1971.

398 Chu D. Clinical Immunology and Immunopathology. 45, p48, 1987.

399 Lisbalchim M & Dean S. Journal of Applied Microbiology 82, 2, p759, 1997.

400 Quattra B. International Journal of Food. Microbial 37, 2. 1997.

401 Fatope M. Planta Medica. p190. 1988.

402 Afaq S & Siddiqui M. Pharmacology and Clinical studies on Unani Medicinal Plants. Vol 1 1984.

403 Bach D. Therapiewoche. 35, p4292. 1985.

404 Bauer H. Urology International. 41, p139. 1986.

405 Marcoli M New trends in Andr. Science. P39 1985.

406 Carani C. Arch Ital Urol. NefrolAndrol 63, 3 1991.

407 Krendal F. Pharmacia. 38 p58. 1989.

408 Wahlstrom M. Adaptogens: Natures Kay to well being. Skandinavisk, Bok. Gothenberg.

409 Bingham Journal of Applied Nutrition. 27 p45. 1975.

410 Werbach M. Nutritional Influences on Disease. Third Line Press. Tarzana USA. 1987.

411 Mills S. The Essential book of Herbal Medicine. 1991 Arcana.

412 Kobayashi, A. Biology & Pharmacology Bulletin. 25 [2] 229-34. 2002.

413 Mills S. The A-Z of Modern Herbalism. Thorsons. 1989.

414 Dwortzan M. Yeasts and fungi: a growing health concern. British Naturopathic Journal Vol 20 No 2. 2003

415 CAM magazine September 2003 Vol 3. Issue 2.

416 Huyghe E. Journal of Urology 170 [1] 5-11 2003.

417 Stern M. Ann Internal Medicine. 136. [8] 2002.

418 Jousilahti P. Archives of Internal Medicine 163 [9] 2003.

Index

Personality, 11, 28, 34, 40, 99, 101, 103, 113, 233, 275
Pertussus, 67
Pessaries, 387
Pharmacokinetics, 392
Pharmacology, 389
Bioavailability, Solubility, absorption, metabolism, 389
Pharmacy, 376
Philosophy, 8, 11, 17, 30, 1013
Physiological disturbance/mechanisms, 76, 96
Physiomedicalism, 7, 8, 11, 12, 16, 30, 52, 70, 72, 96, 111, 337, 1013
Pidoux, 52
Plague, 63, 64
Plasters, 386
Polio, 67, 1010
Polysaccharides, 122
Positive, 32
Posture [*decubitus*], 92
Poultice, 284, 387
Powder, 387

PRACTITIONERS PHARMACOPOEIA
A page 404. B 481. C 500. D 573. E 586. F 612 G page 619. H 642. I 660. J 664. K 668. L 669. M 689. N N page 711. O 716. P 724. Q 782. R 783. S 805. T 855. U page 878. V 886. W 906. Y 907. Z 908.

Precipitation, 396
Predisposition, 14, 38, 42, 99, 113, 354, 357
Pregnancy, 331
Prescribing - Dosage, Elderly, 378
Priest, 9
Primary causative conditions, 98
Primary cause of disease, 29, 56
Principia, 30
Progenitor cryptocides, 53
Prognosis, 111

Prostate tonic, 1009
Prostatitis, Adenoma, Carcinoma, Prostate treatment, 236
Psychoimmunological, 113
Pulse, 60
Pulse test – used to detect allergies., 253
Pyknic, 100, 104, 106
Quality of life, 116
Reconstructive, 30, 111
Redding, 8, 16
Reflex associations, 37
Reich, 54, 354, 1015, 1016
Relaxed conditions, 70, 73
Remission, 93
Rene Dubos, 49
Reserve vitality, 29
Resin, 122
Resistive, 30
Resolution, 59
Resolvent, 96
Respiratory sedatives, 997
Respiratory system, Antiallergic and antihistamine medicines Bronchodilators Formulary, Respiratory conditions, 181
Restorative, 111
RNA, 64, 114
Rosenow, 62
Roy Allen, 53
Rubefacient - warming the skin, 1003
Rubella, 68
Russell, 54, 354
Russell bodies, 51, 54, 62, 354
Saturn, 101
Scientific, 17, 18, 33, 34, 35, 358, 398, 916
Secondary effects/results, 42, 98
Secretions, 60, 72, 73, 81, 85, 88, 98
Secretory organs, 73, 85, 88, 107